T0228360

Extranodal Lymph...

Pathology and Management

Edited by

Franco Cavalli
Director
Institute of Oncology of Southern Switzerland
Bellinzona
Switzerland

Harald Stein
Director
Institut für Pathologie
Charité-Campus Benjamin Franklin
Berlin
Germany

Emanuele Zucca
Head, Lymphoma Unit
Institute of Oncology of Southern Switzerland
Bellinzona
Switzerland

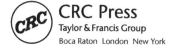

CRC Press
Taylor & Francis Group
Boca Raton London New York

CRC Press is an imprint of the
Taylor & Francis Group, an **informa** business

First published 2008 by Informa UK Ltd

Published 2019 by CRC Press
Taylor & Francis Group
6000 Broken Sound Parkway NW, Suite 300
Boca Raton, FL 33487-2742

© 2008 by Taylor & Francis Group, LLC
CRC Press is an imprint of Taylor & Francis Group, an Informa business

First issued in paperback 2019

No claim to original U.S. Government works

ISBN 13: 978-0-367-45255-1 (pbk)
ISBN 13: 978-0-415-42676-3 (hbk)

This book contains information obtained from authentic and highly regarded sources. Reasonable efforts have been made to publish reliable data and information, but the author and publisher cannot assume responsibility for the validity of all materials or the consequences of their use. The authors and publishers have attempted to trace the copyright holders of all material reproduced in this publication and apologize to copyright holders if permission to publish in this form has not been obtained. If any copyright material has not been acknowledged please write and let us know so we may rectify in any future reprint.

Except as permitted under U.S. Copyright Law, no part of this book may be reprinted, reproduced, transmitted, or utilized in any form by any electronic, mechanical, or other means, now known or hereafter invented, including photocopying, microfilming, and recording, or in any information storage or retrieval system, without written permission from the publishers.

For permission to photocopy or use material electronically from this work, please access www.copyright.com (http://www.copyright.com/) or contact the Copyright Clearance Center, Inc. (CCC), 222 Rosewood Drive, Danvers, MA 01923, 978-750-8400. CCC is a not-for-profit organization that provides licenses and registration for a variety of users. For organizations that have been granted a photocopy license by the CCC, a separate system of payment has been arranged.

Trademark Notice: Product or corporate names may be trademarks or registered trademarks, and are used only for identification and explanation without intent to infringe.

Visit the Taylor & Francis Web site at
http://www.taylorandfrancis.com

and the CRC Press Web site at
http://www.crcpress.com

A CIP record for this book is available from the British Library.
Library of Congress Cataloging-in-Publication Data

Contents

PART III: MAIN ENTITIES/LOCATIONS

Contributors

WY Au
Department of Medicine
Queen Mary Hospital
Hong Kong
China

Tracy T Batchelor
Massachusetts General Hospital
Harvard Medical School
Department of Neurology
Boston, MA
USA

Francesco Bertoni
IOSI
Department of Experimental Oncology
Bellinzona
Switzerland

Atto Billio
Department of Hematology and Bone Marrow
Transplantation
Ospedale Centrale di Bolzano
Bolzano
Italy

Paolo Boffetta
Chief
Unit of Environmental Cancer Epidemiology
International Agency for Research on Cancer
Lyon
France

James J Campbell
Department of Dermatology
Brigham and Women's Hospital
Boston, MA
USA

C Campidelli
Units of Hematopathology and Hematology
Institute of Hematology and Clinical Oncology
L. and A. Seràgnoli
Bologna University School of Medicine
Italy

George P Canellos
Chief Division of Medical Oncology
Dana-Farber Cancer Institute
Boston, MA
USA

Antonino Carbone
Department of Pathology
National Cancer Institute
Milan
Italy

Franco Cavalli
Director
Institute of Oncology
of Southern Switzerland
Bellinzona
Switzerland

David Christie
East Coast Cancer Center
Tugun, Queensland
Australia

Annarita Conconi
Division of Hematology
Department of Medical Science and IRCAD
Amedeo Avogadro
University of Eastern Piedmont
Novara
Italy

Joseph M Connors
Clinical Professor
University of British Columbia
BC Cancer Agency
Vancouver, BC
Canada

Sergio Cortelazzo
Ospedale Centrale di Bolzano
Bolzano
Italy

Christiane Copie-Bergman
Department of Pathology and Inserm U841
Hôpital Henri Mondor
Créteil
France

Francesco d'Amore
Aarhus University Hospital
Aarhus
Denmark

Volker Diehl
Haus LebensWert
University Hospital of Cologne
Cologne
Germany

Claudio Doglioni
San Raffaele Scientific Institute
Milan
Italy

Riccardo Dolcetti
Division of Experimental Oncology
Centro di Riferimento Oncologico
Aviano
Italy

Reinhard Dummer
Dermatologische Klinik
Universitätsspital Zürich
Zürich
Switzerland

Andrés JM Ferreri
Department of Radiochemotherapy
San Raffaele Scientific Institute
Milan
Italy

Michael Fuchs
Internal Medicine 1
University Hospital of Cologne
Cologne
Germany

Randy D Gascoyne
Department of Pathology
BC Cancer Agency
Vancouver, BC
Canada

Philippe Gaulard
Department of Pathology and Inserm U841
Hôpital Henri Mondor
Créteil
France

Mary G Gospodarowicz
Professor and Chair
Department of Radiation Oncology
Princess Margaret Hospital
Toronto, Ontario
Canada

Nancy Lee Harris
James Homer Wright
Pathology Laboratories/Warren 2
Harvard Medical School
Massachusetts General Hospital
Boston, MA
USA

Michael Hummel
Institute of Pathology
Campus Benjamin Franklin
Charité Universitätsmedizin Berlin
Berlin
Germany

Elaine S Jaffe
Laboratory of Pathology
National Cancer Institute
National Institute of Health
Bethesda, MD
USA

Marshall E Kadin
Department of Pathology
Harvard Medical School
and
Department of Dermatology
Brigham Women's Hospital
Boston, MA
and
Department of Dermatology and
Skin Surgery
Roger Williams Hospital
Providence
Rhode Island
USA

Won-Seog Kim
Samsung Medical Center
Sungkyunkwan
Department of Hematology-Oncology
University School of Medicine
Seoul
South Korea

YH Ko
Department of Medicine
Queen Mary Hospital
Hong Kong
China

Katrin Kuscher
Institute for Research in Biomedicine
Bellinzona
Switzerland

Raymond HS Liang
Department of Medicine
Queen Mary Hospital
Hong Kong
China

T Andrew Lister
Department of Medical Oncology
St. Bartholomew's Hospital
London
UK

Christoph Loddenkemper
Institut für Pathologie
Berlin
Germany

Thomas Longerich
Institute of Pathology
University Hospital
Heidelberg
Germany

Armando López-Guillermo
Postgraduate School of Hematology
Hospital Clinic
Villarroel IDIBAPS
Barcelona
Spain

Maurizio Martelli
Department of Cellular
Biotechnology and Hematology
University of Rome "La Sapienza"
Rome
Italy

Giovanni Martinelli
European Institute of Oncology
Milan
Italy

Takuhei Murase
Department of Internal Medicine
Nishio Municipal Hospital
Aichi
Japan

Shigeo Nakamura
Department of Pathology and
Clinical Laboratories
Nagoya University Hospital
Nagoya
Japan

Andreas Neubauer
Klinikum der Philipps-Universität Marburg
für Hämatologie, Onkologie and Immunologie
Marburg
Germany

Peter de Nully Brown
Division of Hematology
Herlev Hospital
Herlev
Denmark

Stefano A Pileri
Units of Hematopathology and Hematology
Institute of Hematology and Clinical Oncology
L. and A. Serágnoli
Bologna University School of Medicine
Bologna
Italy

Miguel A Piris
Centro Nacional de Investigaciones Oncologicas
Department of Molecular Pathology Program
Madrid
Spain

V Poletti
Unit of Lung Diseases Diagnostics and Therapy
G.B. Morgagni-L. Pierontoni Hospital
Forli
Italy

Maurilio Ponzoni
San Raffaela Scientific Institute
Milan
Italy

John Radford
Cancer Research UK Department of Medical
Oncology
Christie Hospital NHS Foundation Trust
Manchester
UK

Daniel Re
Medicine 3
Centre Hospitalier Antibes-Jean les Pins
Antibes
France

Gail Ryan
Peter MacCallum Cancer Institute
Department of Radiation Oncology
Melbourne, Victoria
Australia

Kerry J Savage
Department of Medical Oncology
British Columbia Cancer Agency
University of British Columbia
Vancouver, BC
Canada

John F Seymour
Division of Haematology and Medical Oncology
Peter MacCallum Cancer Institute
Melbourne
Australia

Michele Spina
Divisione Oncologia Medica e AIDS
Centro di Riferimento Oncologico
Aviano
Italy

Harald Stein
Director
Institut für Pathologie
Charité-Campus Benjamin Franklin
Berlin
Germany

Catherine Thieblemont
Department of Hemato-Oncology
Centre Hospitalier Lyon-Sud Hospital Saint-Louis
Paris
France

Umberto Tirelli
Divisione Oncologia Medica e AIDS
Centro di Riferimento Oncologico
Aviano
Italy

Lorenz Trümper
Department of Hematology/Oncology
University Göttingen
Göttingen
Germany

Richard W Tsang
Department of Radiation Oncology
Princess Margaret Hospital
University of Toronto
Toronto, Ontario
Canada

Mariagrazia Uguccioni
Institute for Research in Biomedicine
Bellinzona
Switzerland

Umberto Vitolo
UOA Ematologia 2
Azienda Ospedaliera
Torino
Italy

Julie Vose
Neumann M. and Mildred E. Harris Professor
Chief Section of Oncology
Nebraska Health System
Nebraska Medical Center
Omaha, Nebraska
USA

Luciano Wannesson
Oncology Institute of Southern Switzerland (IOSI)
Ospedale San Giovanni
Bellinzona
Switzerland

Dennis D Weisenburger
Department of Pathology and Microbiology
University of Nebraska
Omaha, Nebraska
USA

Andrew Wotherspoon
Royal Marsden Hospital
Department of Histopathology
London
UK

PL Zinzani
Units of Hematopathology and Hematology
Institute of Hematology and Clinical Oncology
L. and A. Serágnoli
Bologna University School of Medicine
Italy

Emanuele Zucca
Head Lymphoma Unit
Institute of Oncology of Southern Switzerland
Bellinzona
Switzerland

Preface

When two decades ago we began to be interested in the study of the extranodal lymphomas (i.e. those primarily arising outside the lymph nodes), only scanty literature and no textbooks were available on this topic.

At that time, with the exception of cutaneous T-cell lymphomas, whose pathological and clinical features had long been recognized as being clearly different from those of nodal lymphoma, no lymphoma classification was taking into account the site of origin.

The importance of site of origin slowly began to be acknowledged following the description of mucosa-associated lymphoid tissue (MALT) lymphomas in the 1980s, but only in 1994, PG Isaacson and AJ Norton published their textbook on extranodal lymphomas, which (despite being designed to provide a practical help to the hematopathologist for the diagnosis rather than addressing the therapeutic problems) become an important and stimulating reference also for clinicians and biologists involved in the research into this fascinating group of lymphomas. Indeed, that book contributed to the general acceptance of the MALT lymphoma concept, making many clinicians aware of the specific clinical and therapeutical problems posed by the site of origin. In the late 1990s the attitude of the scientific community towards the extranodal lymphomas was changing and a shared interest generated the International Extranodal Lymphoma Study Group (IELSG), with the precise aim of improving our understanding of extranodal lymphomas. The IELSG, by bringing together numerous scientists from different institutions, allowed data to be collected from a sufficient number of patients to successfully study specific extranodal sites of involvement.

Now, more than 10 years later, we believe that the time is right for another textbook on the extranodal lymphoma. The REAL and later the WHO lymphoma classifications have been published, recognizing not only the MALT lymphomas as a specific extranodal entity but also several other peculiar 'extranodal' conditions (e.g. within the group of diffuse large B-cell lymphomas, the intravascular lymphoma and the primary mediastinal lymphoma). Lymphoma treatments have also changed over time.

This book is aimed at providing an overview of today's exceedingly abundant information on this no-longer neglected group of lymphomas, with special attention to the advances that have been most recently reported. Most chapters have been written in collaboration with authors of different institutions or different specialties in order to have the most balanced synopsis of the present knowledge. The authors have tried to address the extranodal lymphoma in the context of the novel acquisitions on the biology and pathology of these entities and also to provide clinical information to help colleagues in the difficult task of choosing the proper treatment for each individual situation.

We must express our sincere and grateful thanks to all the authors, most of them belonging to the IELSG, for their commitment. We are particularly indebted to Olga Jackson for the outstanding secretarial and logistic assistance and gratefully acknowledge our Publishers for their patience in waiting for some very delayed chapters and their ability to complete the task within a very tight time schedule.

Franco Cavalli,
Harald Stein
and Emanuele Zucca

PART I
CONCEPTUAL BASIS

PART I

CONCEPTUAL BASIS

Challenging issues in the management of extranodal lymphomas

1

Emanuele Zucca and Franco Cavalli

INTRODUCTION

The term extranodal lymphoma encompasses a vast assortment of morphologies, molecular alterations, and clinical presentations. Correct diagnosis and appropriate treatment of extranodal lymphoma are often complicated by the variety of lymphoma types and the relative rarity of many of these tumor types. Moreover, in comparison with nodal presentation, B- and T-cell lymphoma diagnosed at extranodal sites may have quite different outcomes and may frequently require different therapeutic approaches due to specific organ-related problems. Indeed, the extranodal lymphomas represent a frequent challenge in routine lymphoma diagnosis, due to the diversity of morphologies, molecular abnormalities, and clinical pictures that can be present.

Until very recently, the literature on many of the specific types and sites of extranodal lymphomas was scant and often contradictory, lacking uniformity in histopathological classification. Many historical series were published before the recognition of mucosa-associated lymphoid tissue (MALT) as the origin of many extranodal lymphomas, and the older classification of non-Hodgkin's lymphomas (NHL) did not take into account peculiar histogenetic features of primary extranodal lymphomas. The first attempt to eliminate this problem was made only in 1994 with the proposal of the REAL classification[1] and afterwards with the World Health Organization (WHO) classification,[2] which definitely recognized the presence of specific extranodal entities such as mycosis

fungoides, enteropathy-associated T-cell lymphoma, nasal type natural killer (NK)/T-cell lymphomas, and the extranodal marginal zone B-cell lymphomas of MALT lymphoma.

This chapter provides an overview of the main challenging questions and controversial issues that one has to tackle when dealing with the management of extranodal lymphomas. Most of these issues are covered in detail in the rest of the book.

CONTROVERSY IN THE DEFINITION OF PRIMARY EXTRANODAL LYMPHOMAS

Approximately one-third of NHL arise from sites other than lymph nodes, spleen, or the bone marrow, and even from sites which normally contain no native lymphoid tissue.[3,4]

The exact designation of extranodal lymphoma is controversial, particularly in the presence of both nodal and extranodal disease. The first definition has been proposed by Dawson for gastrointestinal lymphomas,[5] and later refined by Lewin[6] and Herrmann.[7] The original Dawson criteria defined primary gastric lymphoma, a presentation with main disease manifestation in the stomach, with or without involvement of regional lymph nodes. Later these criteria were relaxed to allow for contiguous involvement of other organs (e.g. liver, spleen), and for distant nodal disease, providing that the extranodal lesion was the presenting site and, after routine staging procedures, constituted the predominant disease bulk, to which primary treatment must be directed.[8]

The designation of stage III and IV lymphomas as primary extranodal lymphomas is also debatable and many authors consider only stage I and II presentation as primary extranodal disease. However, since many extranodal lymphomas have the potential to disseminate, this approach may result in an incomplete picture. On the contrary, extranodal involvement in a disseminated disease may represent a secondary spread. Clearly, any chosen definition inevitably introduces a selection bias; a Dutch study from a population-based registry showed that the frequency of extranodal NHL fluctuated from 20% to 34%, depending on the adopted designation criteria.[9]

The Ann Arbor staging system is sometimes imperfect when dealing with extranodal presentation. As a consequence, the distinction between stage I and stage IV in the case of multifocal involvement of a single organ can be controversial, as well as the stage definition of bilateral involvement of 'paired organs'.

The designation of extranodal vs extralymphatic site can also be questionable and may affect the classification of extranodal lymphomas, since lymphomas of tonsils and Waldeyer's ring, thymus, spleen, appendix, and Peyer's patches can be regarded as originating from lymphatic tissues and not considered as extranodal lesions. Nonetheless, most clinicians separate nodal from extranodal rather than lymphatic from extralymphatic disease, and the term extranodal lymphoma is generally adopted to indicate presentation outside lymph node areas.

VARIABILITY IN THE REPORTED INCIDENCE OF PRIMARY EXTRANODAL LYMPHOMAS

The NHL incidence in Western countries has increased substantially in the last 40 years.[10] This increase appears to be higher in extranodal rather than nodal disease.[11–13] This may in part be due to improved diagnostic procedures (particularly in brain and gastrointestinal

lymphomas) and changes in classification, but much of the change is real and the reasons for it have been the subject of much debate. The acquired immunodeficiency syndrome (AIDS) epidemics in the 1980s does not explain completely this rise[12] and the etiology of extranodal lymphomas appears to be multifactorial and includes immune suppression, infections, both viral and bacterial, and exposure to pesticides and other environmental agents.[10] The differences in the extranodal lymphoma incidence patterns by histological subtype are notable and suggest etiological heterogeneity.[14] However, despite the considerable progress made in the understanding of MALT lymphoma and its relationship to bacterial infections,[15–18] the precise cause of most lymphoid neoplasms remains to be elucidated.

The proportion of NHL presenting at extranodal sites accounts for from one-quarter to more than one-half of new lymphoma cases, with important geographic variations (e.g. USA and Canada 27%, Denmark 37%, Holland 41%, Italy 48%, Hong Kong 29%, Thailand 58%).[3,12,19–24] The reasons for these discrepancies include variable reporting criteria, with diverse definitions of primary extranodal disease, variable inclusion of mycosis fungoides and other T-cell lymphomas, variable inclusion of Waldeyer's ring lymphomas, different types of data source (referral cancer centers vs population-based tumor registry series). Nevertheless, true geographic differences are also present: for example, the higher incidence of Epstein–Barr virus (EBV) and human T-lymphotropic virus 1 (HTLV1)-associated T-cell lymphomas and the lower incidence of follicular and small lymphocytic lymphoma in Asia is most likely affecting the frequency of extranodal presentations.

DIFFERENT CLINICOPATHOLOGICAL FEATURES AT DIFFERENT SITES

Signs and symptoms at presentation depend largely on the lymphoma localization and usually do not differ significantly from those of other malignancies affecting that specific organ. Gastric lymphomas present typically with symptoms of peptic disease, bowel lymphomas with diarrhea or obstruction, bone lymphoma usually with fractures and pain, or central nervous system (CNS) lymphomas with the symptoms associated to an intracranial mass. Especially in the absence of nodal involvement, primary extranodal lymphoma is often not suspected and most often is clinically indistinguishable from a carcinoma arising in the same site. Histological diagnosis with immunophenotypic and histochemical analysis is therefore particularly important.

The histological spectrum of extranodal lymphomas on the whole differs from that of nodal lymphomas. A population-based US study showed that about one-third of diffuse large B-cell lymphomas (the most common histologic subtype in most countries) can primarily present at extranodal sites, while more than three-quarters of peripheral T-cell lymphomas (almost all involving the skin) and less than 10% of follicular lymphoma cases are extranodal. Nearly half of the extranodal cases were of diffuse large cell histology.[12]

Extranodal lymphomas can arise in almost every organ.[3,4] However, most of the extranodal presentations appears to be clustered in a few sites: skin, stomach, brain, small intestine, and – when included in the reports – the Waldeyer's ring, being about one-third of all the extranodal lymphomas found in the gastrointestinal tract.[8,12,25–27]

With respect to histological classification, aggressive subtypes are predominant in NHL of CNS, testis, bone, and liver, whereas, in the gastrointestinal tract, a large spectrum of histological disease entities can be seen, comprising diffuse large B-cell lymphoma, MALT lymphoma (including the immunoproliferative small intestinal disease), Burkitt's lymphoma, enteropathy-associated T-cell lymphoma, mantle cell lymphoma, and follicular lymphoma.

Certain extranodal sites appear to have characteristic patterns of either B- or T-cell disease (e.g. nearly all primary lymphoma of the bone are of B-cell origin, whereas most cutaneous lymphomas are of T-cell lineage).

Regulation of lymphocyte trafficking and homing has been shown to play a major role in the biology of primary extranodal lymphomas of the skin and in MALT lymphomas of the gastrointestinal tract.[28–30] It seems plausible that the ability of mature lymphocytes to recirculate between blood and the lymph can be implicated in the determination of the specific location of extranodal forms.

CLINICAL OUTCOME

Despite the relative prominence of extranodal presentations, the outcomes of extranodal lymphomas are difficult to ascertain. Many reported data are limited to single-institution retrospective reviews and, in prospective therapeutic trials, extranodal lymphomas are often included together with nodal lymphomas. In the late 1990s, the International Extranodal Lymphoma Study Group (IELSG) was created to provide the adequate network for studying the extranodal lymphomas. Although extranodal lymphomas are not rare, the frequency of involvement of any particular site is not high enough for a single institution to answer the major question. Attempting to overcome these difficulties, the IELSG has gathered numerous scientists from different institutions in order to collect the data from a sufficient number of patients to study specific extranodal sites. This effort has originated a number of retrospective and prospective trials aimed to clarify the management issues distinct to extranodal presentations (http://www.ielsg.org/).

Whether or not extranodal lymphomas have an overall survival similar to that of nodal cases as a whole has also been a matter of controversy.[3] However, considering the many variables which influence site-specific outcome in extranodal lymphomas, it is questionable whether such a general distinction has clinical relevance. Indeed, as shown in Figure 1.1, which reports the survival rates of extranodal lymphomas in some large series of the IELSG,[31–38] the clinical outcome vary among all the specific sites of primary extranodal

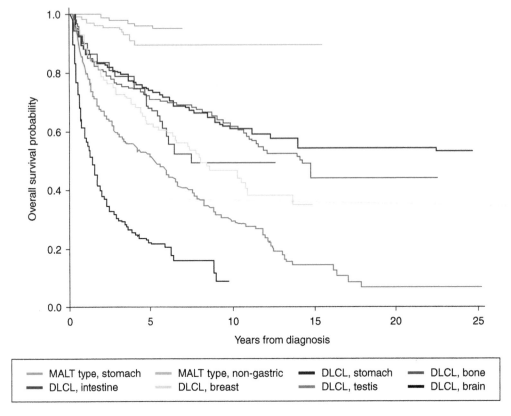

Figure 1.1 Outcome of primary extranodal lymphomas in the studies of the International Extranodal Lymphoma Study Group (IELSG): overall survival by histological subtype and presentation site.[31-38] MALT, mucosa-associated lymphoid tissue; DLCL, diffuse large B-cell lymphoma.

lymphomas. For example, in spite of the other factors being equal, the prognosis of diffuse large B-cell lymphoma in the brain or testis is quite different from that of gastric or bone lymphoma. In fact, in addition to the histological subtype – which is undoubtedly the main predictor of prognosis of either nodal or extranodal lymphomas – the primary organ of origin represents the most significant discriminatory factor among aggressive extranodal lymphomas. This is partially due to differences in natural history, but mainly to differences in management strategy, which are related to organ-specific problems (e.g. the blood–brain barrier). Furthermore, some specific disease localizations require specific staging procedures (such as an ophthalmological examination with slit-lamp in brain lymphoma).

The influence of the localization site on the outcome is less clear in MALT lymphoma, where multifocal lesions are present in 20–40% of patients.[32,39–42] Dissemination is more frequent in non-gastric lymphomas and can occur either to other mucosal sites or to a non-mucosal site such as spleen, bone marrow, or liver. Interestingly, as depicted in Figure 1.2, in MALT lymphoma, at least when limited to mucosal sites, dissemination does not seem to be necessarily associated with a poorer outcome.[32,41]

In conclusion, the pronounced heterogeneities in the pathogenesis, clinicopathological features, and outcome of the various primary extranodal presentations are important reasons for a detailed consideration of the different sites of origin of these lymphomas, which is the aim of the present textbook.

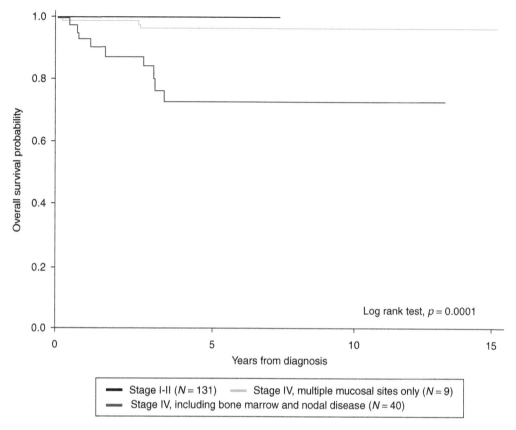

Figure 1.2   Kaplan–Meier estimate of overall survival according to the Ann Arbor stage of disease in a series of primary non-gastric marginal zone B-cell lymphomas of MALT type. Within the category of stage IV disease, the subgroup of patients with involvement of multiple MALT sites had a significantly better survival than the remaining cases with stage IV, comprising those with multiple organ involvement or multifocal involvement of a single organ and additional bone marrow or nodal involvement. This research was originally published in *Blood.*[32] (© the American Society of Hematology.)

REFERENCES

1. Harris NL, Jaffe ES, Stein H, et al. A revised European-American classification of lymphoid neoplasms: a proposal from the International Lymphoma Study Group. Blood 1994; 84: 1361–92.
2. Jaffe ES, Harris NL, Stein H, Vardiman JW. Pathology and genetics of tumours of haematopoietic and lymphoid tissues. World Health Organization Classification of Tumours, 3rd edn. Lyon: IARC Press, 2001: 1–351.
3. Zucca E, Roggero E, Bertoni F, Cavalli F. Primary extranodal non-Hodgkin's lymphomas. Part 1: gastrointestinal, cutaneous and genitourinary lymphomas. Ann Oncol 1997; 8: 727–37.
4. Zucca E, Roggero E, Bertoni F, Conconi A, Cavalli F. Primary extranodal non-Hodgkin's lymphomas. Part 2: Head and neck, central nervous system and other less common sites. Ann Oncol 1999; 10: 1023–33.
5. Dawson IM, Cornes JS, Morson BC. Primary malignant lymphoid tumours of the intestinal tract. Report of 37 cases with a study of factors influencing prognosis. Br J Surg 1961; 49: 80–9.
6. Lewin KJ, Ranchod M, Dorfman RF. Lymphomas of the gastrointestinal tract: a study of 117 cases presenting with gastrointestinal disease. Cancer 1978; 42: 693–707.
7. Herrmann R, Panahon AM, Barcos MP, Walsh D, Stutzman L. Gastrointestinal involvement in non-Hodgkin's lymphoma. Cancer 1980; 46: 215–22.
8. d'Amore F, Christensen BE, Brincker H, et al. Clinicopathological features and prognostic factors in extranodal non-Hodgkin lymphomas. Danish LYFO Study Group. Eur J Cancer 1991; 27: 1201–8.

9. Krol AD, le Cessie S, Snijder S, et al. Primary extran-odal non-Hodgkin's lymphoma (NHL): the impact of alternative definitions tested in the Comprehensive Cancer Centre West population-based NHL registry. Ann Oncol 2003; 14: 131–9.

10. Parkin DM, Bray F, Ferlay J, Pisani P. Global cancer statistics, 2002. CA Cancer J Clin 2005; 55: 74–108.

11. Devesa SS, Fears T. Non-Hodgkin's lymphoma time trends: United States and international data. Cancer Res 1992; 52: 5432s–40s.

12. Groves FD, Linet MS, Travis LB, Devesa SS. Cancer surveillance series: non-Hodgkin's lymphoma inci-dence by histologic subtype in the United States from 1978 through 1995. J Natl Cancer Inst 2000; 92: 1240–51.

13. Chiu BC, Weisenburger DD. An update of the epidemiology of non-Hodgkin's lymphoma. Clin Lymphoma 2003; 4: 161–8.

14. Morton LM, Wang SS, Devesa SS, et al. Lymphoma incidence patterns by WHO subtype in the United States, 1992–2001. Blood 2006; 107: 265–76.

15. Bertoni F, Zucca E. State-of-the-art therapeutics: mar-ginal-zone lymphoma. J Clin Oncol 2005; 23: 6415–20.

16. Guidoboni M, Ferreri AJ, Ponzoni M, Doglioni C, Dolcetti R. Infectious agents in mucosa-associated lymphoid tissue-type lymphomas: pathogenic role and therapeutic perspectives. Clin Lymphoma Myeloma 2006; 6: 289–300.

17. Suarez F, Lortholary O, Hermine O, Lecuit M. Infection-associated lymphomas derived from marginal zone B cells: a model of antigen-driven lymphoproliferation. Blood 2006; 107: 3034–44.

18. Ferreri AJ, Dolcetti R, Du MQ, et al. Ocular adnexal MALT lymphoma: an intriguing model for antigen-driven lymphomagenesis and microbial-targeted therapy. Ann Oncol 2007.

19. Haddadin WJ. Malignant lymphoma in Jordan: a ret-rospective analysis of 347 cases according to the World Health Organization classification. Ann Saudi Med 2005; 25: 398–403.

20. Sukpanichnant S. Analysis of 1983 cases of malignant lymphoma in Thailand according to the World Health Organization classification. Hum Pathol 2004; 35: 224–30.

21. Economopoulos T, Asprou N, Stathakis N, et al. Primary extranodal non-Hodgkin's lymphoma in adults: clinicopathological and survival characteris-tics. Leuk Lymphoma 1996; 21: 131–6.

22. Chang KC, Huang GC, Jones D, et al. Distribution and prognosis of WHO lymphoma subtypes in Taiwan reveals a low incidence of germinal-center derived tumors. Leuk Lymphoma 2004; 45: 1375–84.

23. Isikdogan A, Ayyildiz O, Buyukcelik A, et al. Non-Hodgkin's lymphoma in southeast Turkey: clinico-pathologic features of 490 cases. Ann Hematol 2004; 83: 265–9.

24. Temmim L, Baker H, Amanguno H, Madda JP, Sinowatz F. Clinicopathological features of extranodal lymphomas: Kuwait experience. Oncology 2004; 67: 382–9.

25. Sutcliffe SB, Gospodarowicz MK. Localized extran-odal lymphomas. In: Keating A, Armitage J, Burnett A, Newland A, eds. Hematological Oncology. Cam-bridge: Cambridge University Press, 1992: 189–222.

26. Gospodarowicz MK, Ferry JA, Cavalli F. Unique aspects of primary extranodal lymphomas. In: Mauch PM, Armitage JO, Harris NL, Dalla-Favera R, Coiffier B, eds. Non-Hodgkin's Lymphomas. Philadelphia: Lippincott Williams & Wilkins, 2003: 685–707.

27. Shenkier TN, Connors JM. Primary extranodal non-Hodgkin's lymphomas. In: Canellos GP, Lister TA, Young BD, eds. The Lymphomas, 2nd edn. Philadelphia: Saunders Elsevier, 2006: 325–47.

28. Dogan A, Du M, Koulis A, Briskin MJ, Isaacson PG. Expression of lymphocyte homing receptors and vascular addressins in low-grade gastric B-cell lymphomas of mucosa- associated lymphoid tissue. Am J Pathol 1997; 151: 1361–9.

29. Du MQ, Peng HZ, Dogan A, et al. Preferential dissemination of B-cell gastric mucosa-associated lymphoid tissue (MALT) lymphoma to the splenic marginal zone. Blood 1997; 90: 4071–7.

30. Drillenburg P, van der Voort R, Koopman G, et al. Preferential expression of the mucosal homing recep-tor integrin alpha 4 beta 7 in gastrointestinal non-Hodgkin's lymphomas. Am J Pathol 1997; 150: 919–27.

31. Hancock B, Linch D, Delchier J, et al. Chlorambucil versus observation after anti-Helicobacter therapy in low-grade gastric lymphoma: results of the inter-national LY03 trial (abstract). Ann Oncol 2005: 16(supp 5); 56: abstract 074.

32. Zucca E, Conconi A, Pedrinis E, et al. Nongastric marginal zone B-cell lymphoma of mucosa-associ-ated lymphoid tissue. Blood 2003; 101: 2489–95.

33. Cortelazzo S, Rossi A, Oldani E, et al. The modified International Prognostic Index can predict the out-come of localized primary intestinal lymphoma of both extranodal marginal zone B-cell and diffuse large B-cell histologies. Br J Haematol 2002; 118: 218–28.

34. Cortelazzo S, Rossi A, Roggero F, et al. Stage-modified international prognostic index effectively predicts clini-cal outcome of localized primary gastric diffuse large B-cell lymphoma. International Extranodal Lymphoma Study Group (IELSG). Ann Oncol 1999; 10: 1433–40.

35. Christie D, Gracia E, Gospodarowicz M, et al. Patterns of outcome and prognostic factors in primary bone lymphoma (osteolymphoma): a survey of 499 cases by the International Extranodal Lymphoma Study Group. Haematologica 2007; 92(Suppl 1): Abstract # 0717.

36. Ryan G, Martinelli G, Kuper-Hommel M, et al. Primary diffuse large B-cell lymphoma of the breast: prognostic factors and outcomes of a study by the International Extranodal Lymphoma Study Group. Ann Oncol 2008; 19: 233–41.

37. Zucca E, Conconi A, Mughal TI, et al. Patterns of outcome and prognostic factors in primary large-cell lymphoma of the testis in a survey by the

International Extranodal Lymphoma Study Group. J Clin Oncol 2003; 21: 20–7.

38. Ferreri AJ, Blay JY, Reni M, et al. Prognostic scoring system for primary CNS lymphomas: the International Extranodal Lymphoma Study Group experience. J Clin Oncol 2003; 21: 266–72.

39. Zucca E, Bertoni F, Roggero E, Cavalli F. The gastric marginal zone B-cell lymphoma of MALT type. Blood 2000; 96: 410–19.

40. Pinotti G, Zucca E, Roggero E, et al. Clinical features, treatment and outcome in a series of 93 patients with low-grade gastric MALT lymphoma. Leuk Lymphoma 1997; 26: 527–37.

41. Thieblemont C, Berger F, Dumontet C, et al. Mucosa-associated lymphoid tissue lymphoma is a disseminated disease in one third of 158 patients analyzed. Blood 2000; 95: 802–6.

42. Thieblemont C, Coiffier B. MALT lymphoma: sites of presentations, clinical features and staging procedures. In: Zucca E, Bertoni F, eds. MALT Lymphomas. Georgetown, TX: Landes Bioscience/ Kluwer Academic, 2004: 60–80.

2

Historical prospect for the concept of primary extranodal lymphoma

George P Canellos and T Andrew Lister

Primary extranodal lymphoma was first recognized in the mid-20th century. References in the literature to extranodal presentations of lymphoma, referred to in the Gall–Mallory system of 'lymphosarcoma,' abound from the 1950s, usually in small case series.[1] Primary lymphoma of the lung, gastrointestinal tract, bone, salivary glands, and testis were noted.[2–6] The reality of extranodal lymphoma as an entity was generally formalized in 1961 in an extensive review by Dr Saul Rosenberg that included a detailed review of 1269 cases of 'lymphosarcoma' at Memorial Hospital in New York.[6] Since the treatments employed were rudimentary by today's standards, the distinction between 'extranodal and nodal disease' were not very clear and primary extranodal sites were not enumerated as distinct entities. Given the times and referral patterns to major urban cancer hospitals, it is not surprising that extranodal primary disease was less well defined because of the dissemination that can occur in the late untreated phases of many primary extranodal lymphomas.[7] The limitations of imaging technology also were a factor, since primary extranodal intestinal presentations, by historical analysis, were very rare. In the Gall and Mallory series, only 4% of 389 patients were considered 'localized.' Similarly, the Rosenberg series had only 4.6% presenting in the gastrointestinal tract but up to 50% at autopsy.

In the early 1960s, the etiology of extranodal lymphoma began to emerge. The lymphoid abnormalities complicating the course of Sjögren's syndrome were referred to as 'pseudolymphoma' and serve as an example.[8]

It was noted that in the natural history of the disease, some patients actually died of 'reticulum cell sarcoma,' and to some the histological abnormalities in the extrasalivary lymphoid tissues were considered 'unequivocally lymphomatous.'[9] It remained for the detailed use of immunoperoxidase techniques to identify intracellular heavy chains and kappa, lambda light chains to define the lymphoid disorder in Sjögren's syndrome as a monoclonal B-cell neoplasm.[10] In the early 1970s, one of the pioneering attempts to define extranodal lymphoma as a distinct entity came from the 'End Results Group' of the National Cancer Institute. Of the 6150 reported cases of lymphoma in the USA, 24% (1467 cases) were described as extranodal,[11] a higher percentage than noted in the previous decades. There was variation in reported incidence, according to geographic location, with a higher incidence of primary gastrointestinal lymphomas, for example, in the Middle East. The distribution of extranodal lymphomas according to histological subtype on presentation has been shown to be an aggressive, usually large cell lymphoma (usually B-cell origin) in 56% of cases, with a small minority defined as lymphoblastic or Burkitt-type included. The remainder are divided among the known lower-grade lymphomas: follicular, small lymphocytic, marginal zone, and lymphoplasmacytic.[12] In fact, in the passage of time, it has become apparent that about 40% of all diffuse large B-cell lymphoma present as an extranodal tumors.[13]

The major sites of involvement can vary according to the institutional referral patterns,

Table 2.1   Sites of primary extranodal lymphoma

Majority (65%):
- Gastrointestinal tract
- Waldeyer's ring of lymphoid tissue
- Skin

Minority (35%):
- Central nervous system
- Bone
- Lung
- Testis
- Salivary glands

but in general there is agreement that the gastrointestinal tract, Waldeyer's ring, and skin make up the majority, approximately 65%, with the remainder divided almost equally between central nervous system (CNS), lung, testis, salivary glands, and bone[14,15] (Table 2.1). The generally agreed upon definition of primary extranodal lymphoma is disease confined to a single extranodal site, with or without regional lymph node involvement.

Important biological information as to microbiological etiological factors in lymphoma have emerged from the study of the unique features of some extranodal lymphomas, and indicate the role of chronic antigenic stimulation. Extranodal low-grade lymphomas of the marginal B-cell origin within mucosa-associated lymphoid tissue (MALT) have assumed a special biological importance. It was demonstrated that there were functional if not etiological relationships between these lymphoid abnormalities in the stomach defined as MALTomas and the presence of the bacterium *Helicobacter pylori*.[16] Resolution in many but not all patients following oral antibiotics opened speculation as to the role of bacterial antigens as stimulants to the growth of lymphoma cells in the gastric MALT.[17,18] There is further unconfirmed evidence for a similar relationship of ocular adnexal lymphoma, a non-gastric marginal zone lymphoma, and the presence of *Chlamydia psittaci*.[19,20] Another feature noted in low-grade gastric MALT lymphoma is the unexpectedly high incidence of other tumors.[21] The explanation for this is still unclear.

In the last 20 years, a distinct increase of extranodal large cell lymphoma has been

recognized in association with acquired immunodeficiency syndrome (AIDS) and intense immunosuppression following organ transplantation. In both these circumstances, extranodal presentations such as primary CNS lymphoma were common and associated in many instances with Epstein–Barr virus (EBV) as an etiological factor.[22] Primary lymphoma of the nasal area, usually of natural killer/T-cell origin is more common in Asia but is also associated with EBV.[23] Immune suppressed patients also were rarely noted to develop a primary effusion lymphoma (PEL), an entity found to be associated with the human herpes virus 8 (HHV8), an etiological factor also in Castleman's disease and Kaposi's sarcoma.[24]

Although 25–40% of all lymphomas are now thought to be present as primary extranodal lymphomas, the WHO (World Health Organization) classification of lymphomas has allowed for separate classification of some but not all lymphomas presenting mainly in extranodal sites,[25] including (1) extranodal marginal zone B-cell lymphoma of MALT type, (2) primary effusion lymphoma, and extranodal natural killer/T-cell lymphoma nodal type. The unique biological and therapeutic aspects of the extranodal lymphomas had generated enough international interest to warrant the formation of a cooperative group structure to explore the various clinical/therapeutic aspects of the extranodal lymphomas. In 1997, the International Extranodal Lymphoma Study Group (IELGS) was organized and has been active in promoting natural history studies and therapeutic trials (Table 2.2).

The IELSG's interest in these abovementioned areas has resulted in multiple publications on topics from CNS to testis lymphoma.[26,27] In 1993, an international prognostic model for aggressive lymphomas was developed and used extensively.[28] A modification was adapted by the IELSG for intestinal lymphoma of both low-grade marginal zone and diffuse large B-cell histology.[29]

As a general rule, diffuse large B-cell lymphoma presenting in the gastrointestinal tract and Waldeyer's ring have a more favorable

Table 2.2   Historical evolution of primary extranodal lymphoma

- 1950s – isolated case reports
- 1961 – review of Memorial Hospital series (1267 cases by Rosenberg et al)
- 1964 – lymphomatous evolution in Sjögren's syndrome
- 1972 – 'end results' analysis (1467 cases by Freeman et al)
- 1993 – Association of gastric MALT lymphoma with *Helicobacter pylori*
- 1997 – founding of IELSG (International Extranodal Lymphoma Study Group)
- 2003 – clinical definitions and subsequent survival

outcome than nodal or indeed other extranodal presentations.[14] In addition, controlled trials in the recent past have emphasized an important role of chemotherapy in providing an equivalent outcome to combined radiation–chemotherapy treatment. This observation is especially helpful in the management of localized lymphoma in the elderly.[30,31] Extranodal lymphoma has been demonstrated to have specific therapies designed for initial presentation and relapse. For example, there has been an evolution in the use of drugs which penetrate the blood–brain barrier to treat primary large cell CNS lymphoma. Similarly, testis lymphoma is almost always 'large cell' in type and requires radiotherapy to the contralateral testis as well as CNS prophylaxis because of the higher propensity for relapse in those sites.

The introduction of positron emission tomography (PET) scans in the staging of lymphoma has generated some issues unique to extranodal marginal zone lymphoma of MALT. PET scanning with ^{18}F-2-fluoro-2-deoxy-D-glucose is now widely accepted as a routine investigation. A recent analysis demonstrated that only a MALToma with plasmacytic differentiation showed a distinctly positive PET scan, whereas MALT tumors without it may have a high false-negative rate.[32] This can also be seen in other presentations of low-grade lymphoma. Furthermore, combined PET and CT (computed tomography), rather than separate studies, was noted to better define extranodal disease.[33]

The new wave of molecular science in lymphoma has identified genetic signatures that correlate with prognosis in large cell lymphoma.[34,35] A unique biological association of extranodal lymphoma was noted in studies of amplification of the proto-oncogene REL. About 73% of patients with diffuse large cell lymphoma who show amplification of REL were, in fact, primary extranodal lymphoma.[36] This technology has been applied to primary mediastinal large B-cell lymphoma of presumed thymic origin, which has been shown to share some molecular genetic features with classic Hodgkin's lymphoma.[37] Coordinated clinical and correlative scientific investigations in other extranodal lymphomas are likely to be productive of unique genetic profiles that could be targets for specific inhibitors in the future. The concept of primary extranodal lymphoma is now an accepted phenomenon. It remains for future scientific progress to define molecular uniqueness.

REFERENCES

1. Gall EA, Mallory TB. Malignant lymphoma. A clinicopathologic survey of 618 cases. Am J Pathol 1942; 18: 381–429.
2. Beck WC, Reganis JC. Primary lymphoma of the lung; review of literature, report of one case, and addition of eight other cases. J Thorac Surg 1951; 22: 323–8.
3. Parker JW Jr, Jackson M. Primary reticulum cell sarcoma of bone. Surg Gynecol Obstet 1939; 68: 45–53.
4. Abeshouse BS, Tiongson A, Goldfarb M. Bilateral tumors of the testis – review of the literature of bilateral simultaneous lymphosarcoma. J Urol 1955; 74: 522–32.
5. Dawson IMP, Cornes JS, Morson BC. Primary malignant tumors of the intestinal tract. Report of 37 cases with a study of factors influencing prognosis. Br J Surg 1961; 49: 80–9.
6. Rosenberg SA, Diamond HD, Jaslowitz B, Craver LF. Lymphosarcoma: a review of 1269 cases. Medicine 1961; 40: 31–76.
7. Gospodarowicz MK, Sutcliffe SB, Brown TC, et al. Patterns of disease in localized extranodal lymphomas. J Clin Oncol 1987; 5: 875–80.
8. Talal N, Sokoloff L, Barth WF. Extrasalivary lymphoid abnormalities in Sjögren's syndrome (reticulum cell sarcoma, 'pseudolymphoma,' macroglobulinemia). Am J Med 1967; 43: 50–65.

9. Talal N, Bunim JJ. The development of malignant lymphoma in the course of Sjögren's syndrome. Am J Med 1964; 36: 529–40.

10. Zulman J, Jaffe R, Talal N. Evidence that the malignant lymphoma of Sjögren's syndrome is a monoclonal B-cell neoplasm. N Engl J Med 1978; 299: 1215–20.

11. Freeman C, Berg J, Cutler S. Occurrence and prognosis of extranodal lymphomas. Cancer 1977; 29: 252–60.

12. d'Amore F, Christensen BE, Brincker H, et al. Clinicopathological features and prognostic factors in extranodal non-Hodgkin lymphomas. Eur J Cancer 1991; 27: 1201–8.

13. Mann RB. Are there site-specific differences among extranodal aggressive B-cell neoplasms? Am J Clin Pathol 1999; 111(Suppl 1): S144–50.

14. Krol ADG, le Cessie S, Snijder S, et al. Primary extranodal non-Hodgkin's lymphoma (NHL): the impact of alternative definitions tested in the Comprehensive Cancer Centre West population-based NHL registry. Ann Oncol 2003; 14: 131–9.

15. Lopez-Guillermo A, Colomo L, Jimenez M, et al. Diffuse large B-cell lymphoma: clinical and biological characterization and outcome according to the nodal or extranodal primary origin. J Clin Oncol 2005; 23: 2797–804.

16. Hussell R, Isaacson PG, Crabtree JE, Spencer J. The response of cells from low-grade B-cell gastric lymphomas of mucosa-associated lymphoid tissue to *Helicobacter pylori*. Lancet 1993; 342: 571–4.

17. Bayerdorffer E, Neubauer A, Rudolph B, et al. Regression of primary gastric lymphoma of mucosa-associated lymphoid tissue type after cure of *Helicobacter pylori* infection. Lancet 1995; 345: 1591–4.

18. Lenze D, Berg E, Volkmer-Engert R, et al. Influence of antigen on the development of MALT lymphoma. Blood 2006; 107: 1141–8.

19. Ferreri AJM, Ponzoni M, Guidoboni M, et al. Regression of ocular adnexal lymphoma after Chlamydia psittaci-eradicating antibody therapy. J Clin Oncol 2005; 23: 5067–73.

20. Rosado MF, Byrne GE Jr, Ding F, et al. Ocular adnexal lymphoma: a clinicopathologic study of a large cohort of patients with no evidence for an association with *Chlamydia psittaci*. Blood 2006; 107: 467–72.

21. Zucca E, Pinotti G, Roggero E, et al. High incidence of other neoplasms in patients with low-grade gastric MALT lymphoma. Ann Oncol 1995; 6: 726–8.

22. Navarro WH, Kaplan LD. AIDS-related lymphoproliferative disease. Blood 2006; 107: 13–20.

23. Au WY, Ma SY, Chim CS, et al. Clinicopathologic features and treatment outcome of mature T-cell and natural killer-cell lymphomas diagnosed according to the World Health Organization classification scheme: a single center experience of 10 years. Ann Oncol 2005; 16: 206–14.

24. Horenstein MG, Nador RG, Chadbury A, et al. Epstein-Barr virus latent gene expression in primary effusion lymphomas containing Kaposi's sarcoma-associated herpesvirus/human herpesvirus-8. Blood 1997; 90: 1186–91.

25. Jaffe ES, Harris NL, Stein H, Vardiman JW, eds. Pathology and Genetics of Tumours of Haematopoietic and Lymphoid Tissues. Lyon: IARC Press, 2001.

26. Ferreri AJM, Blay JY, Reni M, et al. Prognostic scoring system for primary CNS lymphomas: the International Extranodal Lymphoma Study Group experience. J Clin Oncol 2003; 21: 266–72.

27. Zucca E, Conconi A, Mughal TI, et al. Patterns of outcome and prognostic factors in primary large-cell lymphoma of the testis in a survey by the International Extranodal Lymphoma Study Group. J Clin Oncol 2003; 21: 20–7.

28. International Non-Hodgkin's Lymphoma Prognostic Factors Project. A predictive model for aggressive non-Hodgkin's lymphoma. N Engl J Med 1993; 329: 987–94.

29. Cortelazzo S, Rossi A, Oldani E, et al. The modified International Prognostic Index can predict the outcome of localized primary intestinal lymphoma of both extranodal marginal zone B-cell and diffuse large B-cell histologies. Br J Haematol 2002; 118: 218–28.

30. Miller TP, Dahlberg S, Cassady JR, et al. Chemotherapy alone compared with chemotherapy plus radiotherapy for localized intermediate and high-grade non-Hodgkin's lymphoma. N Engl J Med 1998; 339: 21–6.

31. Reyes F, Lepage E, Ganem G, et al. ACVBP versus CHOP plus radiotherapy for localized aggressive lymphoma. N Engl J Med 2005; 352: 1197–205.

32. Hoffmann M, Wohrer S, Becherer A, et al. 18F-Fluorodeoxy-glucose positron emission tomography in lymphoma of mucosa-associated lymphoid tissue: histology makes the difference. Ann Oncol 2006; 17: 1761–5.

33. Hernandez-Maraver D, Hernandez-Navarro F, Gomez-Leon N, et al. Positron emission tomography/computed tomography: diagnostic accuracy in lymphoma. Br J Haematol 2006; 13: 293–302.

34. Bea S, Zetti A, Wright G, et al. Diffuse large B-cell lymphoma subgroups have distinct genetic profiles that influence tumor biology and improve gene-expression-based survival prediction. Blood 2005; 106: 3183–90.

35. Monti S, Savage KJ, Kutok JL, et al. Molecular profiling of diffuse large B-cell lymphoma identified robust subtypes including one characterized by host inflammatory response. Blood 2005; 105: 1851–61.

36. Houldsworth J, Mathew S, Rao PH, et al. PEL protooncogene is frequently amplified in extranodal diffuse large cell lymphoma. Blood 1996; 87: 25–9.

37. Savage KJ, Monti S, Kutok JL, et al. The molecular signature of mediastinal large B-cell lymphoma differs from that of other diffuse large B-cell lymphomas and shares features with classical Hodgkin lymphoma. Blood 2003; 102: 3871–9.

Epidemiology of extranodal lymphomas

3

Francesco d'Amore, Peter de Nully Brown, and Dennis D Weisenburger

INTRODUCTION

Although most non-Hodgkin's lymphomas (NHL) originate in lymph nodes, primary localizations in other organs, even in sites which usually do not contain lymphoid tissue, are not uncommon. However, an accurate estimate of the frequency of primary extranodal NHL (PE-NHL) is highly dependent on the criteria used to define this entity. These criteria can either be:

- rigorously limited to extranodal disease at one or multiple anatomical sites in the absence of any nodal manifestation
- allow the existence of a 'minor' nodal component along with 'clinically dominant' extranodal involvement.

The majority of existing reports on PE-NHL are based on the latter definition.

SITES OF DISEASE, LYMPHOMA CLASSIFICATION, AND HISTOLOGICAL SUBTYPES

It has been controversial whether some anatomical sites such as the tonsils/Waldeyer's ring, spleen, and bone marrow should be regarded as extranodal localizations. In recent years, new developments in our knowledge of NHL have allowed the identification of well-defined and biologically distinct new entities. Consequently, a precise recognition of the histopathological entity has become more important than characterization based merely on the site of disease. Hence, splenic marginal zone lymphoma should be recognized as a primary entity affecting the spleen, whereas splenic involvement

by an otherwise disseminated follicular NHL should be regarded as part of generalized disease. On the other hand, in the recent World Health Organization (WHO) lymphoma classification,[1] some of the entities, particularly among the T- and NK-cell neoplasms, have typical anatomical localizations (e.g. liver–spleen, nasal cavity, small intestine, subcutaneous soft tissue) and this clinical information has been included in the definition of these entities (hepatosplenic, nasal-type, enteropathy-type, subcutaneous panniculitis-like).[2] Moreover, for some anatomical manifestations, such as primary central nervous system lymphomas (PCNSL), the site of disease, although not characterized by unique histopathological features, represents crucial information for the choice of treatment. With regard to the common histologies, such as diffuse large B-cell lymphoma (DLBCL) and follicular lymphoma (FL), the reported frequency among all PE-NHL is 40–45% for DLBCL[3] and 15–20% for FL.[3-5] Primary nodal DLBCL is slightly less frequent than PE disease, whereas FL is clearly more frequent as nodal disease. Figure 3.1 shows the different distributions by histological subtype among primary nodal and PE lymphomas, according to the population-based Danish Lymphoma Group (LYFO Registry).

FACTORS INFLUENCING THE ANATOMICAL LOCATION OF THE TUMOR

The site at which lymphoma cells proliferate is probably a reflection of an interaction

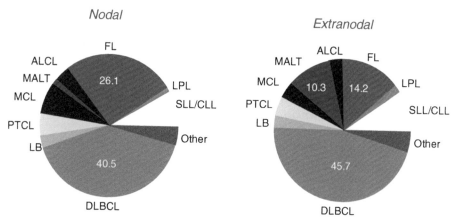

Figure 3.1 Distribution of histological subtypes in primary nodal and PE-NHL (data source: Danish Lymphoma Group – LYFO Registry). ALCL, anaplastic large cell lymphoma; DLBCL, diffuse large B-cell lymphoma; FL, follicular lymphoma; MALT, mucosa-associated lymphoid tissue lymphoma; LB, lymphoblastic lymphoma, including. Burkitt and Burkitt-like; LPL, lymphoplasmacytic lymphoma; PTCL, peripheral T-cell lymphoma; SLL/CLL, small lymphocytic lymphoma/CLL-type; MCL, mantle cell lymphoma.

between tumor cell characteristics (e.g. homing and adhesion molecules, growth factor receptors, etc.) and growth-promoting microenvironmental features (presence of corresponding ligands and growth factors). For example, in Burkitt's lymphoma, cells that have acquired the pathogenetically relevant translocation in the bone marrow will subsequently migrate to sites supportive of tumor growth. Histopathological examination of the jaw, a site often involved in young African children, has demonstrated an intimate association of the lymphoma cells with developing molar teeth, a microenvironment rich in growth factors. In fact, jaw involvement is far less common in older children and adults, in whom molar tooth development and eruption are complete. Similarly, breast involvement in Burkitt's lymphoma is primarily seen in pubertal and lactating women, substantiating the impression that lymphoma cell migration and proliferation is facilitated by the presence of physiological growth factors in the microenvironment of the tumor.

INCIDENCE RATES

Different studies from Western countries have reported the occurrence of PE-NHL in 24–48% of all NHL,[6,7] a figure much higher

than observed in Hodgkin's lymphoma (HL) (2–5%). Homogeneous data reported from large population-based registries (US, Holland, Denmark) seem to agree on a frequency of PE-NHL of 30–35%.[3,8]

Variation by ethnicity and geography

The distribution of the major histological NHL subtypes (e.g. germinal center cell-derived entities such as FL and DLBCL, or natural killer (NK)/T-cell derived entities) differs by geographic location.[9] The incidence of NHL, as a whole, also varies considerably in different parts of the world, with the lowest rates in Asia and Africa, and higher rates in Europe and North America.[10] However, the opposite seems to apply for PE-NHL rates.[11] Registry-based studies from Arabian Gulf countries have demonstrated a particularly high occurrence of extranodal lymphomas (42–45%).[11,12] This is primarily due to a higher frequency of gastrointestinal tract (GIT) involvement. Significant differences in the occurrence of GIT lymphomas have also been reported in Europe. A comparative study revealed a 13-fold higher occurrence of primary gastric lymphoma in northeastern Italy compared to the southern UK. The authors suggested that this difference could be correlated with a higher occurrence of *Helicobacter pylori* infection in the Italian cohort.[13] Enteropathy-type T-cell lymphoma (ETL) involves primarily the small intestine and is seen most frequently in areas with a high prevalence of coeliac sprue, i.e. Northern Europe and particularly Western Ireland.[14] The extranodal NK/T-cell lymphoma of nasal type is a rare Epstein–Barr virus (EBV)-associated NHL that most commonly affects the nasal cavity and upper aerodigestive tract. In Western countries, it accounts for only 1–2% of all PE-NHL, whereas its frequency is considerably higher in the Far East, where it constitutes 25% of all NHL in Thailand and Singapore.[15,16] NK/T-cell lymphoma of nasal type has also been described in native populations of North, Central (Guatemala), and South America (Peru).[17,18] The anatomical distribution of these lymphomas is similar to that seen in Asian countries. Genetic factors associated with ancient populational migration from Asia to the American continent over the Aleutian range may explain the similarities between Asian and native American populations with regard to the epidemiology of NK/T-cell lymphoma of nasal type.

Variation over time

A remarkable increase in the incidence of NHL was observed, at least in Western countries, during the second half of the 20th century,[19–21] with NHL ranking among the most rapidly increasing malignancies in the USA and Europe. In the USA, data from the SEER (Surveillance, Epidemiology, and End Results) program indicate that the incidence of NHL has increased substantially since the early 1970s, from 10.2 per 100 000 in 1973 to 18.5 in 1990, i.e. an overall increase of 81%, with a yearly growth rate of 3.6%.[22] However, recent analyses from the same registry and data from Europe indicate a leveling off of the rate of increase to below 1% per year.[10,23] Although some reports suggest a similar increase in the incidence of PE-NHL in general, and PCNSL in particular,[24] other studies have not confirmed this observation.[25] Updated information from the Danish Lymphoma Group shows an incidence of PE-NHL around 3 in 100 000 during the 1980s and 1990s, with

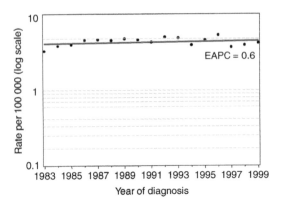

Figure 3.2 Trend in the incidence of PE-NHL, 1983–1999, in Western Denmark (data source: Danish Lymphoma Group – LYFO Registry). EAPC, estimated annual percent change.

a modest 0.6% estimated annual increase.[26] (Figure 3.2). The variability in the proportion of PE-NHL may, to some extent, be explained by differences in the definition of PE-NHL, and other factors such as the occurrence of human immunodeficiency virus (HIV)-associated NHL in the study cohort. The latter may well account for differences in epidemiological figures for PCNSL.[24]

Variation by gender

For most primary extranodal localizations, a predominance of males has been reported. However, some sites, such as the salivary glands and thyroid, seem to have a consistent majority of females. Figure 3.3 shows the site vs gender correlations in the Danish Lymphoma Group.

Variation by age

Reported incidence rates show an exponential rise as a function of age, with a pattern for PE-NHL similar to that seen in nodal NHL, i.e. with a median age in the mid-late 60 year olds. Median age values are slightly higher for females, and peak rates are found in the age group 80–84 years old for both genders.

Variation by anatomical site

The site-specific distribution of PE-NHL in the Danish Lymphoma Group is shown in

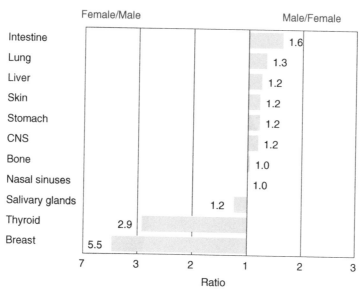

Figure 3.3 Gender distribution for selected anatomical sites of PE-NHL (data source: Danish Lymphoma Group – LYFO Registry).

Figure 3.4. The GIT, with the stomach as the most frequently involved site, represents the most common extranodal localization, followed by the skin (both B- and T-cell tumors), lungs, and central nervous system (CNS). Although many reports have suggested changes of the incidence of PE-NHL for one or several anatomical sites, few population-based studies are available to support such statements. Data from the Danish Lymphoma Group over the period 1983–1999 show that significant changes have taken place during the last two decades. A 2.8-fold increase was observed for the breast. Less-marked increases were observed for NHL of salivary glands and CNS (1.8-fold), testes (1.6-fold), lungs (1.3-fold), and skin (1.2-fold). In contrast, the incidence of PE-NHL of the thyroid and the GIT decreased by 71%, and 15%, respectively (Figure 3.5).[26]

ETIOLOGY AND RISK FACTORS

Genetic susceptibility

Extranodal NK/T-cell lymphoma, nasal type, and ETL are entities with an epidemiology suggestive of an underlying genetic suscepti- bility that probably plays an important role in

the pathogenetic process. Extranodal NK/ T-cell lymphoma, nasal type, is much more prevalent in Asians than in Europeans. Clusters have also been reported in Central and South America in individuals of Native American heritage.[18] These observations strongly suggest that host-related genetic factors play an important role in the pathogenesis of this dis- ease. Extranodal NK/T-cell lymphoma, nasal type, is strongly associated with the intratu- moral presence of EBV, which is likely to be implicated in the pathogenesis of this disease.[18] Genetic susceptibility could therefore reflect an inherited or acquired impaired immunity against EBV.

ETL is associated with specific human leuko- cyte antigen (HLA) types (HLA DQA1*0501, DQB1*0201).[14] This disorder develops in patients with long-standing coeliac sprue and/ or dermatitis herpetiformis. There is substan- tial evidence for a genetic role in this disease, which reflects the genetic background known for coeliac sprue in affected patients and their relatives. Recently, the presence of two distinct groups of ETL has been suggested on morpho- logical and genetic grounds. Type 1 ETL is characterized by a more polymorphic cellular- ity, CD56 negativity, and chromosomal gains of

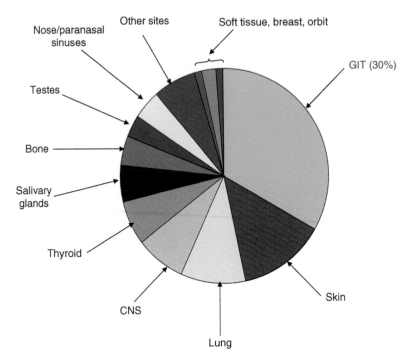

Figure 3.4   Distribution of PE-NHL by anatomical site (data source: Danish Lymphoma Group – LYFO Registry).

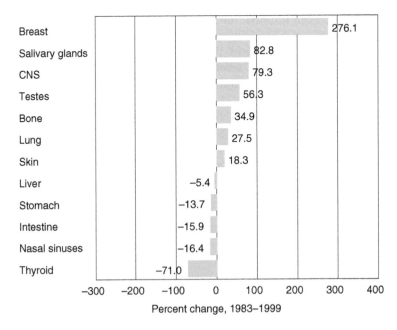

Figure 3.5   Change in incidence of PE-NHL in the period 1983–1999 for selected anatomical sites (data source: Danish Lymphoma Group – LYFO Registry).

1q and 5q, and appears to be linked pathogenetically to coeliac disease, since it shares genetic alterations and HLA-DQB1 genotype patterns with (refractory) coeliac disease. Type 2 ETL shows monomorphic small- to medium-sized tumor cell morphology, is frequently CD56 positive, and frequently displays c-MYC oncogene locus gains. As opposed to type 1 ETL, type 2 ETL shows a HLA-DQB1 genotype pattern closer to that found in the normal Caucasian population.[27]

Post-transplant lymphoproliferative disease

Since the beginning of the 1970s, we know that patients undergoing immunosuppressive therapy to prevent rejection after organ transplantation experience an excessive risk of various neoplasms, in particularly NHL.[28] This particular type of lymphoproliferative disorder has therefore been termed post-transplant lymphoproliferative disease (PTLD). A relative risk (RR) of 20 for developing PTLD following kidney transplantation and of 120 following heart transplantation has been reported, based on population-based transplant registries.[29] However, in more recent reports, the RR of NHL following kidney transplantation was between 8 and 10, and the RR of developing HL was 4.6.[30,31] The RR of NHL is highest in the first-year post-transplantation and declines subsequently. This early-onset PTLD is typically of aggressive histology (mostly DLBCL), often extranodal, and positive for the EBV genome. The RR for PCNSL is more than 1000 and these tumors develop early (mean 29 months), whereas the RR for other NHLs is 7, with a mean time to diagnosis of 69 months.[32,33]

Acquired immunodeficiency syndrome

In population-based record linkages between cancer registries and acquired immunodeficiency syndrome (AIDS) registries in the USA, Italy, and Australia, the RRs of NHL in individuals with AIDS ranged between 15 for indolent and T-cell NHL to 400 for NHL of aggressive histology. The corresponding RR of HL was 10.[34] Risk of developing NHL in individuals with human immunodeficiency virus (HIV) infection is independently predicted by the degree of immunodeficiency (decrease in CD4+ T-cell counts), duration of immunodeficiency, and chronic B-cell stimulation.[35] The majority of HIV-associated NHLs are of aggressive B-cell histology and very often present with extranodal involvement (see Chapter 25). Sites rarely involved in HIV-negative individuals are described. For example, involvement of the anorectal region has been reported in homosexual men with AIDS, suggesting the importance of local etiological factors. Also, the occurrence of primary effusion lymphoma (PEL) is associated with an immunodeficient state and the presence of human herpes virus 8 (HHV-8).

Since the mid 1990s, a marked reduction in the incidence of NHL in general, and PCNSL in particular, has been observed among HIV-positive individuals. This is primarily due to the introduction of highly active antiretroviral therapy (HAART). In the period 1990–2003, the incidence rates of PCNSL declined from 31.3 to 7.7 per 100 000, and for non-CNS NHL from 39 to 15.7 per 100 000. No significant reduction was observed for Burkitt's lymphoma.[36]

Other immunodeficiencies

The pattern of NHL subtypes in congenital immunodeficiency is similar to that occurring in patients with AIDS and solid organ transplants. Exceptions are ataxia-telangiectasia, in which an excess of T-cell tumors occurs, and conditions that only involve antibody deficiency, which in rare cases may lead to PCNSL.[37]

Autoimmune diseases

A number of autoimmune diseases, e.g. rheumatoid arthritis and Wegener's granulomatosis,[38,39] have been linked to an increased risk of NHL in general, and PE-NHL in particular. Primary lymphoma of the thyroid has been often reported in patients with a preceding history of Hashimoto's thyroiditis.[40] The higher frequency of autoimmune thyroid disease in women is, therefore, probably an explanation for the strong female preponderance among thyroid lymphomas (see Figure 3.3). It has been suggested that therapy with immunosuppressive medications such as steroids and azathioprine could cause this increase. However, in polymyalgia rheumatica, where only steroids are used, the RR for NHL is decreased, suggesting that steroids themselves do not lead to increased NHL risk.[41] Systemic lupus erythematosus and Sjögren's syndrome have been associated with a 2–5-fold increased risk of NHL.[42] Studies of patients with autoimmune inflammatory bowel disease have reported variable findings. A recent large population-based linkage study in Sweden showed no increased risk for NHL in individuals with ulcerative colitis or Crohn's disease.[43] In a cohort of 11 650 patients hospitalized with coeliac disease, however, there was an RR of 2.2 for B-cell NHL, an RR of 51 for T-cell NHL, and an RR of 24 for primary GIT lymphoma.[44]

Epstein–Barr virus

There is strong evidence that EBV infection, in conjunction with HIV/AIDS and other forms of immunodeficiency, is associated with an increased risk of NHL. Although most immune deficiency-associated NHLs are of B-cell origin, EBV infection is actually more frequent in T-cell compared with B-cell NHL, and the most striking association is with NK/T-cell lymphoma, nasal type.[18] The presence of intratumoral EBV genome is very often found in endemic African Burkitt's lymphoma and in PCNSL in HIV-positive patients.

Human T-cell lymphotropic virus, type 1

Infection with the retrovirus human T-cell lymphotropic virus, type 1 (HTLV-1) is endemic in southern Japan and in the Caribbean region. Infection in early childhood is associated with a 10-fold increased risk of developing adult T-cell leukemia/lymphoma (ATLL) (primarily bone marrow disease).[45]

Hepatitis C

Infection with hepatitis C virus (HCV) is associated with a 2–4-fold increased risk of B-cell NHL.[46] A causative association between HCV and NHL (including primary hepatic localization) was recently suggested.[47] Morphologically, HCV-associated lymphomas represent a variety of histological subtypes, including marginal zone (splenic, nodal, and extranodal), small lymphocytic, lymphoplasmacytic, and DLBCL. Remarkably, some HCV-associated NHL cases appear to be highly responsive to antiviral therapy.

Human herpes virus-8

Human herpes virus-8 (HHV-8) is widespread in homosexual men. It has been associated with the development of Kaposi's sarcoma (primarily skin) and PEL (primarily thoracic cavity) in adults with acquired immunosuppression secondary to HIV infection or organ transplantation.[48]

Helicobacter pylori and other infections

Helicobacter pylori (HP) infection is associated with a 6-fold increased risk of gastric mucosa-associated lymphoid tissue (MALT) lymphoma and a 3-fold increase in splenic marginal zone NHL.[49] The relationship with gastric NHL is regarded as causal, and eradication of HP results in complete regression in the majority of HP-positive MALT lymphomas. HP infection does not appear to be associated with other NHL subtypes. Other MALT lymphomas have also been associated with specific infections and, in fact, there is growing evidence that the development of extranodal MALT lymphoma is related to antigen-driven B-cell proliferation.[50] Small series have suggested that MALT lymphoma of the ocular adnexa is associated with exposure to *Chlamydia psittaci*.[51]

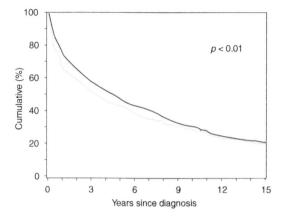

Figure 3.6 Overall survival according to the primary site of disease (data source: Danish Lymphoma Group – LYFO Registry). Nodal NHL (solid line), PE-NHL (dashed line).

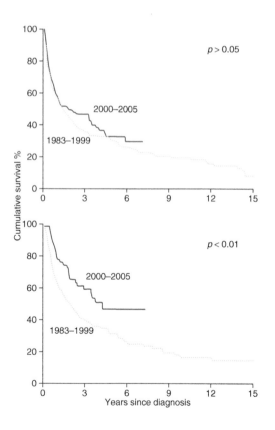

Figure 3.7 Comparison of overall survival for the periods 1983–1999 vs 2000–2005 in PCNSL (upper) and primary testicular NHL (lower). (data source: Danish Lymphoma Group – LYFO Registry).

However, a number of subsequent studies have not confirmed this observation.[52] MALT lymphoma of the small intestine has been associated with *Campylobacter jejuni*[53] and some MALT lymphomas of the skin have been associated with *Borrelia burgdorferi*.[54]

OUTCOME BY SITE

PE-NHL can arise in virtually any organ. The primary organ of origin may influence the outcome (PCNSL, testis, etc.), and the presence of two or more extranodal sites is currently used as an adverse prognostic factor in the International Prognostic Index for aggressive lymphomas.[55] Figure 3.6 shows the overall survival for PE vs primary nodal NHL. PE-NHL, taken as a group, seems to fare slightly worse than its nodal counterpart. However, there are other aspects that need to be considered when evaluating outcome in PE-NHL. For example, some of the localizations are seen predominantly in elderly patients (thyroid, testis, salivary glands, etc.). Some PE-NHL tend to be localized at presentation (salivary glands, thyroid, stomach), whereas others are more often widespread (lungs, liver, bones, testes). Indolent histology is more often seen in PE-NHL of the salivary glands and bone marrow, whereas aggressive histology is more common in the CNS, testes, bones, liver, and lungs. Figure 3.7 shows the overall survival (OS) data from the Danish Lymphoma Group over two decades for two of the most unfavorable localizations, i.e. the CNS and testes. Interestingly, at a median follow-up >10 years, no significant change in OS can be seen for the PCNSL cohort, whereas the opposite is true for the primary testicular cohort. The systematic use of CNS prophylaxis in almost all cases of testicular NHL may have contributed to this improvement in outcome.

CONCLUDING REMARKS

The international adoption of the WHO classification of lymphoid malignancies has provided a common framework to compare subtype-specific lymphoma epidemiology at the country level[56] and on a worldwide scale. However, much of our knowledge of PE-NHL is still based on data collected according to the Working Formulation or the Kiel classification. Future efforts aimed at prospective analysis of PE-NHL epidemiology using the WHO classification are therefore encouraged.

REFERENCES

1. Jaffe ES, Harris NL, Stein H, Vardiman JW, eds. World Health Organization Classification of Tumours: Pathology and Genetics of Tumours of Haematopoietic and Lymphoid Tissues. Lyon: IARC Press, 2001.

2. Harris NL, Jaffe ES, Diebold J, et al. World Health Organization classification of neoplastic diseases of the hematopoietic and lymphoid tissues: report of the Clinical Advisory Committee meeting – Airlie House, Virginia, November 1997. J Clin Oncol 1999; 17(12): 3835–49.

3. d'Amore F, Christensen BE, Brincker H, et al. Clinicopathological features and prognostic factors in extranodal non-Hodgkin lymphomas. Danish LYFO Study Group. Eur J Cancer 1991; 27(10): 1201–8.

4. Kukreti V, Petersen P, Pintilie M, et al. Extranodal follicular lymphoma – a retrospective review and comparison with localized nodal follicular lymphoma. Blood 2004; 104(11): 1375.

5. Newton R, Ferlay J, Beral V, Devesa S. The epidemiology of non-Hodgkin's lymphoma: comparison of nodal and extra-nodal sites. Int J Cancer 1997; 72: 923–30.

6. Zucca E, Roggero E, Bertoni F, Cavalli F. Primary extranodal non-Hodgkin's lymphomas. Part 1: gastrointestinal, cutaneous and genitourinary lymphomas. Ann Oncol 1997; 8(8): 727–37.

7. Zucca E, Roggero E, Bertoni F, Conconi A, Cavalli F. Primary extranodal non-Hodgkin's lymphomas. Part 2: head and neck, central nervous system and other less common sites. Ann Oncol 1999; 10(9): 1023–33.

8. Krol AD, le Cessie S, Snijder S, et al. Primary extranodal non-Hodgkin's lymphoma (NHL): the impact of alternative definitions tested in the Comprehensive Cancer Centre West population-based NHL registry. Ann Oncol 2003; 14(1): 131–9.

9. Anderson JR, Armitage JO, Weisenburger DD, on behalf of the Non-Hodgkin's Lymphoma Classification Project. Epidemiology of the non-Hodgkin's lymphomas: distributions of the major subtypes differ by geographic locations. Ann Oncol 1998; 9: 717–20.

10. Curado MP, Edwards B, Shin HR, et al., eds. Cancer Incidence in Five Continents, Volume IX. IARC Scientific Publications No. 160. Lyon: IARC Press, France.

11. Temmim L, Baker H, Amanguno H, Madda JP, Sinowatz F. Clinicopathological features of extranodal lymphomas: Kuwait experience. Oncology 2004; 67: 382–9.

12. Shome DK, George SM, Al-Hilli F, Satir AA. Spectrum of malignant lymphomas in Bahrain. Leitmotif of a regional pattern. Saudi Med J 2004; 25: 164–7.

13. Doglioni C, Wotherspoon AC, Moschini A, de Boni M, Isaacson PG. High incidence of primary gastric lymphoma in northeastern Italy. Lancet 1992; 339(8797): 834–5.

14. Howell WM, Leung ST, Jones DB, et al. HLA-DRB, -DQA and -DQB polymorphism in celiac disease and enteropathy-associated T-cell lymphoma. Common features and additional risk factors for malignancy. Hum Immunol 1995; 43: 29–37.

15. Ng SB, Lai KW, Murugaya S, et al. Nasal-type extranodal natural killer/T-cell lymphomas: a clinicopathologic and genotypic study of 42 cases in Singapore. Mod Pathol 2004; 17(9): 1097–107.

16. Aozasa K, Yang WJ, Lee YB, et al. Lethal midline granuloma in Seoul (Korea) and Shanghai (China). Int J Cancer 1992; 52(4): 673–4.

17. van de Rijn M, Bhargava V, Molina-Kirsch H, et al. Extranodal head and neck lymphomas in Guatemala: high frequency of EBV-associated sinonasal lymphomas. Hum Pathol 1997: 28(7): 834–9.

18. Arber DA, Weiss LM, Albújar PF, Chen YY, Jaffe ES. Nasal lymphomas in Peru. High incidence of T-cell immunophenotype and Epstein-Barr virus infection. Am J Surg Pathol 1993; 17(4): 392–9.

19. Cartwright R, Brincker H, Carli PM, et al. The rise in incidence of lymphomas in Europe 1985–1992. Eur J Cancer 1999; 35: 627–33.

20. Groves FD, Linet MS, Travis LB, Devesa SS. Cancer surveillance series: non-Hodgkin's lymphoma incidence by histologic subtype in the United States from 1978 through 1995. J Natl Cancer Inst 2000; 92: 1240–51.

21. Zheng T, Mayne ST, Boyle P, et al. Epidemiology of non-Hodgkin lymphoma in Connecticut. 1935–1988. Cancer 1992; 70: 840–9.

22. Ries LAG, Eisner MP, Kosary CL, et al, eds. SEER cancer statistics review, 1973–1999. Bethesda, MD: National Cancer Institute, 2002; http://seer.cancer.gov/csr/1973_1999/

23. Sandin S, Hjalgrim H, Glimelius B, et al. Incidence of non-Hodgkin's lymphoma in Sweden, Denmark, and Finland from 1960 through 2003: an epidemic that was. Cancer Epidemiol Biomarkers Prev 2006; 15(7): 1295–300.

24. Devesa SS, Fears T. Non-Hodgkin's lymphoma time trends: United States and international data. Cancer Res 1992; 52(Suppl): 5432S–440S.

25. Krogh-Jensen M, d'Amore F, Jensen MK, et al. Incidence, clinico-pathological features and outcome of primary central nervous system lymphomas. Ann Oncol 1994; 5: 349–54.

26. d'Amore F, Mortensen LS. Incidence trends for non-Hodgkin's Lymphomas (NHL) in Western Denmark over the last two decades. Ann Oncol 2002; 13(Suppl): 20.

27. Deleeuw RJ, Zettl A, Klinker E, et al. Whole-genome analysis and HLA genotyping of enteropathy-type T-cell lymphoma reveals 2 distinct lymphoma subtypes. Gastroenterology 2007; 132: 1902–11.

28. Hoover R, Fraumeni JF. Risk of cancer in renal-transplant recipients. Lancet 1973; 2: 55–7.

29. Opelz G, Henderson R. Incidence of non-Hodgkin lymphoma in kidney and heart transplant recipients. Lancet 1993; 342: 1514–16.

30. Vajdic CM, McDonald SP, McCredie MR, et al. Cancer incidence before and after kidney transplantation. JAMA 2006; 296(23): 2823–31.

31. Birkeland SA, Storm HH, Lamm LU, et al. Cancer risk after renal transplantation in the Nordic countries, 1964–1986. Int J Cancer 1995; 60: 183–9.

32. Disney AP. Complications of immunosuppressive therapy in transplantation. Neoplasia and infection. Med J Aust 1992; 157: 262–4.

33. Kasiske BL, Snyder JJ, Gilbertson DT, et al. Cancer after kidney transplantation in the United States. Am J Transplant 2004; 4: 905–13.

34. Dal Maso L, Franceschi S. Epidemiology of non-Hodgkin lymphomas and other haemolymphopoietic neoplasms in people with AIDS. Lancet Oncol 2003; 4(2): 110–19.

35. Robotin MC, Law MG, Milliken S, et al. Clinical features and predictors of survival of AIDS-related non-Hodgkin's lymphoma in a population-based case series in Sydney, Australia. HIV Med 2004; 5(5): 377–84.

36. Biggar RJ, Chaturvedi AK, Goedert JJ, Engels EA. AIDS-related cancer and severity of immunosuppression in persons with AIDS. J Natl Cancer Inst 2007; 99: 962–72.

37. Mueller BU, Pizzo PA. Cancer in children with primary or secondary immunodeficiencies. J Pediatrics 1995; 126: 1–10.

38. Gridley G, McLaughlin JK, Ekbom A, et al. Incidence of cancer among patients with rheumatoid arthritis. J Natl Cancer Inst 1993; 85(4): 307–11.

39. Knight A, Askling J, Ekbom A. Cancer incidence in a population-based cohort of patients with Wegener's granulomatosis. Int J Cancer 2002; 100(1): 82–5.

40. Pedersen RK, Pedersen NT. Primary non-Hodgkin's lymphoma of the thyroid gland: a population based study. Histopathology 1996; 28(1): 25–32.

41. Askling J, Klareskog L, Hjalgrim H, et al. Do steroids increase lymphoma risk? A case-control study of lymphoma risk in polymyalgia rheumatica/giant cell arteritis. Ann Rheum Dis 2005; 64(12): 1765–8.

42. Zintzaras E, Voulgarelis M, Moutsopoulos HM. The risk of lymphoma development in autoimmune diseases: a meta-analysis. Arch Intern Med 2005; 165(20): 2337–44.

43. Askling J, Brandt L, Lapidus A, et al. Risk of haematopoietic cancer in patients with inflammatory bowel disease. Gut 2005; 54(5): 617–22.

44. Smedby KE, Kerman M, Hildebrand H, et al. Malignant lymphomas in coeliac disease: evidence of increased risks for lymphoma types other than enteropathy-type T cell lymphoma. Gut 2005; 54: 54–9.

45. Manns A, Cleghorn FR, Falk RT, et al. Role of HTLV-I in development of non-Hodgkin lymphoma in Jamaica and Trinidad and Tobago. The HTLV Lymphoma Study Group. Lancet 1993; 342(8885): 1447–50.

46. Engels E, Chatterjee N, Cerhan JR, et al. Hepatitis C virus infection and non-Hodgkin lymphoma: results of the NCI-SEER multi-center case-control study. Int J Cancer 2004; 111(1): 76–80.

47. Viswanatha DS, Dogan A. Hepatitis C virus and lymphoma. J Clin Pathol 2007; 60(12): 1378–83.

48. Cannon M, Cesarman E. Kaposi's sarcoma-associated herpes virus and acquired immunodeficiency syndrome-related malignancy. Semin Oncol 2000; 27(4): 409–19.

49. Shaye OS, Levine AM. Marginal zone lymphoma. J Natl Compr Canc Netw 2006; 4(3): 311–18.

50. Jaffe ES. Common threads of mucosa-associated lymphoid tissue lymphoma pathogenesis: from infection to translocation. J Natl Cancer Inst 2004; 96(8): 571–3.

51. Ferreri AJ, Guidoboni M, Ponzoni M, et al. Evidence for an association between Chlamydia psittaci and ocular adnexal lymphomas. J Natl Cancer Inst 2004; 96(8): 586–94.

52. Zucca E, Bertoni F. Chlamydia or not Chlamydia, that is the question: which is the microorganism associated with MALT lymphomas of the ocular adnexa? J Natl Cancer Inst 2006; 98(19): 1348–9.

53. Lecuit M, Abachin E, Martin A, et al. Immunoproliferative small intestinal disease associated with Campylobacter jejuni. N Engl J Med 2004; 350(3): 239–48.

54. Cerroni L, Zöchling N, Pütz B, Kerl H. Infection by Borrelia burgdorferi and cutaneous B-cell lymphoma. J Cutan Pathol 1997; 24(8): 457–61.

55. Shipp M. A predictive model for aggressive non-Hodgkin's lymphoma. The International Non-Hodgkin's Lymphoma Prognostic Factors Project. N Engl J Med 1993; 329(14): 987–94.

56. Morton LM, Wang S, Devesa S, et al. Lymphoma incidence patterns by WHO subtype in the United States, 1992–2001. Blood 2006; 107(1): 265–76.

Infectious etiopathogenesis of extranodal lymphomas

4

Paolo Boffetta and Riccardo Dolcetti

INTRODUCTION

Several infectious agents are established causes of non-Hodgkin's lymphoma in humans. They include human immunodeficiency virus (HIV), Epstein–Barr virus (EBV), human herpes virus 8 (HHV-8), hepatitis C virus (HCV), and *Helicobacter pylori*. In addition, a causal role is suspected for hepatitis B virus (HBV), *Borrelia burgdorferi*, *Campylobacter jejuni*, and various *Chlamydia* species. For some of these agents, notably HIV, HHV-8, *H. pylori*, *Chlamydia*, and *B. burgdorferi*, the association seems specific to one or a few types of extranodal lymphomas, while EBV is associated with a variety of nodal and extranodal lymphomas. In the case of HCV, the risk of both nodal and extranodal lymphomas seems increased among chronically infected individuals. No data are available on HBV and risk of extranodal lymphoma. In the following sections, the epidemiological and pathogenetic evidence linking infectious agents to extranodal lymphoma is reviewed. Infectious agents may contribute to lymphomagenesis by two main pathogenetic mechanisms. First, a direct role is played mainly by viruses such as EBV and HHV-8, which infect target cells and express a variety of viral products that promote cell growth and survival. Additional environmental and genetic factors contribute to the malignant phenotype. The virus genome is usually present in all tumor cells. Secondly, infectious agents, mainly bacteria, may indirectly contribute to lymphomagenesis by providing a chronic antigenic stimulus that would drive the development of extranodal lymphomas along a continuum pathway, starting from the development of acquired mucosa-associated lymphoid tissue (MALT), through low-grade lymphoma, and ultimately leading to high-grade tumors. Proliferation of B cells may be dependent on the contact with infiltrating antigen-specific CD4+ helper T cells. Antigens derived from the infectious agent may be cross-reactive with self-antigens, which, in turn, may further sustain B cell growth. This model indicates that infectious agents could trigger autoimmune reactivity and emphasizes the likely relevant role of autoimmune mechanisms in the pathogenesis of some extranodal lymphomas (Figure 4.1).

HUMAN IMMUNODEFICIENCY VIRUS

HIV-associated non-Hodgkin's lymphomas, although histologically heterogeneous, are characterized by an aggressive clinical course. High-grade disease is common and extranodal sites are often involved, with lesions in the central nervous system being virtually unknown except in the immunosuppressed. About one-fifth of lymphomas in HIV-positive patients in Europe and North America are primary brain lymphomas.[1,2] The risk of brain lymphomas in HIV-infected individuals does not change with age, and it is twice as high in men as it is in women, and in Blacks as it is in Whites.[2]

The pattern of HIV-associated lymphoma is changing following the introduction of new therapeutic regimens. This applies also to HIV-associated brain lymphoma. In a combined reanalysis of much of the worldwide data on this issue, the International

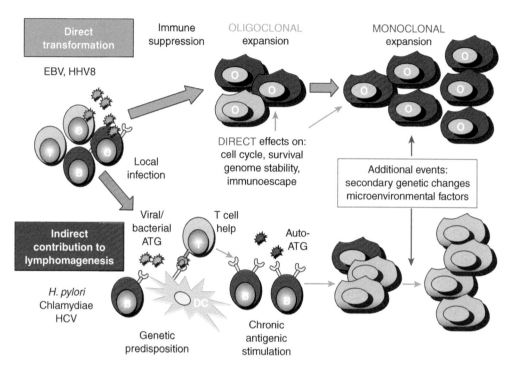

Figure 4.1 Pathogenetic mechanisms underlying infection-driven lymphomagenesis. ATG, antigen; B, B lymphocyte; DC, dendritic cell; T, T lymphocyte.

Collaboration on HIV and Cancer reported a great decline in the incidence of brain lymphoma among HIV-infected individuals.[3] The incidence in 1992–96 was 1.7/1000/year and 0.7/1000/year in 1997–99 (rate ratio = 0.42, standard error = 0.09).

Little is known about the types of extranodal lymphoma that occur in HIV-infected people from African or other low-income countries. The predominant type would appear to be immunoblastic tumors, and cerebral lymphomas have been identified at autopsy.[4]

A study from the USA showed that, subsequent to a diagnosis of acquired immunodeficiency syndrome (AIDS), children were at an increased risk of non-Hodgkin's lymphoma, including lymphoma of the brain.[5]

EPSTEIN–BARR VIRUS

Serological surveys from many different populations consistently reported that more than 90% adults are positive for EBV infection.[6] Transmission occurs mainly during infancy,

childhood, and adolescence, mainly via saliva.[7] Primary infection in infancy and childhood is often asymptomatic, or results in a febrile illness. Seroconversion in adolescence and adulthood often results in the syndrome of infectious mononucleosis.[8] EBV has evolved an elegant strategy to establish a life-long asymptomatic infection in memory B lymphocytes by exploiting cellular pathways that regulate antigen-dependent B-cell differentiation.[9] EBV immortalizes B lymphocytes through the cooperative activity of viral proteins (six nuclear antigens, EBNA1-6, and two membrane proteins, LMP-1 and -2) that derange critical cellular pathways controlling growth and/or survival of B lymphocytes.[9] Full transformation of infected B cells is achieved by the contribution of poorly defined additional cofactors, including microenvironmental stimuli, genetic and epigenetic alterations. The regulation and expression of viral genes and their interactions with host factors are complex, and, although different types of EBV-associated lymphomas present specific patterns of EBV-gene expression (latency patterns), the precise role of viral genes in lymphomagenesis remains poorly understood. EBV infection is a cause of nasopharyngeal carcinoma, in particular its undifferentiated type, and is suspected to play a role in gastric cancer.[9,10] It causes Burkitt's lymphoma, Hodgkin's lymphoma, and nodal B-cell lymphomas, notably diffuse large B-cell lymphoma, in particular in the setting of immune deficiency. In patients receiving solid organ or hematopoietic stem cell transplant, the defect in EBV-specific immune responses may allow the outgrowth of EBV-carrying B lymphocytes that may give rise to a spectrum of different clinicopathological entities encompassed by the term post-transplantation lymphoproliferative disorders (PTLD).[10,11] These lymphoproliferations often arise at or involve extranodal sites. Several risk factors may favor the development of PTLD, including EBV seronegativity before transplant, primary EBV infection post-transplantation, high cumulative levels of immunosuppression, the type of solid organ transplanted, presence of cytomegalovirus disease, and possibly younger age, independently of EBV status.[10,11] In keeping with the notion that the level of immunosuppression varies with the type of organ transplanted, the incidence of PTLD varies widely, ranging from less than 1% to 33%.[10,11]

An additional type of extranodal lymphoma associated with EBV infection comprises natural killer (NK)/T-cell lymphomas, in particular those arising in the nose.[12,13] These disorders are most prevalent in Asia and Latin America. Unlike B cells, T lymphocytes are usually refractory to EBV infection in vitro. Since most of NK/T-cell lymphomas express proteins associated with cytotoxic functions (granzyme B and TIA-1), it has been suggested that EBV infection in these lymphomas may have resulted from the interaction of a cytotoxic effector with an EBV-infected cell.[14] More than half of AIDS-associated primary central nervous system lymphomas are also associated with EBV.[15] Other extranodal lymphomas associated with EBV infection are lymphoid granulomatosis, a B-cell neoplasm which involves the skin, lung, kidney, and brain,[16] and pyothorax-associated

lymphoma, which has been described in tuberculosis patients treated with placement of balls in the pleural space to maintain pneumothorax, leading to chronic inflammation.[17,18] This latter disease is of special interest as a model for the role of inflammation in EBV-related lymphomagenesis.

HUMAN HERPES VIRUS 8

HHV-8, also known as Kaposi's sarcoma-associated virus, shows large variation in its prevalence across populations, ranging from over 60% in areas of Africa, to 10–15% in the Mediterranean area, to 1–3% in Northern Europe, North America, and many parts of Asia. Transmission within families during childhood via a salivary route seems important, as well as sexual practices in adulthood.[19] Primary infection can be asymptomatic or be accompanied by rash, lymphadenopathy, and splenomegaly.[20] HHV-8 genes potentially important in lymphomagenesis include the latent genes, LANA1, LANA2, vCYC, and vFLIP, as well as the lytic genes vIL6 and K1, although it is unclear whether the second group of genes is necessary for transformation and maintenance of the transformed cells.

The main neoplasm caused by HHV-8 is Kaposi's sarcoma: all varieties of the sarcoma are caused by HHV-8, including classic, endemic, post-transplant, and AIDS-related Kaposi's sarcoma.[21] It also causes multicentric Castleman's disease, a polyclonal, non-neoplastic lymphoproliferative disorder.[22] Primary effusion lymphoma of body cavities is the main type of extranodal lymphoma associated with HHV-8: the majority of these neoplasms, however, are coinfected by EBV.[23,24]

HEPATITIS C VIRUS

HCV is an RNA virus belonging to the family of flaviviruses. Approximately 170 million people are infected with HCV worldwide, making HCV a major public health problem.[25,26] HCV is hepatotropic and causes hepatitis, liver cirrhosis, and hepatocellular carcinoma.[27] HCV is also lymphotropic and is involved in the etiology of mixed cryoglobulinemia (MC),

Table 4.1 Case-control studies of extranodal lymphoma and hepatitis C virus infection

Reference	Country	Type of controls	Cases HCV+/HCV–	Controls HCV+/HCV–	RR (95% CI)
Zuckerman et al[29]	USA	Hospital	10/15	6/108	12 (3.8, 38)
Mizorogi et al[34]	Japan	Hospital	9/40	34/482	3.2 (1.4, 7.1)
Montella et al[30]	Italy	Hospital	16/38	17/209	5.0 (2.3, 11)
Engels et al[33]	USA	Population	10/263	14/670	1.8 (0.7, 4.2)
Talamini et al[32]	Italy	Hospital	14/56	45/459	2.6 (1.3, 5.3)
Seve et al[35]	France	Hospital	3/14	20/954	9.9 (2.6, 38)

CI, confidence interval; HCV, hepatitis C virus; RR, relative risk.

a lymphoproliferative disease that can evolve into B-cell lymphoma.[28]

Some early studies found that HCV infection was more strongly related to extranodal lymphoma,[29,30] or to involvement of specific organs (e.g. liver[31]), than to nodal lymphoma. However, two large case-control studies[32,33] did not confirm these results and showed a similar strength of association between HCV infection and nodal and extranodal lymphoma (Table 4.1). The pooled relative risk (RR) of studies of HCV infection and risk of extranodal lymphoma was 3.7 (95% confidence interval [CI] 2.6, 4.3), based on 488 cases included in six case-control studies from France, Italy, Japan, and the USA.

Six distinct but related HCV genotypes and multiple subtypes have been identified; however, no consistent difference in excess risk of extranodal lymphoma emerged between different genotypes in the available studies.[29,32] Although HCV may directly contribute to B-cell transformation, several lines of evidence indicates that HCV is mainly associated with antigen-driven lymphomagenesis. In fact, similar to other pathogen-driven lymphoproliferations, HCV-associated lymphomas express distinct sets of stereotyped immunoglobulins.[36] Moreover, HCV-associated splenic lymphomas with villous lymphocytes, a subset of splenic marginal zone lymphomas, are constantly associated with MC, show a close correlation between viral load and tumor burden, and undergo complete hematological responses with antiviral therapy.[37]

HELICOBACTER PYLORI

H. pylori is a bacterium that infects the human gastric mucosa. The prevalence of *H. pylori* is strongly correlated to socioeconomic conditions, and is higher than 80% in middle-aged adults in many low-income countries, compared to 20% in high-income countries.[38] *H. pylori* infection in adults is usually chronic and does not heal without specific antimicrobical treatment.[38] *H. pylori* causes continuous gastric inflammation in virtually all infected individuals and induces a vigorous humoral and cellular immune response that contributes to tissue damage. MALT lymphoma of the stomach is among the possible long-term outcomes of *H. pylori* infection.

The first large study to address the evaluation of *H. pylori* as a risk factor for gastric lymphoma was a case-control study nested in two cohorts from the USA and Norway[39] (Table 4.2). A total of 33 gastric lymphomas were matched to 134 controls. *H. pylori* prevalence, tested by enzyme-linked immunosorbent assay (ELISA), was 85% among the cases, compared to 55% among the controls (RR = 6.3; 95% CI 2.0, 20). In a parallel series of cases of non-gastric non-Hodgkin's lymphoma, the prevalence of *H. pylori* was 65%. Xue and colleagues conducted a meta-analysis of Chinese studies on the association between *H. pylori*, non-Hodgkin's lymphoma, and gastric cancer.[40] Three case-control studies included 83 gastric lymphomas and 143 controls. The overall *H. pylori* prevalence was 88% among cases and 56% among controls (RR = 5.7; 95% CI 2.7, 12).

Table 4.2   Epidemiological studies of gastric lymphoma and *Helicobacter pylori* infection

Reference	Country	Study design	Cases Hp+/Hp−	Controls Hp+/Hp−	RR (95% CI)
Parsonnet et al[39]	USA	Cohort study	28/5	74/60	6.3 (2.0, 20)
Xue et al[40]	China	Meta-analysis of three case-control studies	73/10	80/63	5.7 (2.7–12)

CI, confidence interval; Hp, *Helicobacter pylori*; RR, relative risk.

The mechanism by which *H. pylori* infection contributes to the development of gastric MALT lymphoma is relatively well understood.[41] Colonization of the gastric mucosa by *H. pylori* induces and sustains an actively proliferating B-cell population through direct (autoantigen) and indirect (intratumoral T cells specific for *H. pylori*) immunological stimulation. Moreover, the bacterial infection provokes a neutrophilic response, which causes the release of oxygen free radicals. These reactive species may promote the acquisition of genetic abnormalities and malignant transformation of reactive B lymphocytes. A transformed clone carrying the translocation t(11;18)(q21;q21) can give origin to MALT lymphoma.[41] In its early stages, the tumor can be successfully treated by eradication of the bacterium, whereas at later stages the tumor may escape its growth dependency through acquisition of additional genetic abnormalities. Further genetic abnormalities, such as inactivation of the tumor suppressor genes p53 and p16, can lead to high-grade transformation.[41]

Over 70% of patients with gastric MALT lymphoma can achieve complete remission after *H. pylori* eradication.[41] In 50% of patients, the tumor clone can be detected by polymerase chain reaction (PCR) clonality analysis on material obtained from post-remission biopsy samples, even though no histological tumor lesion is detectable. The monoclonal tumor cell population decreases during long-term follow-up. Relapse after complete remission occurs in less than 10% of cases, and it is unclear whether this is caused by *H. pylori* reinfection. In cases of *H. pylori* reinfection, the tumor can again be cured by the eradication of the organism. In the absence of *H. pylori*, relapse is frequently a transient self-limiting event.[41,42]

BORRELIA BURGDORFERI

Lyme borreliosis is a multiorgan infection caused by tick-borne spirochetes of the *Borrelia burgdorferi* (BB). Using phylogenetic studies, BB can be subdivided into multiple genospecies (i.e., *B. burgdorferi sensu stricto*, *B. garinii*, and *B. afzelii*), with different distribution worldwide.[43]

Common skin manifestations of Lyme borreliosis include erythema migrans, acrodermatitis chronica atrophicans, and lymphocytoma, a benign B-cell lymphoproliferative process.[43] A few reports have suggested a positive association between BB and primary cutaneous B-cell lymphoma.[44]

Results on prevalence of BB in cutaneous lymphoma in studies reporting at least 20 cases are summarized in Table 4.3. In a series of 50 cutaneous lymphomas, Cerroni and colleagues identified DNA sequences for BB in 18% of cases, compared to a reported prevalence of 15% in the region where the study was carried out.[45] In case-series from the USA (including 38 cutaneous lymphoma) and from Taiwan (24 cases), no BB-specific DNA was detected in any of the cases.[46,47]

Jelic and colleagues reported 55% of antibody positivity for BB among B-cell cutaneous lymphoma cases (12/22) from the former Yugoslavia, while the prevalence was 0% (10 cases) in T-cell cutaneous lymphomas, and 5% (4/75) in other B-cell non-Hodgkin lymphomas.[48] The RR for BB positivity was 26 (95% CI 7.0, 95) using a control group comprising 30 breast cancer patients and 60 blood donors, among whom the prevalence to BB was 4%. In a further study conducted in Scotland, which included 20 cutaneous B-cell lymphomas and a control group of 40 dermatological patients

Table 4.3   Case-series and case-control studies of cutaneous lymphoma and *Borrelia burgdorferi* infection

Study design and references	Country	Type of controls	Type of lymphoma	Cases BB+/BB–	Controls BB+/BB–	RR (95% CI)
Case series						
Cerroni et al[45]	Austria	–	CBCL	9/41	–	–
Wood et al[46]	USA	–	CBCL	0/38	–	–
Li et al[47]	Taiwan	–	CMZL	0/24	–	–
Case-control studies						
Jelic et al[48]	Former	Blood donors	CBCL	12/10	2/58	35 (6.7, 179)
	Yugoslavia		CTCL	0/10	2/58	0 (0–12)
Goodlad et al[49]	Scotland	Dermatology patients	CBCL	7/13	1/40	21 (2.4, 187)

BB, *Borrelia burgdorferi*; CBCL, cutaneous B-cell lymphoma; CI, confidence interval; CMZL, cutaneous marginal zone B-cell lymphoma; CTCL, cutaneous T-cell lymphoma; RR, relative risk.

(20 with melanoma and 20 with inflammatory dermatosis), BB DNA, detected by nested PCR assay, was present in seven (35%) of the cases compared to one (2.5%) control (RR = 21; 95% CI 2.4, 187).[49]

Some caveats are needed in the interpretation of the findings on BB and cutaneous B-cell lymphoma. First, no clear association has been found between incidence of Lyme disease and that of this type of lymphoma.[50] In addition, the distinction between cutaneous B-cell non-Hodgkin's lymphoma and B-cell lymphocytoma that is clearly related to BB infections, is difficult[51] and may produce histological misclassification between benign and malignant lymphoid neoplasms.

CAMPYLOBACTER JEJUNI

Campylobacter jejuni (CJ) is probably the most prevalent cause of bacteria-mediated diarrheal disease worldwide and is considered an initiating factor in chronic autoimmune diseases, such as the Guillain–Barré syndrome and reactive arthritis.[52] Recent evidence has suggested a possible link between CJ infection and immunoproliferative small intestinal disease (IPSID), a distinct form of MALT lymphoma that is mainly prevalent in the Middle East and Africa.[53] Involvement of proximal small intestine results in malabsorption, diarrhea, and abdominal pain, which are associated with an abnormal production of truncated α heavy chain proteins lacking both the light chains and the first constant domain. The geographic variations in incidence, the low socioeconomic status of affected individuals, and the therapeutic efficacy of antibiotics have previously suggested that environmental factors such as an infectious agent could contribute to the pathogenesis of IPSID.

CJ infection was first demonstrated by PCR, DNA sequencing, fluorescent in situ hybridization (FISH), and immunohistochemistry in intestinal tissues obtained from a patient with IPSID who had a dramatic clinical and pathological response to antibiotics.[53] A retrospective analysis of archival intestinal biopsy specimens disclosed *Campylobacter* species in four of six additional patients with IPSID.[53] Similar to *H. pylori*-associated gastric MALT lymphoma, if diagnosed early, IPSID may regress after treatment with broad-spectrum antibiotics. This strategy results in response rates ranging between 33% and 71% in early-stage disease.[54]

The association between IPSID and CJ, however, needs to be substantiated by further investigation. It should be considered, in fact, that some of the characteristics of CJ infection make this pathogen an unlikely cause of cancer. In particular, unlike other microorganisms involved in lymphomagenesis, CJ is not a persistent colonizer of humans, and while this infection is a common but transient condition, IPSID is a rare malignancy that arises only in endemic areas. Moreover, the temporal relationship between CJ infection and IPSID development has not been elucidated so far. IPSID patients frequently show an impairment of both humoral and cellular responses, which may result in a defective control of persistent or chronic (re-)infections, also including CJ.[55] Sustained proliferation of immunoglobulin A (IgA)-producing plasma cells may then favor the accumulation of genetic alterations that contribute to malignant transformation and immune evasion (elimination of antigenic idiotypes).[55]

CHLAMYDIA SPECIES

An Italian study explored the association between *Chlamydia* infection and the rare lymphoma of the ocular adnexa (OAL).[56] About 60–80% of these lymphomas are of MALT-type and share some clinicopathological features with gastric MALT lymphoma. In fact, both lymphomas display similar somatic hypermutation rates of the immunoglobulin genes with a pattern of ongoing mutations, indicating that the development of these disorders is probably favored by a chronic antigen stimulation.[57,58] Moreover, OAL is often preceded by a chronic conjunctivitis that may be induced by chlamydial infections.[56] The presence of DNA of *C. pneumoniae*, *C. trachomatis*, and *C. psittaci* was initially investigated among 40 histologically proven OAL. PCR assay was performed in tissue and peripheral blood mononuclear cell samples. None of the samples were positive for *C. pneumoniae* or *C. trachomatis*, while 32 (80%) of the cases were positive for *C. psittaci*.[56] Of 46 control subjects (20 with non-neoplastic conjunctival/orbital diseases and 26 with reactive lymphoadenopathies), only three (7%) were *C. psittaci* DNA-positive (RR = 57; 95% CI 14, 233). In OAL biopsies, immunohistochemical analyses identified infiltrating macrophages as the cells harboring this microorganism.[56] *C. psittaci* is the etiological agent of psittacosis, a human infection caused by exposure to infected birds, cats, and other household animals.[59] Notably, half of OAL patients reported close contacts with household animals.[60] In OAL patients, *C. psittaci* establishes a systemic infection, as demonstrated by the detection of the DNA of the bacterium in peripheral blood mononuclear cells of 40% of the cases.[56] Such a systemic infection persists over time in a high proportion of cases, even more than 5 years, further supporting the possible involvement of *C. psittaci* in sustaining lymphoma cell growth.[56]

The prevalence of *C. psittaci* infection in OAL patients varies widely among the different series investigated so far. Although there may be differences in the sensitivity of the detection methods used, a large study with centralized molecular analysis recently confirmed the existence of geographical variations in the prevalence of the *C. psittaci*–OAL association.[61] The virtual absence of *C. psittaci* in OAL patients from some countries, particularly from North America, seems to suggest the involvement of other etiopathogenetic agents in these areas. Further studies using standardized detection methods on large OAL series from different countries will allow a better definition of the epidemiology of this intriguing association.

Notably, *C. psittaci* eradication with the antibiotic doxycycline induced objective clinical response in a substantial fraction of OAL patients, further supporting a likely causal role for this infection, and resulted in a safe, cheap, and effective therapeutic strategy for this lymphoma.[62,63] Tumor remission was observed even in patients with multiple failures, with involvement of regional lymph nodes and lesions arisen in previously irradiated areas. Moreover, lymphoma regression was recently observed also in one-third of *Chlamydia*-negative OAL after doxycycline treatment.[63] This could be due to false-negative results, as a consequence of sampling biases or, more likely, to the presence of chlamydial DNA loads below the threshold of PCR detection. This latter occurrence could be more frequent than expected, particularly in the light of the frequent use of broad-spectrum local antibiotics immediately before biopsy. A further possibility is related to the presence of sequence variations in the DNA of *C. psittaci* strains preventing amplification of the target DNA. On the other hand, OAL may be associated with the infection by other bacteria responsive to doxycycline, an attractive possibility that deserves further investigation.

More recently, the same bacterial strain was detected in a woman with two distinct metachronous *C. psittaci*-related lymphomas and in her household canary.[64] Evidence has been also provided indicating that prolonged exposure to the infected bird resulted in continuous reinfection. It is well established that *C. psittaci* transmission from animals to humans mainly occurs through aerosols of fecal or feather dust where infectious bacteria may remain viable for months. Notably, both lymphomas of this patient arose in organs (ocular adnexa, bronchus) considered as 'first barriers' to exposure to air-transported antigens. In patients with *C. psittaci*-related lymphomas, cohabitation with potentially infected animals should therefore be investigated. The finding that doxycycline successfully induced clinical remission of a diffuse large B-cell lymphoma in this patient[64] suggest that, at least in early phases, even histologically aggressive lymphomas may be still dependent on the stimulation by bacterial antigenic stimulation.

REFERENCES

1. Human immunodeficiency viruses. IARC Monographs on the Evaluation of Carcinogenic Risks to Humans. Volume 67, Human Immunodeficiency Viruses and Human T-Cell Lymphotropic Viruses. Lyon, France: IARC, 1996: 31–259.
2. Beral V, Peterman TA, Berkelman R, Jaffe H. AIDS-associated non-Hodgkin lymphoma Lancet 1991; 337: 805–9.
3. International Collaboration on HIV and Cancer. The impact of highly active anti-retroviral therapy on the incidence of cancer in people infected with the human immunodeficiency virus. J Natl Cancer Inst 2000; 92: 1823–30.
4. Lucas SB, Diomande M, Hounnou A, et al. HIV-associated lymphoma in Africa: an autopsy study on Côte D'Ivoire. Int J Cancer 1994; 59: 20–4.
5. Biggar RJ, Frisch M, Goedert JJ. Risk of cancer in children with AIDS. AIDS-Cancer Match Registry Study Group. JAMA 2000; 284: 205–9.
6. Henle W, Henle G, Lennette ET. The Epstein–Barr virus. Sci Am 1979; 241: 48–59.
7. Koelle DM, Huang ML, Chandran B, et al. Frequent detection of Kaposi's sarcoma-associated herpesvirus (human herpesvirus 8) DNA in saliva of human immunodeficiency virus-infected men: clinical and immunological correlates. J Infect Dis 1997; 176: 94–102.
8. Cohen JL. Epstein–Barr virus infection. N Engl J Med 2000; 343: 481–92.
9. Dolcetti R, Masucci MG. Epstein-Barr virus: induction and control of cell transformation. J Cell Physiol 2003; 196: 207–18.
10. Epstein–Barr virus. IARC Monographs on the Evaluation of Carcinogenic Risks to Humans. Volume 70, Epstein–Barr Virus and Kaposi's Sarcoma Virus/Human Herpesvirus 8. Lyon, France: IARC, 1997: 47–373.
11. Dolcetti R. B lymphocytes and Epstein–Barr virus: the lesson of post-transplant lymphoproliferative disorders. Autoimmun Rev 2007; 7: 96–101.
12. Chiang AK, Tao Q, Srivastava G, Ho FC. Nasal NK- and T-cell lymphoma share the same type of Epstein–Barr virus latency as nasopharyngeal carcinoma and Hodgkin's disease. Int J Cancer 1996; 68: 285–90.
13. Cheung MM, Chan JK, Wong KF. Natural killer cell neoplasms: a distinctive group of highly aggressive lymphomas/leukemias. Semin Hematol 2003; 40: 221–32.
14. Mitarnun W, Suwiwat S, Pradutkanchana J, et al. Epstein–Barr virus-associated peripheral T-cell and NK-cell proliferative disease/lymphoma: clinicopathologic, serologic, and molecular analysis. Am J Hematol 2002; 70: 31–8.
15. MacMahon EM, Glass JD, Hayward SD, et al. Epstein–Barr virus in AIDS-related primary central nervous system lymphoma. Lancet 1991; 338: 969–73.
16. Beaty MW, Toro J, Sorbara L, et al. Cutaneous lymphomatoid granulomatosis: correlation of clinical and biologic features. Am J Surg Pathol 2001; 25: 1111–20.
17. Copie-Bergman C, Niedobitek G, Mangham DC, et al. Epstein–Barr virus in B-cell lymphomas associated with chronic suppurative inflammation. J Pathol 1997; 183: 287–92.
18. Aozasa K, Takakuwa T, Nakatsuka S. Pyothorax-associated lymphoma: a lymphoma developing in chronic inflammation. Adv Anat Pathol 2005; 12: 324–31.
19. Martin JN, Ganem DE, Osmond DH, et al. Sexual transmission and the natural history of human herpesvirus 8 infection. N Engl J Med 1998; 338: 948–54.
20. Casper C, Wald A, Pauk J, et al. Correlates of prevalent and incident Kaposi's sarcoma-associated herpesvirus infection in men who have sex with men. J Infect Dis 2002; 185: 990–3.
21. Kaposi's sarcoma virus/human herpesvirus 8. IARC Monographs on the Evaluation of Carcinogenic

Risks to Humans. Volume 70, Epstein–Barr Virus and Kaposi's Sarcoma Virus/Human Herpesvirus 8. Lyon, France: IARC, 1997: 375–492.

22. Soulier J, Grollet L, Oksenhendler E, et al. Kaposi's sarcoma associated herpesvirus-like DNA sequences in multicentric Castleman's disease. Blood 1995; 86: 1276–80.

23. Cesarman E, Chang Y, Moore PS, et al. Kaposi's sarcoma-associated herpesvirus-like DNA sequences in AIDS-related body-cavity-based lymphomas. N Engl J Med 1995; 332: 1186–91.

24. Chadburn A, Hyjek E, Mathew S, et al. KSHV-positive solid lymphomas represent an extra-cavitary variant of primary effusion lymphoma. Am J Surg Pathol 2004; 28: 1401–16.

25. Poynard T, Yuen MF, Ratziu V, Lai CL. Viral hepatitis C. Lancet 2003; 362: 2095–100.

26. Alter MJ, Kruszon-Moran D, Nainan OV, et al. The prevalence of hepatitis C virus infection in the United States, 1988 through 1994. N Engl J Med 1999; 341: 556–62.

27. Lauer GM, Walker BD. Hepatitis C virus infection. N Engl J Med 2001; 345: 41–52.

28. Gasparotto D, De Re V, Boiocchi M. Hepatitis C virus, B-cell proliferation and lymphomas. Leuk Lymphoma 2002; 43: 747–51.

29. Zuckerman E, Zuckerman T, Levine AM, et al. Hepatitis C virus infection in patients with B-cell non-Hodgkin lymphoma. Ann Intern Med 1997; 127: 423–8.

30. Montella M, Crispo A, Frigeri F, et al. HCV and tumors correlated with immune system: a case-control study in an area of hyperendemicity. Leuk Res 2001; 25: 775–81.

31. De Vita S, Zagonel V, Russo A, et al. Hepatitis C virus, non-Hodgkin's lymphomas and hepatocellular carcinoma. Br J Cancer 1998; 77: 2032–5.

32. Talamini R, Montella M, Crovatto M, et al. Non-Hodgkin's lymphoma and hepatitis C virus: a case-control study from northern and southern Italy. Int J Cancer 2004; 110: 380–5.

33. Engels EA, Chatterjee N, Cerhan JR, et al. Hepatitis C virus infection and non-Hodgkin lymphoma: results of the NCI-SEER multi-center case-control study. Int J Cancer 2004; 111: 76–80.

34. Mizorogi F, Hiramoto J, Nozato A, et al. Hepatitis C virus infection in patients with B-cell non-Hodgkin's lymphoma. Intern Med 2000; 39: 112–17.

35. Seve P, Renaudier P, Sasco AJ, et al. Hepatitis C virus infection and B-cell non-Hodgkin's lymphoma: a cross-sectional study in Lyon, France. Eur J Gastroenterol Hepatol 2004; 16: 1361–5.

36. De Re V, De Vita S, Marzotto A, et al. Sequence analysis of the immunoglobulin antigen receptor of hepatitis C virus-associated non-Hodgkin lymphomas suggests that the malignant cells are derived from the rheumatoid factor-producing cells that occur mainly in type II cryoglobulinemia. Blood 2000; 96: 3578–84.

37. Hermine O, Lefrère F, Bronowicki JP, et al. Regression of splenic lymphoma with villous lymphocytes after treatment of hepatitis C virus infection. N Engl J Med 2002; 347: 89–94.

38. Suerbaum S, Michetti P. Helicobacter pylori infection. N Engl J Med 2002; 347: 1175–86.

39. Parsonnet J, Hansen S, Rodriguez L, et al. Helicobacter pylori infection and gastric lymphoma. N Engl J Med 1994; 330: 1267–71.

40. Xue FB, Xu YY, Wan Y, et al. Association of H. pylori infection with gastric carcinoma: a meta-analysis. World J Gastroenterol 2001; 7: 801–4.

41. Du MQ, Isaccson PG. Gastric MALT lymphoma: from aetiology to treatment. Lancet Oncol 2002; 3: 97–104.

42. Stolte M, Bayerdorffer E, Morgner A, et al. Helicobacter and gastric MALT lymphoma. Gut 2002; 50(Suppl 3): III19–24.

43. Hengge UR, Tannapfel A, Tyring SK, et al. Lyme borreliosis. Lancet Infect Dis 2003; 3: 489–500.

44. Slater DN. Borrelia burgdorferi-associated primary cutaneous B-cell lymphoma. Histopathology 2001; 38: 73–7.

45. Cerroni L, Zochling N, Putz B, Kerl H. Infection by Borrelia burgdorferi and cutaneous B-cell lymphoma. J Cutan Pathol 1997; 24: 457–61.

46. Wood GS, Kamath NV, Guitart J, et al. Absence of Borrelia burgdorferi DNA in cutaneous B-cell lymphomas from the United States. J Cutan Pathol 2001; 28: 502–7.

47. Li C, Inagaki H, Kuo TT, et al. Primary cutaneous marginal zone B-cell lymphoma: a molecular and clinicopathologic study of 24 Asian cases. Am J Surg Pathol 2003; 27: 1061–9.

48. Jelic S, Filipovic-Ljeskovic I. Positive serology for Lyme disease borrelias in primary cutaneous B-cell lymphoma: a study in 22 patients; is it a fortuitous finding? Hematol Oncol 1999; 17: 107–16.

49. Goodlad JR, Davidson MM, Hollowood K, et al. Primary cutaneous B-cell lymphoma and Borrelia burgdorferi infection in patients from the Highlands of Scotland. Am J Surg Pathol 2000; 24: 1279–85.

50. Munksgaard L, Frisch M, Melbye M, Hjalgrim H. Incidence patterns of lyme disease and cutaneous B-cell non-Hodgkin's lymphoma in the United States. Dermatology 2000; 201: 351–2.

51. Grange F, Wechsler J, Guillaume JC, et al. Borrelia burgdorferi-associated lymphocytoma cutis simulating a primary cutaneous large B-cell lymphoma. J Am Acad Dermatol 2002; 47: 530–4.

52. Young KT, Davis LM, Dirita VJ. Campylobacter jejuni: molecular biology and pathogenesis. Nat Rev Microbiol 2007; 5: 665–79.

53. Lecuit M, Abachin E, Martin A, et al. Immunoproliferative small intestinal disease associated with Campylobacter jejuni. N Engl J Med 2004; 350: 239–48.

54. Guidoboni M, Ferreri AJ, Ponzoni M, et al. Infectious agents in mucosa-associated lymphoid tissue-type lymphomas: pathogenic role and therapeutic perspectives. Clin Lymphoma Myeloma 2006; 6: 289–300.

55. Al-Saleem T, Al-Mondhiry H. Immunoproliferative small intestinal disease (IPSID): a model for mature B-cell neoplasms. Blood 2005; 105: 2274–80.

56. Ferreri AJ, Guidoboni M, Ponzoni M, et al. Evidence for an association between Chlamydia psittaci and ocular adnexal lymphomas. J Natl Cancer Inst 2004; 96: 586–94.

57. Coupland SE, Foss HD, Anagnostopoulos I, et al. Immunoglobulin VH gene expression among extranodal marginal zone B-cell lymphomas of the ocular adnexa. Invest Ophthalmol Vis Sci 1999; 40: 555–62.

58. Hara Y, Nakamura N, Kuze T, et al. Immunoglobulin heavy chain gene analysis of ocular adnexal extranodal marginal zone B-cell lymphoma. Invest Ophthalmol Vis Sci 2001; 42: 2450–7.

59. Peeling RW, Brunham RC. Chlamydiae as pathogens: new species and new issues. Emerg Infect Dis 1996; 2: 307–19.

60. Nasisse MP, Guy JS, Stevens JB, et al. Clinical and laboratory findings in chronic conjunctivitis in cats: 91 cases (1983–1991). J Am Vet Med Assoc 1993; 203: 834–7.

61. Chanudet E, Zhou Y, Bacon CM, et al. Chlamydia psittaci is variably associated with ocular adnexal MALT lymphoma in different geographical regions. J Pathol 2006; 209: 344–51.

62. Ferreri AJ, Ponzoni M, Guidoboni M, et al. Regression of ocular adnexal lymphoma after Chlamydia psittaci-eradicating antibiotic therapy. J Clin Oncol 2005; 23: 5067–73.

63. Ferreri AJ, Ponzoni M, Guidoboni M, et al. Bacteria-eradicating therapy with doxycycline in ocular adnexal MALT lymphoma: a multicenter prospective trial. J Natl Cancer Inst 2006; 98: 1375–82.

64. Ferreri AJ, Dolcetti R, Magnino S, et al. A woman and her canary: a tale of chlamydiae and lymphomas. J Natl Cancer Inst 2007; 99: 1418–19.

5

Lymphocyte homing and immunology of extranodal lymphoid tissues

Mariagrazia Uguccioni, James J Campbell, Katrin Kuscher, and Marshall E Kadin

INTRODUCTION

The trafficking concept

Although all cells migrate during embryogenesis, most cells are relatively stationary after they have been organized into solid organs and tissues in the fully developed mammal. The cells within many solid tissues, such as the heart and liver, are linked to each other via permanent junctions.

In contrast, hematopoietic cells are seldom stationary. Hematopoietic cells travel continually through the circulatory and lymph systems. Leukocytes transit into and out of the interstitial spaces of a variety of tissues. This constant movement is known as trafficking. Trafficking increases the chances that leukocytes will encounter foreign antigens, which is necessary for imunosurveillance, an important function of these cells.

Innate and adaptive immunity

Two types of immunity, known as innate and adaptive immunity, involve different types of leukocytes. Innate immunity is the first line of defense against foreign pathogens and does not require prior exposure to antigen. Granulocytes and some types of mononuclear cells, including monocytes, dendritic cells (DCs), and natural killer (NK) lymphocytes, contribute to innate immunity. The immune system's adaptive function depends on memory acquired during prior exposure to a given antigen. T and B lymphocytes are responsible for adaptive immunity.

The various subsets of T and B lymphocytes have functional differences. Some lymphocyte subsets constitute 'naive' cells that have not encountered 'non-self' antigen, whereas others are 'memory' cells that have been exposed to cognate antigens. These lymphocyte subsets also differ in their state of activation and in the specialized homing molecules they bear, which determines the category of tissues through which they can move.

Mechanisms of leukocyte trafficking

Leukocyte trafficking can be considered as having two basic components: *entry* into tissues from the blood and *exit* from the tissues. These two basic but very different processes combine to determine the total number of leukocytes within a given tissue. The specific set of tissues through which each subtype of leukocytes moves is unique and depends on the adhesion molecules and chemoattractant receptors expressed by that specific cellular subtype.

While a large repertoire of adhesion molecules and chemoattractant receptors is expressed by the various types of leukocytes, each subtype of leukocytes expresses a specific subset of these molecules and receptors. The specific adhesion molecules and chemoattractant receptors expressed and the degree of expression of these molecules varies greatly among leukocyte subtypes. The expression pattern possessed by each leukocyte subtype determines the tissues through which that subtype will traffic. Here we review our current understanding of leukocyte trafficking by detailing some of the best-described examples of each of the basic components of trafficking.

ENTRY FROM BLOOD

Leukocytes enter tissues from the blood via a multistep process involving interactions with endothelial cells followed by migration through tissues.[1,2] This multistep process involves *rolling, activation, adhesion,* and *diapedesis.* In step 1, leukocytes in the bloodstream initiate contact with endothelium (tether) and slow down as they *roll* along endothelial cells. In step 2, leukocytes are *activated* by chemoattractants produced by the endothelium which signal the leukocytes to rapidly transform their leukocyte adhesion molecules into high-affinity states. In step 3, activated leukocytes *adhere* to endothelial cells and stop rolling. The adhesion occurs when the adhesion molecules expressed by the leukocytes bind to their ligands residing on the endothelial cell surfaces. In step 4, *diapedesis,* the leukocytes pass through the endothelium into tissue. The chemoattractants, receptors, and adhesion molecules that mediate this multistep process are referred to as '*homing molecules*'.

Trafficking of lymphocytes from blood into lymphoid organs

The transit of lymphocytes from circulation into secondary lymphoid organs, e.g. lymph nodes (LNs) and Peyer's patches (PPs), is the best understood example of leukocyte trafficking from blood into solid tissues. Leukocyte trafficking occurs differently in LNs and PPs. All secondary lymphoid organs serve as 'clearing houses' to expose antigens to lymphocytes, but LNs and PPs accumulate antigens by different routes. PPs have direct access to the intestinal lumen and accumulate antigens present in the lumen. LNs do not have direct access to tissues but instead accumulate antigens from lymph fluid draining from tissues.

Lymphocytes enter secondary lymphoid organs primarily through specialized postcapillary venules called 'high endothelial venules'

(HEVs), which are named for the unique tall (or 'high') endothelial cells lining these specialized venules. Stamper and Woodruff first recognized the unique adhesive properties of these vessels by demonstrating that viable lymphocytes bind preferentially to the HEVs (but not other areas) of human tonsil sections ex vivo.[3–5] More recent research has utilized real-time observation of lymphocyte–HEV interactions in living animals, allowing the process to be studied in greater detail.[6,7]

Lymphocyte trafficking is concentrated at the HEVs in large part because the endothelial cells in the HEVs express large numbers of homing molecules. While most *naive* lymphocytes can enter all secondary lymphoid organs, peripheral LNs and PPs selectively allow the entry of peripheral or intestinal *memory* lymphocytes, respectively. T and B cells utilize similar homing cascades to enter LNs and PPs, but the specific molecules involved vary, depending on the type of lymphocyte and the type of secondary lymphoid organ.[8]

Trafficking of T cells from blood into lymphoid organs

L-selectin/CD62L (expressed by most lymphocytes) mediates the initial recognition of LN HEV by lymphocytes passing through their lumens. L-selectin reversibly binds members of a complex family of carbohydrates, collectively called 'peripheral node addressins' (PNAds),[2,8] which are O-linked to a variety of proteins on the HEV luminal surface.[9,10] L-selectin has evolved to perform the highly specialized task of slowing down fast-moving blood cells as they pass through specific regions of vessels.[11,12] Although L-selectin cannot by itself mediate the full homing event, the downstream components of the homing cascade (as will be discussed below) are unable to interact with high-velocity cells. Thus, in the absence of functional L-selectin or PNAd, lymphocyte–HEV interactions are not initiated. This has been dramatically illustrated by in-vivo experiments: Disrupting the L-selectin–PNAd interaction with monoclonal antibodies to L-selectin prevents nearly all lymphocyte homing through LN. This occurs even though the components of the cascade downstream of L-selectin are fully functional.[6]

PNAd is not expressed at the same high levels in the PPs as it is in the LNs.[13,14] This lower amount of PNAd on the HEV in PP is sufficient to support L-selectin-mediated tethering, and some rolling. However, it is not sufficient to support rolling that is slow enough to enable the subsequent downstream events.[14] Thus, homing through PP HEV requires an additional class of molecular interactions between lymphocytes and PP HEV endothelial cells that is not necessary in lymph nodes. Interactions of this class slow down lymphocytes that are rolling along endothelium.

In the PPs an interaction between the integrin heterodimer $\alpha_4\beta_7$ on lymphocytes with its ligand, mucosal addressin cell adhesion molecule 1 (MAdCAM-1), slows lymphocyte rolling.[14-16] The $\alpha_4\beta_7$ heterodimer (composed of the α_4 integrin chain [CD49d] paired with the β_7 integrin chain) is expressed at low levels by essentially all naive T and B cells.[15] In contrast, memory T and B populations contain subsets that do not express any detectable levels of $\alpha_4\beta_7$, as well as other subsets that express high levels of $\alpha_4\beta_7$.[2,8] Thus (as mentioned above), some memory subsets that are capable of homing to peripheral LN (i.e. those lymphocytes lacking $\alpha_4\beta_7$) are not equipped to interact successfully with PP HEV. In a fascinating example of evolutionary economy, PNAd carbohydrates (the ligand for L-selectin) are often functionally presented by MAdCAM-1 molecules (the ligand for $\alpha_4\beta_7$) in lymphoid organs associated with intestinal tissue, including the PPs and mesenteric LNs.[13] The interaction between $\alpha_4\beta_7$ and MAdCAM-1 is discussed further in intestinal-specific trafficking.

Once a lymphocyte has successfully tethered and begun to roll within HEV, the downstream components can begin to initiate firm adhesion. The firm adhesion step is mediated by interactions between LFA-1 (lymphocyte function-associated antigen 1) and ICAM (intracellular adhesion molecule) for both LN and PP HEV.[14,17] Like $\alpha_4\beta_7$, LFA-1 is an integrin dimer, but LFA-1 is expressed by most leukocyte subsets. LFA-1 is composed of the α_L integrin chain (CD11a) paired with the β_2 integrin chain (CD18).[12] Under the proper conditions, LFA-1 binds to members of the ICAM family located on the luminal surface of HEV. Intravital microscopy shows that blocking the interaction between LFA-1 and ICAM has little or no effect on the tethering and rolling speed of lymphocytes on HEV, but can completely prevent such cells from coming to a stop.[6,14] Thus, without LFA-1/ICAM interactions, rolling cells continue to roll until they pass through the PNAd- or PNAd/MAdCAM-expressing areas of the HEV, to re-enter the general circulation downstream.[6,14]

LFA-1 exists on most circulating lymphocytes in a 'low affinity' or 'resting' state that cannot firmly bind the ICAM molecules on the HEV.[18] For such adhesion to occur, the cell must be activated by factors present on (or in the vicinity of) the HEV. Such factors act through the $G\alpha_i$ subfamily of G-protein-coupled receptors (GPCRs), whose ability to transduce intracellular signaling is inhibited by pertussis toxin (PTX).[19] Intravital microscopy shows that lymphocytes treated with PTX can engage normally in the early tethering and rolling stages in both LN and PP.[6,7] The PTX effect appears to directly inhibit the signals that trigger increased affinity of LFA-1 for ICAM, because experimental blocking of LFA-1/ICAM interactions has no additional effect on PTX-treated cells on HEV.[14] Crystallography studies of LFA-1 demonstrate that the molecule folds like a closed jackknife when in its low-affinity state, but opens straight when it is activated.[20,21]

Although each step of the homing cascade makes an essential contribution to successful and efficient lymphocyte–HEV interaction, the GPCR-mediated activation step is clearly the most important for imparting specificity to the process. This is elegantly demonstrated by the fact that neutrophils have all the adhesion molecules necessary for HEV interaction (i.e. L-selectin and LFA-1) but they rarely enter secondary lymphoid organs. This is because neutrophils do not bear the proper GPCRs to respond to the HEV-associated factors that trigger LFA-1 activation in lymphocytes.[22]

The importance of PTX-inhibitable GPCRs in triggering adhesion of rolling lymphocytes in the HEV has been understood since the early 1990s.[7] However, it was not until 1998 that members of the chemokine and chemokine receptor families[23] were formally implicated in this role. The first breakthrough came when it was discovered that only three of the more than 40 known chemokines (including CCL21/SLC) had the unique ability to trigger rapid and robust (~30 ms) adhesion of rolling lymphocytes to ICAM-1 in vitro.[17] The receptor that is present on lymphocytes, and shown to be responsible for this effect, was identified as CCR7.[24,25] The second breakthrough came when in-situ hybridization studies revealed that in the mouse CCL21 was produced directly by the endothelial cells of HEV.[26,27] Thus, circumstantial evidence strongly implicated CCL21/CCR7 interactions as key components of the process by which lymphocytes home to LNs and PPs from the blood.

Subsequent studies have demonstrated that CCR7 and CCL21 are important for homing of T lymphocytes into LNs and PPs in homeostatic conditions. The majority of T cell homing through HEVs require interaction of CCR7 with CCL21 and/or CCL19, which are both normally available on the HEV lumen, to trigger integrin-mediated adhesion.

In summary, it seems clear that successful homing of T cells to secondary lymphoid organs from the circulation requires:

- tethering and rolling mediated by L-selectin on lymphocytes interacting with PNAd on HEV (with the help of $\alpha_4\beta_7$/MAdCAM interactions in the PP)
- activation of LFA-1 via a G-protein-mediated signal through CCR7 via CCL21 and/or CCL19 on the HEV.

The scenario above clearly describes the vast majority of interactions between T cells and HEVs. However, a small percentage of T cells can still interact with HEVs in the absence of CCR7.[28] This small subset of interactions is eliminated in the absence of another chemokine receptor, CXCR4. The ligand for CXCR4, CXCL12, can be found on HEVs, although it does not appear to be produced by the HEVs directly. Thus, there is a potential role for CXCR4–CXCL12 interactions in homing of a small subset of T cells to lymphoid organs, an intriguing possibility that must be explored through future experiments.

Trafficking of B cells from blood into lymphoid organs

Homing of B cells to LNs and PPs through HEV involves largely the same combinations of adhesion molecules discussed above for T cells. However, B cells are able to interact with regions of the HEV where T cells interactions are rare. HEV zones in which B interactions greatly outnumber T interactions are located at sites where the HEVs pass through B cell follicles in PPs.[22] This difference in T vs B localization in HEV is apparently due to the usage of different chemokine-receptor combinations by each cell type.[28–30]

As discussed above, the vast majority of T cell–HEV interactions require CCR7.[8] However, B cell–HEV interactions are largely unaffected by the absence of functional CCR7.[22] B-cell homing to LNs and PPs is not affected by disruption of signaling through any single chemokine/receptor pair tested. However, simultaneous absence of both CXCR4 and CCR7 function eliminates most B-cell homing to secondary lymphoid organs.[28] Elimination of CXCR4 alone does not significantly affect the number of B cells entering LNs but no studies have determined whether elimination of CXCR4 signaling changes the location of B cell–HEV interactions.

PPs have an additional level of control for B-cell homing. In addition to CXCR4 and CCR7 signaling, CXCR5 contributes to B-cell homing to PPs.[28] The CXCR5 ligand, CXCL13, is found on the luminal surfaces of HEV in the vicinity of B follicles in PPs, where B-cell homing dominates over T-cell homing. Thus, it is likely that CXCR5 plays a major role in directing B cells to B-specific regions of the PPs. It should be noted that CXCL13 is also found in the HEVs of human tonsils,[31] so that CXCR5 may play a similar role in B-cell homing to this organ.

Trafficking of lymphocytes from blood into non-lymphoid tissues

Lymphocyte homing to LNs and PPs through HEVs occurs constantly and at a very high rate, which has led to our intricate knowledge of these processes (discussed above) gained through intravital microscopy. Homing to non-lymphoid tissues, although less amenable to such direct study, holds hope for medical usefulness in the future. Such hope lies in tissue-specific lymphocyte-mediated autoimmune diseases, such as psoriasis (selective for skin) or Crohn's disease (selective for intestine). The access of memory lymphocytes to non-lymphoid tissues is even more tissue-specific than that of LNs and PPs. The vast majority of epidermal or intestinal memory lymphocytes express an adhesion molecule repertoire that preferentially directs them to that particular tissue. Thus, if lymphocyte homing to skin or intestine could be manipulated pharmacologically, there would be great potential for controlling tissue-specific autoimmune diseases.

In the absence of direct intravital microscopy data, circumstantial evidence for tissue-specific homing cascades is provided through association of a given lymphocyte subset with a particular tissue. It is rare to find naive lymphocytes in non-lymphoid tissues. Thus, homing to such tissues is largely restricted to memory lymphocytes.

Although the mechanism is not completely understood, antigen stimulation of naive lymphocyes generates memory cells with homing properties that guide them back to tissues containing the stimulatory antigen.[32] This happens despite the fact that the naive lymphocytes rarely if ever enter the tissue containing the antigen. Instead, naive lymphocytes enter draining lymph nodes and are stimulated by antigen-presenting cells (dendritic cells DCs) in the lymph nodes. Apparently, these DCs carry information indicating the type of tissue from which the antigen was obtained, which is used to instruct the differentiation of naive cells into tissue-specific memory cells. In this way, DCs perform a type of 'imprinting' on lymphocytes.[33]

While all naive cells share the same repertoire of adhesion molecules and chemoattractant receptors expressed on their surfaces, various subsets of memory cells express different repertoires of such homing molecules. The homing properties of memory cells are dependent upon the repertoire of homing molecules that they express.[2,8] For example, approximately 20% of memory Th2 lymphocytes from human peripheral blood express the cutaneous lymphocyte antigen (CLA). CLA is a carbohydrate that allows lymphocytes to roll on E-selectin-expressing blood vessels. A separate ~20% of memory Th2 lymphocytes from blood express the $\alpha_4\beta_7$-integrin (Figure 5.1).[2,8] As discussed in the previous section, $\alpha_4\beta_7$ allows rolling and adhesion within vessels expressing the mucosal addressin MAdCAM-1.[14-16] There are essentially no Th2 cells that express both CLA and $\alpha_4\beta_7$ together, so these markers define distinct populations. Similar contrasts are found for expression of chemokine receptors: CCR4 is found primarily on $\alpha_4\beta_7$-negative Th2 cells,[34-36] whereas CCR9 is found only on a subset of $\alpha_4\beta_7$-positive Th2 cells.[37] To complete the picture, cutaneous and intestinal tissues have differential expression of the ligands for these chemokine receptors and homing molecules.[34,38] Study of lymphocytes isolated from surgical samples of such tissues confirm that co-expression of CLA and CCR4 defines the population of memory Th2 lymphocytes that is specialized to home through cutaneous sites.[34-36] CCR10 is also expressed on a subset of cutaneous lymphocytes, and may also play a role in cutaneous homing.[39] Co-expression of $\alpha_4\beta_7$ and CCR9 defines a population of memory Th2 cells dedicated to homing to the small intestine.[37,38,40]

The intestinal lamina propria (LP) contains numerous previously activated/memory CD4+ T-cells involved in intestinal immunity and the induction and maintenance of chronic

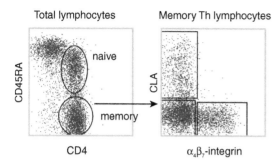

Total lymphocytes   Memory Th lymphocytes

Figure 5.1   *Flow cytometric analysis (subsets) of human periph-eral blood CD4 lymphocytes.*

intestinal inflammation.[41] T-cell entry into the intestinal mucosa is mediated by distinct sets of cell adhesion molecules expressed on the T-cell and intestinal microvascular endothelial surface. Interaction between the gut-associated integrin $\alpha_4\beta_7$, on the T cell surface, with its ligand MAdCAM-1, on intestinal microvascular endothelium cells, is important for T-cell entry into the LP.[42–44] Moreover, antibody neutralization studies suggest a role for P-selectin and P-selectin glycoprotein ligand 1 (PSGL-1) in effector CD4+ T-cell entry to this site. The chemokine receptor CCR9 is required for efficient effector CD8+ T-cell localization to the small intestinal epithelium.[40,45]

B-cell subsets can also express homing receptors that may allow their selective homing to particular types of tissue. A recent discovery concerns B cells that produce the immunoglobulin isotype IgA. IgA is an immunoglobulin type that is specialized to be present in fluids that are secreted by the body (e.g. tears, breast milk, intestinal mucus, lung mucus). The small subset of differentiated B cells that secrete IgA express the chemokine receptor CCR10, which is only rarely expressed by B cells that secrete other immunoglobulin isotypes.[46,47] A ligand for CCR10, CCL28, is preferentially expressed by mucosal tissues from which IgA is secreted.[44,48,49] Thus, CCR10 may be a homing receptor that allows IgA-secreting B cells to home to the tissues where IgA would be the most useful.

Recent studies have demonstrated a critical role of the LN environment for the induction

of certain chemokine receptors. Thus, CD8+ and CD4+ T cells are induced to express CCR9 or respond to the CCR9 ligand CCL25, respectively, after activation in mesenteric lymph nodes (MLNs) but not peripheral lymph nodes (PLNs).[40,45] The induction of CCR9 and additional chemokine receptors during CD4+ T-cell priming in MLNs and the role of the LN environment in regulating induction of these receptors remain largely uncharacterized.

Given the large number of lymphocyte subtypes that are constantly being identified in human blood over time (at least 50 non-overlapping subtypes of lymphocytes in human blood at the time of this writing), it is likely that many more such associations between homing receptors and tissue specificities will be uncovered. Great promise for the future of medical and pharmaceutical practice lies within such findings.

EXIT FROM TISSUES

The preceding section shows that there is a great deal of detailed knowledge concerning the mechanisms by which lymphocytes enter tissues. However, much less is known about the exit of lymphocytes from tissues. Except during times of escalating inflammation, the number of cells within a given tissue remains relatively constant.[2]

Two examples of leukocytes exiting from tissues are discussed: eosinophils, which are stored in great numbers in the bone marrow, can be rapidly triggered to enter the blood; DCs, after spending time gathering antigens within tissues, leave the tissues, and migrate to secondary lymphoid organs, where they present these antigens to lymphocytes entering the organ from blood.

Rapid release of eosinophils into circulation from bone marrow

Eosinophils are a specialized subset of granulocytes that has evolved to assist in the expulsion of helminth infestations from tissues.[50,51] In asthma, where eosinophils have been best studied, these granulocytes play a destructive role, leading to characteristic airway constriction.

Allergic insult of the lung leads to a coordinated recruitment of eosinophils. Upon such insult, lung tissue produces the cytokine interleukin-5 (IL-5), along with eotaxin chemokines, which are three closely related chemokines, CCL11,[52,53] CCL24,[54] and CCL26,[55,56] whose only known receptor (as agonists) is CCR3. Eosinophils express CCR3 and specific receptors for IL-5, and functional blockade of either the IL-5 receptor or CCR3 inhibits eosinophil accumulation in lung.[57]

As chemoattractants, eotaxins are likely to function by attracting eosinophils, as well as basophils[58] and Th2 lymphocytes,[59,60] from the blood as part of a lung-homing cascade, as discussed for lymphocytes above. Thus, the finding that inhibition of these leukocytes' accumulation occurs through eotaxin-CCR3 blockade is logical.[57] However, the influence of IL-5 on eosinophil accumulation was less obvious when discovered, as IL-5 is not a chemoattractant for eosinophils. Further investigation revealed that IL-5 treatment in the absence of eotaxin causes a rapid increase in blood eosinophil count, without accumulation in lung. This increase was accompanied by a corresponding decrease in bone marrow eosinophil number.[50]

The mechanism was revealed by a series of elegant experiments in which cells exiting bone marrow could be captured and studied directly. Our current understanding of the process is as follows. Lung tissue synthesizes both IL-5 and eotaxin. IL-5 is carried via the blood to the bone marrow. Eosinophils in the bone marrow are stimulated by IL-5, and enter the blood. The greatly increased population of eosinophils then circulates in the blood until they enter a venule passing through inflamed lung tissue. In such a venule, the eosinophil encounters eotaxin, which participates in attracting the eosinophil into the lung tissue.[50]

In conclusion, IL-5 acts at a distance (in the bone marrow), whereas eotaxins act locally. This mechanism allows eosinophils, which can be potentially destructive in the circulation,[50] to be more safely stored until needed. Release of eosinophils from the bone marrow is the best-understood example of coordinated leukocyte release from any tissue.

Reprogramming dendritic cells to exit tissues towards secondary lymphoid organs

As mentioned earlier, DCs move throughout all tissues, patrolling for foreign antigens. Immature DCs express a variety of chemokine receptors, including CCR1, CCR5, and CCR6. These receptors are thought to help keep immature DCs within tissues, where ligands for these receptors are abundant.[61] Immature DCs continue to collect antigen until they are stimulated by a 'danger signal', which indicates that recently collected antigens may belong to a foreign invader. Examples of such danger signals include lipopolysaccharide, bacterial lipoproteins, peptidoglycans, and CpG dinucleotides often originating from bacteria. Danger signals, acting through toll-like receptors, induce DCs to mature. Mature DCs lose expression and function of CCR1, CCR5, and CCR6 and gain functional expression of CCR7.[62,63] The loss of 'immature' chemokine receptors thus removes the signals thought to keep the DCs within the tissue. Lymphatic endothelium expresses CCR7 ligands,[64-66] so the gain of CCR7 function induces the mature DC to exit the tissue via the lymph. The lymph ultimately transports the DCs to a downstream secondary lymphoid organ, which allows their antigens to be presented to T cells to induce a cognate response.

These are two very different mechanisms by which leukocytes exit tissues: eosinophils, stored in the bone marrow, are poised for rapid release into the blood upon receipt of the necessary signal; by contrast, dendritic cells must be entirely reprogrammed to exit tissue.

Trafficking of lymphocytes from lymphoid tissues into circulation

Lymphocytes continuously traffic from the blood through secondary lymphoid organs, where they search for their cognate antigen.

The mechanism of entrance via blood is well understood also thanks to the generation of gene-targeted mice lacking central molecules required for entry.[25,67–69] In contrast, the egress of lymphocytes from spleen or lymph nodes is recently starting to be elucidated. Retention and exit from lymphoid tissues is fundamental, because lymphocytes should be trapped in secondary lymphoid organs for receiving appropriate priming signals before leaving into medullary sinuses. Lymphocytes exit the spleen into the blood, and the LNs and PPs into the lymph. The mechanism of egression has been ascribed to the family of the sphingosine 1-phosphate (S1P) receptors. S1P, the ligand of $S1P_1$ receptor, is found in high concentrations in blood and lymph, and is certainly implicated in the egression of lymphocytes, expressing the $S1P_1$ receptor, from secondary lymphoid organs.[70] Of note, FTY720, a small molecule agonist acting on several S1P receptor types, causes a reduction of lymphocytes in blood and tissues and their sequestration into lymphoid organs, which is independent of the chemokine receptors CCR7 and CXCR5.[71–73] However, the detailed mechanisms of lymphocyte egression from lymphoid tissues remain to be clarified.

LYMPHOCYTE TRAFFICKING IN NK/T-CELL LYMPHOMAS

The World Health Classification of Tumors of Hematopoietic and Lymphoid Tissues recognizes cutaneous T-cell lymphomas, leukemic/disseminated NK/T-cell lymphomas, other extranodal NK/T-cell lymphomas, and several types of nodal T-cell lymphomas, including angioimmunoblastic T-cell lymphoma (AILD), anaplastic T-cell lymphoma (ALCL), and peripheral T-cell lymphoma, unspecified (PTCL-U) (WHO Classification of Tumors of Hematopoietic and Lymphoid Tissues, Lyon, 2001). The latter category includes T-zone lymphoma, lymphoepithelioid (Lennert's) lymphoma, pleomorphic T-cell lymphoma, small, medium, and large cell types, and T-immunoblastic lymphoma. As might be expected, the localization of tumor cells to lymph nodes, gut, skin, and other extranodal sites is largely determined by the homing receptors on the tumor cells and their ligands expressed on the vascular endothelium of the target organs (Table 5.1). The following section will summarize the literature on this subject.

Cutaneous T-cell lymphomas

Cutaneous T-cell lymphomas (CTCLs) have been divided into several distinct subtypes.[74,75] The most common type is mycosis fungoides (MF) and its leukemic variant, the Sezary syndrome (SS). Tumor cells are CD4+ Th2 cells in 95% of MF and SS cases.

In CTCL, tumor cells home to the skin because of binding to endothelial cells of dermal capillaries. Circulating CTCL cells expressing CLA roll along endothelial cells expressing E-selectin. CCR4 on MF cells recognize CCL17 or CCL22 on the luminal side of endothelial cells, facilitating binding of LFA-1 on MF cells to ICAM-1 on endothelial cells and subsequent extravasation into the dermis. Ferenczi et al found co-expression of CCR4 and CLA characterized tumor cells in the blood and skin lesions of patients with MF and SS.[76] In early MF, tumor cells commonly migrate into the epidermis, a phenomenon known as epidermotropism. Epidermotropism is associated with epidermal keratinocyte secretion of human IFN-inducible protein 10 (CXCL10), which is chemotactic for CD4+ lymphocytes. CXCL10 is confined to basal layer keratinocytes of normal skin but was found to be markedly increased and extended to the superbasal keratinocytes of 17 of 18 CTCL patients.[77] CXCL10 expression was not increased in any of 4 patients with B cell lymphoma involving the dermis. Yamaguchi et al reported that CXCR3, the receptor for CXCL10, was especially present in epidermotropic small lymphoma cells of MF.[78] MF was distinguished from adult T-cell leukemia/lymphoma (ATLL) by expression of CLA in MF but not ATLL cells.[78] Lu found that the CXCR3 was expressed by a subset of tumor lymphocytes in all 25 cases of low-grade MF, with most cells positive in 20 cases.[79] In progressed or transformed MF, CXCR3 expression was present in only 5 of 22 cases and in 4 of 5 cases with sequential biopsies, large cell transformation was accompanied by loss of CXCR3. In early MF, tumor cells cluster around Langerhans' cells in the epidermis, forming Pautrier's microabscesses which are virtually diagnostic of MF. This process is facilitated by interactions of integrin $\alpha_E\beta_7$, CCR4, and the T-cell receptor complex on MF cells with E-cadherin, CCL22, and major histocompatibility complex class II antigens, respectively, on Langerhans' cells. In progressed or transformed MF, CXCR3 is lost, a finding consistent with loss of epidermotropism and downward migration of tumor cells in plaque and tumor stage MF.[79]

Skin homing of Sezary cells involves CXCL12–CXCR4 signaling and down-regulation of CD26/depeptidlypeptidase IV.[80] Although CXCL12 is constitutively expressed in a number of tissues, including bone marrow and lung, Sézary cells rarely enter these tissues. This might be explained by the coexistence of specific skin-homing receptors such as CLA and CCR4, and of CXCR4, in SS cells. On the contrary, the lack of SS spreading into other tissues may be dictated by the absence of additional signals. In this regard, Xu et al recently demonstrated that lymphocyte homing to bronchus-associated lymphoid tissue (BALT) is dependent on CD49d–VCAM1 interaction. Interestingly, CD49d is not present on the SS cell surface.[81]

Anaplastic large cell lymphoma

ALCL consists of two major subtypes: a primary cutaneous type, which includes lymphomatoid papulosis (LyP); a systemic type, which involves lymph nodes primarily. Most cutaneous ALCL are anaplastic lymphoma kinase (ALK)-negative, whereas most nodal ALCL are ALK+ (ALK-negative nodal ALCL occurs in patients over age 30 years old). Vermeer et al found CCR4 to be expressed by neoplastic cells in 9/9 primary cutaneous ALCL, and in 9/15 nodal ALK-negative ALCL, but in only one of four ALK+ nodal

ALCL.[82] CCL17 was expressed by neoplastic cells in 12/27 ALK-negative ALCL but in none of 12 ALK+ ALCL. Ishida et al also found usual absence of CCR4 in ALK+ ALCL and preferential expression of CCR4 in ALK-negative ALCL.[83] These results are in contrast to the earlier detection of CCR4 in 5/5 ALK+ ALCL by Jones et al.[84] The authors also found that CXCR3 was present in only 1 of 15 ALK+ ALCL. Weng et al found that CXCR4/CD184 is expressed in tumors with markers of Th2 differentiation, including 88% of ALCL.[85]

Kleinhans et al detected the CCR3 ligand, CCL11, in tumor cells in primary cutaneous ALCL. Functional activity of CCR3 was demonstrated in a CD30+ ALCL line clonally derived from LyP by actin polymerization and migration in response to CCL11. The results suggest that CCR3 and its ligand play a role in the recruitment and retention of CD30+ ALCL cells in the skin.[86]

About one-half of cases of primary cutaneous ALCL express CLA. We found expression of CLA by the CD30+ cells in each of 12 cases of LyP. CLA expression was lost with extracutaneous spread of disease in 2 LyP cases and was low in expression of two ALCL lines derived from tumor cells in the peripheral blood and a skin tumor in one of these cases. Systemic ALCL are usually CLA-negative (Figure 5.2). The results are consistent with the established role of CLA in homing of T lymphocytes to the skin.

Peripheral T-cell lymphoma, unspecified

PTCL-U is a heterogeneous group of tumors. Patients present with nodal involvement but often have infiltrates of extranodal tissues such as bone marrow, liver, spleen, and skin. Japanese investigators attempted to understand patterns of organ involvement by analysis of chemokine receptors. They assigned distinct patterns of chemokine receptors and activated T-cell receptor OX40/CD134 to AILD and ALCL.[87] Nearly all cases of AILD expressed OX40/CD134 (96%) and Th1-associated CXCR3. In contrast, ALCL cases were negative for OX40/CD134 and only

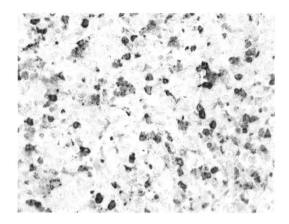

Figure 5.2 *Expression of cutaneous lymphocyte antigen (CLA) in ALCL detected by immunohistochemistry.* Tumor cells in extracutaneous ALCL are unstained while intervening small non-malignant lymphocytes and macrophages are strained in brown.

infrequently positive for CXCR3 (24%) but positive for Th2-associated ST2(L) in 94% of cases. Cases of PTCL-U, were divided into two groups: group 1 (cases positive for either ST2(L), CCR5, or CXCR3) tended to show a favorable prognosis compared with group 2 (cases negative for ST2(L), CCR5, and CXCR3). Ishida et al found CCR4 to be a significant unfavorable prognostic marker in PTCL-U.[83] They found a significant correlation between mRNA expression of CCR4 and Foxp3, suggesting an association with the immunocompromised states of these patients.

Leukemic/disseminated T-cell lymphoma – Adult T-cell leukemia/lymphoma

ATLL is a tumor caused by human T-cell leukemia virus type 1 (HTLV-1) and is endemic to Japan, the Caribbean, and parts of Central Africa. Several clinical variants are recognized: acute, lymphomatous, chronic, and smoldering. The acute variant is characterized by a leukemic phase, skin rash, and generalized lymphadenopathy. The lymphomatous variant is characterized by prominent lymphadenopathy without peripheral blood involvement. ATLL cells from patients with lymphoid organ involvement express significantly more CCR7 than ATL cells from

patients without lymphoid organ involvement.[88] ATLL cells were found to be positive for ST2(L) in 23 of 47 (49%) of cases and negative for OX40/CD134, CXCR3, and CCR5 in cases of the lymphomatous type.[87]

Nasal type NK/T-cell lymphoma

These lymphomas are associated with Epstein–Barr virus infection and expression of EBV-latent membrane protein (LMP)-1 and EB nuclear antigen (EBNA)-1. Angioinvasion by neoplastic cells is characteristic, but the mechanism is unknown. To investigate the mechanism, Liu et al studied expression of cell adhesion and chemokine receptor levels in 17 cases of nasal NK/T-cell lymphoma and compared them with 10 diffuse large B-cell lymphomas and non-neoplastic nasal mucosa as controls. They found mRNA levels of integrin subunits α_4, α_2, α_M, and β_2 to be significantly elevated in nasal NK/T-cell lymphomas. Immunohistochemistry highlighted α_M in cases with LMP-1 expression, and the investigators suggested that angioinvasion is mediated through up-regulation of α_M by LMP-1.[89] Yagi et al found epidermotropism in 4 of 5 cases and infiltration of subcutaneous tissues in nasal extranodal NK/T-cell lymphomas. Tumor cells expressed CXCR3 in all cases.[90] Yoshino et al examined expression of CLA in 52 cases of nasal NK/T-cell lymphoma and found that CLA was highly expressed in 29 cases with cutaneous involvement ($n = 29$) compared with the CLA-negative group ($n = 23$). CLA was associated with a worse prognosis in a multivariate analysis.[91]

Enteropathy-type T-cell lymphoma

Little is known about expression of chemokine receptors in enteropathy-type T-cell lymphoma (EATCL). Drillenburg et al demonstrated mucosal homing receptor integrin $\alpha_4\beta_7$ in 56% of mucosal T-cell lymphomas, but only 17% or nodal T-cell lymphomas and no cutaneous T-cell lymphoma. This receptor mediates binding to MAdCAM-1, a vascular adhesion molecule (addressin) selectively expressed on mucosal

Table 5.1 Expression of chemokine receptors and their ligands in NK/T-cell lymphomas

Chemokine receptor/ligand	Lymphoma type
CCR4	Mycosis fungoides, primary cutaneous ALCL and ALK-ALCL, ATLL
Cutaneous lymphocyte antigen (CLA)	Mycosis fungoides, Sezary syndrome, primary cutaneous ALCL, lymphomatoid papulosis, unfavorable nasal NK/T-cell lymphomas
CCL17, CCL22	ALK-negative ALCL
CCL11	Primary cutaneous ALCL
CXCR3	Present in AILD, favorable PTCL-U, nasal NK/T-cell lymphomas, and epidermotropic MF but not in progressed MF or dermal based T-cell tumors
$\alpha_4\beta_7$ integrin	Mucosal T-cell lymphomas
ST2(L)	Lymphomatous type of ATLL

endothelium. Further studies are needed to determine the role of $\alpha_4\beta_7$ in EATCL.[92]

Hepatosplenic T-cell lymphoma

Hepatosplenic T-cell lymphoma is distinguished by hepatosplenomegaly, minimal or no lymphadenopathy, frequent bone marrow involvement, and a distinctive pattern of intrasinusoidal infiltration of tumor cells. The tumor cells appear to be adjacent to endothelial cells within sinuses of the liver, spleen, and bone marrow.[82] Although this tumor exemplifies a curious and distinctive pattern of lymphocyte trafficking, there are no published studies which have determined the molecules responsible for these phenomena.

Angioimmunoblastic T-cell lymphoma

AITCL, which has a composite Th1-like immunophenotype, has a low expression of CXCR4/CD184.[85]

LYMPHOCYTE TRAFFICKING IN B-CELL LYMPHOMAS

Our knowledge of the molecules guiding malignant B cells to extranodal sites, as well as of the function of chemokines in the tumor environment, is at a very early stage. Hereafter, we report the information available so far on molecules involved in migration and on chemokine receptor expression in B-cell lymphoma developing at extranodal sites.

Large B-cell lymphomas are a heterogeneous group, accounting for about 40% of adult non-Hodgkin's lymphomas. In contrast to T-cell lymphomas, the anatomical site of B-cell lymphoma has not been one of the major features defining these tumors. Recently, the location of large B-cell lymphomas has been considered more carefully, as the clinical outcome can depend on the sites of involvement. This feature is due to the fact that different organs are able to produce different chemoattractants as well as express different endothelial-associated proteins able to recruit different cell subpopulations. Recent evidence demonstrates that large B-cell lymphomas can recruit monocytes via CCL5 for supporting, by the production of several factors, B-cell survival and proliferation.[93]

Malignant B cells can express chemokine receptors, which might be involved not only in their capacity to migrate but also to survive at tumor sites. CXCL13 has been the first chemokine described to selectively attract B lymphocytes.[94] For its characteristics, it was immediately investigated in pathological conditions with a typical B-cell infiltrate and in malignancies of B-cell origin.[95]

Mature B-cell neoplasms are clonal proliferations of B cells at various stages of differentiation, ranging from naive B cells to mature plasma cells. The major risk factor of mature B-cell neoplasia appears to be an abnormality of the immune system, either immunodeficiency or autoimmune disease. Some autoimmune diseases are also associated with an

Figure 5.3 *mRNA expression of CXCL13 in large B-cell lymphomas of the stomach detected by in-situ hybridization.* Several tumor cells express CXCL13 and are stained in black. Magnification 100×.

increased risk of lymphoma, particularly extranodal marginal zone/mucosa-associated lymphoid tissue (MALT) lymphoma in patients with Hashimoto's thyroiditis, and lymphoepithelial sialadenitis associated with Sjögren's syndrome. Bacteria or immune responses to bacterial antigens have been implicated in the pathogenesis of B-cell lymphomas of extranodal MALT type. Treatment of *Helicobacter pylori* infection causes regression of the lymphoma in many patients with associated gastric MALT lymphomas. Similarly, *borrelia burgdorferi* has been implicated in the pathogenesis of cutaneous MALT lymphoma. MALT lymphomas are the most studied with regard to chemokine expression. Many reports have shown the expression of the B-cell-attracting chemokine, CXCL13. Inducible expression of CXCL13 was first described in relation to gastric lymphomas of the MALT type (Figure 5.3), arising in association with an *H. pylori*-induced gastritis and mucosal lymphoid aggregates.[95]

The analysis of a small series of patients with cutaneous lymphomas confirmed the findings in gastric MALT lymphoma, adding further evidence of the close similarities between this type of lymphoma and MALT lymphomas.[96] CXCL12 and CXCL13 have been identified in primary intraocular B-cell lymphoma, suggesting that the two chemokines might be involved in the recruitment of malignant B cells to the retinal pigment epithelium from the choroidal circulation.[97,98]

Many publications have shown CXCL13 and its selective receptor CXCR5, in different extranodal B-cell lymphomas, as the primary central nervous system lymphoma (PCNSL).[99] PCNSL is a rare, but often rapidly fatal form of non-Hodgkin's B-cell lymphomas which arises in the CNS, involves the brain, spinal cord, meninges, and/or eye, and has a low propensity to metastasize. Gene expression profiling, using cDNA microarrays for cytokines/chemokines and their receptors, has been utilized to assess the role of the dysregulation of the endogenous immune system in PCNSL, extranodal and nodal lymphomas. This study, although employing few cases of each subtype, has underlined the importance of CXCL13, in addition to the chemokines active on monocytes and T lymphocytes.[100] CXCL13, a B-cell-attracting chemokine, has been the first chemokine identified in malignant B lymphocytes of PCNSL.[99] The protein, but not its mRNA, has been detected also on vascular endothelium, within the tumor mass. It has been hypothesized that there is an active mechanism of transport from the source to endothelial cells. Indeed, an active transport from the stroma to endothelial cells has been reported for other chemokines.[101] In addition, malignant B cells express CXCR5, the selective CXCL13 receptor.[99] This latter feature suggests a role for CXCL13 in the pathogenesis of PCNSL. Recent publications report that malignant B lymphocytes in PCNSL express CXCL12, as well as its selective receptor CXCR4.[102–104] These data need confirmation at the mRNA level, but corroborate the need for thoughtful studies to assess the role of chemokines in PCNSL development and localization.

To date we still need information on mediastinal and intravascular B-cell lymphomas, as well as on the large B-cell lymphoma, leg type and acquired immunodeficiency syndrome (AIDS)-associated B-cell lymphomas. It remains to investigate if chemokines and other selective molecules are fundamental in determining these unique and important clinical entities. Moreover, the involvement of selective chemokine receptors or adhesion molecules has not been analyzed so far in the precursor B lymphoblastic lymphoma (B-LBL), a rare neoplasm composed of immature lymphocytes that display lymphoblastic morphology and express precursor and B-cell marker. The analysis of skin homing molecules, such as CCR4 and its agonists, together with B-cell-attracting chemokines, would shed light on its preferential homing to the skin, in addition to lymph nodes and bone marrow.

Our understanding and appreciation of the complexity of the network of chemokines and chemokine receptors in tumor development, maintenance, and inflammation is still at its infancy. New therapeutic opportunities will emerge from a better understanding of the milieu of chemokines expressed at different sites, and of the accessory molecules involved in cell migration. Nevertheless, chemokines and chemokine receptors might represent appropriate molecular targets to optimize anticancer therapies.

REFERENCES

1. Baggiolini M. Chemokines and leukocyte traffic. Nature 1998; 392: 565–8.
2. Butcher EC, Williams M, Youngman K, Rott L, Briskin M. Lymphocyte trafficking and regional immunity. Adv Immunol 1999; 72: 209–53.
3. Stamper HB Jr, Woodruff JJ. Lymphocyte homing into lymph nodes: in vitro demonstration of the selective affinity of recirculating lymphocytes for high-endothelial venules. J Exp Med 1976; 144: 828–33.
4. Stamper HB Jr, Woodruff JJ. An in vitro model of lymphocyte homing. I. Characterization of the interaction between thoracic duct lymphocytes and specialized high-endothelial venules of lymph nodes. J Immunol 1977; 119: 772–80.
5. Woodruff JJ, Katz M, Lucas LE, Stamper HB Jr. An in vitro model of lymphocyte homing. II. Membrane and cytoplasmic events involved in lymphocyte adherence to specialized high-endothelial venules of lymph nodes. J Immunol 1977; 119: 1603–10.
6. Warnock RA, Askari S, Butcher EC, Von Andrian UH. Molecular mechanisms of lymphocyte homing to peripheral lymph nodes. J Exp Med 1998; 187(2): 205–16.
7. Bargatze RF, Butcher EC. Rapid G protein-regulated activation event involved in lymphocyte binding to high endothelial venules. J Exp Med 1993; 178: 367–72.
8. Campbell JJ, Butcher EC. Chemokines in tissue-specific and microenvironment-specific lymphocyte homing. Curr Opin Immunol 2000; 12: 336–41.
9. Berg EL, Robinson MK, Warnock RA, Butcher EC. The human peripheral lymph node vascular addressin is a ligand for LECAM-1, the peripheral lymph node homing receptor. J Cell Biol 1991; 114(2): 343–9.
10. van Zante A, Rosen SD. Sulphated endothelial ligands for L-selectin in lymphocyte homing and inflammation. Biochem Soc Trans 2003; 31(2): 313–17.
11. Butcher EC. Leukocyte-endothelial cell recognition: three (or more) steps to specificity and diversity. Cell 1991; 67: 1033–6.
12. Springer TA. Traffic signals for lymphocyte recirculation and leukocyte emigration: the multistep paradigm. Cell 1994; 76: 301–14.
13. Berg EL, McEvoy LM, Berlin C, Bargatze RF, Butcher EC. L-selectin-mediated lymphocyte rolling on MAdCAM-1. Nature 1993; 366(6456): 630–1.
14. Bargatze RF, Jutila MA, Butcher EC. Distinct roles of L-selectin and integrins alpha 4 beta 7 and LFA-1 in lymphocyte homing to Peyer's patch-HEV in situ: the multistep model confirmed and refined. Immunity 1995; 3(1): 99–108.
15. Berlin C, Berg EL, Briskin MJ, et al. Alpha 4 beta 7 integrin mediates lymphocyte binding to the mucosal vascular addressin MAdCAM-1. Cell 1993; 74: 185–95.
16. Berlin C, Bargatze RF, Campbell JJ, et al. α4 integrins mediate lymphocyte attachment and rolling under physiologic flow. Cell 1995; 80: 413–22.
17. Campbell JJ, Hedrick J, Zlotnik A, et al. Chemokines and the arrest of lymphocytes rolling under flow conditions. Science 1998; 279: 381–4.
18. Dustin ML, Springer TA. T-cell receptor cross-linking transiently stimulates adhesiveness through LFA-1. Nature 1989; 341(6243): 619–24.
19. Kurose H, Katada T, Amano T, Ui M. Specific uncoupling by islet-activating protein, pertussis toxin, of negative signal transduction via alpha-adrenergic, cholinergic, and opiate receptors in neuroblastoma x glioma hybrid cells. J Biol Chem 1983; 258: 4870–5.
20. Takagi J, Petre BM, Walz T, Springer TA. Global conformational rearrangements in integrin extracellular domains in outside-in and inside-out signaling. Cell 2002; 110: 599–11.
21. Shimaoka M, Xiao T, Liu JH, et al. Structures of the alpha L I domain and its complex with ICAM-1 reveal a shape-shifting pathway for integrin regulation. Cell 2003; 112: 99–111.
22. Warnock RA, Campbell JJ, Dorf ME, et al. The role of chemokines in the micro environmental control of T versus B cell arrest in Peyer's patch high endothelial venules. J Exp Med 2000; 191: 77–88.
23. Zlotnik A, Yoshie O. Chemokines: a new classification system and their role in immunity. Immunity 2000; 12: 121–7.
24. Yoshida R, Nagira M, Kitaura M, et al. Secondary lymphoid-tissue chemokine is a functional ligand for the CC chemokine receptor CCR7. J Biol Chem 1998; 273: 7118–22.
25. Förster R, Schubel A, Breitfeld D, et al. CCR7 coordinates the primary immune response by

establishing functional microenvironments in secondary lymphoid organs. Cell 1999; 99: 23–33.

26. Gunn MD, Tangemann K, Tam C, et al. A chemokine expressed in lymphoid high endothelial venules promotes the adhesion and chemotaxis of naive T lymphocytes. Proc Natl Acad Sci USA 1998; 95: 258–63.

27. Willimann K, Legler DF, Loetscher M, et al. The chemokine SLC is expressed in T cell areas of lymph nodes and mucosal lymphoid tissues and attracts activated T cells via CCR7. Eur J Immunol 1998; 28: 2025–34.

28. Okada T, Ngo VN, Ekland EH, et al. Chemokine requirements for B cell entry to lymph nodes and Peyer's patches. J Exp Med 2002; 196(1): 65–75.

29. Forster R, Mattis AE, Kremmer E, et al. A putative chemokine receptor, BLR1, directs B cell migration to defined lymphoid organs and specific anatomic compartments of the spleen. Cell 1996; 87: 1037–47.

30. Sallusto F, Lenig D, Forster R, Lipp M, Lanzavecchia A. Two subsets of memory T lymphocytes with distinct homing potentials and effector functions. Nature 1999; 401: 708–12.

31. Schaerli P, Willimann K, Lang AB, et al. CXC chemokine receptor 5 expression defines follicular homing T cells with B cell helper function. J Exp Med 2000; 192: 1553–62.

32. Campbell DJ, Butcher EC. Rapid acquisition of tissue-specific homing phenotypes by CD4(+) T cells activated in cutaneous or mucosal lymphoid tissues. J Exp Med 2002; 195: 135–41.

33. Mora JR, Bono MR, Manjunath N, et al. Selective imprinting of gut-homing T cells by Peyer's patch dendritic cells. Nature 2003; 424(6944): 88–93.

34. Campbell JJ Haraldsen G, Pan J, et al. The chemokine receptor CCR4 in vascular recognition by cutaneous but not intestinal memory T cells. Nature 1999; 400: 776–80.

35. Kunkel EJ, Boisvert J, Murphy K, et al. Expression of the chemokine receptors CCR4, CCR5, and CXCR3 by human tissue-infiltrating lymphocytes. Am J Pathol 2002; 160: 347–55.

36. Soler D, Humphreys TL, Spinola SM, Campbell JJ. CCR4 versus CCR10 in human cutaneous TH lymphocyte trafficking. Blood 2003; 101: 1677–82.

37. Zabel BA, Agace WW, Campbell JJ, et al. Human G protein-coupled receptor GPR-9-G/CC chemokine receptor 9 is selectively expressed on intestinal homing T lymphocytes, mucosal lymphocytes, and thymocytes and is required for thymus-expressed chemokine-mediated chemotaxis. J Exp Med 1999; 190: 1241–55.

38. Kunkel EJ, Campbell JJ, Haraldsen G, et al. Lymphocyte CC chemokine receptor 9 and epithelial thymus-expressed chemokine (TECK) expression distinguish the small intestinal immune compartment: epithelial expression of tissue-specific chemokines as an organizing principle in regional immunity. J Exp Med 2000; 192: 761–8.

39. Homey B, Alenius H, Muller A, et al. CCL27-CCR10 interactions regulate T cell-mediated skin inflammation. Nat Med 2002; 8: 157–65.

40. Svensson M, Marsal J, Ericsson A, et al. CCL25 mediates the localization of recently activated CD8alpha-beta(+) lymphocytes to the small-intestinal mucosa. J Clin Invest 2002; 110: 1113–21.

41. Bouma G, Strober W. The immunological and genetic basis of inflammatory bowel disease. Nat Rev Immunol 2003; 3(7): 521–33.

42. Lefrancois L, Parker CM, Olson S, et al. The role of beta7 integrins in CD8 T cell trafficking during an antiviral immune response. J Exp Med 1999; 189: 1631–8.

43. Hamann A, Andrew DP, Jablonski-Westrich D, Holzmann B, Butcher EC. Role of alpha 4-integrins in lymphocyte homing to mucosal tissues in vivo. J Immunol 1994; 152(7): 3282–93.

44. Haddad W, Cooper CJ, Zhang Z, et al. P-selectin and P-selectin glycoprotein ligand 1 are major determinants for Th1 cell recruitment to nonlymphoid effector sites in the intestinal lamina propria. J Exp Med 2003; 198: 369–77.

45. Johansson-Lindbom B, Svensson M Wurbel MA, et al. Selective generation of gut tropic T cells in gut-associated lymphoid tissue (GALT): requirement for GALT dendritic cells and adjuvant. J Exp Med 2003; 198: 963–9.

46. Lazarus NH, Kunkel EJ, Johnston B, et al. A common mucosal chemokine (mucosae-associated epithelial chemokine/CCL28) selectively attracts IgA plasmablasts. J Immunol 2003; 170: 3799–805.

47. Kunkel EJ, Kim CH, Lazarus NH, et al. CCR10 expression is a common feature of circulating and mucosal epithelial tissue IgA Ab-secreting cells. J Clin Invest 2003; 111: 1001–10.

48. Pan J, Kunkel EJ, Gosslar U, et al. A novel chemokine ligand for CCR10 and CCR3 expressed by epithelial cells in mucosal tissues. J Immunol 2000; 165(6): 2943–9.

49. Hieshima K, Kawasaki Y, Hanamoto H, et al. CC chemokine ligands 25 and 28 play essential roles in intestinal extravasation of IgA antibody-secreting cells. J Immunol 2004; 173: 3668–75.

50. Rankin SM, Conroy DM, Williams TJ. Eotaxin and eosinophil recruitment: implications for human disease. Mol Med Today 2000; 6(1): 20–7.

51. Palframan RT, Collins PD, Severs NJ, et al. Mechanisms of acute eosinophil mobilization from the bone marrow stimulated by interleukin 5: the role of specific adhesion molecules and phosphatidylinositol 3-kinase. J Exp Med 1998; 188: 1621–32.

52. Jose PJ, Griffiths-Johnson DA, Collins PD, et al. Eotaxin: a potent eosinophil chemoattractant cytokine detected in a guinea pig model of allergic airways inflammation. J Exp Med 1994; 179: 881–7.

53. Ponath PD, Qin SX, Ringler DJ, et al. Cloning of the human eosinophil chemoattractant, eotaxin–expression, receptor binding, and functional properties suggest a mechanism for the selective recruitment of eosinophils. J Clin Invest 1996; 97: 604–12.

54. Forssmann U, Uguccioni M, Loetscher P, et al. Eotaxin-2, a novel CC chemokine that is selective for

the chemokine receptor CCR3, and acts like eotaxin on human eosinophil and basophil leukocytes. J Exp Med 1997; 185: 2171–6.

55. Kitaura M, Suzuki N, Imai T, et al. Molecular cloning of a novel human CC chemokine (Eotaxin-3) that is a functional ligand of CC chemokine receptor 3. J Biol Chem 1999; 274: 27975–80.

56. Shinkai A, Yoshisue H, Koike M, et al. A novel human CC chemokine, eotaxin-3, which is expressed in IL-4-stimulated vascular endothelial cells, exhibits potent activity toward eosinophils. J Immunol 1999; 163: 1602–10.

57. Collins PD, Marleau S, Griffiths-Johnson DA, Jose PJ, Williams TJ. Cooperation between interleukin-5 and the chemokine eotaxin to induce eosinophil accumulation in vivo. J Exp Med 1995; 182: 1169–74.

58. Uguccioni M, Mackay CR, Ochensberger B, et al. High expression of the chemokine receptor CCR3 in human blood basophils. Role in activation by eotaxin, MCP-4, and other chemokines. J Clin Invest 1997; 100: 1137–43.

59. Gerber BO, Zanni MP, Uguccioni M, et al. Functional expression of the eotaxin receptor CCR3 in T lymphocytes co-localizing with eosinophils. Curr Biol 1997; 7: 836–43.

60. Sallusto F, Mackay CR, Lanzavecchia A. Selective expression of the eotaxin receptor CCR3 by human T helper 2 cells. Science 1997; 277: 2005–7.

61. Sozzani S, Allavena P, D'Amico G, et al. Differential regulation of chemokine receptors during dendritic cell maturation: a model for their trafficking properties. J Immunol 1998; 161: 1083–6.

62. Sallusto F, Schaerli P, Loetscher P, et al. Rapid and coordinated switch in chemokine receptor expression during dendritic cell maturation. Eur J Immunol 1998; 28: 2760–9.

63. Sallusto F, Palermo B, Lenig D, et al. Distinct patterns and kinetics of chemokine production regulate dendritic cell function. Eur J Immunol 1999; 29: 1617–25.

64. Saeki H, Moore AM, Brown MJ, Hwang ST. Secondary lymphoid-tissue chemokine (SLC) and CC chemokine receptor 7 (CCR7) participate in the emigration pathway of mature dendritic cells from the skin to regional lymph nodes. J Immunol 1999; 162: 2472–5.

65. Serra HM, Eberhard Y, Martin AP, et al. Secondary lymphoid tissue chemokine (CCL21) is upregulated in allergic contact dermatitis. Int Arch Allergy Immunol 2004; 133: 64–71.

66. Martin-Fontecha A, Sebastiani S, Hopken UE, et al. Regulation of dendritic cell migration to the draining lymph node: impact on T lymphocyte traffic and priming. J Exp Med 2003; 198: 615–21.

67. Arbones ML, Ord DC, Ley K, et al. Lymphocyte homing and leukocyte rolling and migration are impaired in L-selectin-deficient mice. Immunity 1994; 1: 247–60.

68. Von Andrian UH, Mempel TR. Homing and cellular traffic in lymph nodes. Nat Rev Immunol 2003; 3: 867–78.

69. Guarda G, Hons M, Soriano SF, et al. L-selectin-negative CCR7-effector and memory CD8+ T cells enter reactive lymph nodes and kill dendritic cells. Nat Immunol 2007; 8: 743–52.

70. Matloubian M, Lo CG, Cinamon G, et al. Lymphocyte egress from thymus and peripheral lymphoid organs is dependent on S1P receptor 1. Nature 2004; 427: 355–60.

71. Henning G, Ohl L, Junt T, et al. CC chemokine receptor 7-dependent and -independent pathways for lymphocyte homing: modulation by FTY720. J Exp Med 2001; 194: 1875–81.

72. Muller G, Reiterer P, Hopken UE, Golfier S, Lipp M. Role of homeostatic chemokine and sphingosine-1-phosphate receptors in the organization of lymphoid tissue. Ann N Y Acad Sci 2003; 987: 107–16.

73. Schwab SR, Cyster JG. Finding a way out: lymphocyte egress from lymphoid organs. Nat Immunol 2007; 8: 1295–301.

74. Willemze R, Jaffe ES, Burg G, et al. WHO-EORTC classification for cutaneous lymphomas. Blood 2005; 105: 3768–85.

75. Burg G, Kempf W, Cozzio A, et al. WHO/EORTC classification of cutaneous lymphomas 2005: histological and molecular aspects. J Cutan Pathol 2005; 32: 647–74.

76. Ferenczi K, Fuhlbrigge RC, Pinkus J, Pinkus GS, Kupper TS. Increased CCR4 expression in cutaneous T cell lymphoma. J Invest Dermatol 2002; 119: 1405–10.

77. Sarris AH, Esgleyes-Ribot T, Crow M, et al. Cytokine loops involving interferon-gamma and IP-10, a cytokine chemotactic for CD4+ lymphocytes: an explanation for the epidermotropism of cutaneous T-cell lymphoma. Blood 1995; 86: 651–8.

78. Yamaguchi T, Ohshima K, Tsuchiya T, et al. The comparison of expression of cutaneous lymphocyte-associated antigen (CLA), and Th1- and Th2-associated antigens in mycosis fungoides and cutaneous lesions of adult T-cell leukemia/lymphoma. Eur J Dermatol 2003; 13: 553–9.

79. Lu D, Duvic M, Medeiros LJ, et al. The T-cell chemokine receptor CXCR3 is expressed highly in low-grade mycosis fungoides. Am J Clin Pathol 2001; 115: 413–21.

80. Narducci MG, Scala E, Bresin A, et al. Skin homing of Sézary cells involves SDF-1-CXCR4 signaling and down-regulation of CD26/dipeptidylpeptidase IV. Blood 2006; 107: 1108–15.

81. Xu B, Wagner N, Pham LN, et al. Lymphocyte homing to bronchus-associated lymphoid tissue (BALT) is mediated by L-selectin/PNAd, alpha4beta1 integrin/VCAM-1, and LFA-1 adhesion pathways. J Exp Med 2003; 197: 1255–67.

82. Vermeer MH, Dukers DF, ten Berge RL, et al. Differential expression of thymus and activation regulated chemokine and its receptor CCR4 in nodal and cutaneous anaplastic large-cell lymphomas and Hodgkin's disease. Mod Pathol 2002; 15(8): 838–44.

83. Ishida T, Inagaki H, Utsunomiya A, et al. CXC chemokine receptor 3 and CC chemokine receptor

4 expression in T-cell and NK-cell lymphomas with special reference to clinicopathological significance for peripheral T-cell lymphoma, unspecified. Clin Cancer Res 2004; 10: 5494–500.

84. Jones D, O'Hara C, Kraus MD et al. Expression pattern of T-cell-associated chemokine receptors and their chemokines correlates with specific subtypes of T-cell non-Hodgkin lymphoma. Blood 2000; 96(2): 685–90.

85. Weng AP, Shahsafaei A, Dorfman DM. CXCR4/CD184 immunoreactivity in T-cell non-Hodgkin lymphomas with an overall Th1- Th2+ immunophenotype. Am J Clin Pathol 2003; 119: 424–30.

86. Kleinhans M, Tun-Kyi A, Gilliet M et al. Functional expression of the eotaxin receptor CCR3 in CD30+ cutaneous T-cell lymphoma. Blood 2003; 101(4): 1487–93.

87. Tsuchiya T, Ohshima K, Karube K et al. Th1, Th2, and activated T-cell marker and clinical prognosis in peripheral T-cell lymphoma, unspecified: comparison with AILD, ALCL, lymphoblastic lymphoma, and ATLL. Blood 2004; 103: 236–41.

88. Hasegawa H, Nomura T, Kohno M et al. Increased chemokine receptor CCR7/EBI1 expression enhances the infiltration of lymphoid organs by adult T-cell leukemia cells. Blood 2000; 95: 30–8.

89. Liu A, Nakatsuka S, Yang WI, Kojya S, Aozasa K. Expression of cell adhesion molecules and chemokine receptors: angioinvasiveness in nasal NK/T-cell lymphoma. Oncol Rep 2005; 13: 613–20.

90. Yagi H, Seo N, Ohshima A et al. Chemokine receptor expression in cutaneous T cell and NK/T-cell lymphomas: immunohistochemical staining and in vitro chemotactic assay. Am J Surg Pathol 2006; 30: 1111–19.

91. Yoshino T, Nakamura S, Suzumiya J et al. Expression of cutaneous lymphocyte antigen is associated with a poor outcome of nasal-type natural killer-cell lymphoma. Br J Haematol 2002; 118: 482–7.

92. Drillenburg P, Van der Voort R, Koopman G, et al. Preferential expression of the mucosal homing receptor integrin alpha 4 beta 7 in gastrointestinal non-Hodgkin's lymphomas. Am J Pathol 1997; 150: 919–27.

93. Mueller CG, Boix C, Kwan WH et al. Critical role of monocytes to support normal B cell and diffuse large B cell lymphoma survival and proliferation. J Leukoc Biol 2007; 82(3): 567–75.

94. Legler DF, Loetscher M, Roos RS et al. B cell-attracting chemokine 1, a human CXC chemokine expressed in lymphoid tissues, selectively attracts B lymphocytes via BLR1/CXCR5. J Exp Med 1998; 187: 655–60.

95. Mazzucchelli L, Blaser A, Kappeler A et al. BCA-1 is highly expressed in *Helicobacter pylori*-induced mucosa-associated lymphoid tissue and gastric lymphoma. J Clin Invest 1999; 104: R49–54.

96. Mori M, Manuelli C, Pimpinelli N et al. BCA-1, A B-cell chemoattractant signal, is constantly expressed in cutaneous lymphoproliferative B-cell disorders. Eur J Cancer 2003; 39: 1625–31.

97. Chan CC, Shen D, Hackett JJ, Buggage RR, Tuaillon N. Expression of chemokine receptors, CXCR4 and CXCR5, and chemokines, BLC and SDF-1, in the eyes of patients with primary intraocular lymphoma. Ophthalmology 2003; 110: 421–6.

98. Falkenhagen KM, Braziel RM, Fraunfelder FM, Smith JR. B-Cells in ocular adnexal lymphoproliferative lesions express B-cell attracting chemokine 1 (CXCL13). Am J Ophthalmol 2005; 140: 335–7.

99. Smith JR, Braziel RM, Paoletti S, et al. Expression of B-cell-attracting chemokine 1 (CXCL13) by malignant lymphocytes and vascular endothelium in primary central nervous system lymphoma. Blood 2003; 101: 815–21.

100. Fujii A, Ohshima K, Hamasaki M, et al. Differential expression of chemokines, chemokine receptors, cytokines and cytokine receptors in diffuse large B cell malignant lymphoma. Int J Oncol 2004; 24: 529–38.

101. Middleton J, Neil S, Wintle J, et al. Transcytosis and surface presentation of IL-8 ky venular endothelial cells. Cell 1997; 91: 385–95.

102. Smith JR, Falkenhagen KM, Coupland SE, et al. Malignant B cells from patients with primary central nervous system lymphoma express stromal cell-derived factor-1. Am J Clin Pathol 2007; 127: 633–41.

103. Jahnke K, Coupland SE, Na IK, et al. Expression of the chemokine receptors CXCR4, CXCR5, and CCR7 in primary central nervous system lymphoma. Blood 2005; 106: 384–5.

104. Brunn A, Montesinos-Rongen M, Strack A, et al. Expression pattern and cellular sources of chemokines in primary central nervous system lymphoma. Acta Neuropathol 2007; 114(3): 271–6.

Specific management problems posed by the primary extranodal presentations: Part I – staging and response evaluation

6

Richard W Tsang, Joseph M Connors, and Mary G Gospodarowicz

DEFINITION OF PRIMARY EXTRANODAL LYMPHOMA

Primary extranodal lymphomas are common, and account for approximately 20–45% of all non-Hodgkin's lymphomas (NHL).[1-6] The presenting sites are diverse and many have unique clinical and pathological characteristics, and distinct biological behavior, thereby requiring a different management approach as compared with nodal lymphomas of similar histology. The World Health Organization (WHO) classification[7] includes the following diagnoses where extranodal involvement is the salient feature: splenic marginal zone lymphoma, extranodal marginal zone lymphoma of mucosa-associated lymphoid tissue (MALT) type, primary mediastinal (thymic) large B-cell lymphoma, primary effusion lymphoma, and intravascular lymphoma. In addition, in case of T-cell lymphoma, enteropathy type T-cell lymphoma, extranodal natural killer (NK)/T-cell lymphoma of nasal type, hepatosplenic T-cell lymphoma, mycosis fungoides, primary cutaneous CD30+ T-cell lymphoma, and subcutaneous panniculitis-like T-cell lymphoma are included.

The primary extranodal lymphomas often present in a localized fashion (stage IE–IIE) and, therefore, traditionally, have involved the use of some form of local therapy, either surgery or radiation therapy.

Most clinicians consider the designation of primary extranodal lymphoma to be appropriate, as defined by Dawson et al, who, in the context of gastrointestinal lymphoma, proposed that a patient must present with disease principally affecting an extranodal site, may only have regional lymph node involvement, with no distant peripheral lymph node involvement, and no liver or spleen involvement.[8] Others later proposed that these criteria be relaxed to allow for contiguous involvement of organs such as the liver and spleen, and allowed for distant nodal disease providing that the extranodal lesion was the presenting site and constituted the predominant disease bulk.[9] However, most clinicians consider such patients, especially those presenting with aggressive histology lymphoma, clearly to have stage IV disease and would not consider them as having primary extranodal presentations, especially if there are multiple extranodal sites of involvement; but, rather, advanced stage disease with extranodal involvement. The prognosis of patients with extranodal involvement as part of disseminated lymphoma is worse, particularly if more than one extranodal site is involved by disease, as supported by the International Prognostic Index (IPI) data.[10] However, patients with MALT lymphoma, by definition, have extranodal involvement, and disseminated disease does not necessarily imply a short survival.[11] This special topic will be discussed elsewhere in this book.

STAGING OF PRIMARY EXTRANODAL LYMPHOMA

The AJCC (American Joint Committee on Cancer) and UICC (International Union Against Cancer) have endorsed the use of the Ann Arbor classification for staging of NHL. The Ann Arbor staging classification originally created for Hodgkin's lymphoma, has been used for the NHL as well for over 40 years.[12,13] In the Ann Arbor system, Waldeyer's ring, thymus, spleen, appendix, and Peyer's patches of the small intestine are considered to be lymphatic tissues, and involvement of these areas does not constitute an 'E' lesion, originally defined as extralymphatic involvement. However, because of the unique pathological and clinical characteristics of primary lymphoma affecting extranodal sites, most clinicians consider them as special entities and report their involvement as an extranodal presentation, with the possible exception of the spleen. The Ann Arbor classification differentiates locoregional from widespread lymphoma and documents overall anatomical extent of disease and B-symptoms, but it is not optimal for describing the extent of local disease, invasion of adjacent organs, tumor bulk, or multiple sites of involvement within one organ: e.g. skin, or gastrointestinal tract. Several modifications to the Ann Arbor classification have been proposed in the past. In head and neck lymphoma, the size of the primary tumor has been classified according to the TNM classification for squamous cell carcinoma of that region.[14] In gastric lymphoma, substaging of stage I to reflect the depth of the stomach wall penetration has been suggested. These proposals reflect local tumor bulk and/or invasiveness but do not add substantially to the overall value of staging classification. Therefore these systems are seen to complicate matters unnecessarily and have not received widespread adoption for clinical use. For gastric lymphoma, in stage II disease, distinction of involvement of the immediate nodal region (II_1) vs more extensive regional lymph node involvement (II_2) has been found to be of prognostic significance.[1,15]

There is also difficulty with how an 'extranodal organ' is defined in assigning the stage. For example, the Waldeyer's ring structures consist of the tonsils in the lateral oropharyngeal wall (palatine tonsils), the nasopharyngeal lymphatic tissue, and the lingual tonsil. Therefore, involvement of both the nasopharynx and the palatine tonsil is still considered as stage IE. A problem arises also with the paired organs: for example, the parotid glands, or orbital adnexal tissue. Lymphoma involving bilateral orbital adnexa has been considered as stage IE, similar to the bilateral parotid gland involvement. Other areas of involvement, such as multiple lesions in the skin, raise additional difficulty. On the one hand, most clinicians consider a cluster of skin lesions within a well-defined area (e.g. part of an extremity) to be stage IE, whereas for widely separated cutaneous lesions, even when the disease is still confined to the skin, most would assign stage IV. On the other hand, even closely contiguous separate lesions in the liver are always considered stage IV disease. How far apart lesions have to be before one classifies them as stage IV rather than stage I, and why different rules apply to different organs, remain unresolved at present. Multiple lung lesions are in the same difficult category and pose the complexity added by bilaterality. The Ann Arbor classification originally regarded multiple nodules in the lung as localized extralymphatic disease, provided that it was limited to one lobe.[16] Do these distinctions matter biologically and prognostically? Obviously, they do if one wishes to compare results of clinical trials or series between different centers, and for eligibility considerations for clinical trials. Some clinicians use an 'operational' definition of assessing the ability to encompass the disease within acceptable radiation fields, therefore defining cases treatable with localized radiation as stage IE. This is obvious in some cases but in general is an unsatisfactory approach, particularly with changing radiation therapy practice.

In general, there are some organs and tissues where the occurrence of multiple distinct lesions is commonly assigned the Ann Arbor stage IV. Examples include diffuse lung involvement, diffuse gastrointestinal tract involvement, or leptomeningeal disease. Where there is difficulty, the principle of distinguishing stage IE and stage IV should be based on the most plausible route of spread: for contiguous extensions of disease, use stage I/II E, and for hematogenous spread, assign stage IV. Such an approach is usually helpful: for example, justifying the assignment of stage IE to a closely clustered set of skin nodules, but stage IV for widely separated nodules, or stage IE for a nodule in one kidney, but stage IV for a nodule in each kidney, and so on. A similar approach is helpful to distinguish differing types of associated nodal involvement. Thus, a bone lesion in the proximal humerus with closeby ipsilateral axillary nodal involvement is stage IIE disease, but the same bone lesion with mediastinal and retroperitoneal nodal involvement is stage IV disease.

CLINICAL ASSESSMENT OF SPECIFIC EXTRANODAL SITES

There are specific anatomical, histological, and phenotypical patterns of disease that are consistently observed in the primary extranodal lymphomas. There are also associated or predisposing conditions which are characteristic for certain extranodal lymphomas. Examples are infectious agents or autoimmune diseases in certain marginal zone lymphomas of the extranodal type (*Helicobacter pylori* in gastric MALT lymphoma, and Sjögren's syndrome in salivary gland MALT lymphomas). Lymphomas arising in the context of immunodeficiency, including human immunodeficiency virus (HIV) infection, are often extranodal. Examples include primary effusion lymphoma (related to the human herpes virus 8) and plasmablastic lymphoma of the oral cavity (related to the Epstein–Barr virus). Diffuse large B-cell lymphomas arising in immunodeficient individuals also tend to involve extranodal organs such as the brain and the gastrointestinal tract.

In terms of histological correlations with specific extranodal sites, one of the commonest extranodal lymphomas is skin lymphoma, with the majority being T-cell in origin.[4] Within the dermatotropic T-cell lymphomas are diseases such as mycosis fungoides, primary cutaneous anaplastic large cell lymphoma, and other rare types with unique clinical features. Most common among the B-cell lymphomas are gastric lymphoma, Waldeyer's ring lymphoma (tonsil lymphoma being most frequent),[5] and others less frequent sites. Whereas some lymphomas commonly spread to lymph nodes, e.g. Waldeyer's ring, others such as brain or orbital adnexal lymphoma almost never do. Some histological types are associated with certain extranodal tissues: extranodal NK/T-cell lymphoma of nasal type, Burkitt's lymphoma in the mandible, or terminal ileum/ovary, mantle cell lymphoma disseminating to the gastrointestinal tract (colonic polyposis). In addition, some entities have geographic or ethnic predisposition, such as extranodal NK/T-cell lymphoma of nasal type in individuals of eastern Asian derivation or endemic Burkitt's lymphoma in equatorial Africa. Other unusual anatomical associations include predisposing sites of spread, e.g. testis lymphoma and relapse in the central nervous system. Some extranodal lymphomas have distinct prognosis by virtue of the site of diagnosis or histology, with traditional prognostic factors having a secondary or minimal impact. Examples of this include stage IE primary diffuse large B-cell lymphoma of the brain, or testis, and stage IE extranodal NK/T-cell lymphoma of nasal type, all carrying a poor prognosis despite the absence of initial evidence of dissemination or association with the adverse features such as those used in the IPI.

Given these various unusual characteristics, the clinical assessment and management of the extranodal lymphomas must be individualized, taking account of the clinical context, appropriate work-up, and management of the associated conditions (e.g. HIV infection) and including special investigations in addition to the standard work-up for nodal lymphoma (Table 6.1). Examples of these additional investigations include:

- endoscopy for upper aerodigestive lesions, i.e. nasopharynx, tonsil
- endoscopy (with or without ultrasound) and bowel series for stomach or gastro-intestinal lymphomas
- magnetic resonance imaging (MRI) and nuclear bone scan for bone lymphoma
- MRI for central nervous system (CNS), head and neck, and paraspinal lesions
- slit lamp eye examination for CNS lymphomas.

Surgical management may become necessary for airway compromise (e.g. temporary tracheostomy for bulky thyroid lymphoma), or rapidly progressive spinal cord compression.

RESPONSE ASSESSMENT

The investigations that revealed lymphoma-associated abnormalities during initial staging should be repeated after treatment to document response (see Table 6.1). It is common to find residual abnormalities in some extranodal sites, particularly if the initial disease was bulky. This includes primary mediastinal (thymic) lymphoma and bone lymphoma, among other sites. The original National Cancer Institute sponsored International Workshop on response criteria[17] included the category of complete remission unconfirmed/ uncertain (CRu), to describe circumstances in which a patient has no clinical evidence of lymphoma, but some residual imaging abnormality, persisting at a site of previous disease. Further investigation of residual computed tomography (CT) abnormalities in order to distinguish persistent disease from residual scar tissue is done only if further treatment is being considered. Whole-body FDG-PET (positron emission tomography with [18F]-fluoro-2-deoxy-D-glucose) is a useful tool in evaluating disease regression, and has been incorporated in the revised response criteria for malignant lymphoma summarized by the International Harmonization Project.[18] The former CRu category is no longer recognized, and cases with residual mass lesions are classified into complete response (CR) if the FDG-PET is

negative and partial response (PR) if the FDG PET is positive.[18] FDG-PET is especially useful in the group of patients who would have been assigned PR status, using the original International Workshop Criteria,[15] While FDG-PET negativity allows assignment of CR status and implies a prognosis similar to CR patients.[19] Guidelines on the performance and proper interpretation of FDG-PET scans for lymphoma response assessment have also been published as part of the same project.[19] Whereas a negative post-treatment FDG-PET is strongly predictive, great care is required to use and incorporate positive FDG-PET information in decision making, because false-positive FDG-PET scans are common in lymphoma patients, observed in up to 23% of positive scans in one review of 706 patients.[20] The most common false-positive conditions are brown fat uptake, thymic rebound, muscle contraction, and non-specific inflammation in mediastinum, lymph nodes, mucosa, or bowel.[20] Radiation pneumonitis may also lead to abnormalities on FDG-PET following mediastinal radiation therepy (RT).[21,22] To avoid false positives, some clinicians recommend that FDG-PET re-evaluation should be delayed until 2–3 months following completion of mediastinal RT.[19,21–23] Re-biopsy may be warranted to evaluate persistent FDG-PET and/ or CT imaging abnormalities, depending on the degree of suspicion, the morbidity of biopsy, and whether salvage treatment will significantly alter outcome.

EVOLVING ROLE OF FDG-PET AND ITS CAVEATS

The intensity of FDG uptake, as reflected in the standardized uptake values (SUV), for indolent lymphomas is generally lower than that of aggressive histology lymphomas, or relapsed disease.[24] However, there is no cut-off value that will reliably distinguish the two groups of lymphomas. T-cell lymphomas have a lower probability of FDG avidity, particularly for lesions of the skin, where the positivity rate is only 50% for tumorous lesions.[25] Marginal zone lymphomas of MALT type also have a lower likelihood of FDG avidity, approximately 80%,[26,27]

Table 6.1 Primary extranodal lymphoma – clinical characteristics

Site	Histology	Frequency	Age	Additional investigations
Gastrointestinal				
Stomach	MALT	50–60%	Older	Endoscopy, *H. pylori*
Stomach	Large B-cell	20%	Older	Endoscopy
IPSID	MALT	<5%	Young adult	Endoscopy
Intestinal	B-cell	10%	Older	Small bowel series
Intestinal	T-cell	<5%	Young adult	Small bowel series
Waldeyer's ring				
Tonsil	Large B-cell	70–80%	Older	Endoscopy, MRI
Nasopharynx	B-cell	20%	Older	Endoscopy, MRI
Tongue, oropharynx	B-cell	10%	Older	Endoscopy, MRI
Paranasal sinuses and nasal cavities				
Maxillary sinus	Large B-cell	80%	Older	MRI, CSF cytology
Nasal cavity	T-cell	<10%	Middle	MRI
Other sinuses	B-cell	Rare	Older	MRI, CSF cytology
Salivary gland				
Parotid	MALT	80%	Older	Rheumatic serology
Thyroid	MALT	50%	Older	
	Large B-cell	50%	Older	
Orbital				
Conjunctiva	MALT	50–70%	Older	MRI, *Chlamydia*
Orbit	MALT	20%	Older	MRI
Orbit	Large B-cell	Rare	Older	MRI
Lung	BALT	50–70%	Older	Bronchoscopy
	Large B-cell	10–20%	Older	
	T-cell	<5%		
Breast	MALT	70–80%	Older	MRI, mammography
	Large B-cell	10–15%	Young, pregnant	
Bone	Large B-cell	80–90%	Middle	MRI, bone scan
Extradural	Large B-cell	90%	Middle	MRI, CSF cytology
Genitourinary				
Testis	Large B-cell	80–90%	Older	CSF cytology
Bladder	MALT	<5%	Older	Cystoscopy
Prostate	Large cell	Very rare		
Central nervous system				
Brain	Large B-cell	90%	Middle	MRI, CSF cytology
Ocular, meningeal, spinal		Very rare		Slit lamp eye exam lumbar puncture
Skin	B-cell	20–30%	Older	
	T-cell CD30−ve		Older	
	ALCL CD30+ve		Middle/older	

MALT, mucosa-associated lymphoid tissue; BALT, bronchus-associated lymphoid tissue; MRI, magnetic resonance imaging; CSF, cerebrospinal fluid; IPSID, immunoproliferative small intestinal disease; ALCL, anaplastic large cell lymphoma.

especially in the stomach, or with early-stage disease.[28] It must also be emphasized that an FDG-PET negative scenario does not imply the absence of microscopic disease. In primary cases treated with chemotherapy, achieving an FDG-PET-negative CR implies a good prognosis, but, although the risk of recurrence is low (10–25%), it is not negligible.[29,30] There is emerging literature that an FDG-PET scan after a limited number (1–4) of cycles of chemotherapy is predictive of excellent disease control when the same chemotherapy is being continued,[31–35] raising the future prospects of treatment adaptation by completing planned treatment for FDG-PET negative cases and switching to an alternate treatment incorporating intensification approaches for the FDG-PET-positive patients. Similarly, FDG-PET scans performed following salvage chemotherapy, before autologous hematopoietic stem cell transplantation (ASCT), is also prognostic. Schot et al studied 46 patients following two courses of salvage chemotherapy with DHAP-VIM.[36] A negative PET-FDG was observed in 15 patients (33%), and with subsequent ASCT, their 2-year PFS was 62%, compared with 32% for FDG-PET-positive patients.[36] Similar results were obtained by other investigators,[37–39] indicating a high specificity (positive FDG-PET reliably predicts presence of persistent disease that will not be cured by the high-dose chemotherapy and ASCT), but only moderate sensitivity (negative FDG-PET results are still followed by failure rates of 12–38%) for FDG-PET scans performed just prior to ASCT. Therefore, if there is an indication to give local radiation therapy to enhance local control because of initially bulky disease, or significant residual mass following salvage chemotherapy, it should still be considered despite a negative FDG-PET scan.

SUMMARY

The principles behind proper staging of extranodal lymphoma can be straightforwardly summarized. In addition to the standard tests employed with all lymphomas, including history, physical examination, total body CT, screening blood tests of bone marrow, liver, and renal function, protein electrophoresis, and unilateral bone marrow biopsy, special tests are appropriate, depending on initial site of presentation and type of lymphoma, as described in Table 6.1 (last column). Distinction between an E lesion (stage IE or IIE) and stage IV disease can be made by considering the most likely mode of spread. Lesions best understood as having spread hematogenously (e.g. bilateral disease in paired organs or nodal involvement on both sides of the diaphragm in addition to the extranodal site) should be considered stage IV. Lesions such as a localized cluster of skin nodules or nodal plus extranodal involvement in close proximity reflecting typical lymphatic flow (e.g. a thyroid mass with ipsilateral nodal involvement) should be considered stage IE (disease confined to a single extranodal site) or stage IIE (disease confined to locally confined nodal and extranodal tissue). By convention, some sites of involvement such as the bone marrow or liver are always considered stage IV even when involvement can only be demonstrated to be local. Finally, post-treatment assessment of response requires repetition of all tests initially abnormal due to lymphoma, applying the rules described in the recent response assessment harmonization publications.[18,19] FDG-PET scanning can be particularly helpful in the assessment of residual masses still evident by CT or MRI scanning.

REFERENCES

1. d'Amore F, Brincker M, Gronbaek K, et al. Non-Hodgkin's lymphoma of the gastrointestinal tract: a population-based analysis of incidence, geographic distribution, clinicopathologic presentation features, and prognosis. J Clin Oncol 1994; 12: 1673–84.
2. Economopoulos T, Asprou N, Stathakis N, et al. Primary extranodal non-Hodgkin's lymphoma in adults: clinicopathological and survival characteristics. Leuk Lymphoma 1996; 21: 131–6.
3. Newton R, Ferlay J, Beral V, et al. The epidemiology of non-Hodgkin's lymphoma: comparison of nodal and extra-nodal sites. Int J Cancer 1997; 72: 923–30.
4. Groves FD, Linet MS, Travis LB, et al. Cancer surveillance series: non-Hodgkin's lymphoma incidence by histologic subtype in the United States from 1978 through 1995. J Natl Cancer Inst 2000; 92: 1240–51.

5. Lopez-Guillermo A, Colomo L, Jimenez M, et al. Diffuse large B-cell lymphoma: clinicobiological characterization and outcome according to the nodal or extranodal primary origin. J Clin Oncol 2005.

6. Muller AM, Ihorst G, Mertelsmann R, et al. Epidemiology of non-Hodgkin's lymphoma (NHL): trends, geographic distribution, and etiology. Ann Hematol 2005; 84: 1–12.

7. Jaffe ES, Harris NL, Stein H, et al. Pathology and genetics of tumours of haematopoietic and lymphoid tissues. In: Kleihues P, Sobin LH, eds. World Health Organization Classification of Tumours. Lyon, France: IARC Press, 2001.

8. Dawson I, Cornes J, Morson B. Primary malignant lymphoid tumours of the intestinal tract: report of 37 cases with a study of factors influencing prognosis. Br J Surg 1961; 49: 80–9.

9. Lewin K, Ranchod M, Dorfman R. Lymphomas of the gasatrointestinal tract: a study of 117 cases presenting with gastrointestinal disease. Cancer 1978; 42: 693–707.

10. The International non-Hodgkin's Lymphoma Prognostic Factors Project. A predictive model for aggressive Non-Hodgkin's lymphoma. N Engl J Med 1993; 329: 987–94.

11. Zucca E, Conconi A, Pedrinis E, et al. International Extranodal Lymphoma Study Group. Nongastric marginal zone B-cell lymphoma of mucosa-associated lymphoid tissue. Blood 2003; 101(7): 2489–95.

12. UICC. TNM Classification of Malignant Tumours, 6th edn. New York: John Wiley & Sons, 2002.

13. Fleming ID, Cooper JS, Henson DE, et al. AJCC Cancer Staging Manual, 5th edn. Philadelphia: Lippincott-Raven, 1997.

14. Logsdon MD, Ha CS, Kavadi VS, et al. Lymphoma of the nasal cavity and paranasal sinuses: improved outcome and altered prognostic factors with combined modality therapy. Cancer 1997; 80: 477–88.

15. Rohatiner A, d'Amore F, Coiffier B, et al. Report on a workshop convened to discuss the pathological and staging classifications of gastrointestinal tract lymphoma. Ann Oncol 1994; 5: 397–400.

16. Carbone PP, Kaplan HS, Musshoff K, et al. Report of the Committee on Hodgkin's Disease Staging Classification. Cancer Res 1971; 31: 1860–1.

17. Cheson BD, Horning SJ, Coiffier B, et al. Report of an international workshop to standardize response criteria for non-Hodgkin's lymphomas. J Clin Oncol 1999; 17: 1244–53.

18. Cheson BD, Pfistner B, Juweid ME, et al. Revised response criteria for malignant lymphoma. J Clin Oncol 2007; 25: 579–86.

19. Juweid ME, Stroobants S, Hoekstra OS, et al. Use of positron emission tomography for response assessment of lymphoma: consensus of the Imaging Subcommittee of International Harmonization Project in Lymphoma. J Clin Oncol 2007; 25: 571–8.

20. Castellucci P, Nanni C, Farsad M, et al. Potential pitfalls of 18F–FDG PET in a large series of patients treated for malignant lymphoma: prevalence and scan interpretation. Nucl Med Commun 2005; 26: 689–94.

21. Jerusalem G, Hustinx R, Beguin Y, et al. Positron emission tomography imaging for lymphoma. Curr Opin Oncol 2005; 17: 441–5.

22. Kazama T, Faria SC, Varavithya V, et al. FDG PET in the evaluation of treatment for lymphoma: clinical usefulness and pitfalls. Radiographics 2005; 25: 191–207.

23. Castellucci P, Zinzani P, Nanni C, et al. 18F-FDG PET early after radiotherapy in lymphoma patients. Cancer Biother Radiopharm 2004; 19: 606–12.

24. Schoder H, Noy A, Gonen M, et al. Intensity of 18fluorodeoxyglucose uptake in positron emission tomography distinguishes between indolent and aggressive non-Hodgkin's lymphoma. J Clin Oncol 2005; 23: 4643–51.

25. Kako S, Izutsu K, Ota Y, et al. FDG-PET in T-cell and NK-cell neoplasms. Ann Oncol 2007; 18: 1685–90.

26. Beal KP, Yeung HW, Yahalom J. FDG-PET scanning for detection and staging of extranodal marginal zone lymphomas of the MALT type: a report of 42 cases. Ann Oncol 2005; 16: 473–80.

27. Alinari L, Castellucci P, Elstrom R, et al. 18F-FDG PET in mucosa-associated lymphoid tissue (MALT) lymphoma. Leuk Lymphoma 2006; 47: 2096–101.

28. Perry C, Herishanu Y, Metzer U, et al. Diagnostic accuracy of PET/CT in patients with extranodal marginal zone MALT lymphoma. Eur J Haematol 2007; 79: 205–9.

29. Lavely WC, Delbeke D, Greer JP, et al. FDG PET in the follow-up management of patients with newly diagnosed Hodgkin and non-Hodgkin lymphoma after first-line chemotherapy. Int J Radiat Oncol Biol Phys 2003; 57: 307–15.

30. Juweid ME, Wiseman GA, Vose JM, et al. Response assessment of aggressive non-Hodgkin's lymphoma by integrated International Workshop Criteria and fluorine-18-fluorodeoxyglucose positron emission tomography. J Clin Oncol 2005; 23: 4652–61.

31. Mikhaeel NG, Timothy AR, O'Doherty MJ, et al. 18-FDG-PET as a prognostic indicator in the treatment of aggressive Non-Hodgkin's Lymphoma – comparison with CT. Leuk Lymphoma 2000; 39: 543–53.

32. Spaepen K, Stroobants S, Dupont P, et al. Early restaging positron emission tomography with (18)F-fluorodeoxyglucose predicts outcome in patients with aggressive non-Hodgkin's lymphoma. Ann Oncol 2002; 13: 1356–63.

33. Kostakoglu L, Coleman M, Leonard JP, et al. PET predicts prognosis after 1 cycle of chemotherapy in aggressive lymphoma and Hodgkin's disease. J Nucl Med 2002; 43: 1018–27.

34. Haioun C, Itti E, Rahmouni A, et al. [18F]fluoro-2-deoxy-D-glucose positron emission tomography (FDG-PET) in aggressive lymphoma: an early prognostic tool for predicting patient outcome. Blood 2005; 106: 1376–81.

35. Fruchart C, Reman O, Le Stang N, et al. Prognostic value of early 18 fluorodeoxyglucose positron emission tomography and gallium-67 scintigraphy in aggressive lymphoma: a prospective comparative study. Leuk Lymphoma 2006; 47: 2547–57.

36. Schot B, van Imhoff G, Pruim J, et al. Predictive value of early 18F-fluoro-deoxyglucose positron emission tomography in chemosensitive relapsed lymphoma. Br J Haematol 2003; 123: 282–7.

37. Spaepen K, Stroobants S, Dupont P, et al. Prognostic value of pretransplantation positron emission tomography using fluorine 18-fluorodeoxyglucose in patients with aggressive lymphoma treated with high-dose chemotherapy and stem cell transplantation. Blood 2003; 102: 53–9.

38. Filmont JE, Czernin J, Yap C, et al. Value of F-18 fluorodeoxyglucose positron emission tomography for predicting the clinical outcome of patients with aggressive lymphoma prior to and after autologous stem-cell transplantation. Chest 2003; 124: 608–13.

39. Cremerius U, Fabry U, Wildberger JE, et al. Pretransplant positron emission tomography (PET) using fluorine-18-fluoro-deoxyglucose (FDG) predicts outcome in patients treated with high-dose chemotherapy and autologous stem cell transplantation for non-Hodgkin's lymphoma. Bone Marrow Transplant 2002; 30: 103–11.

7

Specific management problems posed by the primary extranodal presentations: Part II – local control of localized disease

Mary G Gospodarowicz, Richard W Tsang, and Joseph M Connors

INTRODUCTION

Primary extranodal lymphomas are a group of very diverse but very interesting presentations of malignant lymphoma. Although the majority of lymphomas present in lymph nodes, primary extranodal presentations represent approximately 20–45% of new cases.[1,2] There is considerable controversy about the appropriate definition of primary extranodal lymphoma when stage III or IV disease is present; therefore, most authors confine the term 'primary extranodal lymphoma' to patients who present with stage I and II disease.[2]

PATTERN OF PRESENTATION

Of those who have stage I–II at diagnosis, approximately 50% have extranodal disease at presentation.[2] Almost all the organs in the body have been reported as presenting sites of primary extranodal lymphoma. The common sites include skin, stomach, Waldeyer's ring structures including tonsil, nasopharynx and oropharynx, and small bowel.[2-6] The less common, but not infrequent, presenting sites are bone, orbital adnexae, thyroid gland, brain, paranasal sinuses, and testis.[2,3,7-16] The uncommon presentations include breast, lung, female genital tract, urinary bladder, and extradural soft tissue.[17-21] The very rare presentations include dura, heart, pleura, and intravascular lymphoma.[22-25]

Although the specific pathological entities represent the full spectrum of the World Health Organization (WHO) classification, the majority of patients with extranodal lymphomas present with diffuse large B-cell lymphoma. In contrast, follicular lymphomas, a very common form of non-Hodgkin's lymphoma (20–30% of all cases), infrequently present in extranodal sites (9%), other than the bone marrow.[1] In addition to diffuse large B-cell lymphoma, a number of very specific disease entities affect extranodal sites. They fall into two distinct groups. The first group, indolent lymphomas, include marginal zone lymphomas of extranodal type, also called the mucosa-associated lymphoid tissue (MALT) lymphomas and the small cell cutaneous lymphomas of both B-cell and T-cell type.[6,26,27] The second group, aggressive lymphomas, include rare but very important entities of nasal type natural killer (NK)/T-cell lymphoma, and the enteropathy-associated intestinal lymphoma.[28-30]

A knowledge of the patterns of spread and typical outcomes using modern treatment techniques for primary extranodal lymphomas is important for the appropriate decision making. In patients with aggressive lymphomas, complete response and local control are the most important goals of treatment. Whereas chemotherapy has a high likelihood of eradicating systemic microscopic disease, local extranodal disease is best controlled with the addition of some form of local therapy. Treatment failure carries a very high risk of death. By contrast, for patients with indolent extranodal lymphomas who may survive for decades, it is important to minimize treatment-related morbidity.

MANAGEMENT

The natural history of a disease and its management are related to the histological type and to the presenting site. Since a number of histopathological entities have only been recognized in the last 15 years, and since these new entities are rare, large case series of uniformly treated patients with long-term outcomes are largely unavailable.[31,32] The approach to the management of primary extranodal lymphomas is based on the principles that govern the approach to nodal lymphomas. The most important factors are the histological type and the anatomical disease extent (Table 7.1). Because localized disease (stage IE–IIE) is an important part of the spectrum of presentation of extranodal lymphomas, the issue of local control is very important since it represents a cure in a number of disease entities.[2,33–35] As such, it is particularly important in the scenarios where systemic chemotherapy does not offer a curative potential or where cure with systemic therapy is rare.

Recent progress in defining the etiological agents in MALT lymphoma has opened the door to new therapeutic interventions that address the source of antigenic stimulation. Attempts to extend the success in eradicating gastric low-grade MALT lymphoma with antibiotics to the management of conjunctival MALT lymphoma[36,37] has met with some success. It is expected that such approaches may be extended to the other MALT presentations as additional etiological organisms are discovered.

The management of localized marginal zone primary extranodal lymphomas is usually with involved field radiation therapy.[10,16,26,38,39] Doses in the range of 25–30 Gy result in local control rates approaching 100%. The most reported experience is with antibiotic refractory gastric MALT lymphoma, MALT lymphoma of orbital adnexae, thyroid, and other stage IE MALT lymphomas. In gastric and thyroid MALT lymphoma, relapse is very rare.[26] In the other sites, approximately 30–40% of patients develop recurrent disease in distant non-irradiated sites.

Single alkylating agent chemotherapy and rituximab therapy are also effective in producing regression in indolent B-cell extranodal lymphomas, but are less likely to achieve durable local control. Since the management of localized presentation usually involves radiation therapy, large series with long-term outcomes will be needed to evaluate the ability of systemic treatments to produce durable local disease control. Given the rarity of each specific site of MALT lymphomas, long-term data are not available for many of the disease entities.

As in nodal counterparts, the patients who present with diffuse large B-cell lymphoma are managed with R-CHOP (CHOP regimen + rituximab) chemotherapy, usually followed by involved field radiation to secure local disease control.[40] The role of involved field radiation is controversial in patients who receive full-course (i.e. six courses of) R-CHOP chemotherapy. To date, there are no randomized trials to guide practice in the era of R-CHOP chemotherapy. It is known that low-risk presentations of diffuse large cell lymphoma can be successfully treated with 3 cycles of R-CHOP and involved field radiation therapy.[33] It is also accepted that adjuvant moderate-dose radiation therapy of about 30–35 Gy results in almost universal local control, especially in patients with chemotherapy-responsive diffuse large B-cell lymphoma. In patients who have partial response to R-CHOP chemotherapy, local control can still be obtained with the addition of radiation therapy (40 Gy).[34] Such patients can be cured with standard-dose chemotherapy (CHOP × 8) alone but 6-year failure-free survival is lower (56% in the E1484 trial of the ECOG). Furthermore, for those with lymphoma progression after chemotherapy alone, the local control rate was only 52% (15 local failures in 31 patients).[34] By contrast, the use of radiotherapy with 30 Gy results in a lower overall failure rate, and the local control rate of 82%.[34]

Generally, surgery is not part of the management of non-Hodgkin's lymphomas, other than to establish the diagnosis. However, there are specific management circumstances where surgery is of benefit. It is of benefit in presentations with impending airway obstruction which may need airway preservation with tracheostomy, spinal cord compression requiring laminectomy, and splenic mass or primary splenic lymphoma, which may benefit from a splenectomy. Orchiectomy is both a diagnostic and therapeutic procedure in primary testicular lymphoma. Patients who present with bone fracture may require surgical stabilization. Although surgical management is frequently a supportive measure, it may also be therapeutic, as in primary testicular and primary splenic lymphoma. For MALT lymphomas, surgery also plays a role in primary presentations in the lung and skin where complete excision may be possible. Resection may also be helpful as part of the combined modality therapy of intestinal lymphoma, testicular lymphoma, and other sites. However, overtly aggressive surgery should be avoided because it may compromise cosmesis (mastectomy, parotidectomy) or function (gastrectomy, cystectomy) and is, therefore, not recommended as a combination of chemotherapy and radiotherapy is very effective in securing local disease control.

The role of radiotherapy in the management of primary extranodal lymphoma has changed from that of sole curative therapy, defined by the body region, to a precision radiotherapy management where modern techniques such as 3D conformal radiotherapy and intensity-modulated radiation therapy (IMRT) offer unprecedented opportunity for normal tissue sparing while achieving a high level of local control of the disease.[41–43] The sparing of the organ at risk is often more difficult in patients who present with primary extranodal lymphomas than nodal lymphomas, as the extranodal site may be in proximity to critical organs. For example, radiotherapy of the head and neck region may compromise salivary gland function or vision. In lymphomas of the Waldeyer's ring, the current approaches with IMRT can both routinely identify and spare the parotid gland, resulting in dose exposure of one-third to one-half of the prescribed dose of 30–40 Gy, and thereby significantly reducing the incidence and severity of xerostomia. Treatment of the lung must respect lung tolerance to radiotherapy, particularly if the lesion is large. The limited tolerance of lung limits the applicability of radiotherapy to relatively small lesions, as tissue exposed to a dose of ≥30 Gy will likely be permanently fibrosed on computed tomography (CT) scan. Treatment of the abdomen must ensure the protection of the heart, lungs, and kidneys, which are the main radiosensitive organs, as well as the small bowel. Even though traditional dose constraints for the normal organs are always respected, the principles in radiotherapy planning is to achieve dose exposure to as low as reasonably achievable (ALARA principle). The current practice utilizes high-precision technologies and, additionally, where appropriate, techniques to deal with respiratory motion, such as 4D CT and/or respiratory gating, in order to arrive at appropriate margins.

In the case of stage III or IV presentations, primary treatment is chemotherapy and there is no role for the routine use of adjuvant radiation therapy. An exception to the rule is the role of adjuvant scrotal radiotherapy in testicular lymphoma.[9] It is important to note that the scrotal radiotherapy in testis lymphoma is not aimed at improving the control or cure of disease evident at presentation, but rather to prevent new lymphoma developing in the other testicle, presumably from dormant tumor stem cells remaining after chemotherapy in a sanctuary site. In such scenario, low-dose (25–30 Gy) adjuvant scrotal radiotherapy is very effective in preventing relapse in the contralateral testis.[9]

The issue of a sanctuary site is also relevant to another presentation. In a similar but quite distinct scenario, extranodal lymphomas presenting in parameningeal sites require additional treatment. It has been observed that lymphomas presenting in paranasal sinuses and nasopharynx are associated with a significant risk of isolated central nervous system (CNS) relapse (usually meningeal).[9,15] The hypothesis is similar to that above: i.e. residual microscopic disease may be present in the CNS (sanctuary site) after the successful management of the presenting disease. In such cases, CNS prophylaxis with intrathecal chemotherapy rather than radiotherapy is indicated (Table 7.1).

Table 7.1   Examples of management schemas in primary extranodal lymphoma

Presentation	Histology	Management
Skin	All	RT ± local excision
Stomach	MZL DLBCL	Antibiotics, if resistant RT R-CHOP + RT
Thyroid	MZL DLBCL	RT R-CHOP + RT
Paranasal sinuses (adjacent to base of the skull)	DLBCL	R-CHOP + RT + CNS pr
Breast	MZL DLBCL Burkitt's lymphoma[44,45]	RT R-CHOP + RT LMB or similar regimens
Testis	DLBCL	R-CHOP + scrotal RT + CNS pr
Spleen	MZL DLBCL	Splenectomy or RT R-CHOP + RT or splenectomy
Intestine	MZL DLBCL	Resection + RT R-CHOP ± resection ± RT
Lung	MZL	Resection, RT
Orbital adnexae	MZL	Antibiotics, if resistant RT
Bone	DLBCL	R-CHOP + RT
Nasal	NK/T cell	CHOP + RT ± ASCT
Extradural	DLBCL	R-CHOP + RT ± CNS pr

MZL, marginal zone lymphoma; DLBCL, diffuse large B-cell lymphoma; NK, natural killer; RT, radiation therapy; LMB, lymphoma malignancy B protocol from the French Society of Paediatric Oncology; CHOP, cyclophosphamide + doxorubicin hydrochloride + vincristine (aka Oncovin) + prednisolone; R-CHOP, CHOP regimen + rituximab; ASCT, autologous stem cell transplantation, CNS pr., CNS prophylaxis.

OUTCOMES

The outcomes in localized primary extranodal lymphoma mirror those in nodal lymphomas. However, the outcomes vary greatly, depending on histology and the presenting site. For example, the outcomes in primary orbital lymphomas are excellent, primarily because marginal zone lymphoma represents the majority of cases. On the other hand, stage IE and IIE bone lymphomas have similar outcomes to stage I and II nodal lymphomas, since diffuse large B-cell pathology predominates in both cases. However, even within the specific histological type, differences in outcome are observed, depending on the presenting site. For example, diffuse large cell lymphomas presenting in skin have much better outcome than those presenting in bone, cervix, or breast. On the other hand, diffuse large cell lymphomas presenting in the CNS or in testis have inferior outcomes to those presenting in other sites. The exact reasons for these differences are under investigation, but it is believed that differences in gene expression patterns in lymphoma cells and the gene characterizing the microenvironment may be responsible.

SUMMARY

Primary extranodal lymphomas present the clinician with an opportunity to provide curative treatment to the majority of patients. Radiation, given with the guidance of modern imaging techniques and careful dosimetry, is a cornerstone of modern treatment of extranodal lymphomas. For those presentations involving the indolent lymphomas, especially the various MALT lymphomas such as those involving skin, orbital soft tissue, and thyroid, radiation can be curative with minimal toxicity. For more aggressive presentations, such as those associated with large B-cell lymphoma, the major modality of treatment is multiagent chemotherapy; however, radiation, and occasionally surgery, often proves very helpful in assuring local control. Knowledge of the need for systemic chemotherapy, the typical modes of spread of the lymphoma, and the potential for cure or at least enhanced local control available with well-tolerated irradiation is important for the clinician wishing to provide the extranodal lymphoma patient the best chance of cure with the least long-term toxicity.

REFERENCES

1. Muller AM, Ihorst G, Mertelsmann R, et al. Epidemiology of non-Hodgkin's lymphoma (NHL): trends, geographic distribution, and etiology. Ann Hematol 2005; 84: 1–12.
2. Gospodarowicz MK, Sutcliffe SB. The extranodal lymphomas. Semin Radiat Oncol 1995; 5: 281–300.
3. Zucca E, Roggero E, Bertoni F, et al. Primary extranodal non-Hodgkin's lymphomas. Part 2: Head and neck, central nervous system and other less common sites. Ann Oncol 1999; 10: 1023–33.
4. Zucca E, Roggero E, Bertoni F, et al. Primary extranodal non-Hodgkin's lymphomas. Part 1: Gastrointestinal, cutaneous and genitourinary lymphomas. Ann Oncol 1997; 8: 727–37.
5. Zucca E, Cavalli F. Extranodal lymphomas. Ann Oncol 2000; 11(Suppl 3): 219–22.
6. Smith BD, Wilson LD. Cutaneous lymphomas. Semin Radiat Oncol 2007; 17: 158–68.
7. Batchelor T, Loeffler JS. Primary CNS lymphoma. J Clin Oncol 2006; 24: 1281–8.
8. Rathmell AJ, Gospodarowicz MK, Sutcliffe SB, et al. Localised lymphoma of bone: prognostic factors and treatment recommendations. The Princess Margaret Hospital Lymphoma Group. Br J Cancer 1992; 66: 603–6.
9. Zucca E, Conconi A, Mughal TI, et al. Patterns of outcome and prognostic factors in primary large-cell lymphoma of the testis in a survey by the International Extranodal Lymphoma Study Group. J Clin Oncol 2003; 21: 20–7.
10. Zhou P, Ng AK, Silver B, et al. Radiation therapy for orbital lymphoma. Int J Radiat Oncol Biol Phys 2005; 63: 866–71.
11. Tsang RW, Gospodarowicz MK, Sutcliffe SB, et al. Non-Hodgkin's lymphoma of the thyroid gland: prognostic factors and treatment outcome. The Princess Margaret Hospital Lymphoma Group. Int J Radiat Oncol Biol Phys 1993; 27: 599–604.
12. Vega F, Lin P, Medeiros LJ. Extranodal lymphomas of the head and neck. Ann Diagn Pathol 2005; 9: 340–50.
13. Iwamoto FM, DeAngelis LM. An update on primary central nervous system lymphoma. Hematol Oncol Clin North Am 2006; 20: 1267–85.
14. Frata P, Buglione M, Grisanti S, et al. Localized extranodal lymphoma of the head and neck: retrospective analysis of a series of 107 patients from a single institution. Tumori 2005; 91: 456–62.
15. Laskin JJ, Savage KJ, Voss N, et al. Primary paranasal sinus lymphoma: natural history and improved outcome with central nervous system chemoprophylaxis. Leuk Lymphoma 2005; 46: 1721–7.
16. Tsang RW, Gospodarowicz MK. Radiation therapy for localized low-grade non-Hodgkin's lymphomas. Hematol Oncol 2005; 23: 10–17.
17. Wannesson L, Cavalli F, Zucca E. Primary pulmonary lymphoma: current status. Clin Lymphoma Myeloma 2005; 6: 220–7.
18. Ganjoo K, Advani R, Mariappan MR, et al. Non-Hodgkin lymphoma of the breast. Cancer 2007; 110: 25–30.
19. Kosari F, Daneshbod Y, Parwaresch R, et al. Lymphomas of the female genital tract: a study of 186 cases and review of the literature. Am J Surg Pathol 2005; 29: 1512–20.
20. Al-Maghrabi J, Kamel-Reid S, Jewett M, et al. Primary low-grade B-cell lymphoma of mucosa-associated lymphoid tissue type arising in the urinary bladder: report of 4 cases with molecular genetic analysis. Arch Pathol Lab Med 2001; 125: 332–6.
21. Rathmell AJ, Gospodarowicz MK, Sutcliffe SB, et al. Localized extradural lymphoma: survival, relapse pattern and functional outcome. The Princess Margaret Hospital Lymphoma Group. Radiother Oncol 1992; 24: 14–20.
22. Ceresoli GL, Ferreri AJ, Bucci E, et al. Primary cardiac lymphoma in immunocompetent patients: diagnostic and therapeutic management. Cancer 1997; 80: 1497–506.
23. Iwamoto FM, Abrey LE. Primary dural lymphomas: a review. Neurosurg Focus 2006; 21: E5.
24. Ponzoni M, Ferreri AJ. Intravascular lymphoma: a neoplasm of 'homeless' lymphocytes? Hematol Oncol 2006; 24: 105–12.
25. Ponzoni M, Ferreri AJ, Campo E, et al. Definition, diagnosis, and management of intravascular large B-cell lymphoma: proposals and perspectives from an international consensus meeting. J Clin Oncol 2007; 25: 3168–73.
26. Tsang RW, Gospodarowicz MK, Pintilie M, et al. Stage I and II MALT lymphoma: results of treatment with radiotherapy. Int J Radiat Oncol Biol Phys 2001; 50: 1258–64.
27. Zucca E, Conconi A, Pedrinis E, et al. Nongastric marginal zone B-cell lymphoma of mucosa-associated lymphoid tissue. Blood 2003; 101: 2489–95.

28. Gale J, Simmonds PD, Mead GM, et al. Enteropathy-type intestinal T-cell lymphoma: clinical features and treatment of 31 patients in a single center. J Clin Oncol 2000; 18: 795–803.

29. Greer JP. Therapy of peripheral T/NK neoplasms. Hematology Am Soc Hematol Educ Program 2006: 331–7.

30. Isobe K, Uno T, Tamaru J, et al. Extranodal natural killer/T-cell lymphoma, nasal type: the significance of radiotherapeutic parameters. Cancer 2006; 106: 609–15.

31. Harris NL, Jaffe ES, Diebold J, et al. World Health Organization classification of neoplastic diseases of the hematopoietic and lymphoid tissues: report of the Clinical Advisory Committee meeting-Airlie House, Virginia, November 1997. J Clin Oncol 1999; 17: 3835–49.

32. Chan JK. The new World Health Organization classification of lymphomas: the past, the present and the future. Hematol Oncol 2001; 19: 129–50.

33. Shenkier TN, Voss N, Fairey R, et al. Brief chemotherapy and involved-region irradiation for limited-stage diffuse large-cell lymphoma: an 18-year experience from the British Columbia Cancer Agency. J Clin Oncol 2002; 20: 197–204.

34. Horning SJ, Weller E, Kim K, et al. Chemotherapy with or without radiotherapy in limited-stage diffuse aggressive non-Hodgkin's lymphoma: Eastern Co-operative Oncology Group study 1484. J Clin Oncol 2004; 22: 3032–8.

35. Miller TP, Dahlberg S, Cassady JR, et al. Chemotherapy alone compared with chemotherapy plus radiotherapy for localized intermediate- and high-grade non-Hodgkin's lymphoma. N Engl J Med 1998; 339: 21–6.

36. Zucca E, Cavalli F. Are antibiotics the treatment of choice for gastric lymphoma? Curr Hematol Rep 2004; 3: 11–6.

37. Ferreri AJ, Ponzoni M, Dognini GP, et al. Bacteria-eradicating therapy for ocular adnexal MALT lymphoma: questions for an open international prospective trial. Ann Oncol 2006; 17: 1721–2.

38. Gospodarowicz M, Tsang R. Mucosa-associated lymphoid tissue lymphomas. Curr Oncol Rep 2000; 2: 192–8.

39. Briggs JH, Algan O, Miller TP, et al. External beam radiation therapy in the treatment of patients with extranodal stage IA non-Hodgkin's lymphoma. Am J Clin Oncol 2002; 25: 34–7.

40. Pfreundschuh M, Trumper L, Osterborg A, et al. CHOP-like chemotherapy plus rituximab versus CHOP-like chemotherapy alone in young patients with good-prognosis diffuse large-B-cell lymphoma: a randomised controlled trial by the MabThera International Trial (MInT) Group. Lancet Oncol 2006; 7: 379–91.

41. Nieder C, Schill S, Kneschaurek P, et al. Influence of different treatment techniques on radiation dose to the LAD coronary artery. Radiat Oncol 2007; 2: 20.

42. Della Biancia C, Hunt M, Furhang E, et al. Radiation treatment planning techniques for lymphoma of the stomach. Int J Radiat Oncol Biol Phys 2005; 62: 745–51.

43. Girinsky T, Ghalibafian M. Radiotherapy of Hodgkin lymphoma: indications, new fields, and techniques. Semin Radiat Oncol 2007; 17: 206–22.

44. Yustein JT, Dang CV. Biology and treatment of Burkitt's lymphoma. Curr Opin Hematol 2007; 14: 375–81.

45. Gerecitano J, Straus DJ. Treatment of Burkitt lymphoma in adults. Expert Rev Anticancer Ther 2006; 6: 373–81.

PART II

PATHOBIOLOGY AND CLINICOPATHOLOGICAL CORRELATIONS

Pathobiology and molecular basis of MALT lymphoma

8

Francesco Bertoni and Randy D Gascoyne

INTRODUCTION

As described in other chapters, extranodal marginal zone B-cell lymphoma (EMZL) of the mucosa-associated lymphoid tissue (MALT) type (MALT lymphoma) is a well-defined lymphoma subtype showing distinctive features. The prototypical MALT lymphoma involves the gastric mucosa and is specifically associated with an infectious agent, *Helicobacter pylori*.

In the mid-1990s, MALT lymphomas were classified together with two other related entities, the nodal marginal zone lymphomas (MZL) and splenic MZL.[1] The MZL subtypes share common characteristics in terms of morphology, immunophenotype, and genetics.[2] More recently, a series of specific chromosomal translocations have been exclusively identified in EMZL,[3–6] identifying EMZL as a separate entity.

CHROMOSOMAL TRANSLOCATIONS

The four main recurrent chromosomal translocations associated with the pathogenesis of EMZLs are the t(11;18)(q21;q21), t(1;14) (p22;q32), t(14;18)(q32;q21), and t(3;14) (p14;q32)[3–7] (Table 8.1). The translocations appear as mutually exclusive events and with a different pattern of anatomical localization (Table 8.2). Similar to the reported prevalence of infectious agents in EMZL,[8] there might also be geographic differences in terms of prevalence of the chromosomal translocations,[7] suggesting that the genetic background of the host or unique features of the pathogens are somehow responsible for specific chromosomal translocations.[9–11]

Interestingly, at least three [t(11;18), t(1;14), t(14;18)] of these seemingly disparate translocations affect the same signaling pathway, resulting in the constitutive activation of nuclear factor kappa B (NF-κB), a lymphoid transcription factor with a central role in immunity, inflammation, and apoptosis.[12,13]

The t(11;18)(q21;q21) translocation is the most common translocation, occurring in 15–40% of cases.[3,7,12,14–18] It results in the reciprocal fusion of two genes, comprising the cellular inhibitor of apoptosis protein 2 (*API2*; official gene symbol is now *BIRC3*) on chromosome 11q21 with *MALT1* on chromosome 18q21. The creation of a fusion protein encoded by *API2/MALT1* on the derivative chromosome 11 is the key pathogenetic event. *API2* belongs to the inhibitor of apoptosis proteins (IAP) family, characterized by the presence of one to three baculovirus IAP repeat (BIR) domains.[19] *API2* contains three N-terminal BIR domains, a middle caspase recruitment domain (CARD), and a C-terminal zinc binding RING finger domain (Figure 8.2). *MALT1*, a paracaspase, is composed of an N-terminal Death Domain (DD), followed by two Ig-like C2 domains and a caspase-like domain. All the breakpoints in the *API2* gene occur downstream of the third BIR domain but upstream of the C-terminal RING, with over 90% of them just proximal to the CARD domain. In contrast, the breakpoints involving the *MALT1* gene are more variable, but always upstream of the caspase-like domain. Thus, the resulting fusion gene *API2/MALT1* always includes the N-terminal region of *API2* gene with three intact BIR domains and the

Table 8.1 Clinical and biological features associated with the four main recurrent chromosomal translocations described in MALT lymphomas

	Translocation			
	t(11;18)(q21,q21)	*t(14;18)(q32,q21)*	*t(1;14)(p22;q32)*	*t(3;14)(p14;q32)*
Involved genes	cIAP2 (11q21), MALT1 (18q21)	IGH (14q32), MALT1 (18q21)	BCL10 (1p22), IGH (14q32)	FOXP1 (3p14), IGH (14q32)
Consequence	cIAP2–MALT1 fusion protein	Overexpression of MALT1	Overexpression of BCL10	Overexpression of FOXP1
Percent of cases[a]	15–40%	5–20%	<5%	5–10%
MALT1 expression	Cytoplasmic, weak	Cytoplasmic, strong	Cytoplasmic, weak	Unknown
BCL10 expression	Nuclear, strong	Cytoplasmic, strong	Nuclear, strong	Unknown
NF-κB activation	Yes	Yes	Yes	Unknown
Additional genomic abnormalities	Infrequent	Yes	Yes	Yes
Histological transformation	No	Yes	Yes	Yes

[a] There might be a geographical variability in the prevalence of translocations. The t(11;18) is particularly common in the lung (~50%).

Table 8.2 Anatomical localization, common chromosomal translocations, and implicated infectious agents in MALT lymphomas

Anatomical localization	Most common translocation	Known infectious agent
Stomach	t(11;18), t(1;14)	*Helicobacter pylori*
Intestine	t(11;18), t(1;14)	*Campylobacter jejuni*
Ocular adnexa	t(3;14), t(14;18)	*Chlamydia psittaci*
Skin	t(14;18) t(3;14)	*Borrelia burgdorferi*
Lung	t(11;18), t(1;14)	??
Salivary gland	t(14;18)	??
Thyroid	t(3;14)	??
Liver	t(14;18)	??

C-terminal portion of the *MALT1* gene containing an intact caspase-like domain. The specific selection of certain functional domains of API2 and MALT1 to form a fusion product strongly suggests the importance and synergy of these domains in oncogenic activities.[20]

The t(1;14)(p22;q32)[4,21] and the variant translocation t(1;2)(p22;p12)[22] juxtapose *BCL10* to the immunoglobulin heavy chain (*IGH*) and Ig light kappa chain genes, respectively. The t(1;14)(p22;q32) translocation is rare and leads to an overexpression of the *BCL10* gene as a result of its juxtaposition to

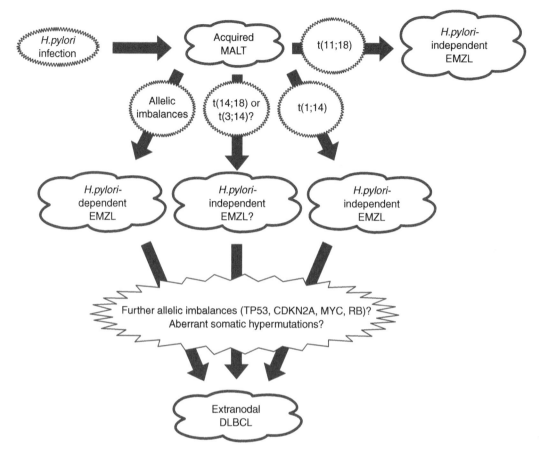

Figure 8.1   Possible pathways of EMZL pathogenesis and progression.

the promoter region of the immunoglobulin heavy chain gene.

The t(14;18)(q32;q21) translocation, described in approximately 20% of EMZL cases, is cytogenetically identical to the t(14;18) (q32;q21) involving the *BCL2* gene, characteristic of follicular lymphoma. However, in MALT lymphomas that harbor a t(14;18)(q32;q21), the breakpoints on chromosome 18 lie approximately 5 megabases downstream of the *BCL2* gene and involve the *MALT1* gene. The resultant translocation juxtaposes the *MALT1* gene to the *IGH* promoter region with subsequent MALT1 overexpression.[5,23] The MALT1 locus can also be overexpressed as a result of increased gene copy number, as it is amplified in up to 30% of the MALT lymphomas.[23,24]

NF-κB activation (Figure 8.3) is one of the main downstream effects of the stimulation of cell-surface receptors on lymphoid cells, such as the B-cell receptor. In unstimulated cells, NF-κB molecules are sequestered in the cytoplasm, due to their binding with inhibitory κB (IκB) proteins. The IκBα protein is phosphorylated by the IκB kinase (IKK) heterodimer; the phosphorylation leads to ubiquitylation and degradation of IκBα, leaving NF-κB protein to freely translocate into the nucleus where it functions as an important transcription factor

(a)

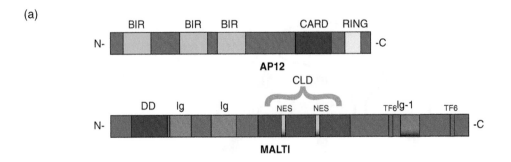

(b)

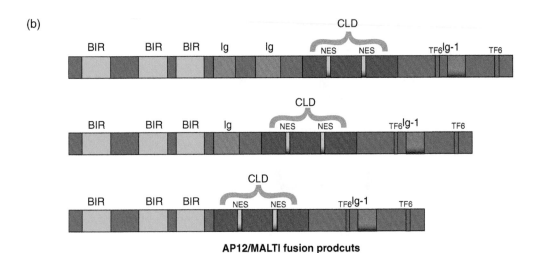

Figure 8.2 Functional domains of wild-type *API2, MALT1* (a) and of three possible API2/MALT1 fusion products (b). The API2/MALT1 products are the most common variants. BIR, Baculovirus IAP Repeat; CARD, CAspase Recruitment Domain; RING, Really Interesting New Gene; DD, Death Domain; Ig, Immunoglobulin-like; CLD, Caspase-Like Domain; NES, Nuclear Export Signal; TF6, TRAF6 binding domain; Ig-l, Immunoglobulin-like domain; N-, N-terminal; -C, C-terminal. Drawn with data from the Conserved Domains Database of the National Center for Biotechnology Information (NCBI) (http: //www.ncbi.nlm.nih.gov/), from the Expert Protein Analysis System (ExPASy) proteomics server of the Swiss Institute of Bioinformatics (http://www.expasy.org) and from References 15, 20, 32, 80, and 81.

targeting a number of genes involved in diverse cellular functions including immunity, inflammation, and apoptotic signaling. The IKK complex comprises two catalytically active kinases (IKKα and IKKβ) and a regulatory component (IKKγ, also known as NEMO). *MALT1, BCL10,* and *API2,* the three genes involved in the above-mentioned translocations, all act upstream of the IKK complex.[20,25–30] After receptor stimulation, CARMA1 (also known as CARD11) recruits BCL10, MALT1, and TRAF6 and the

IKK heteodimer to the lipid rafts surrounding the receptor. Here, IKKγ degradation induced by the complex CARMA1-BCL10-MALT1-TRAF6 activates NF-κB.[26–32] API2 and the API2/MALT1 fusion protein localize to the lipid rafts via their BIR domains. MALT1 and the fusion product API2/MALT1 can directly bind to TRAF6 via the Ig-like domains of MALT1, and this leads to the direct activation of TRAF6, which subsequently activates NF-κB.[32] Wild-type API2 might represent a physiological regulator of

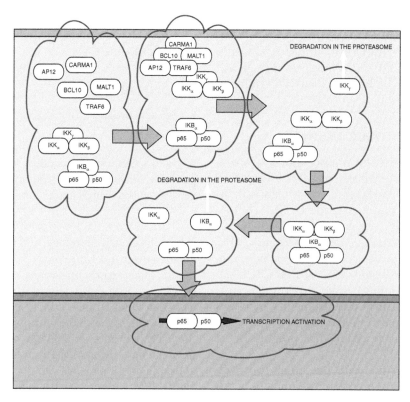

Figure 8.3   Activation of NF-κB pathway. Yellow, cytoplasm; magenta, nucleus; purple line, cell membrane; brown line, nuclear membrane.

this process.[20] Similar to other IAPs,[33] the API2 RING domain has ubiquitin ligase (E3) activity.[20] Owing to the BIR-mediated binding, API2 leads to BCL10 ubiquitylation and thus regulates BCL10 response after antigen receptor stimulation.[20] The API2/MALT1 fusion protein created by the t(11;18) translocation always contains the BIR domains, while it always lacks the API2 RING domain. The result might be that API2/MALT1 binds BCL10 but can no longer ubiquitylate the molecule.[20]

The presence of the t(11;18) translocation can predict the therapeutic response of gastric MALT lymphoma to *H. pylori* eradication.[34] The translocation is absent in gastric MALT lymphomas showing complete regression,[35] but is present in the large majority of non-responsive tumors.[36] Additionally,

nuclear expression of BCL10 or NF-κB is also predictive of *H. pylori*-independent status of EMZL with or without t(11;18)(q21;q21).[37–39] The presence of the t(11;18) does not seem to correlate with response to chemotherapy or rituximab.[40,41]

The t(3;14)(p14;q32) is the most recently described translocation and results in the juxtaposition of the transcription factor *FOXP1* located on chromosome 3p14 next to the enhancer region of the *IGH* genes.[6] The pathogenetic relevance of this translocation is still unclear. FOXP1 is normally expressed by a fraction of mantle zone B cells and of germinal center and pregerminal center B cells[42] and it is necessary for the transition from pro-B cell to pre-B cell.[43] Strong nuclear expression of FOXP1 is associated with a poor clinical outcome and appears associated with an elevated risk of transformation to diffuse large B-cell lymphoma (DLBCL).[44] Indeed, FOXP1 expression and translocations or gains/amplification of FOXP1 locus determine a poor prognosis in de-novo DLBCL.[45–47]

OTHER GENOMIC LESIONS

EMZL are devoid of translocations involving BCL2, CCND1(cyclin D1), or MYC.[48] The BCL6 gene can be rearranged, but usually only in the presence of a high-grade DLBCL component.[49] The BCL6 gene, together with other genes such as MYC, PAX5, RHOH and PIM1, are targeted by aberrant somatic hypermutation in approximately 30% of EMZL.[50,51] The significance of the aberrant hypermutations is not clear, but since their frequency increases from EMZL to extranodal DLBCL, they might play a role in the histological progression of typical EMZL.[51]

EMZL, together with the other two MZL subtypes, share recurrent genomic aberrations at a frequency higher than other B-cell tumors. For example, gains of chromosome 3/3q, 7q deletions (although more frequent among SMZL), gains of chromosome 18/18q, and gains of chromosome 12/12q are all common to MZLs.[2,52] To underscore the possible relevance to MZL pathogenesis, the presence of trisomy 3 has also been associated with a marginal zone differentiation in follicular lymphomas.[53]

Gastric EMZL bearing the t(11;18) have a lower number of genomic aberrations than t(11;18)-negative cases.[54,55] A recent comparative genomic hybridization (CGH) study identified chromosomal gains in 5/9 t(11;18)-positive cases and in 17/17 t(11;18)-negative cases.[55] Gains were usually whole chromosomes or chromosome arms, most commonly involving chromosome 3, 12, 18, and 22.[55] Indeed, this study shows that t(11;18)-positive cases have additional genomic aberrations, and thus the detection of the t(11;18) does not necessarily preclude additional genomic abnormalities.

In small retrospective series, trisomy 3 and trisomy 18 have been associated with a poorer clinical outcome.[56–59]

TRANSFORMATION

EMZL can progress to a high-grade morphology, usually DLBCL.[60,61] The true frequency of transformation is largely unknown, but appears to be less common than other low-grade lymphomas. Moreover, the relationship between the low- and the high-grade components is still unclear. In some cases the DLBCL is likely to have arisen from the low-grade EMZL, but others may be clonally unrelated and thus represent a de-novo second lymphoma. A study comparing the gene expression profiles of eight MALT lymphomas with those derived from 14 de-novo gastrointestinal DLBCL and 10 gastrointestinal DLBCL with a low-grade component indicates the likely derivation of the large cell lymphoma from the underlying MALT lymphoma.[61] Kuo et al examined 18 patients with coexistent MALT and DLBCL and showed that in five cases (28%) the two entities were clonally unrelated.[62]

Factors clearly associated with the risk of transformation are still lacking. EMZL bearing the t(11;18) translocation seem to carry a lower burden of additional genomic aberrations when compared to t(11;18)-negative cases, and indeed they seldom progress to aggressive lymphoma. In contrast, cases expressing nuclear FOXP1 have an increased tendency to transform.[44]

In a polymerase chain reaction (PCR)-based study, genomic DNA gains at 3q27 region, and DNA losses at 5q21, 13q14, and 17p13, have been associated with transformation of EMZL to DLBCL.[63] Importantly, genome-wide strategies may be more informative to delineate the complete list of loci associated with histological transformation.

PATTERN OF IMMUNOGLOBULIN GENE REARRANGEMENTS

B cells undergo proliferation, somatic hypermutation within the Ig variable (V) regions and isotype class switch recombination in the germinal centers of secondary lymphoid organs, under the influence of antigen-specific CD4+ T cells and antigen-presenting cells known as follicular dendritic cells. The accumulation of somatic mutations within *IGH* and *IGL* V–region genes greatly increases the affinity of antibodies for antigens and defines the process of affinity maturation. By examining the somatic mutation pattern of the *IG* gene rearrangements expressed by lymphoma cells, normal B-cell counterparts have been hypothesized for individual lymphoma subtypes.

EMZL cells almost always bear a pattern of somatic hypermutation and rearrangement suggesting that the cell of origin appears to be a postgerminal center marginal zone B cell. The tumor cell has undergone antigen selection in germinal centers and can continue to be at least partially driven by direct antigen stimulation.[64-68] Lymphoma cells often bear autoreactive immunoglobulins[69,70] and the role of antigen selection is also suggested by the demonstration of individual lymphoma clones derived from individual patients sharing almost the same CDR3 amino acid sequence.[71] However, the notion of antigen dependency has more recently been put partially in doubt with the demonstration that immunoglobulins derived from MALT lymphoma clones seem not to recognize antigen.[72]

It is interesting that among the three MZLs, EMZL is the only one to present consistently a unique pattern with somatically mutated *IGH* genes. Both splenic and nodal MZLs can be subdivided in two groups based upon their *IGH* status, perhaps reflecting the different normal B-cell populations resident within the marginal zone that comprise both naive and postgerminal center B cells.[73]

UNIFYING PATHOGENESIS

In 'early' gastric MALT lymphomas that lack the characteristic translocations, the presence of *H. pylori* provides the antigenic stimulus that signals through the B-cell receptor (BCR) and maintains NF-κB signaling.[74]

In this scenario, removing the antigen by antibiotic therapy reduces signaling through the BCR and can result in spontaneous regression of even clonal MALT lymphomas.[18] When the lymphoma B cells acquire one of the three characteristic translocations [t(11;18), t(1;14) or t(14;18)], NF-κB signaling is now constitutively turned on and is no longer dependent on *H. pylori*-induced signaling through the BCR.[12,13] In this situation, removing the stimulating antigen by antibiotic therapy has little effect on the lymphoma cells, and thus additional treatment modalities are required. Importantly, documenting the presence of one of these MALT-related translocations does not preclude antibiotic therapy in addition to other agents because of the known association of the microorganism with chronic gastritis and gastric adenocarcinoma.

MOLECULAR MARKERS IN PRACTICE

All the above-described chromosomal translocations that characterize EMZLs can be detected by fluorescent in-situ hybridization (FISH) strategies using locus-specific probes, a technique that can be applied to both fresh and formalin-fixed paraffin embedded tissues. The latter can be performed using whole sections, but may be hampered by difficulties interpreting the signal constellations. A strategy that uses tissue cores from the paraffin block followed by disaggregation of the nuclei produces interphase nuclei of a quality similar to fresh material.[75]

Since the demonstration that the presence of the t(11;18) or the t(1;14) predicts a poor response to antibiotics, their routine detection is advisable.[76,77] As noted above, *H. pylori* eradication is recommended in t(11;18)-positive or t(11;14)-positive gastric EMZL, since sporadic cases can achieve durable remissions and the improvement of the chronic gastritis might reduce the risk of additional gastric lymphomas or adenocarcinoma.[77] Concerning the presence of the t(11;18), it is worthy of reminder that although the t(11;18)-positive cases do not achieve sustained responses to antibiotics, they appear at lower risk of high-grade transformation.[77]

The detection of the t(14;18) and of the t(3;14) should still be considered investigational for prognostic or therapeutic purposes at this time.

Since the four translocations are highly specific for EMZL, their demonstration can be useful in the differential diagnosis of MALT lymphomas vs other small cells lymphomas involving extranodal sites.[78]

Similarly, extra copies of chromosomes 3 and 18 have been associated with poor outcome and with decreased response to antibiotics,[56–59] and also the detection of these abnormalities may be useful tools to help in the differential diagnosis of EMZL vs other low-grade lesions.[78] However, their prognostic relevance is based on small and/or retrospective series[56–59] and the specificity has to be questioned since follicular lymphomas with marginal zone differentiation seem to carry an increased frequency of similar chromosome gains.[53]

Differently from chronic lymphocytic leukemia,[79] the analysis of the *IGH* mutational status has no prognostic role in EMZL.

REFERENCES

1. Harris NL, Jaffe ES, Stein H, et al. A revised European-American classification of lymphoid neoplasms: a proposal from the International Lymphoma Study Group. Blood 1994; 84: 1361–92.
2. Dierlamm J, Pittaluga S, Wlodarska I, et al. Marginal zone B-cell lymphomas of different sites share similar cytogenetic and morphologic features. Blood 1996; 87: 299–307.
3. Dierlamm J, Baens M, Wlodarska I, et al. The apoptosis inhibitor gene API2 and a novel 18q gene, MLT, are recurrently rearranged in the t(11;18)(q21;q21) associated with mucosa-associated lymphoid tissue lymphomas. Blood 1999; 93: 3601–9.
4. Willis TG, Jadayel DM, Du MQ, et al. Bcl10 is involved in t(1;14)(p22;q32) of MALT B cell lymphoma and mutated in multiple tumor types. Cell 1999; 96: 35–45.
5. Streubel B, Lamprecht A, Dierlamm J, et al. T(14;18)(q32;q21) involving IGH and MALT1 is a frequent chromosomal aberration in MALT lymphoma. Blood 2002; 101: 2335–9.
6. Streubel B, Vinatzer U, Lamprecht A, et al. T(3;14)(p14.1;q32) involving IGH and FOXP1 is a novel recurrent chromosomal aberration in MALT lymphoma. Leukemia 2005; 19: 652–8.
7. Remstein ED, Dogan A, Einerson RR, et al. The incidence and anatomic site specificity of chromosomal translocations in primary extranodal marginal zone B-cell lymphoma of mucosa-associated lymphoid tissue (MALT lymphoma) in North America. Am J Surg Pathol 2006; 30: 1546–53.
8. Zucca E, Bertoni F. Chlamydia or not Chlamydia, that is the question: which is the microorganism associated with MALT lymphomas of the ocular adnexa? J Natl Cancer Inst 2006; 98: 1348–9.
9. Rollinson S, Levene AP, Mensah FK, et al. Gastric marginal zone lymphoma is associated with polymorphisms in genes involved in inflammatory response and antioxidative capacity. Blood 2003; 102: 1007–11.
10. Cheng TY, Lin JT, Chen LT, et al. Association of T-cell regulatory gene polymorphisms with susceptibility to gastric mucosa-associated lymphoid tissue lymphoma. J Clin Oncol 2006; 24: 3483–9.
11. Mager D. Bacteria and cancer: cause, coincidence or cure? A review. J Transl Med 2006; 4: 14.
12. Isaacson PG, Du MQ. MALT lymphoma: from morphology to molecules. Nat Rev Cancer 2004; 4: 644–53.
13. Jost PJ, Ruland J. Aberrant NF-{kappa}B signaling in lymphoma: mechanisms, consequences and therapeutic implications. Blood 2007; 109: 2700–7.
14. Farinha P, Gascoyne RD. Molecular pathogenesis of mucosa-associated lymphoid tissue lymphoma. J Clin Oncol 2005; 23: 6370–8.
15. Bertoni F, Zucca E. Delving deeper into MALT lymphoma biology. J Clin Invest 2006; 116: 22–6.
16. Murga Penas EM, Hinz K, Roser K, et al. Translocations t(11;18)(q21;q21) and t(14;18)(q32;q21) are the main chromosomal abnormalities involving MLT/MALT1 in MALT lymphomas. Leukemia 2003; 17: 2225–9.
17. Ye H, Liu H, Attygalle A, et al. Variable frequencies of t(11;18)(q21;q21) in MALT lymphomas of different sites: significant association with CagA strains of H. pylori in gastric MALT lymphoma. Blood 2003; 102: 1012–18.
18. Zucca E, Bertoni F, Cavalli F. Marginal zone B-cell lymphomas. In: Canellos GP, Lister TA, Young B, eds. The Lymphomas, 2nd edn. Philadelphia: Saunders Elsevier, 2006: 381–96.
19. Reed JC. Mechanisms of apoptosis. Am J Pathol 2000; 157: 1415–30.
20. Hu S, Du MQ, Park SM, et al. Ubiquitination of Bcl10 by c-IAP2 and its dysregulation in mucosa-associated lymphoid tissue lymphomas. J Clin Invest 2006; 116: 174–81.

21. Zhang Q, Siebert R, Yan M, et al. Inactivating mutations and overexpression of BCL10, a caspase recruitment domain-containing gene, in MALT lymphoma with t(1;14)(p22;q32). Nat Genet 1999; 22: 63–8.

22. Achuthan R, Bell SM, Leek JP, et al. Novel translocation of the BCL10 gene in a case of mucosa associated lymphoid tissue lymphoma. Genes Chromosomes Cancer 2000; 29: 347–9.

23. Sanchez-Izquierdo D, Buchonnet G, Siebert R, et al. MALT1 is deregulated by both chromosomal translocation and amplification in B-cell non-Hodgkin lymphoma. Blood 2003; 101: 4539–46.

24. Dierlamm J, Rosenberg C, Stul M, et al. Characteristic pattern of chromosomal gains and losses in marginal zone B cell lymphoma detected by comparative genomic hybridization. Leukemia 1997; 11: 747–58.

25. Ho L, Davis RE, Conne B, et al. MALT1 and the API2-MALT1 fusion act between CD40 and IKK and confer NF-kappa B-dependent proliferative advantage and resistance against FAS-induced cell death in B cells. Blood 2005; 105: 2891–9.

26. Zhou H, Wertz I, O'Rourke K, et al. Bcl10 activates the NF-kappaB pathway through ubiquitination of NEMO. Nature 2004; 427: 167–71.

27. Lynch OT, Gadina M. Ubiquitination for activation: new directions in the NF-kappaB roadmap. Mol Interv 2004; 4: 144–6.

28. Che T, You Y, Wang D, et al. MALT1/paracaspase is a signaling component downstream of CARMA1 and mediates T cell receptor-induced NF-kappaB activation. J Biol Chem 2004; 279: 15870–6.

29. Thome M. CARMA1, BCL-10 and MALT1 in lymphocyte development and activation. Nat Rev Immunol 2004; 4: 348–59.

30. Lucas PC, McAllister-Lucas LM, Nunez G. NF-kappaB signaling in lymphocytes: a new cast of characters. J Cell Sci 2004; 117: 31–9.

31. Baens M, Fevery S, Sagaert X, et al. Selective expansion of marginal zone B cells in Emicro-API2-MALT1 mice is linked to enhanced IkappaB kinase gamma polyubiquitination. Cancer Res 2006; 66: 5270–7.

32. Noels H, van Loo G, Hagens S, et al. A novel TRAF6 binding site in MALT1 defines distinct mechanisms of NF-kappa B activation by API2-MALT1 fusions. J Biol Chem 2007; 282: 10180–9.

33. Vaux DL, Silke J. IAPs, RINGs and ubiquitylation. Nat Rev Mol Cell Biol 2005; 6: 287–97.

34. Liu H, Ye H, Ruskone-Fourmestraux A, et al. T(11;18) is a marker for all stage gastric MALT lymphomas that will not respond to H. pylori eradication. Gastroenterology 2002; 122: 1286–94.

35. Alpen B, Neubauer A, Dierlamm J, et al. Translocation t(11;18) absent in early gastric marginal zone B-cell lymphoma of MALT type responding to eradication of Helicobacter pylori infection. Blood 2000; 95: 4014–15.

36. Liu H, Ruskon-Fourmestraux A, Lavergne-Slove A, et al. Resistance of t(11; 18) positive gastric mucosa-associated lymphoid tissue lymphoma to Helicobacter pylori eradication therapy. Lancet 2001; 357: 39–40.

37. Yeh KH, Kuo SH, Chen LT, et al. Nuclear expression of BCL10 or nuclear factor kappa B helps predict Helicobacter pylori-independent status of low-grade gastric mucosa-associated lymphoid tissue lymphomas with or without t(11;18)(q21;q21). Blood 2005; 106: 1037–41.

38. Ye H, Gong L, Liu H, et al. Strong BCL10 nuclear expression identifies gastric MALT lymphomas that do not respond to H pylori eradication. Gut 2006; 55: 137–8.

39. Kuo SH, Chen LT, Yeh KH, et al. Nuclear expression of BCL10 or nuclear factor kappa B predicts Helicobacter pylori-independent status of early-stage, high-grade gastric mucosa-associated lymphoid tissue lymphomas. J Clin Oncol 2004; 22: 3491–7.

40. Streubel B, Ye H, Du MQ, et al. Translocation t(11;18)(q21;q21) is not predictive of response to chemotherapy with 2CdA in patients with gastric MALT lymphoma. Oncology 2004; 66: 476–80.

41. Martinelli G, Laszlo D, Ferreri AJ, et al. Clinical activity of rituximab in gastric marginal zone non-Hodgkin's lymphoma resistant to or not eligible for anti-Helicobacter pylori therapy. J Clin Oncol 2005; 23: 1979–83.

42. Banham AH, Beasley N, Campo E, et al. The FOXP1 winged helix transcription factor is a novel candidate tumor suppressor gene on chromosome 3p. Cancer Res 2001; 61: 8820–9.

43. Hu H, Wang B, Borde M, et al. Foxp1 is an essential transcriptional regulator of B cell development. Nat Immunol 2006; 7: 819–26.

44. Sagaert X, de Paepe P, Libbrecht L, et al. Forkhead box protein P1 expression in mucosa-associated lymphoid tissue lymphomas predicts poor prognosis and transformation to diffuse large B-cell lymphoma. J Clin Oncol 2006; 24: 2490–7.

45. Wlodarska I, Veyt E, De Paepe P, et al. FOXP1, a gene highly expressed in a subset of diffuse large B-cell lymphoma, is recurrently targeted by genomic aberrations. Leukemia 2005; 19: 1299–305.

46. Barrans SL, Fenton JA, Banham A, et al. Strong expression of FOXP1 identifies a distinct subset of diffuse large B-cell lymphoma (DLBCL) patients with poor outcome. Blood 2004; 104: 2933–5.

47. Banham AH, Connors JM, Brown PJ, et al. Expression of the FOXP1 transcription factor is strongly associated with inferior survival in patients with diffuse large B-cell lymphoma. Clin Cancer Res 2005; 11: 1065–72.

48. Gaidano G, Volpe G, Pastore C, et al. Detection of BCL-6 rearrangements and p53 mutations in Malt-lymphomas. Am J Hematol 1997; 56: 206–13.

49. Gaidano G, Capello D, Gloghini A, et al. Frequent mutation of bcl-6 proto-oncogene in high grade, but not low grade, MALT lymphomas of the gastrointestinal tract. Haematologica 1999; 84: 582–8.

50. Capello D, Vitolo U, Pasqualucci L, et al. Distribution and pattern of BCL-6 mutations throughout the spectrum of B-cell neoplasia. Blood 2000; 95: 651–9.

51. Deutsch AJ, Aigelsreiter A, Staber PB, et al. MALT lymphoma and extranodal diffuse large B-cell lymphoma are targeted by aberrant somatic hypermutation. Blood 2007; 109: 3500–4.

52. Callet-Bauchu E, Baseggio L, Felman P, et al. Cytogenetic analysis delineates a spectrum of chromosomal changes that can distinguish non-MALT marginal zone B-cell lymphomas among mature B-cell entities: a description of 103 cases. Leukemia 2005; 19: 1818–23.

53. Torlakovic EE, Aamot HV, Heim S. A marginal zone phenotype in follicular lymphoma with t(14;18) is associated with secondary cytogenetic aberrations typical of marginal zone lymphoma. J Pathol 2006; 209: 258–64.

54. Starostik P, Greiner A, Schultz A, et al. Genetic aberrations common in gastric high-grade large B-cell lymphoma. Blood 2000; 95: 1180–7.

55. Zhou Y, Ye H, Martin-Subero JI, et al. Distinct comparative genomic hybridisation profiles in gastric mucosa-associated lymphoid tissue lymphomas with and without t(11;18)(q21;q21). Br J Haematol 2006; 133: 35–42.

56. Krugmann J, Tzankov A, Dirnhofer S, et al. Unfavourable prognosis of patients with trisomy 18q21 detected by fluorescence in situ hybridisation in t(11;18) negative, surgically resected, gastrointestinal B cell lymphomas. J Clin Pathol 2004; 57: 360–4.

57. Krugmann J, Tzankov A, Dirnhofer S, et al. Complete or partial trisomy 3 in gastro-intestinal MALT lymphomas co-occurs with aberrations at 18q21 and correlates with advanced disease stage: a study on 25 cases. World J Gastroenterol 2005; 11: 7384–5.

58. Taji S, Nomura K, Matsumoto Y, et al. Trisomy 3 may predict a poor response of gastric MALT lymphoma to Helicobacter pylori eradication therapy. World J Gastroenterol 2005; 11: 89–93.

59. Tanimoto K, Sekiguchi N, Yokota Y, et al. Fluorescence in situ hybridization (FISH) analysis of primary ocular adnexal MALT lymphoma. BMC Cancer 2006; 6: 249.

60. Chan JK, Ng CS, Isaacson PG. Relationship between high-grade lymphoma and low-grade B-cell mucosa- associated lymphoid tissue lymphoma (MALToma) of the stomach. Am J Pathol 1990; 136: 1153–64.

61. Barth TF, Barth CA, Kestler HA, et al. Transcriptional profiling suggests that secondary and primary large B-cell lymphomas of the gastrointestinal (GI) tract are blastic variants of GI marginal zone lymphoma. J Pathol 2007; 211: 305–13.

62. Kuo SH, Chen LT, Wu MS, et al. Differential response to H. pylori eradication therapy of co-existing diffuse large B-cell lymphoma and MALT lymphoma of stomach-significance of tumour cell clonality and BCL10 expression. J Pathol 2007; 211: 296–304.

63. Starostik P, Patzner J, Greiner A, et al. Gastric marginal zone B-cell lymphomas of MALT type develop along 2 distinct pathogenetic pathways. Blood 2002; 99: 3–9.

64. Qin Y, Greiner A, Trunk MJ, et al. Somatic hypermutation in low-grade mucosa-associated lymphoid tissue-type B-cell lymphoma. Blood 1995; 86: 3528–34.

65. Du M, Diss TC, Xu C, et al. Ongoing mutation in MALT lymphoma immunoglobulin gene suggests that antigen stimulation plays a role in the clonal expansion. Leukemia 1996; 10: 1190–7.

66. Dono M, Ferrarini M. Immunoglobulin gene mutation patterns and heterogeneity of marginal zone lymphoma. Methods Mol Med 2005; 115: 173–96.

67. Bertoni F, Cazzaniga G, Bosshard G, et al. Immunoglobulin heavy chain diversity genes rearrangement pattern indicates that MALT-type gastric lymphoma B cells have undergone an antigen selection process. Br J Haematol 1997; 97: 830–6.

68. Bahler DW, Miklos JA, Swerdlow SH. Ongoing Ig gene hypermutation in salivary gland mucosa-associated lymphoid tissue-type lymphomas. Blood 1997; 89: 3335–44.

69. Greiner A, Marx A, Heesemann J, et al. Idiotype identity in a MALT-type lymphoma and B cells in Helicobacter pylori associated chronic gastritis. Lab Invest 1994; 70: 572–8.

70. Zucca E, Bertoni F, Roggero E, et al. Autoreactive B cell clones in marginal-zone B cell lymphoma (MALT lymphoma) of the stomach. Leukemia 1998; 12: 247–9.

71. Bertoni F, Cotter FE, Zucca E. Molecular genetics of extranodal marginal zone (MALT-type) B-cell lymphoma. Leuk Lymphoma 1999; 35: 57–68.

72. Lenze D, Berg E, Volkmer-Engert R, et al. Influence of antigen on the development of MALT lymphoma. Blood 2006; 107: 1141–8.

73. Martin F, Kearney JF. Marginal-zone B cells. Nat Rev Immunol 2002; 2: 323–35.

74. Ohmae T, Hirata Y, Maeda S, et al. Helicobacter pylori activates NF-kappaB via the alternative pathway in B lymphocytes. J Immunol 2005; 175: 7162–9.

75. Paternoster SF, Brockman SR, McClure RF, et al. A new method to extract nuclei from paraffin-embedded tissue to study lymphomas using interphase fluorescence in situ hybridization. Am J Pathol 2002; 160: 1967–72.

76. Gascoyne RD. Hematopathology approaches to diagnosis and prognosis of indolent B-cell lymphomas. Hematology (Am Soc Hematol Educ Program) 2005; 299–306.

77. Du MQ, Atherton JC. Molecular subtyping of gastric MALT lymphomas: implications for prognosis and management. Gut 2006; 55: 886–93.

78. Campo E, Chott A, Kinney MC, et al. Update on extranodal lymphomas. Conclusions of the Workshop held by the EAHP and the SH in Thessaloniki, Greece. Histopathology 2006; 48: 481–504.

79. Crespo M, Bosch F, Villamor N, et al. ZAP-70 expression as a surrogate for immunoglobulin-variable-region mutations in chronic lymphocytic leukemia. N Engl J Med 2003; 348: 1764–75.

80. Nakagawa M, Hosokawa Y, Yonezumi M, et al. MALT1 contains nuclear export signals and regulates cytoplasmic localization of BCL10. Blood 2005; 106: 4210–16.

81. Sagaert X, De Wolf-Peeters C, Noels H, et al. The pathogenesis of MALT lymphomas: where do we stand? Leukemia 2007; 21: 389–96.

Principles of the WHO classification with special reference to aggressive extranodal lymphomas

9

Harald Stein, Michael Hummel, Lorenz Trümper, and Nancy Lee Harris

WHO CLASSIFICATION OF LYMPHOID NEOPLASMS

The World Health Organization (WHO) Classification of Neoplasms of the Hematopoietic and Lymphoid Tissues represents the first true worldwide consensus classification of hematological malignancies.[1,2] The WHO classification is based on the principles defined in the 'Revised European–American Classification of Lymphoid Neoplasms' (REAL) classification, originally published by the International Lymphoma Study Group (ILSG) in 1994.[3] The classification is a consensus list of lymphoid neoplasms that pathologists can recognize using a combination of available morphological, immunological, and genetic information, and that appear to be distinct clinical entities (Table 9.1). Their frequencies and the clinical features are described in Tables 9.2 and 9.3. This approach to lymphoma classification uses *all* available information – morphology, immunophenotype, genetic features, and clinical features – to define a disease entity. The relative importance of each of these features varies among diseases, and there is no one 'gold standard'. Morphology is always important, and some diseases are primarily defined by morphology, with immunophenotype as backup in difficult cases. Some diseases have a virtually specific immunophenotype, such that one would hesitate to make the diagnosis in the absence of the immunophenotype. In some lymphomas, a specific genetic abnormality is an important

defining criterion, whereas others lack specific known genetic abnormalities. Still others require knowledge of clinical features as well – nodal vs extranodal presentation, or specific anatomical site. The REAL/WHO classification has been shown to have good reproducibility when used by expert hematopathologists, and the entities that are included have distinctive clinical features, making it a useful and practical classification, despite the large number of entities.[4,5]

The WHO classification of hematological malignancies stratifies neoplasms primarily according to lineage: myeloid, lymphoid, mast cell, and histiocytic/dendritic cell. Within each category, distinct diseases are defined according to a combination of morphology, immunophenotype, genetic features, and clinical syndromes. The classification recognizes three major categories of lymphoid neoplasms: B-cell neoplasms, T- and natural killer (NK)-cell neoplasms, and Hodgkin's lymphoma (HL). Both lymphomas and lymphoid leukemias are included, since both solid and circulating phases are present in many lymphoid neoplasms, and distinction between them is artificial. Thus, B-cell chronic lymphocytic leukemia and B-cell small lymphocytic lymphoma are simply different manifestations of the same neoplasm, as are lymphoblastic lymphomas and acute lymphoid leukemias. Within the B- and T/NK-cell categories, two major categories are recognized: precursor neoplasms, corresponding to the earliest stages of differentiation; and

Table 9.1 Lymphoid neoplasms in the WHO 4th edn[2]

Mature B-cell neoplasms	Extranodal localization[a]
Chronic lymphocytic leukemia/small lymphocytic lymphoma	Rare, any site, secondary
B-cell prolymphocytic leukemia	
Splenic marginal zone lymphoma	
Hairy cell leukemia	Liver, skin (rare, secondary)
Splenic lymphoma/leukemia, unclassifiable	
Lymphoplasmacytic lymphoma	Rare, any site, secondary
Waldenström macroglobulinemia	
Heavy-chain diseases	
Alpha heavy-chain disease	Small intestine (immunoproliferative small intestinal disorder)
Gamma heavy-chain disease	
Mu heavy-chain disease	
Plasma cell myeloma	
Solitary plasmacytoma of bone	Bone
Extraosseous plasmacytoma	Head and neck; skin/subcutis (rule out MALT lymphoma)
Extranodal marginal zone B-cell lymphoma of mucosa-associated lymphoid tissue (MALT lymphoma)	Stomach, salivary gland, thyroid, ocular adnexae, skin (trunk, limbs), breast, other sites
Nodal marginal zone B-cell lymphoma	
Follicular lymphoma	Small bowel (duodenum); testis
Primary cutaneous follicle center lymphoma	Skin (head, trunk)
Mantle cell lymphoma	Waldeyer's ring, gastrointestinal tract
Diffuse large B-cell lymphoma, not otherwise specified	
T-cell/histiocyte-rich large B-cell lymphoma	
Primary DLBCL of the CNS	Central nervous system, eye, nerve roots
DLBCL associated with chronic inflammation	Pleural cavity
BV-positive + DLBCL (age-related)	
Primary mediastinal (thymic) large B-cell lymphoma	Thymus, gastrointestinal tract, ovary, kidney, CNS
Intravascular large B-cell lymphoma	CNS, kidney, skin, lung
Primary cutaneous DLBCL, leg type	Skin: leg (typically lower leg) but may occur on trunk
ALK-positive DLBCL	
Plasmablastic lymphoma	Oral cavity, gastrointestinal tract, soft tissue, bone
Primary effusion lymphoma	Pleural and peritoneal cavities, lung, gastrointestinal tract
Large B-cell lymphoma arising in HHV8-associated multicentric Castleman's disease	
Lymphomatoid granulomatosis	Lung, CNS, kidney
Burkitt's lymphoma	Gastrointestinal tract, ovary, jaws
B-cell lymphoma, with features intermediate between DLBCL and BL	
B-cell lymphoma with features intermediate between DLBCL and cHL	

(Continued)

Table 9.1   (Continued)

Mature T-cell and NK-cell neoplasms	*Extranodal localization*[a]
T-cell prolymphocytic leukemia	
T-cell large granular lymphocytic leukaemia	
Chronic lymphoproliferative disorder of NK cell	
Aggressive NK-cell leukemia	
Systemic EBV+ T-cell lymphoproliferative disease of childhood *(associated with chronic active EBV infection)*	
Hydroa vaccineforme-like lymphoma	Skin of face
Adult T-cell leukemia/lymphoma	
Extranodal NK/T-cell lymphoma, nasal type	Nasal cavity, testis, gastrointestinal tract, skin
Enteropathy-associated T-cell lymphoma	Gastrointestinal tract, skin
Hepatosplenic T-cell lymphoma	Liver, spleen
Subcutaneous panniculitis-like T-cell lymphoma	Subcutis (any site)
Mycosis fungoides	Skin (any site)
Sézary syndrome	Skin, blood
Primary cutaneous anaplastic large cell lymphoma	Skin
Primary cutaneous aggressive epidermotropic CD8-positive cytotoxic T-cell lymphoma	Skin
Cutaneous gamma-delta T-cell lymphoma	Skin, subcutis, mucosae
Primary cutaneous small/medium CD4-positive T-cell lymphoma (provisional)	Skin
Peripheral T-cell lymphoma, not otherwise specified	May occur in extranodal sites
Angioimmunoblastic T-cell lymphoma	Skin rash may occur (secondary)
Anaplastic large cell lymphoma (ALCL), ALK-positive	Bone, soft tissue, skin, gastrointestinal tract
Anaplastic large cell lymphoma (ALCL), ALK-negative	Bone, soft tissue, skin, gastrointestinal tract

Hodgkin's lymphoma	*Extranodal localization*
Nodular lymphocyte predominant Hodgkin's lymphoma	
Classical Hodgkin's lymphoma	Bone; secondary skin/soft tissue, epidural, gastrointestinal tract, lung, CNS involvement may occur
Nodular sclerosis classical Hodgkin's lymphoma	
Lymphocyte-rich classical Hodgkin's lymphoma	
Mixed cellularity classical Hodgkin's lymphoma	
Lymphocyte-depleted classical Hodgkin's lymphoma	

[a] Other than bone marrow, spleen.

peripheral or mature neoplasms, corresponding to more differentiated stages. Within the category of 'non-Hodgkin's' lymphomas, there are a large number of distinct diseases. These are associated with distinctive epidemiology, etiology, clinical features, and, often, distinctive responses to therapy. One of the corollaries of defining distinct entities is that it is neither possible nor helpful to sort them precisely according to histological grade or clinical aggressiveness. Histological grade is just one of many prognostic factors that should be applied *within* a disease entity and not across the whole range of lymphoid neoplasms. Both

Table 9.2 Frequency of lymphoid neoplasms: the non-Hodgkin's lymphoma classification project[4]

Lymphoma	Percent
B-cell lymphomas	88
Diffuse large B-cell	31
Follicular	22
Marginal zone (MALT)	8
B-CLL/SLL	7
Mantle cell	6
Mediastinal large B-cell	2
Marginal zone (nodal)	2
Burkitt-like	2
Lymphoplasmacytic	1
Burkitt's	<1
Marginal zone (splenic)	<1
T-cell lymphomas	12
Peripheral T-cell NOS	4
Anaplastic large-cell	2
Precursor T-LBL	2
Nasal (angiocentric)	1
Angioimmunoblastic	1
Mycosis fungoides	<1
Intestinal	<1
ATL/L	<1

the pathologist and the oncologist must 'get to know' each disease entity and its spectrum of morphology and clinical behavior.[6]

The lymphoid neoplasms can be sorted according to various principles, including their postulated normal counterpart in the immune system, their morphological features, or their clinical features. Attempting to understand the normal counterpart of the neoplastic cell is an important component of any tumor classification. At present, the normal counterpart, both lineage and differentiation stage, of many hematological malignancies can be postulated with reasonable certainty. However, our understanding of the immune system is insufficient to permit this to be done in all cases, and therefore rigid adherence to classification by normal counterpart is not feasible at this time.

PRIMARY EXTRANODAL LYMPHOMAS

There are several lymphomas that virtually always present in extranodal sites, and appear to correspond to normal lymphoid cells specific for extranodal immunological reactions (see Table 9.1). Primary extranodal B-cell lymphomas include extranodal marginal zone B-cell lymphoma of mucosa-associated lymphoid tissue (MALT) type, primary cutaneous follicle center lymphoma (PCFCL), primary cutaneous diffuse large B-cell lymphoma (DLBCL) of the type commonly found on the lower legs (leg type), plasmablastic lymphoma, primary mediastinal DLBCL (PMBL), primary effusion lymphoma (PEL), intravascular DLBCL, DLBCL associated with chronic inflammation, primary central nervous system DLBCL, and lymphomatoid granulomatosis. Primary extranodal T- and NK-cell lymphomas include hydroa-vacciniforme-like T-cell lymphoma, nasal-type NK/T-cell lymphoma, intestinal (enteropathy-associated) T-cell lymphoma, hepatosplenic T-cell lymphoma, mycosis fungoides, primary cutaneous aggressive CD8+ cytotoxic T-cell lymphoma, primary cutaneous small/medium-sized CD4+ T-cell lymphoma, cutaneous gamma/delta T-cell lymphoma, subcutaneous panniculitis-like T-cell lymphoma, and primary cutaneous anaplastic large-cell lymphoma.

Because their clinical presentation and treatment options differ from the more common nodal or leukemic lymphoid neoplasms, primary extranodal lymphomas are considered a distinct clinical category. They are less likely to disseminate than primary nodal lymphomas, and, when they do, it is more often to other extranodal sites than to lymph nodes and bone marrow. Exposure to antigen, as has been demonstrated for MALT lymphoma, may play a part in the pathogenesis of many of these neoplasms.

LYMPHOMAS THAT MAY PRESENT IN OR INVOLVE EXTRANODAL SITES

Several other indolent or aggressive lymphomas often present in or involve extranodal sites, typically in the setting of widespread disease. Mantle cell lymphoma, while it usually presents with widespread nodal disease, often involves Waldeyer's ring and the gastrointestinal tract. Follicular lymphoma may rarely

Table 9.3 Presenting features of common B- and T-cell neoplasms[5]

Neoplasm	Frequency (%)	Age	Male	Stage				BSx	EN	BM	GI	IPI		
				I	II	III	IV					0/1	2/3	4/5
Diffuse large B-cell	31	64	55	25	29	13	33	33	71	16	18	35	46	9
Primary mediastinal B-cell	2	37	34	10	56	3	31	38	56	3	0	52	37	11
Follicular	22	59	42	18	15	16	51	28	64	42	4	45	48	7
Small lymphocytic lymphoma/chronic lymphocytic leukemia	6	65	53	4	5	8	83	33	80	72	3	23	64	13
MALT	8	60	48	39	28	2	31	19	98	14	50	44	48	8
Mantle cell	6	63	74	13	7	9	71	28	81	51	9	23	54	23
Peripheral T-cell	7	61	55	8	12	15	65	50	82	36	15	17	52	31
Anaplastic large cell	2	34	69	19	32	10	39	53	59	13	9	61	18	21

BSx, B symptoms; EN, any extranodal site, including bone marrow; BM, bone marrow; GI, gastrointestinal tract; IPI, International Prognostic Index.

present in and be confined to extranodal sites, particularly the small intestine/duodenum. Diffuse large B-cell lymphoma (not otherwise specified/NOS) may present with extranodal disease, which may be either localized or disseminated; in addition to the central nervous system (CNS), common sites of extranodal DLBCL are gastrointestinal tract, bone, soft tissue, lung, and testis. Burkitt's lymphoma often presents with extranodal disease of the jaws ileocecal region, often with adjacent nodal involvement. Anaplastic lymphoma kinase (ALK)-positive anaplastic large cell lymphoma (ALCL) may present with extranodal disease, such as bone, soft tissue, and skin. Staging may reveal widespread disease.

The pathological features of many specific types of extranodal lymphomas are described in detail in other chapters, including MALT lymphoma (Chapter 19), intravascular lymphoma (Chapter 13), primary mediastinal large B-cell lymphoma (Chapter 18), and cutaneous (Chapter 22) and pulmonary (Chapter 17) lymphomas. In this chapter, we will focus on the pathology and pathobiology of selected aggressive B-cell and T/NK-cell lymphomas.

EXTRANODAL AGGRESSIVE B-CELL NEOPLASMS

Extranodal aggressive B-cell neoplasms comprise (DLBCL), Burkitt's lymphoma, and lymphomatoid granulomatosis. (LYG) DLBCL arise primarily in extranodal sites in 40%, Burkitt's lymphoma and lymphomatoid granulomatosis in nearly 100% of the cases.

In addition, several variants, subgroups and subtypes/entities of DLBCL have been recognized. Only those categories and entities are described in detail which are not covered in other chapters of this book.

Diffuse large B-cell lymphoma

Characteristics

DLBCL is a diffuse proliferation of large neoplastic B-lymphoid cells with nuclear size equal to or exceeding normal macrophage nuclei or more than twice the size of a normal lymphocyte.

Subclassification

DLBCL has proved to be morphologically, biologically, and clinically very heterogeneous. Therefore, this lymphoma category has been further subdivided into morphological variants, molecular genetic and immunophenotypical subgroups, and distinct disease entities (Table 9.4).

Diffuse large B-cell lymphoma, not otherwise specified (DLBCL NOS)

Characteristics

This category comprises all DLBCL cases that cannot be allocated to specific subtypes or disease entities mentioned in Table 9.4.

Table 9.4 Diffuse large B-cell lymphoma: variants, subgroups, and subtypes/entities

---

Diffuse large B-cell lymphoma, not otherwise specified (NOS)

Common morphological variants:
  Centroblastic
  Immunoblastic
  Anaplastic
Rare morphological variants
Molecular subgroups
  Germinal-center B-cell-like (GCB)
  Activated B-cell-like (ABC)
Immunohistochemical subgroups
  CD5-positive DLBCL
  Germinal-center B-cell-like (GCB)
  Non-germinal center B-cell-like (non-GCB)

Diffuse large B-cell lymphoma subtypes/entities
Primary mediastinal (thymic) large B-cell lymphoma
T-cell/histiocyte-rich large B-cell lymphoma
Intravascular large B-cell lymphoma
Primary DLBCL of the CNS
Primary cutaneous DLBCL, leg type
ALK-positive DLBCL
DLBCL associated with chronic inflammation
EBV+ DLBCL of the elderly
Lymphoma arising in HHV8-associated multicentric
  Castleman's disease
Plasmablastic lymphoma
Primary effusion lymphoma

Borderline cases
B-cell lymphoma, unclassifiable, with features
  intermediate between DLBCL and BL
B-cell lymphoma, unclassifiable, with features
  intermediate between DLBCL
  and classical Hodgkin's lymphoma

Epidemiology: geographic and age distribution

DLBCL NOS account for 25–30% of all non-Hodgkin's lymphomas, one of the most frequent malignant lymphoma types. It is most common in the elderly, with a median age in the 7th decade but can occur at any age. Males are slightly more often affected than females.[4,5]

Sites of involvement

Up to 40% of DLBCL NOS are at least initially confined to extranodal sites.[3] The gastrointestinal tract (stomach and ileocecal region) is the most common extranodal location (Chapter 21), but virtually any extranodal site may be primarily affected. Other common extranodal sites include skin (Chapter 22), brain (Chapter 11), bone (Chapter 16), bone marrow, testis (Chapter 12), spleen, Waldeyers's ring, salivary glands, thyroid gland, liver (Chapter 24), kidney, and adrenal glands. Blood may also be affected (in 3–10% of the cases).

Histology and immunophenotype

The affected extranodal tissues show a diffuse proliferation of large B cells. Their cytomorphology is diverse. This led to the distinction of common and uncommon morphological variants. In some instances, the involvement may be morphologically discordant; i.e. there are (in addition to the manifestations of DLBCL) infiltrates consisting of a low-grade B-cell lymphoma. This is most commonly seen when the DLBCL is associated with neoplastic infiltrates in the bone marrow.[7]

Common morphological variants

Three common variants have been distinguished: centroblastic, immunoblastic, and anaplastic. In these morphological variants, a large number of T cells and/or histiocytes may be present. This histological pattern may lead to confusion with T-cell rich B-cell lymphoma if not all diagnostic criteria are drawn into consideration.

Centroblastic variant

The centroblastic variant represents the most common morphological DLBCL pattern. Its neoplastic cells resemble centroblasts of reactive germinal centers, but there is cytological heterogeneity. A common feature is that the centroblastic cells are medium-sized to large cells with oval to round, vesicular nuclei containing open chromatin. There are usually two nucleoli located near or at the nuclear membrane. The cytoplasm is usually scanty and amphophilic to basophilic (Fig 9.1a). If most of the neoplastic cells very closely resemble reactive centroblasts, the term *monomorphic centroblastic DLBCL* has been applied. More frequently, the centroblastic cells are *polymorphic* and admixed with immunoblasts (<90%).[8,9] In some cases the majority of centroblastic cells may contain multilobated nuclei, which led to the designation *DLBCL, multilobated*.

Immunoblastic variant

This variant differs from the centroblastic variant by a predominance of cells with features of immunoblasts (>90%). These cells contain a single prominent centrally located nucleolus and usually an abundant basophilic cytoplasm (Fig 9.1b). The distinction of the immunoblastic variant from the common centroblastic variant is much more reliably possible in well Giemsa-stained sections than in hematoxylin and eosin (H&E) stained sections. The cytoplasm of the immunoblastic tumor may be eccentric, have a hof, and thus resemble that of plasma cells.[3,8,9]

Anaplastic variant

The cells of this variant are usually larger in size and much more pleomorphic than those present in the centroblastic and immunoblastic variants. They may resemble in part Hodgkin's and/or Reed–Sternberg cells or the cells of anaplastic large cell lymphoma.[10,11]

Rare morphological variants

These cases may demonstrate a myxoid stroma or a fibrillary matrix or a pseudorosette formation. The tumor cells may be spindle-shaped or have features of signet ring cells.[2]

Immunophenotypical features

So far no antigen profiles have been reported that allow distinguishing between DLBCL NOS

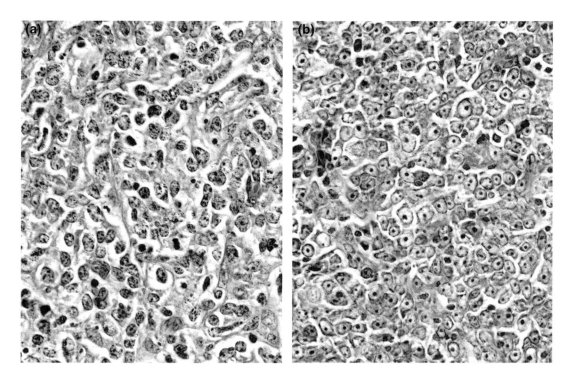

Figure 9.1   Diffuse large B-cell lymphoma: (a) centroblastic variant; (b) immunoblastic variant.

arising in extranodal sites and those arising in lymph nodes. The DLBCL cells are generally characterized by the expression of pan B-cell antigens, including CD19, CD20, CD22, and CD79a. One or more of these antigens may be lost. Surface and/or cytoplasmic immunoglobulin is detectable in 50–75% of the cases.[12] The immunoglobulin heavy-chain class is IgM in most instances, which is located at the surface membrane and/or the cytoplasm. There is no correlation between the presence of cytoplasmic immunoglobulin and a strong expression of the plasma cell characteristic antigens such as CD38 and/or CD138. A co-expression of CD138 and CD20 is only rarely seen. CD30 is often expressed in the anaplastic variant[11,13] but is usually absent from the centroblastic and immunoblastic variant. The expression of CD5 is encountered in approximately 10% of the cases.[14] Most of theses cases are de-novo DLBCL. They can be distinguished from CLL/SLL or mantle cell lymphoma by the presence of CD23 and/or absence of cyclin D1.[15,16] The incidence of CD10, BCL6, MUM1/IRF4, and BCL2 expression varies greatly from study to

study: CD10 expression is detectable in 30% (most frequently) to 60%, BCL6 expression in 60–90%, MUM1/IRF4 expression, in 35–65%, and BCL2 expression in 47–84%.[17–19,44,53,96] An expression of FOXP1 by most tumor cells has been observed in DLBCL cases that lack the germinal center markers CD10 and/or BCL6 and express MUM1/IRF4 and BCL2 in the absence of t(14;18).[20]

The growth fraction, as assessed by the Ki-67 staining, ranges from 40% to 100%, with values between 60% and 90% being most frequently seen.[21,22] P53 is expressed in 20–60% of cases.[23–26]

Subgrouping DLBC NOS by immunophenotyping

Several research groups have proposed to subdivide DLBCL NOS into germinal center-like (GCB) and non-germinal center-like (non-GCB) subgroups by using a panel of three antibodies; i.e. CD10, BCL6, and MUM1/ IRF4.[27,28,44] One proposal was to regard cases with a CD10 expression in 30% or more cells as well cases with the profile CD10–, BCL6+ MUM1/IRF4– as GCB,

Table 9.5   Characteristics of the molecular DLBCL subgroups/types

Characteristics[a]	ABC	GCB	PMBL
Chromosomal aberrations			
t(14;18)	0	35%	0
3q gain	26%	0	5%
9p gain	6%	0	35%
12q12 gain	5%	20%	5%
6q12 loss	40%	19%	0%
Molecular genetic features			
Ongoing Ig somatic hypermutations	No	Mostly	No
Rel amplification	0	15%	
NFκB activation	Yes	No	Yes
Clinical features			
5-year survival	15–30%	50–60%	65%
Disease hallmarks	–	Late relapses	Predominantly woman < 35 years

ABC, activated B cell-like; GCB, germinal center B cell-like; PMBL, primary mediastinal large B-cell lymphoma.
[a] Genetic alterations according to fluorescence in-situ hybridization (FISH) and comparative genomic hybridization (CGH).

and to regard all the remaining cases as non-GCB.[50] A further proposal is to improve the immunophenotypical subgrouping by adding BCL2 and cyclin D2 to the mentioned antibody panel (see also under prognosis).[53]

Pathogenesis, genetics, and molecular genetic findings

Extranodal and nodal DLBCL NOS are not only heterogeneous in their morphology and their immunophenotype but also in their molecular genetic properties (Table 9.5). Gene expression profiling by means of high-density arrays revealed, however, common features which were detectable irrespective of the differences in morphology and/or site of involvement. One of these gene expression groups showed a profile characteristic for activated B cells (ABC), whereas another group was related to germinal center B cells (GCB). The remaining cases without ABC- or GCB-like profiles displayed an inhomogeneous pattern without a common gene expression signature. When compared to the clinical outcome, the patients with a GCB-like signature do clinically significantly better than patients with an ABC-like profile. The correlation of the gene expression to genomic alteration revealed that a substantial number of DLBCL with an ABC-like profile are associated

with gains of 3q, 12q12, 18q21-q22, and losses of 6q21-q22.[14,29] Interestingly, translocations involving the BCL2 gene are exclusively found in the GCB-like DLBCL, whereas translocations affecting the BCL6 gene were equally present in both DLBCL gene expression groups.[30,31] Chromosomal breaks in the MYC gene are found to be accumulated in non-ABC/non-GCB cases. In these cases the MYC breakpoints are frequently not fused to immunoglobulin (Ig) heavy- or light-chain genes but to various non-Ig partners. The patients of these non-ABC/non-GCB cases with MYC breaks display an adverse clinical outcome.

Nuclear factor Kappa B (NF-κB) expression and, as a consequence, the up-regulation of many NF-κB target genes is a hallmark of ABC-like DLBCL cases. Although constitutive NF-κB up-regulation is also found in several other lymphoma entities, the mechanism for this activity appears to be different among the various lymphoma types. In ABC-like DLBCL, the activation of NF-κB is mediated by the upstream molecules CARMA1, BCL10, and/or MALT1, which, in turn, activate the IKKs, leading to degradation of the NF-κB inhibitors.[32] This leads to the release of NF-κB into the nucleus and to the expression of the NF-κB target genes.

The ABC/GCB signatures are not the only gene expression profiles detectable in DLBCL.

Whereas the ABC/GCB profile describes the gene expression status of the DLBCL tumor cells, the lymph node (LN) signature and the major histocompatibility complex (MHC) class II signature is derived from the non-malignant immune cells of the microenvironment. Although there is no overlap in the different gene expression signatures, they are all able to separate patients with different clinical outcomes.[33] The finding that this also holds true for the LN and MHC class II signature underlines the fact that the response to treatment is not only based on the molecular characteristics of the tumor cells but is also dependent on the composition of the microenvironment.

In addition to these common features between nodal and extranodal DLBCL, there are further molecular genetic characteristics which are typical for certain anatomical sites. Primary mediastinal large B-cell lymphoma is distinguished by gains on 9p21 and 2p14 as well as overexpression of JAK2.[29,34] In DLBCL of the gastrointestinal tract, deletions of chromosome 7q22 and gains of 5, 15, and 16 are more frequent than in nodal DLBCL.[35] Translocation (3;14) involving FoxP1 is almost exclusively found in gastric DLBCL.[36] Primary DLBCL of the CNS are frequently associated with losses of 6p21 (HLA locus), which are also detectable in DLBCL occurring in the testis.[37] Primary cutaneous DLBCL, leg type, which are usually of the ABC type, in many cases display additional amplifications of 18q21, affecting BCL2 and MALT1.[38]

Clinical features (including presentation, stage, prognosis, and therapy)

Presentation

Many patients with extranodal involvement are asymptomatic, but when symptoms are present they are highly dependent on the site of involvement.[4,5] A tumor mass at single or multiple extranodal sites, as recognized by palpation and/or diagnostic imaging systems, is usually enlarging rapidly. Almost half the patients have stage I or II disease.

Prognosis and therapy

With the introduction of the CHOP regimen in the 1970s, a complete remission could be achieved in 50–70% and a cure in 30–50% of the DLBCL patients.[39] Attempts to improve outcome with more intensive chemotherapy failed.[40] However, the addition of the anti-CD20 monoclonal antibody Rituximab to CHOP (R-CHOP) increased the rate of complete remissions by 13% and the overall survival from 57% to 70% at an observation time of 2 years. Of note: surgery has its place only in the acquisition of biopsy material sufficient in size for a reliable diagnostic assessment by a hematopathologist. A radical surgical resection of lymphoma masses is not justified because this does not usually improve the outcome.

Predictive factors

A highly predictive parameter is the *International Prognostic Index (IPI)*, which defines four different risk groups with differing prognosis. The IPI is based on five pretherapeutic parameters (Table 9.6). However, the IPI seems to lose some of its predictive value in patients treated with rituximab.[41]

There are numerous reports on *morphological and immunophenotypical features* described to predict the clinical course of DLBCL. Immunoblastic morphology, the expression of BCL2, X-linked inhibitor of apoptosis (XIAP), IRF4/MUM1, cyclin D2, cyclin D3, P53, CD5, FOXP1, PKC-beta, ICAM1. HLA-DR, c-FLIP, etc., have been associated with an adverse prognosis, and the expression of BCL6, CD10, LMO2, etc., with a favorable outcome.[20,42-49] The problem with these data is that different studies are often controversial, that many data are based only on one single investigation and that the follow-up data usually stem from differently designed retrospective clinical studies.

Table 9.6 Prognostic factors and risk score constituting the International Prognostic Index

Prognostic factors	Risk score	
• Age (>60 years old)	Low	0, 1
• LDH (> nl)	Low, Int	2
• Performance status (2–4)	High, Int	3
• Stage (III, IV)	High	4, 5
• Extranodal (>1 site)		

A strong proposal for predicting the clinical outcome is not to use only one single but a *combination of markers*. Hans et al[50] reported that the antibody panel consisting of CD10, BCL6, and MUM1 can subdivide DLBCL patients into long- and short-term survivors. This result has been confirmed by some studies but not by others.[51,52] The inclusion of two additional antibodies (cyclin D2, BCL2, or LMO2) to the Hans classifier was found to increase its predictive power, even in patients treated with R-CHOP.[49,53] However, this study needs to be confirmed.

So far, the use of single immunohistochemical markers or a combination of them to define prognostic groups has not played a role in routine clinical practice. One major reason is that the reproducibility in the performance and interpretation of several immunohistochemical stains is limited.[54] Another reason is how this information can be translated into therapeutic consequences.

Gene expression profiling studies identified two subgroups in DLBCL NOS with different clinical outcome: a favorable GCB subgroup and an adverse ABC subgroup. Whether the difference in survival between these two subgroups persists in patients treated with Rituximab remains to be seen. There is good evidence that the presence of an MYC break is linked with a very unfavorable outcome.[102] The impact of *TP53* mutations on outcome is controversial.[23] However, a recent study convincingly demonstrated that mutations in the *TP53* DNA binding domain are associated with an unfavorable prognosis.[23]

The *immune response* appears to have a strong impact on the clinical outcome after chemotherapy, e.g. the loss of MHC class II genes and the MHC class II proteins in patients with DLBCL is associated with a poor outcome.[55]

Plasmablastic lymphoma

Characteristics

Plasmablastic lymphoma (PBL) is a diffuse proliferation of neoplastic cells, most of which resemble B immunoblasts morphologically but plasma cells immunophenotypically. PBL was originally described as occurring in the oral cavity, but subsequent studies showed that it may also occur in other extranodal sites.[56]

Epidemiology: geographic and age distribution

PBL is a rare B-cell neoplasm that predominantly affects HIV-positive males. The age range is broad, with a median around 50 years old. The disease also occurs in HIV-negative patients, but much less often.[52]

Sites of involvement

PBL typically presents in extranodal sites. Most frequently, it is encountered in the oral cavity, but it may arise at any other site, including the sinonasal cavity, orbit, skin, bone, soft tissues, and the gastrointestinal tract. Nodal involvement is seen but is rare.[57]

Histology and immunophenotype

PBL demonstrates a diffuse and cohesive proliferation of immunoblast-like cells (Fig 9.2). Cells with obvious plasmacytic differentiation may be intermingled but don't predominate. The growth fraction is high, as indicated by a high number of mitotic figures and a Ki-67 index usually >90%.[56,57]

Apoptotic cells and tingible body macrophages may be present. The monomorphic cases composed nearly exclusively of immunoblast-like cells occur more commonly in the oral, nasal, and paranasal mucosa (oral type), whereas cases in which cells with a plasmacytic differentiation are seen tend to occur more commonly in other extranodal sites as well as lymph nodes.[57] Cases containing plasmacytically differentiated cells should not be confused with anaplastic or plasmablastic plasma cell myeloma. The presence of a high proliferation fraction, extranodal localization, a history of immune deficiency, and the presence of Epstein–Barr virus (EBV) by in-situ hybridization for EBER are useful in establishing the diagnosis of PBL. LMP-1 is rarely expressed. All cases of PBL express a plasma cell phenotype, including positivity for CD138, CD38, VS38c,

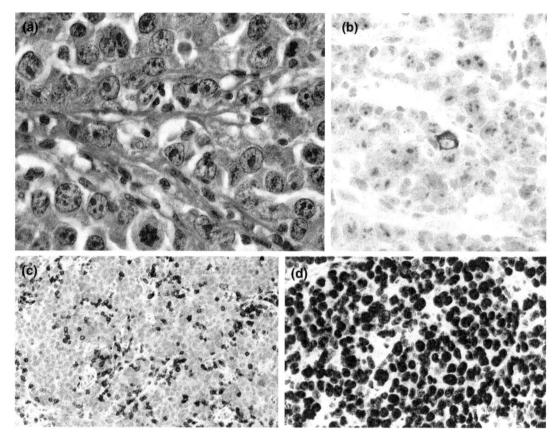

Figure 9.2 Plasmablastic lymphoma: (a) H&E staining; (b) CD20 (APAAP); all tumor cells are negative; (c) CD3 (APAAP); all tumor cells are negative; (d) Ki-67 (APAAP); nearly 100% of the tumor cells show a strong nuclear positivity.

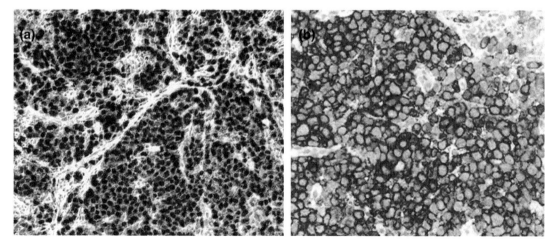

Figure 9.3 Plasmablastic lymphoma: (a) IRF4/MUM1 (APAAP); the nuclei of all tumor cells are positive; (b) CD138 (APAAP); the neoplastic are strongly positive.

and IRF4/MUM1 (Fig 9.3). Immunostainings for CD45, CD20, and PAX5 are negative or only weakly positive. CD79a is positive in approximately 50–85% of the cases.[56,57]

Cytoplasmic immunoglobulins are detectable in 50–70% of the cases, most frequently IgG and either kappa or lambda light chain. CD56 is usually negative in monomorphic PBL cases but may be seen in cases with plasmacytic differentiation. Expression of EMA and CD30 are frequently seen. Human herpes virus 8 (HHV-8) is consistently absent.[56,57]

Pathogenesis, genetics, and molecular genetic findings

The frequent association between PBL and human immunodeficiency virus (HIV) infection suggests that immunodeficiency predisposes to the development of PBL. This is supported by the observation that PBL is also seen in patients suffering from immunodeficiency caused by other reasons, such as iatrogenic immunosuppression for autoimmune disease or prevention of allograft rejection. EBV may also play an oncogenic role, since the majority of this neoplasm is EBV-infected.[56,57]

Clinical features

The majority of patients present with an advanced stage (III or IV).[57] The International Prognostic Index (IPI) is of intermediate or high-risk score. Computed tomography (CT) and positron emission tomography (PET) may show disseminated bone involvement. The clinical course is very aggressive, with most of the patients dying in the first year after diagnosis, although the outcome may have improved more recently, possibly due to a better management of HIV infection.

ALK-positive DLBCL

Characteristics

This neoplasm has the morphological and immunophenotypical features of PBL but differs from the common PBL by a consistent expression of the kinase unit of the anaplastic lymphomakinase (ALK) protein and the presence of a genetic alteration that causes the ALK expression.

Epidemiology: geographic and age distribution

This type of DLBCL is very rare (<1% of DLBCL).[58] It is encountered in all age groups, with a median age of 36 years and a male predominance of 3:1.[58]

Sites of involvement

The most frequent extranodal site of involvement is the mediastinum.[59,60] Other extranodal sites are the nasopharynx,[61] the tongue,[59] the stomach,[62] the bone,[61] and soft tissues.[63] Lymph nodes are also frequently affected.[58,59,64]

Histology and immunophenotype

The tumor cells usually demonstrate the morphological features of monomorphic plasmablasts. The nuclei have an open chromatin, with large central nucleoli. The usually abundant cytoplasm is basophilic and often contains a perinuclear hof. In some tumors atypical multinucleated neoplastic giant cells may be encountered.[65]

A strong expression of the ALK protein is detectable in all cases. The pattern of the immunostaining is most frequently granular in the cytoplasm, which is highly suggestive of a fusion protein formed by ALK and clathrin. In a few cases the ALK protein is present in the nucleus, the nucleoli, and the cytoplasm, which is indicative of the presence of a fusion protein consisting of nucleoplosmin (NPM) and ALK. A further highly characteristic but not specific marker profile is the strong co-expression of the plasma cell markers CD138 and VS38c in the absence the B-cell marker CD20,[65] indicating that the neoplastic cells of this lymphoma usually have the features of plasmablasts and not of B cells.

In addition, the tumor cells also characteristically strongly express EMA but are negative for lineage-associated leukocyte antigens (CD3, CD20, CD79a).[65] CD45 is weak or negative.[65] CD30 is negative,[65] although focal and weak staining has been reported in few cases.[66] Most tumors express cytoplasmic Ig (usually IgA, more rarely IgG) with light-chain restriction.[65] As described in some plasma cell tumors, occasional cases are positive for cytokeratin, which, in addition to EMA positivity and weak/negative staining for CD45, may lead to the mistaken diagnosis of carcinoma.[66] The tumors may be also positive for CD4, CD57, MUM-1/IRF4,[66] focally for CD43, and perforin.[66] These tumors should be distinguished from CD30-positive ALK-positive T/Null ALCL and DLBCL with plasmablastic features lacking the expression of the ALK.[57]

Genetics

The defining oncogenic factor is the expression of ALK fusion protein due to a genetic alteration of the *ALK* locus on chromosome 2 at p23. The most frequent fusion partner is *CLATHRIN*, which is located on chromosome 17 at q23.[59,64,67] In a few cases, the ALK protein is fused with NPM, like in ALK-positive ALCL T/Null.[61,68] A cryptic insertion of 3′*ALK* gene sequences into chromosome 4q22-24 has also been reported.[66]

Clinical features

Most patients present with advanced stage III/IV. The overall median survival of patients with stage III/IV patients is 11 months.[58] Long survival (more than 156 months) has been reported in children.[61,65] Since this tumor is usually negative for CD20 antigen, it is insensitive to Rituximab.

DLBCL associated with chronic inflammation

Characteristics

Permanent activation and proliferation of lymphoid cells (e.g. chronic inflammation) over long periods of time always bear the risk of developing into malignant disorders. Pyothorax-associated lymphoma might serve as an example for such a setting, where, after many years, EBV-associated DLBCL evolve on the basis of a persistent chronic inflammation. However, it may also arise in association with inflammation caused by chronic osteomyelitis, metallic implants, or chronic skin ulcer.

Epidemiology: geographic and age distribution

Although initially described for patients in Japan, pyothorax-associated lymphoma and related lymphoma may also arise in other parts of the world.[69] Owing to the longstanding course of the disease, the real incidence might be underestimated. Strikingly, males are much more affected than females (12:1), and the median age at presentation of the disease is in the late 7th decade of life.[70]

Sites of involvement

DLBCL associated with chronic inflammation might potentially develop at any site. Patients suffering from pyothorax-associated lymphoma show, at presentation, tumor masses in the pleura and, to a less extent, and/or in the lung.

Histology and immunophenotype

DLBCL associated with chronic inflammation, including pyothorax-associated lymphoma, are composed of tumor cells with the morphology of centroblasts, which are often admixed with a significant number of immunoblasts. The immunophenotype of the tumor cells is consistent with a derivation from activated late B cells, demonstrating positivity for CD20, CD79a, and IRF4 and, in some cases, CD138, and negativity for CD10 and BCL-6. In some cases CD20 or CD79a are missing or weakly expressed due to an advanced plasmocytic differentiation of the tumor cells.[71] The proliferation rate, as evidenced by Ki-67 immunostaining, is usually as high as in other DLBCL variants. Interestingly, an aberrant co-expression of T-cell typical antigens such as CD2, CD3, and CD4 is observed in a substantial number of DLBCL cases associated with chronic inflammation[73] and CD30 is found to be expressed in some cases.[74]

Since EBV infection is present in most cases of DLBCL associated with chronic inflammation, EBER in-situ hybridization reveals positivity in the majority of tumor cells. In addition, the EBV-encoded proteins LMP-1 and EBNA-2 are expressed by the tumor cells indicative for a type III latency infection.[74]

Pathogenesis, genetics, and molecular genetic findings

The frequent EBV infection of the tumor cells with a type III latency pattern suggests an important role of the virus in the pathogenesis of DLBCL associated with chronic inflammation. However, it is unlikely that EBV alone might be the sole cause for tumor development. Instead, active EBV infection might help non-functional B cells to survive that would otherwise be eliminated by apoptosis. This assumption is supported by the observation that the immunoglobulin genes from cell lines and tissue specimens derived from DLBCL associated with chronic inflammation may harbor crippling mutations that prevent the expression of functional immunoglobulin genes.[74] It might well be that EBV rescues these cells from apoptosis. The prolonged survival of these cells allows the acquisition of additional aberrations that finally lead to the development of a DLBCL. This hypothesis fits quite nicely to the cytogenetic findings, which describe a complex karyotype in many pyothorax-associated lymphoma cases.[73]

Gene expression profiling of pyothorax-associated lymphoma led – in line with the immunophenotype – to the identification of an ABC-like pattern. However, in comparison to nodal DLBCL cases, pyothorax-associated lymphoma showed several differently expressed genes, underscoring the notion that DLBCL associated with chronic inflammation represents a distinct DLBCL subtype.[75] Notably, among the differently expressed genes, IFI27 (interferon α-inducible protein 27) shows the strongest up-regulation.

Clinical features

DLBCL associated with chronic inflammation is an aggressive disease. Patients suffering from pyothorax-associated lymphoma show, at presentation, tumor masses in the pleura and, to less extent, and/or in the lung. A treatment with CHOP or related regimens was administered in most published cases, and was supplemented in some cases with radiotherapy. The clinical outcome is mainly based on lactate dehydrogenase (LDH) level, performance status, and clinical stage. In particular, advanced pyothorax-associated lymphoma has a very poor prognosis, with a 5-year survival rate of merely 15%, whereas patients with early clinical stages may achieve stable complete remission.[73] The addition of Rituximab might improve the treatment success, and early-stage patients appear to benefit from surgical removal of the tumor.

Lymphomatoid granulomatosis

Characteristics

Lymphomatoid granulomatosis (LYG) is an angiocentric and angiodestructive EBV-driven B-cell lymphoproliferative disorder associated with an exuberant T-cell reaction. It exclusively involves extranodal sites, most commonly the lung.

Epidemiology: geographic and age distribution

LYG is a rare disease that affects adults, but may occur in children suffering from immunodeficiency disorders. The male/female ratio is at least 2:1.[76]

Sites of involvement

The lung is (with over 90%) the most common site of primary manifestation. The lesions are most often bilateral in distribution, involving mid and lower lung fields. Brain, kidney, liver, and skin are also frequently involved, but at a much lower rate, ranging between 25 and 50%. Lymph nodes and spleen are usually spared.[76]

Morphology and immunophenotype

LYG lesions vary in size and can reach several centimeters in diameter. Larger nodules are usually associated with central necrosis.[1,76,77]

Histologically, LYG is characterized by an angocentric and angiodestructive polymorphous lymphoid infiltrate consisting of EBV-positive large B cells a prominent inflammatory

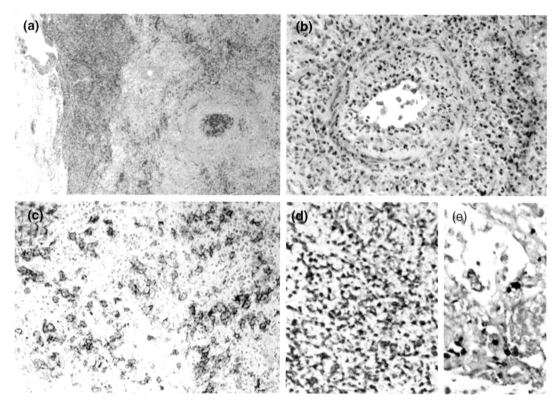

Figure 9.4 Lymphomatoid granulomatosis: (a) H&E staining, lung; (b) grade I lesion (lung), showing a polymorphous infiltrate in the vascular wall (H&E); (c) CD20, grade II lesion – note the large polymorphic B-cells; (d) CD3, grade II lesion with dense T-cell background; (e) EBER in-situ hybridization demonstrating an EBV infection of the polymorphic B cells. Photographs courtesy of Dr Judith Ferry, Boston, MA, USA.

background of small T cells.[76] The EBV-infected B cells vary in shape, ranging from immunoblast-like morphology to a more pleomorphic appearance. Hodgkin-like cells and multinucleated cells may be present. These are usually positive for CD20 and CD30, but not for CD15.[1,78,79] LMP1 is detectable in a variable fraction of the EBV-infected B cells. The most sensitive technique for the detection of EBV-infected cells is the EBER in-situ hybridization. This technique identifies all EBV-infected cells. Most of the background cells are CD3+, with CD4+ cells being more frequent than CD8+ of small cells (Fig 9.4).[76] A further characteristic feature is the infiltration of the vascular walls by lymphoid cells, frequently associated with fibrinoid necrosis. The vascular damage leads to the frequently seen infarct-like tissue necrosis. A prominent granulomatous reaction is typically seen in the subcutis of the skin.[80]

Grading

Three grades are distinguished, based on the relation of EBV-infected B cells to the amount of reactive T cells.[76,78] If the EBV-positive immunoblast-like B cells form uniform sheets, the lesion should be classified as diffuse large B-cell lymphoma.

- Grade 1 lesions: the lymphoid background predominates. The EBER in-situ hybridization demonstrates only few EBV-infected B cells (<5 per high power field).[81]
- Grade 2 lesions contain readily identifiable EBV-infected large lymphoid B cells or B immunoblasts in a polymorphous background (5–20/high power field). Areas of tissue necrosis are more frequently seen than in grade 1 lesions.
- Grade 3 lesions are characterized by larger aggregates of pleomorphic and

Hodgkin-cell-like EBV-infected B cells (>50/high power filed) in a less pronounced inflammatory background. Necrotic areas are prominent.

Pathogenesis, genetics, and molecular genetic findings

EBV obviously plays a dominant pathogenetic role because there is good evidence that the virus drives the B cells to proliferate. Genetic alterations have not been identified. Underlying immunodeficiency appears to predispose to the development of LYG. It is suggested that either the EBV-infected B cells induce the cellular background or the cellular background is an expression of an immune response against the EBV-infected B cells or it is a combination of both.

Clinical features

The most common symptom is cough, followed by dyspnea and chest pain. In addition, there are often general symptoms, including fever, malaise, weight loss, neurological symptoms, arthralgias, and symptoms from the gastrointestinal tract. The symptoms in patients with CNS involvement depend on the site of involvement and include hearing loss, diplopia, dysarthria, ataxia, and altered mental status.[82,83]

In most patients LYG is associated with an aggressive clinical course. The median survival is reported to be <2 years. However, this value is based on a historical series.[77] More recent clinical studies have demonstrated favorable responses to chemotherapy with Rituximab for grade 3 lesions,[84,85] but there are adverse exceptions.[86] Durable remissions are seen in grade 1 and 2 lesions following an interferon-α 2b treatment.[79] LYG may progress to an EBV-positive diffuse large B-cell lymphoma.

Burkitt's lymphoma

Characteristics

Burkitt's lymphoma (BL) is a highly proliferating monomorphic B-cell lymphoma that usually occurs at extranodal sites. An *MYC* translocation is present in the vast majority of cases.

However, this translocation is not sufficient for the diagnosis of Burkitt's lymphoma, because it is also encountered in other types of lymphoma. Three variants of BL are recognized.

Epidemiology: geographic and age distribution

Burkitt's lymphoma in its endemic form is mainly found in equatorial Africa and some other subtropical areas (Asia, South America) and is usually associated with an EBV infection.[3] The sporadic variant of Burkitt's lymphoma as well as the immunodeficiency (acquired immunodeficiency syndrome [AIDS]-related) variant occurs throughout the world. Whereas endemic Burkitt's lymphoma arises almost exclusively in children, predominantly male, the sporadic and immunodeficiency-associated Burkitt's lymphoma develops in children and adults. Sporadic Burkitt's lymphoma accounts for 40% of all pediatric lymphoma in Western countries[87] and endemic Burkitt's lymphoma represents the most common malignancy in childhood in equatorial Africa.[88]

Sites of involvement

Endemic Burkitt's lymphoma occurs primarily in the jaws, facial bones and gastrointestinal tract in the majority of cases. Sporadic Burkitt's lymphoma predominantly arises in the ileocecal region and only seldom in the jaws. Immunodeficiency-associated Burkitt's lymphoma may arise at various anatomical sites, including the lymph nodes.[92]

Histology and immunophenotype

The characteristic morphology of Burkitt's lymphoma is a monomorphic and cohesive growth pattern consisting of medium-sized cells. The cytoplasm of the tumor cells is basophil and the nuclei show a dispersed chromatin, with several paracentrally located nucleoli (Fig 9.5a). Many mitotic and apoptotic cell figures are indicative of an extremely high rate of proliferation, which is accompanied by extensive cell death. To remove the cell debris, many huge macrophages are intermingled in the cohesive sheets of tumor cells, and thus cause the very characteristic starry

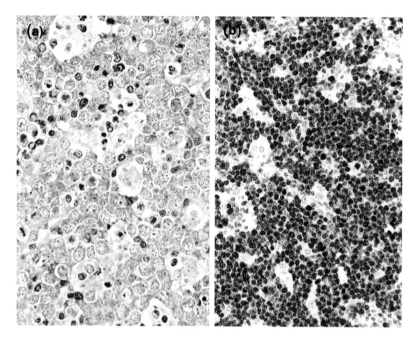

Figure 9.5   Burkitt's lymphoma: (a) Giemsa; (b) Ki-67 (APAAP). Nearly 100% of the BL cells show a stong nuclear expression.

sky impression when viewed at low microscopic magnification.[3] In a substantial number of cases, the morphology of the tumor cells resembles that of centroblasts, making a clear-cut delineation from DLBCL difficult or impossible.

Typically, the immunophenotype of Burkitt's lymphoma is suggestive for a germinal center origin of the tumor cells, with a positivity for CD10, BCL-6, CD38, and CD77. The tumor cells are always negative for TdT, but may express BCL-2 in some cases of sporadic and immunodeficiency Burkitt's lymphoma. In line with the many mitotic cell figures, the growth fraction, as evidenced by means of Ki-67 immunostaining, is extremely high and usually reaches almost 100% (Fig 9.5b).[89]

Pathogenesis, genetics, and molecular genetic findings

Despite the overlapping morphological and immunophenotypical features of endemic, sporadic, and immunodeficiency-associated Burkitt's lymphoma, there is a marked difference in their association with EBV. Whereas EBV is found in almost all cases of endemic Burkitt's lymphoma, EBV is present in only a minority of the non-endemic Burkitt's lymphomas (about 20% in sporadic Burkitt's lymphoma;[90] about 30% in immunodeficiency-associated Burkitt's lymphoma).[91] This sheds some doubt on the pathogenic role of EBV as a cause for this disease.

The translocation involving the *c-MYC* gene is found in the vast majority of Burkitt's lymphoma cases. In most cases the chromosomal translocation partner of the *c-MYC* gene is the immunoglobulin heavy-chain gene causing into a translocation t(8;14). As a result of this translocation, the *MYC* expression is brought under the control of the immunoglobulin promoter, leading to a constant up-regulation of the *MYC* gene activity. In a smaller number of cases, the *MYC* translocation includes the immunoglobulin light-chains genes (Ig κ [15%] or Ig λ [5%]; t(8;22 or t(2;8)), which also leads to a constant overexpression of the *MYC* gene due to the transcriptional control of the immunoglobulin expression. Cases of Burkitt's lymphoma without *MYC* translocations or with *MYC* translocation involving non-immunoglobulin partners are extremely rare.[92] Although *MYC* gene translocations are present in the vast majority of cases, this chromosomal aberration is not specific for Burkitt's lymphoma. In addition to Burkitt's lymphoma, *MYC* translocations are also detectable in other types of lymphoma, including DLBCL, follicular lymphoma, and plasmacytoma.[93]

Interestingly, the location of breakpoints in the immunoglobulin heavy-chain gene that occur in the course of the *MYC* translocation differ in the Burkitt's lymphoma variants. Whereas in endemic Burkitt's lymphoma the break mainly occurs in the VDJ region of the immunoglobulin gene, in sporadic and immunodeficiency-associated Burkitt's lymphoma the breakpoint is located in the immunoglobulin switch region.[94] This clearly indicates that the translocational event occurs at two different stages of the B-cell development. In endemic Burkitt's lymphoma, the translocation occurs early in the B-cell development, during VDJ recombination in the bone marrow, whereas in sporadic and immunodeficiency-associated Burkitt's lymphoma the translocation happens in the course of the germinal center reaction as an accident of the class switch recombination.

In addition to the different immunoglobulin breakpoints, the pattern of somatic immunoglobulin gene mutations is also different among the Burkitt's lymphoma variants. Endemic Burkitt's lymphoma harbors significantly more somatic Ig hypermutations than sporadic Burkitt's lymphoma cases.[95]

In an attempt to better discriminate Burkitt's lymphoma from other types of aggressive mature B-cell lymphomas, global gene expression profiling was performed.[96,97] By this approach, a molecular Burkitt's lymphoma expression signature was developed which was able to identify Burkitt's lymphoma among other aggressive mature B-cell lymphomas with high reliability. These molecularly defined Burkitt's lymphoma cases share a highly homogeneous gene expression profile, usually with only few chromosomal losses and gains. All cases display a gene expression pattern compatible with a germinal center origin of the tumor cells, including positivity for CD10 and BCL-6. However, not all molecular Burkitt's lymphoma cases display an *MYC* breakpoint and some cases demonstrated an expression of BCL-2. Strikingly, different molecular Burkitt's lymphoma signatures are able to identify the same set of cases in independent case selections.

Clinical features

The Burkitt's lymphoma variants differ not only with regard to EBV infection, *MYC* breakpoint characteristics, and Ig somatic mutation pattern but also in the anatomical sites of involvement.

Owing to its extremely high proliferation rate, Burkitt's lymphoma often presents as a bulky disease with a high tumor burden. Despite (or because) of this rapid tumor cells growth, chemotherapeutic intervention is successful in the majority of cases.[98] This holds especially true when the patients are very young (<16 years old) and when short and very intensive chemotherapeutic protocols (e.g. the BFM protocol) are applied. In these cases, a cure rate of >90% can be reached.[99] Owing to the rapid and effective killing of tumor cells, the patients have to be carefully monitored to avoid tumor cell lysis syndrome. Adverse clinical outcome in children as well as in adults is associated with advanced-stage, and/or bulky disease and bone marrow/CNS involvement.

B-cell lymphoma with features intermediate between diffuse large B-cell lymphoma and Burkitt's lymphoma

Characteristics

Lymphomas with features of both DLBCL and Burkitt's lymphoma cannot be reliably allocated to one of these entities based on current diagnostic potentials. Previously, these cases were lumped together as atypical Burkitt's lymphomas. Gene expression profiling studies[96] reveal that most of these cases are more related to DLBCL than to Burkitt's lymphoma, but there are exceptions since some of the cases with a specific molecular Burkitt's lymphoma signature display the morphology of the centroblastic variant of DLBCL. In order to maintain the homogeneity of the category of BL and yet permit further characterization of these borderline cases, the 4th edition of the WHO classification has added a category of B-cell lymphoma with features intermediate between DLBCL and Burkitt's lymphoma.

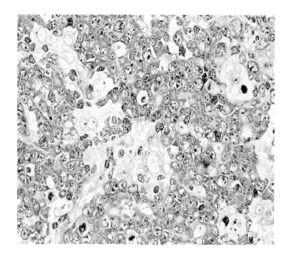

Figure 9.6   B-cell lymphoma with features intermediate between diffuse large B-cell lymphoma and Burkitt's lymphoma: Giemsa.

Epidemiology: geographic and age distribution

Lymphomas intermediate between Burkitt's lymphoma and DLBCL arise mainly at various extranodal sites without preferential localization, and bone marrow and peripheral blood are involved in a substantial number of cases. In contrast to Burkitt's lymphoma, adults are almost exclusively affected by these intermediate cases.

Sites of involvement

There are no dedicated anatomical sites at which B-cell lymphoma with features intermediate and Burkitt's lymphoma arise.

Histology and immunophenotype

The size of tumor cells range between those of DLBCL and Burkitt's lymphoma (Fig 9.6). Even in the same tissue specimen, areas with predominant Burkitt's lymphoma morphology may be present in parallel to areas with doubtless centroblastic tumor cells. Sometimes they may even resemble lymphoblastic lymphoma. The proliferation is usually high, as indicated by numerous mitotic figures, and is frequently accompanied by a starry sky appearance.[100]

The immunophenotype of the tumor cells is usually CD10 and BCL-6 positive and approximately half of the cases express in addition BCL-2. Of course, the tumor cells demonstrate the ordinary B-cell immunophenotype with expression of all pan B-cell markers. As expected from the presence of many mitotic figures, the percentage of Ki-67-positive cells is clearly higher than 60% in most cases.[101–103]

Pathogenesis, genetics, and molecular genetic findings

Cases with overlapping morphological features between Burkitt's lymphoma and DLBCL frequently demonstrate chromosomal breaks of the *MYC* gene (about 40%). In many of these cases the *MYC* gene is not fused to the immunoglobulin heavy- or light-chain gene but, instead, to other chromosomes involving non-immunoglobulin genes.[96] Strikingly, in a substantial number of cases, additional chromosomal translocation (such as t(14;18), involving the *BCL-2* gene) are detectable ('double hit'). These 'double hit' cases appear to be more susceptible for an overall higher genetic complexity.[104] Interestingly, these morphologically intermediate cases display a gene expression profile that is also in between molecularly defined Burkitt's lymphoma (mBL) and DLBCL lacking the *mBL* gene signature.[96]

Clinical features

Cases with intermediate features between Burkitt's lymphoma and DLBCL represent a clinically aggressive lymphoma. This holds especially true for cases with the presence of *MYC* breaks and/or double hit, which are associated with a fatal clinical outcome. Currently established therapeutic regimens are insufficient to treat the patients satisfactory.[96,102]

B-cell lymphoma with features intermediate between diffuse large B-cell lymphoma and classical Hodgkin's lymphoma

Characteristics

This category of neoplasms comprises large B-cell lymphomas with overlapping morphological

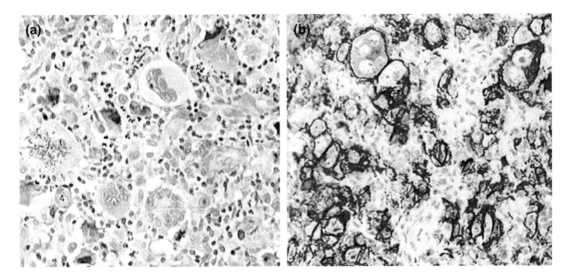

Figure 9.7   B-cell lymphoma with features intermediate between diffuse large B-cell lymphoma and classical Hodgkin's lymphoma: (a) H&E staining; (b) CD30 (APAAP).

and/or immunophenotypical and clinical features between classical Hodgkin's lymphoma (cHL) and DLBCL, especially primary mediastinal DLBCL (PMBL) and anaplastic variant. These lymphomas occur most frequently in the anterior mediastinum, but similar cases have been reported to arise in peripheral lymph nodes as a primary site as well as in the mediastinum.

Epidemiology: geographic and age distribution

Most commonly, young men between 20 and 40 years old are affected. However, this lymphoma category has also been reported to occur in individuals as young as 13 years old and older than 70 years old.[105,106] Most reports on these cases are from Western countries.

Sites of involvement

Patients present most commonly with a large anterior mediastinal mass with or without involvement of supraclavicular lymph nodes.[105,106] Other lymph node groups are less commonly affected. This lymphoma may spread to the lung, liver, spleen, and bone marrow. Other non-lymphoid organs are rarely involved.

Histology and immunophenotype

Typical for this lymphoma category is a confluent, sheet-like growth of pleomorphic tumor cells in a diffusely fibrotic stroma (Fig 9.7a).[105,106] Focal fibrous bands may occur and occasionally with features of nodular sclerosis. The majority of the neoplastic cells are larger and more pleomorphic than in typical DLBCL, including PMBL. The pleomorphic cells may resemble lacunar cells and Hodgkin's cells. The cytological appearance is broad and may vary in different areas, ranging from cHL-like to more DLBCL-like. The amount of admixed inflammatory cells is usually low but scattered eosinophils, lymphocytes, and histiocytes may be present.

The immunophenotype of the lymphoma cells is characterized by features between cHL and PMBL.[105,107] In contrast to cHL, the B-cell program is often preserved, with CD20 being strongly expressed but with immunoglobulin and CD10 being absent. In contrast to cHL, the transcription factors PAX5, OCT-2, and

BOB.1 are usually expressed. Unlike typical DLBCL, the tumor cells usually express CD30 (Fig 9.7b) and CD15. ALK is consistently absent.

Pathogenesis, genetics, and molecular genetic findings

On the whole, little is known about the pathogenesis. Since the morphological and immunophenotypical appearance can vary within the same or in subsequent tumor biopsies, it is speculated that epigenetic factors rather than genetic alterations are responsible for the change in morphology and immunophenotype. EBV may act as cofactor in up to 20% of the cases.

Clinical features

At diagnosis, the disease is advanced (stage III-IV) in most instances. A superior vena cava syndrome or respiratory distress is often seen in patients with a large mediastinal mass. The clinical course is more aggressive and the outcome is worse when compared with cHL or PMBL. There is no consensus about treatment modalities and clinical trial data are not available.

Anaplastic large cell lymphoma

Anaplastic large cell lymphoma (ALCL) was originally defined by Stein et al on the basis of its characteristic morphology of a frequent cohesive proliferation of large pleomorphic blasts, a constant expression of the CD30 molecule on all neoplastic cells,[108] and a consistent T-cell genotype.[109]

In the late 1980s and 1990s a cutaneous type of ALCL and an ALCL type with a translocation between chromosome 2 and 5 were recognized, leading to the distinction of three types of ALCL: systemic ALCL t(2;5)+; systemic ALCL t(2;5)−; and cutaneous ALCL. Cloning of the t(2;5) identified a fusion gene consisting of the nucleophosmin (*NPM*) gene at the breakpoint of chromosome 5 and a novel gene at the breakpoint of chromosome 2, which was designated anaplastic lymphoma kinase (*ALK*).[110] A

reliable detection of the t(2;5) in archival biopsies became possible when a formol-resistant monoclonal antibody directed to the ALK protein was generated.[111] The immunohistological investigation of several hundreds of ALCL cases revealed that 40–60% of this lymphoma category express the ALK protein and thus carry the t(2;5) or its variants (see below). Since the ALK+ ALCL did not only differ from the ALK– ALCL by the presence of the t(2;5) but also in age distribution and response to therapy, it was concluded that the ALCL with the t(2;5) represents an own disease entity, distinct from the ALCL lacking the t(2;5). On the basis of these findings and conclusions, the following subclassification of ALCL and terminology was generally accepted and will be included in the WHO classification of 2008:

- systemic ALCL ALK+
- systemic ALCL ALK–
- cutaneous ALCL.

In this chapter the two types of systemic ALCL are described. The cutaneous type of ALCL is discussed in Chapter 22.

Anaplastic large cell lymphoma, ALK positive

Characteristics

ALCL ALK+ is a T-cell lymphoma composed of CD30+ large pleomorphic cells with a translocation involving the *ALK* gene and expression of the ALK protein.

Epidemiology

ALCL ALK+ is a rare disease in adults (2–3% of adult non-Hodgkin's lymphomas) but is relatively common in children (10–20% of all childhood lymphomas).[112,113] Males predominate, with a ratio 1.7:1.

Sites of involvement

ALCL ALK+ arises in lymph nodes and extranodal sites (Tables 9.7 and 9.8). In extranodal

Table 9.7 Clinical and laboratory characteristics of
ALCL ($n = 159$)[164]

Symptoms/findings	ALK+ ALCL(%)	ALK− ALCL(%)
Age < 60 years old	86	58
Median age	34 years old	57 years old
Male:female	1.7:1	1.5:1
Stage III/IV	65	58
IPI 0/1	41	49
IPI 2/3	44	37
IPI 4/5	15	15
LDH	37	46
Bulky disease	20	1
B symptoms	60	57

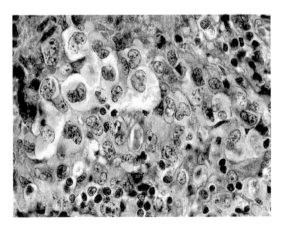

Figure 9.8 Anaplastic large cell lymphoma (ALK+):
Giemsa.

sites, skin, bone, soft tissues, lung, and liver are most commonly involved.[108,113,114] The bone marrow is affected in approximately 30% of cases. The small cell variant of ALCL tends to disseminate into the blood.[115,116]

Histology and immunophenotype

The morphology is heterogeneous. Five different patterns have been described.[3,112,115,117–121] The *common pattern*, with an incidence of 60%, is most common. It demonstrates the 'classic' morphology of ALCL. All tumor cells are large. The cytoplasm is abundant and ranges from clear to basophilic or eosinophilic. Most cells are mononuclear, but mutlinucleated cells may occur. Typically, the nuclei are eccentrically located, horseshoe- or kidney-shaped, and often have an eosinophilic region near the nucleus. The nuclei have an open chromatin with multiple small, basophilic nucleoli (Fig 9.8). These cells have been designated *hallmark cells*.[112] In some instances the nuclei are more prominent. Immunophenotypically, all of the tumor cells are strongly positive for CD30 and perforin. CD30 is expressed on the cell membrane and in the Golgi region, whereas the perforin expression is restricted to the cytoplasm. The T-cell

expression program is often only partially present or may be even totally extinct. B-cell markers, including PAX5, are consistently absent. In lymph nodes the tumor cells may disseminate in sinuses and thus resemble metastatic non-lymphoid malignancy.

The second most frequent pattern is the *lymphohistiocytic pattern* (10%). In this variant, the tumor cells are admixed with an exuberant number of reactive histiocytes.[112,119,120] The tumor cells are usually smaller than in the common pattern and may be masked by the predominance of histiocytes. The tumor cells are easily identifiable by immunostaining with antibodies to CD30, perforin, and/or ALK. The tumor cells may cluster around vessels. Erythrophagocytosis by the reactive histiocytes, but never by the tumor cells, may be seen. (Fig 9.9)

The *small cell pattern* (5–10%) is characterized by a predominance of small to medium-sized neoplastic cells with irregular nuclei (Fig 9.10a).[112,115,119,121] Hallmark cells are intermingled as single cells or in clusters in all instances. The expression of CD30 is weak to absent in the smaller cells but strong in the hallmark cells, whereas perforin is detectable in all tumor cells.

The *Hodgkin-like pattern* (3%) is characterized by the presence of Hodgkin-like and Reed–Sternberg-like cells associated within a nodular sclerosis.[122]

The fifth variant is the *composite pattern* (15%). It shows more than one of the above patterns.[112]

It is important to note that an EBV infection of the tumor cells has not been reported yet.[123]

Expression pattern of anaplastic lymphoma kinase

The ALK staining of large neoplastic cells is both cytoplasmic and nuclear in ALK+ ALCL cases carrying the typical t(2;5), which results in the formation of a fusion protein consisting of NPM-ALK.[112,119,124] In the small cell variant (Fig 9.10a), the ALK positivity is restricted to the nucleus of the smaller tumor cells.[111,112,119,124] In approximately 20% of the ALK+ cases, the ALK protein is detectable only outside of the nucleus, either in the cytoplasm or on the membrane. This is indicative of a variant chromosomal translocation (see below).[111,112,119,124]

Pathogenesis, genetics, and molecular genetic findings

Ninety percent of the ALK+ ALCL cases carry a clonal T-cell genotype. Whether in the remainder a clonal rearrangement of the T-cell receptor genes is really absent or whether this is due to technical reasons remains to be seen.[109]

In all ALK+ ALCL cases, a chromosomal translocation involving the *ALK* gene is present. The most frequent translocation juxtaposes the *ALK* gene on chromosome 2 to the *NPM* gene on chromosome 5. In the remainder of cases the *ALK* gene is fused with genes present on chromosomes 1, 2, 3, 17, 19, 22, or X.[120,124–135] All translocations result in an up-regulation of ALK, but the subcellular distribution of the ALK protein varies, dependent on the type of the translocation and the morphologic variant of the ALK+ ALCL.

The *ALK* gene encodes a tyrosine kinase receptor belonging to the insulin receptor superfamily, which is normally silent in lymphoid cells.[110] In the t(2;5)(p23;35), the catalytic domain of the ALK protein is activated by all the proteins with which ALK is fused. The ALK protein activation obviously plays a crucial role in the development of ALK+ ALCL, since its down-regulation results in a massive apoptosis.[136]

ALK+ ALCLs demonstrate frequent secondary chromosomal imbalances, including losses of chromosomes 4, 11q, and 13q and gains of 7, 17p, and 17q, which might contribute to the pathogenesis of this lymphoma type.[2]

Clinical features

The prognosis of ALK+ ALCL is much more favorable (5-year survival rate close to 80%) than that of ALK– ALCL (5-year survival rate 40%). The outcome does not differ between the cases with the standard t(2;5) and the variant translocation.[113,120,137,138] However, it seems that the small cell variant has a worse prognosis, maybe because patients with this variant often present with disseminated disease at diagnosis. Relapses have been observed in 30% of cases. These patients often remain sensitive to chemotherapy. Allogeneic bone marrow transplantation may be effective in refractory cases.[139]

Anaplastic large cell lymphoma, ALK negative

Characteristics

ALK- ALCL is a CD30+ large cell pleomorphic T-cell neoplasm that is morphologically indistinguishable from the common variant of the ALK+ ALCL. It has to be distinguished from primary cutaneous ALCL and other CD30+ T-cell and B-cell neoplasms with anaplastic/pleomorphic features and cHL. In the 3rd edition of the WHO Classification ALK– ALCL and ALK+ ALCL were not separated from each other. However, this will be done in the 4th edition of the WHO Classification because the ALK– ALCL does not only differ from ALK+ ALCL by the chromosomal translocation consistently involving the *ALK* gene but also by a different age distribution and a different clinical outcome.[1]

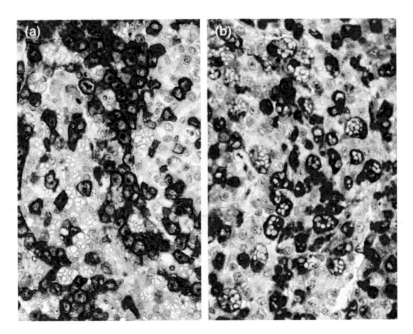

Figure 9.9   Anaplastic large cell lymphoma: (a) CD30 (APAAP); all tumor cells are strongly positive (b) CD68 (APAAP); all tumor cells are negative whereas the erythrophagocytosing histiocytes are strongly labelled. The anaplastic tumor cells express CD30, whereas the histocytes, which have phagocytosed erythrocytes, are CD30 negative.

Epidemiology: geographic and age distribution

ALK– ALCL mainly affects adults, with a peak incidence between 40 and 65 years old, in contrast to ALK+ ALCL, which most frequently arises in children and young adults. The male/female ratio is 1.5:1.[108,140]

Sites of involvement

Sites of primary development are lymph nodes or extranodal tissues. The latter include bone, soft tissues, gastrointestinal tract, and skin. Cases with skin involvement must be distinguished from primary cutaneous ALCL. This is not possible in all instances.

Histology and immunophenotype

The tumor cells are morphologically indistinguishable from those seen in the common variant of ALK+ ALCL. The neoplastic cells are large and pleomorphic and have an abundant cytoplasm, which might be clear to basophilic or eosinophilic. Most neoplastic cells are mononuclear, but multinucleated cells may be encountered. Typically, the nuclei are eccentrically located, horseshoe- or kidney-shaped, and often have an eosinophilic region near the nucleus. The nuclei have an open chromatin with multiple small, basophilic nucleoli. In some instances the nuclei are more prominent. In extranodal tissues, the tumor cells grow in cohesive sheets. In partially involved lymph nodes, there is – apart from a growth in cohesive sheets – a tumor cell growth in sinuses like in ALK+ ALCL. In contrast to ALK+ ALCL, a small cell or a lymphohistiocytic variant has not yet been identified in ALK- ALCL.[124]

A key and defining feature of ALK- ALCL is a strong expression of CD30 at the membrane and in the Golgi area of all tumor cells. This, in connection with all tumor cells being of large size, distinguishes ALK- ALCL from

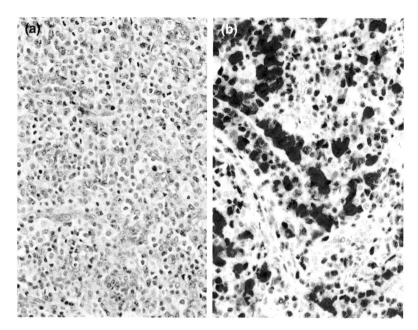

Figure 9.10   Anaplastic large cell lymphoma, small cell variant: (a) H&E staining and (b) ALK-1 (APAAP). The large tumor cells express ALK in the cytoplasm and the nucleus, whereas in the small tumor cells the expression of ALK is restricted to the nucleus.

peripheral T-cell lymphoma. In contrast to ALK+ ALCL, cytotoxic molecules, including perforin, are not found in the majority (but not in all of the cases). The T-cell expression program is only partially preserved and is less often extinct when compared with ALK+ positive ALCL.[124] This is also a feature in which ALK- ALCL differs from peripheral T-cell lymphoma NOS. There are no reports about the detection of EBV in ALK- ALCL tumor cells.

Pathogenesis, genetics, and molecular genetic findings

The majority of cases carry a clonal T-cell genotype,[109] irrespective of whether the neoplastic cells express T-cell antigens or not.

Two studies point to a tendency of ALK–ALCL to differ (e.g. in terms of chromosome losses or gains), both from peripheral T-cell lymphoma, NOS and from ALK-positive ALCL, although overlapping features can also be found.[141] However, recurrent primary genetic aberrations have not yet been reported, indicating that the pathogenesis of ALK– ALCL is still totally obscure.

Clinical features

The prognosis or response to current therapy is worse than for ALK+ ALCL.[142]

AGGRESSIVE EXTRANODAL NATURAL KILLER CELL LEUKEMIA/ LYMPHOMA

NK cells represent lymphocytes of the innate immune system which are localized in peripheral blood, bone marrow, lymph node, and spleen, and which patrol non-lymphoid organs. In the case of inflammation, the NK cells are ready to extravasate to tissues. The constitutive expression of a lytic gene expression machinery enables the NK cells to directly destroy infected or transformed cells without further activation. This activity is mediated by NK-cell receptors, which interact especially with MHC class I negative cells. Aggressive NK-cell leukemia and extranodal NK/T-cell lymphoma, nasal type, represent two highly aggressive extranodal neoplasms derived from NK cells.

Aggressive NK-cell leukemia

Characteristics

Aggressive NK-cell leukemia represents a systemic neoplastic proliferation of NK cells which are almost always infected by EBV. The clinical course is extremely aggressive. The systemic distribution of the NK cells means that the development and establishment of aggressive NK-cell leukemia is not restricted to lymphoid organs but also occurs at any anatomical site.

Epidemiology: geographic and age distribution

Males and females are equally affected, and the median age at presentation is in the third decade of life.[143] Aggressive NK-cell leukemia is a rare disease that is found predominantly in Asian countries.[144]

Sites of involvement

In contrast to other types of leukemias, the number of tumor cells in the peripheral blood is highly variable in aggressive NK-cell leukemia. In addition, liver and spleen as well as bone marrow are often found to be affected at presentation.[156]

Histology and immunophenotype

The morphology of the circulating tumor cells resembles large granular lymphocytes with a slightly immature appearance (Fig 9.11). At presentation, a distinction from extranodal NK/T-cell lymphoma and from chronic NK-cell lymphocytosis may be difficult in some cases. The cytoplasm is broad and pale, with azurophilic granules and occasional nucleoli.[145] Organ-infiltrating tumor cells display a usually diffuse growth pattern, often accompanied by extended necrosis with or without angiocentricity and angiodestruction. The immunophenotype of aggressive NK-cell leukemia is characterized by an expression of CD2, CD56, and cytoplasmatic expression of CD3e (in the absence of surface CD3 expression).[153] In addition, an expression of cytotoxic molecules such as TIA1, perforin, and granzyme B is found. Finally, infection by EBV, as demonstrated by EBER in-situ hybridization, is a hallmark feature of aggressive NK-cell leukemia.[146]

Pathogenesis, genetics, and molecular findings

Besides the constant finding of EBV infection in aggressive NK-cell leukemia, which suggests a pathogenetic role of this virus, there is only very limited knowledge regarding molecular aberration leading to this disease. In some reports, deletions of chromosome 6q21-q25 are described as a recurrent genetic feature in aggressive NK-cell leukemia, as well as in extranodal NK/T-cell lymphoma.[147] However, more recent studies emphasize gains of 1q and loss of 7p15.1-p22.3 and 17p13.1 as genetic alterations more frequently found in aggressive NK-cell leukemia than in extranodal NK/T-cell lymphoma.[148]

Multiorgan involvement is usually found in patients suffering from aggressive NK-cell leukemia and indicates a specific role for chemokine receptors. Indeed, the up-regulation of the expression of CXCR1 and of CCR5 in the tumor cells of aggressive NK-cell leukemia might contribute to the multiorgan involvement, especially in the light of high levels of their ligands in these patients.[149–151]

In line with the NK cell nature of the tumor cells, rearrangements of the T-cell receptor genes are not detectable in aggressive NK-cell leukemia.[152]

Clinical features

Aggressive NK-cell leukemia displays a disastrous clinical course, with a survival after initial diagnosis of several weeks or a few months

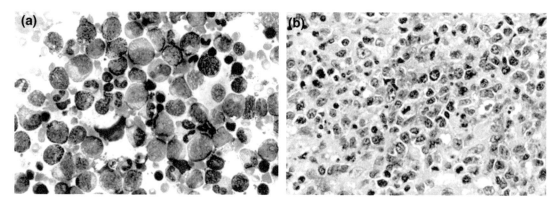

Figure 9.11   Aggressive NK-cell leukemia: (a) Giemsa, bone marrow aspirate; (b) H&E, histologic features of an aggressive NK-cell leukemia. Photographs courtsey of Dr Judith Ferry, Boston, MA, USA.

(median overall survival of 2 months).[153,154] The patients are usually already very ill at presentation, showing high fever, weight loss, and jaundice. Because of the highly variable number of circulating tumor cells, the white cell count is usually increased, but may vary dramatically among the patients. Because of early bone marrow infiltration, the patients suffer from anemia and thrombocytopenia.[155] The disease is mostly accompanied by hepatosplenomegaly and sometimes by lymphadenopathy and, at a later stage of the disease, dysfunction of the liver, dissemination of intravascular coagulates, and hemophagocytic syndrome are frequently observed. Most patients pass away very rapidly, despite intensive therapeutic intervention, and even bone marrow transplantation is unable to expand survival of the patients significantly.[153]

Extranodal NK/T-cell lymphoma, nasal type

Characteristics

Extranodal NK/T-cell lymphoma, nasal type, is mostly derived from NK cells but cytotoxic T cells represent the cell of origin in a few cases. As per definition, the nasal cavity is the primary location at presentation, but this disease may occasionally also arise at other anatomical sites. The strong association with EBV infections suggests a pathogenetic role of the virus. The clinical course is aggressive.

Epidemiology: geographic and age distribution

Extranodal NK/T-cell lymphoma, nasal type, occurs predominantly in Asian countries and, to a less extent, in Central and South America.[156,157] Males are significantly more often affected and the median age is in the 5th decade of life.

Sites of involvement

The nasal cavity is most frequently involved but the disease has also been encountered at other sites, e.g. testis, gastrointestinal tract, skin. At presentation, extranodal NK/T-cell lymphoma is often locally invasive, affecting surrounding tissues. Midfacial destructions (so-called midline granuloma) are frequently developed in the course of the disease. Dissemination into various organs such as intestine, liver, skin, and, at a lower frequency, involvement of bone marrow and nerve tissue, is a common characteristic of the disease.[158]

Histology and immunophenotype

The histological pattern of extranodal NK/T-cell lymphoma is broad, ranging from small to large, sometimes anaplastic, cells.[156] Especially in the early stages, the tumor cells might be inconspicuous and admixed with inflammatory cells causing diagnostic difficulties.[156] More advanced stages show extensive necrosis and ulceration accompanied by angiodestructive growth.[159]

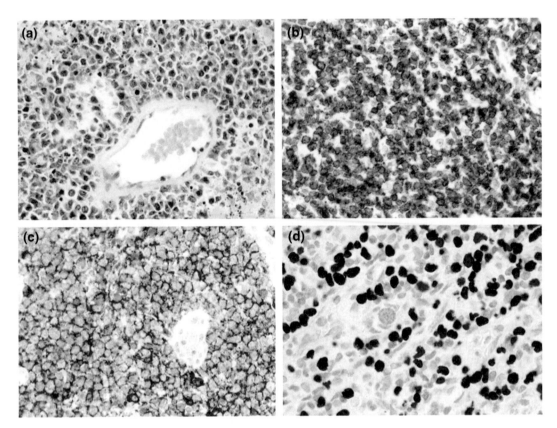

Figure 9.12   Extranodal NK/T-cell lymphoma, nasal type: (a) Giemsa staining; (b) CD30 (APAAP); (c) CD56 (APAAP); (d) EBER in-situ hybridization; EBV-infection of the tumor cells.

Based on the cell of origin, extranodal NK/T-cell lymphoma, nasal type, usually display an NK-cell immunophenotype, with expression of CD2, cytoplasmatic CD3e, and CD56. Whereas most other T-cell characteristic markers are negative, the presence of cytotoxic molecules such as TIA-1, perforin, and granzyme B is a consistent features.[156] A clonal episomal infection of all tumor cells by the EBV is found in almost all cases with rare exceptions. EBER in-situ hybridization, which is able to detect even small numbers of EBV-infected tumor cells, is an important ancillary characteristic, especially at the early stages of the disease (Fig 9.12).[160]

Pathogenesis, genetics, and molecular genetic findings

Little is known regarding the pathogenesis of extranodal NK/T-cell lymphoma, nasal type.

Some observations suggest that – in addition to a pathogenetic role of the EBV – mutations in the tumor suppressor genes such as p53, p16INK4A, p15INK4B, p14ARF, and Rb, or their promoter methylation, prevent proper functionality and/or expression.[161] Recurrent chromosomal aberrations are gains of 2q, and losses of 6q, 11q, 5p14.1-p14.3, 5q34-q35.3, 1p36.23-p36.33, 2p16.1-p16.3, 4q12, and 4q31.3-q32.1.[148] Some of the chromosomal losses may also be associated with the loss of function of important factors that are known to be involved in cell cycle control or DNA repair, such as TP53, β-catenin, K-RAS, or C-KIT.

T-cell receptor genes are in germline configuration in the vast majority of cases of extranodal NK/T-cell lymphoma, nasal type. In a few cases, clonal T-cell receptor rearrangements are detectable, which points to a derivation of the tumor cells from cytotoxic T cells in these cases.[152]

Clinical features

Advanced stages of the disease have a poor survival rate, with approximately 20% 5-year overall survival when CHOP-based regimens are applied. As a main complication at later stages hemophagocytic syndrome are experienced in extranodal NK/T-cell lymphoma.[162] An improvement of the outcome is described by combined radiotherapy and CMED (cyclophosphamide, methotrexate, etoposide, and dexamethasone) chemotherapy.[163] Although the identification of prognostic factors is difficult, owing to the rarity of the disease, the LDH level, B symptoms, performance status, and stage appear to be promising for the prediction of clinical outcome.

REFERENCES

1. Jaffe ES, Harris NL, Stein H, Vardiman JW. Pathology and genetics of tumors of hematopoietic and lymphoid tissues. In: Kleihues P, Sobin L, eds. World Health Organization Classification of Tumours, 3rd edn. Lyon: IARC Press, 2001.
2. Swerdlow SH, et al. Pathology and genetics of tumors of hematopoietic and lymphoid tissues. In: xx, eds. World Health Organization Classification of Tumours, 4th edn. Lyon: IARC Press (in press)
3. Harris NL, Jaffe ES, Stein H, et al. A revised European-American classification of lymphoid neoplasms: a proposal from the International Lymphoma Study Group. Blood 1994; 84: 1361–92.
4. A clinical evaluation of the International Lymphoma Study Group classification of non-Hodgkin's lymphoma. Blood 1997; 89: 3909–18.
5. Armitage JO, Weisenburger DD. New approach to classifying non-Hodgkin's lymphomas: clinical features of the major histologic subtypes. J Clin Oncol 1998; 16: 2780–95.
6. Harris NL, Jaffe ES, Diebold J, et al. The World Health Organization Classification of Hematological Malignancies. Report of the Clinical Advisory Committee Meeting – Airlie House, Virginia, November, 1997. Ann Oncol 1999; 10: 1419–32.
7. Chung R, Lai R, Wei P, et al. Concordant but not discordant bone marrow involvement in diffuse large B-cell lymphoma predicts a poor clinical outcome independent of the International Prognostic Index. Blood 2007; 110(4): 1278–82.
8. Engelhard M, Brittinger G, Huhn D, et al. Subclassification of diffuse large B-cell lymphomas according to the Kiel classification: distinction of centroblastic and immunoblastic lymphomas is a significant prognostic risk factor. Blood 1997; 89(7): 2291–7.
9. Lennert K, Feller AC. Histopathology of Non-Hodgkin's Lymphoma, 2nd edn. New York: Springer Verlag, 1992.
10. Haralambieva E, Pulford KA, Lamant L, et al. Anaplastic large-cell lymphomas of B-cell phenotype are anaplastic lymphoma kinase (ALK) negative and belong to the spectrum of diffuse large B-cell lymphomas. Br J Haematol 2000; 109(3): 584–91.
11. Stein H, Foss HD, Dürkop H, et al. CD30(+) anaplastic large cell lymphoma: a review of its histopathologic, genetic, and clinical features. Blood 2000; 96(12): 3681–95.
12. Loddenkemper C, Anagnostopoulos I, Hummel M, et al. Differential Emu enhancer activity and expression of BOB.1/OBF.1, Oct2, PU.1, and immunoglobulin in reactive B-cell populations, B-cell non-Hodgkin lymphomas, and Hodgkin lymphomas. J Pathol 2004; 202(1): 60–9.
13. Piris M, Brown DC, Gatter KC, Mason DY. CD30 expression in non-Hodgkin's lymphoma. Histopathology 1990; 17(3): 211–18.
14. Tagawa H, Suguro M, Tsuzuki S, et al. Comparison of genome profiles for identification of distinct subgroups of diffuse large B-cell lymphoma. Blood 2005; 106(5): 1770–7.
15. Yamaguchi M, Seto M, Okamoto M, et al. De novo CD5+ diffuse large B-cell lymphoma: a clinicopathologic study of 109 patients. Blood 2002; 99(3): 815–21.
16. Matolcsy A, Chadburn A, Knowles DM. De novo CD5-positive and Richter's syndrome-associated diffuse large B cell lymphomas are genotypically distinct. Am J Pathol 1995; 147(1): 207–16.
17. de Leval L, Harris NL. Variability in immunophenotype in diffuse large B-cell lymphoma and its clinical relevance. Histopathology 2003; 43(6): 509–28.
18. Muris JJ, Meijer CJ, Vos W, et al. Immunohistochemical profiling based on Bcl-2, CD10 and MUM1 expression improves risk stratification in patients with primary nodal diffuse large B cell lymphoma. J Pathol 2006; 208(5): 714–23.
19. Gascoyne RD, Adomat SA, Krajewski S, et al. Prognostic significance of Bcl-2 protein expression and Bcl-2 gene rearrangement in diffuse aggressive non-Hodgkin's lymphoma. Blood 1997; 90(1): 244–51.
20. Barrans SL, Fenton JA, Banham A, Owen RG, Jack AS. Strong expression of FOXP1 identifies a distinct subset of diffuse large B-cell lymphoma (DLBCL) patients with poor outcome. Blood 2004; 104(9): 2933–5.
21. Weiss LM, Strickler JG, Medeiros LJ, et al. Proliferative rates of non-Hodgkin's lymphomas as assessed by Ki-67 antibody. Hum Pathol 1987; 18(11): 1155–9.

22. Miller TP, Grogan TM, Dahlberg S, et al. Prognostic significance of the Ki-67-associated proliferative antigen in aggressive non-Hodgkin's lymphomas: a prospective Southwest Oncology Group trial. Blood 1994; 83(6): 1460–6.

23. Young KH, Weisenburger DD, Dave BJ, et al. Mutations in the DNA-binding codons of TP53, which are associated with decreased expression of TRAILreceptor-2, predict for poor survival in diffuse large B-cell lymphoma. Blood 2007; 110(13): 4396–405.

24. Leroy K, Haioun C, Lepage E, et al; Groupe d'Etude des Lymphomes de l'Adulte. p53 gene mutations are associated with poor survival in low and low-intermediate risk diffuse large B-cell lymphomas. Ann Oncol 2002; 13(7): 1108–15.

25. Chilosi M, Doglioni C, Magalini A, et al. p21/WAF1 cyclin-kinase inhibitor expression in non-Hodgkin's lymphomas: a potential marker of p53 tumor-suppressor gene function. Blood 1996; 88(10): 4012–20.

26. Koduru PR, Raju K, Vadmal V, et al. Correlation between mutation in P53, p53 expression, cytogenetics, histologic type, and survival in patients with B-cell non-Hodgkin's lymphoma. Blood 1997; 90(10): 4078–91.

27. Colomo L, López-Guillermo A, Perales M, et al. Clinical impact of the differentiation profile assessed by immunophenotyping in patients with diffuse large B-cell lymphoma. Blood 2003; 101(1): 78–84.

28. Bai M, Skyrlas A, Agnantis NJ, et al. Cluster analysis of apoptosis-associated bcl2 family proteins in diffuse large B-cell lymphomas. Relations with the apoptotic index, the proliferation profile and the B-cell differentiation immunophenotypes. Anticancer Res 2004; 24(5A): 3081–8.

29. Bea S, Zettl A, Wright G, et al; Lymphoma/Leukemia Molecular Profiling Project. Diffuse large B-cell lymphoma subgroups have distinct genetic profiles that influence tumor biology and improve gene-expression-based survival prediction. Blood 2005; 106(9): 3183–90.

30. De Paepe P, Achten R, Verhoef G, et al. Large cleaved and immunoblastic lymphoma may represent two distinct clinicopathologic entities within the group of diffuse large B-cell lymphomas. J Clin Oncol 2005; 23(28): 7060–8.

31. Huang JZ, Sanger WG, Greiner TC, et al. The t(14;18) defines a unique subset of diffuse large B-cell lymphoma with a germinal center B-cell gene expression profile. Blood 2002; 99(7): 2285–90.

32. Jost PJ, Ruland J. Aberrant NF-kappaB signaling in lymphoma: mechanisms, consequences, and therapeutic implications. Blood 2007; 109(7): 2700–7.

33. Staudt LM, Dave S. The biology of human lymphoid malignancies revealed by gene expression profiling. Adv Immunol 2005; 87: 163–208.

34. Melzner I, Weniger MA, Menz CK, Möller P. Absence of the JAK2 V617F activating mutation in classical Hodgkin lymphoma and primary mediastinal B-cell lymphoma. Leukemia 2006; 20(1): 157–8.

35. Barth TF, Döhner H, Werner CA, et al. Characteristic pattern of chromosomal gains and losses in primary large B-cell lymphomas of the gastrointestinal tract. Blood 1998; 91(11): 4321–30.

36. Haralambieva E, Adam P, Ventura R, et al. Genetic rearrangement of FOXP1 is predominantly detected in a subset of diffuse large B-cell lymphomas with extranodal presentation. Leukemia 2006; 20(7): 1300–3.

37. Jordanova ES, Riemersma SA, Philippo K, et al. Hemizygous deletions in the HLA region account for loss of heterozygosity in the majority of diffuse large B-cell lymphomas of the testis and the central nervous system. Genes Chromosomes Cancer 2002; 35(1): 38–48.

38. Dijkman R, Tensen CP, Jordanova ES, et al. Array-based comparative genomic hybridization analysis reveals recurrent chromosomal alterations and prognostic parameters in primary cutaneous large B-cell lymphoma. J Clin Oncol 2006; 24(2): 296–305.

39. McKelvey EM, Gottlieb JA, Wilson HE, et al. Hydroxyldaunomycin (Adriamycin) combination chemotherapy in malignant lymphoma. Cancer 1976; 38(4): 1484–93.

40. Fisher RI, Gaynor ER, Dahlberg S, et al. Comparison of a standard regimen (CHOP) with three intensive chemotherapy regimens for advanced non Hodgkin's lymphoma. N Engl J Med 1993; 328(14): 1002–6.

41. Sehn LH, Berry B, Chhanabhai M, et al. The revised International Prognostic Index (R-IPI) is a better predictor of outcome than the standard IPI for patients with diffuse large B-cell lymphoma treated with R-CHOP. Blood 2007; 109(5): 1857–61.

42. Winter JN, Weller EA, Horning SJ, et al. Prognostic significance of Bcl-6 protein expression in DLBCL treated with CHOP or R-CHOP: a prospective correlative study. Blood 2006; 107(11): 4207–13.

43. Shivakumar L, Armitage JO. Bcl-2 gene expression as a predictor of outcome in diffuse large B-cell lymphoma. Clin Lymphoma Myeloma 2006; 6(6): 455–7.

44. Berglund M, Thunberg U, Amini RM, et al. Evaluation of immunophenotype in diffuse large B-cell lymphoma and its impact on prognosis. Mod Pathol 2005; 18(8): 1113–20.

45. Iqbal J, Neppalli VT, Wright G, et al. BCL2 expression is a prognostic marker for the activated B-cell-like type of diffuse large B-cell lymphoma. J Clin Oncol 2006; 24(6): 961–8.

46. Hans CP, Weisenburger DD, Greiner TC, et al. Expression of PKC-beta or cyclin D2 predicts for inferior survival in diffuse large B-cell lymphoma. Mod Pathol 2005; 18(10): 1377–84.

47. Leroy K, Haioun C, Lepage E, et al; Groupe d'Etude des Lymphomes de l'Adulte. p53 gene mutations

are associated with poor survival in low and low-intermediate risk diffuse large B-cell lymphomas. Ann Oncol 2002; 13(7): 1108–15.

48. Muris JJ, Cillessen SA, Vos W, et al. Immunohistochemical profiling of caspase signaling pathways predicts clinical response to chemotherapy in primary nodal diffuse large B-cell lymphomas. Blood 2005; 105(7): 2916–23.

49. Natkunam Y, Farinha P, Hsi ED, et al. LMO2 protein expression predicts survival in patients with diffuse large B-cell lymphoma treated with anthracycline-based chemotherapy with and without rituximab. J Clin Oncol 2008; 26(3): 447–54.

50. Hans CP, Weisenburger DD, Greiner TC, et al. Confirmation of the molecular classification of diffuse large B-cell lymphoma by immunohistochemistry using a tissue microarray. Blood 2004; 103(1): 275–82.

51. Nyman H, Adde M, Karjalainen-Lindsberg ML, et al. Prognostic impact of immunohistochemically defined germinal center phenotype in diffuse large B-cell lymphoma patients treated with immunochemotherapy. Blood 2007; 109(11): 4930–5.

52. Lossos IS, Morgensztern D. Prognostic biomarkers in diffuse large B-cell lymphoma. J Clin Oncol 2006; 24(6): 995–1007.

53. Amen F, Horncastle D, Elderfield K, et al. Absence of cyclin-D2 and Bcl-2 expression within the germinal centre type of diffuse large B-cell lymphoma identifies a very good prognostic subgroup of patients. Histopathology 2007; 51(1): 70–9.

54. de Jong D, Rosenwald A, Chhanabhai M, et al; Lunenburg Lymphoma Biomarker Consortium. Immunohistochemical prognostic markers in diffuse large B-cell lymphoma: validation of tissue microarray as a prerequisite for broad clinical applications – a study from the Lunenburg Lymphoma Biomarker Consortium. J Clin Oncol 2007; 25(7): 805–12.

55. Rimsza LM, Roberts RA, Miller TP, et al. Loss of MHC class II gene and protein expression in diffuse large B-cell lymphoma is related to decreased tumor immunosurveillance and poor patient survival regardless of other prognostic factors: a follow-up study from the Leukemia and Lymphoma Molecular Profiling Project. Blood 2004; 103(11): 4251–8.

56. Delecluse HJ, Anagnostopoulos I, Dallenbach F, et al. Plasmablastic lymphomas of the oral cavity: a new entity associated with the human immunodeficiency virus infection. Blood 1997; 89(4): 1413–20.

57. Colomo L, Loong F, Rives S, et al. Diffuse large B-cell lymphomas with plasmablastic differentiation represent a heterogeneous group of disease entities. Am J Surg Pathol 2004; 28(6): 736–47.

58. Reichard KK, McKenna RW, Kroft SH. ALK-positive diffuse large B-cell lymphoma: report of four cases and review of the literature. Mod Pathol 2007; 20(3): 310–19.

59. De Paepe P, Baens M, van Krieken H, et al. ALK activation by the CLTC-ALK fusion is a recurrent event in large B-cell lymphoma. Blood 2003; 102(7): 2638–41.

60. Gesk S, Gascoyne RD, Schnitzer B, et al. ALK-positive diffuse large B-cell lymphoma with ALK–clathrin fusion belongs to the spectrum of pediatric lymphomas. Leukemia 2005; 19(10): 1839–40.

61. Onciu M, Behm FG, Downing JR, et al. ALK-positive plasmablastic B-cell lymphoma with expression of the NPM-ALK fusion transcript: report of 2 cases. Blood 2003; 102(7): 2642–4.

62. McManus DT, Catherwood MA, Carey PD, Cuthbert RJ, Alexander HD. ALK-positive diffuse large B-cell lymphoma of the stomach associated with a clathrin–ALK rearrangement. Hum Pathol 2004; 35(10): 1285–8.

63. Chikatsu N, Kojima H, Suzukawa K, et al. ALK+, CD30-, CD20- large B-cell lymphoma containing anaplastic lymphoma kinase (ALK) fused to clathrin heavy chain gene (CLTC). Mod Pathol 2003; 16(8): 828–32.

64. Gascoyne RD, Lamant L, Martin-Subero JI, et al. ALK-positive diffuse large B-cell lymphoma is associated with clathrin–ALK rearrangements: report of 6 cases. Blood 2003; 102(7): 2568–73.

65. Delsol G, Lamant L, Mariame B, et al. A new subtype of large B-cell lymphoma expressing the ALK kinase and lacking the 2; 5 translocation. Blood 1997; 89(5): 1483–90.

66. Stachurski D, Miron PM, Al Homsi S, et al. Anaplastic lymphoma kinase-positive diffuse large B-cell lymphoma with a complex karyotype and cryptic 3' ALK gene insertion to chromosome 4 q22–24. Hum Pathol 2007; 38(6): 940–5.

67. Isimbaldi G, Bandiera L, d'Amore ES, et al. ALK-positive plasmablastic B-cell lymphoma with the clathrin-ALK gene rearrangement. Pediatr Blood Cancer 2006; 46(3): 390–1.

68. Adam P, Katzenberger T, Seeberger H, et al. A case of a diffuse large B-cell lymphoma of plasmablastic type associated with the t(2;5)(p23; q35) chromosome translocation. Am J Surg Pathol 2003; 27(11): 1473–6.

69. Martin A, Capron F, Liguory-Brunaud MD. Epstein–Barr virus-associated primary malignant lymphomas of the pleural cavity occurring in longstanding pleural chronic inflammation. Hum Pathol 1994; 25(12): 1314–18.

70. Iuchi K, Ichimiya A, Akashi A, et al. Non-Hodgkin's lymphoma of the pleural cavity developing from long-standing pyothorax. Cancer 1987; 60: 1771–5.

71. Petitjean B, Jardin F, Joly B, et al. Pyothorax-associated lymphoma: a peculiar clinicopathologic entity derived from B cells at late stage of differentiation and with occasional aberrant dual B- and T-cell phenotype. Am J Surg Pathol 2002; 26(6): 724–32.

72. Androulaki A, Drakos E, Hatzianastassiou D, et al. Pyothorax-associated lymphoma (PAL): a western case with marked angiocentricity and review of the literature. Histopathology 2004; 44(1): 69–76.

73. Narimatsu H, Ota Y, Kami M, et al. Clinicopathological features of pyothorax-associated lymphoma; a retrospective survey involving 98 patients. Ann Oncol 2007; 18(1): 122–8.

74. Takakuwa T, Tresnasari K, Rahadiani N, et al. Cell origin of pyothorax-associated lymphoma: a lymphoma strongly associated with Epstein–Barr virus infection. Leukemia 2007; [Epub ahead of print].

75. Nishiu M, Tomita Y, Nakatsuka S, et al. Distinct pattern of gene expression in pyothorax-associated lymphoma (PAL), a lymphoma developing in long-standing inflammation. Cancer Sci 2004; 95(10): 828–34.

76. Jaffe ES, Wilson WH. Lymphomatoid granulomatosis: pathogenesis, pathology and clinical implications. Cancer Surv 1997; 30: 233–48.

77. Katzenstein AL, Carrington CB, Liebow AA. Lymphomatoid granulomatosis: a clinicopathologic study of 152 cases. Cancer 1979; 43(1): 360–73.

78. Guinee DG Jr, Perkins SL, Travis WD, et al. Proliferation and cellular phenotype in lymphomatoid granulomatosis: implications of a higher proliferation index in B cells. Am J Surg Pathol 1998; 22(9): 1093–100.

79. Wilson WH, Kingma DW, Raffeld M, Wittes RE, Jaffe ES. Association of lymphomatoid granulomatosis with Epstein–Barr viral infection of B lymphocytes and response to interferon-alpha 2b. Blood 1996; 87(11): 4531–7.

80. Beaty MW, Toro J, Sorbara L, et al. Cutaneous lymphomatoid granulomatosis: correlation of clinical and biologic features. Am J Surg Pathol 2001; 25(9): 1111–20.

81. Sebire NJ, Haselden S, Malone M, Davies EG, Ramsay AD. Isolated EBV lymphoproliferative disease in a child with Wiskott–Aldrich syndrome manifesting as cutaneous lymphomatoid granulomatosis and responsive to anti-CD20 immunotherapy. J Clin Pathol 2003; 56(7): 555–7.

82. Whelan HT, Moore P. Central nervous system lymphomatoid granulomatosis. Pediatr Neurosci 1987; 13(3): 113–17.

83. Kapila A, Gupta KL, Garcia JH. CT and MR of lymphomatoid granulomatosis of the CNS: report of four cases and review of the literature. AJNR Am J Neuroradiol 1988; 9(6): 1139–43.

84. Robak T, Kordek R, Urbanska-Rys H, et al. High activity of rituximab combined with cladribine and cyclophosphamide in a patient with pulmonary lymphomatoid granulomatosis and bone marrow involvement. Leuk Lymphoma 2006; 47(8): 1667–9.

85. Hu YH, Liu CY, Chiu CH, Hsiao LT. Successful treatment of elderly advanced lymphomatoid granulomatosis with rituximab–CVP combination therapy. Eur J Haematol 2007; 78(2): 176–7.

86. Oosting-Lenstra SF, van Marwijk Kooy M. Failure of CHOP with rituximab for lymphomatoid granulomatosis. Neth J Med 2007; 65(11): 442–7.

87. Murphy SB, Fairclough DL, Hutchison RE, Berard CW. Non-Hodgkin's lymphomas of childhood: an analysis of the histology, staging, and response to treatment of 338 cases at a single institution. J Clin Oncol 1989; 7: 186–93.

88. Van den Bosch CA. Is endemic Burkitt's lymphoma an alliance between three infections and a tumour promoter? Lancet Oncol 2004; 5: 738–46.

89. Hecht JL, Aster JC. Molecular biology of Burkitt's lymphoma. J Clin Oncol 2000; 18(21): 3707–21.

90. Magrath I. The pathogenesis of Burkitt's lymphoma. Adv Cancer Research 1990; 55: 133–270.

91. Powles T, Matthews G, Bower M. AIDS related systemic non-Hodgkin's lymphoma. Sex Transm Infect 2000; 76: 335–41.

92. Ferry JA. Burkitt's lymphoma: clinicopathologic features and differential diagnosis. Oncologist 2006; 11(4): 375–83.

93. Sigaux F, Berger R, Bernheim A, et al. Malignant lymphomas with band 8q24 chromosome abnormality: a morphologic continuum extending from Burkitt's to immunoblastic lymphoma. Br J Haematol 1984; 57: 393–405.

94. Shiramizu B, Barriga F, Neequaye J, et al. Patterns of chromosomal breakpoint locations in Burkitt's lymphoma: relevance to geography and Epstein–Barr virus association. Blood 1991; 77: 1516–26.

95. Bellan C, Lazzi S, Hummel M, et al. Immunoglobulin gene analysis reveals 2 distinct cells of origin for EBV-positive and EBV-negative Burkitt lymphomas. Blood 2005; 106(3): 1031–6.

96. Hummel M, Bentink S, Berger H, et al. Molecular Mechanisms in Malignant Lymphomas Network Project of the Deutsche Krebshilfe. A biologic definition of Burkitt's lymphoma from transcriptional and genomic profiling. N Engl J Med 2006; 354(23): 2419–30.

97. Dave SS, Fu K, Wright GW, et al. Lymphoma/Leukemia Molecular Profiling Project. Molecular diagnosis of Burkitt's lymphoma. N Engl J Med 2006; 354(23): 2431–42.

98. Diebold J. Burkitt lymphoma. In: Jaffe E, Harris N, Stein H et al, eds. Pathology and Genetics of Tumours of Haematopoietic and Lymphoid Tissues. Washington, DC: IARC Press, 2001: 181–4.

99. Kasamon YL, Swinnen LJ. Treatment advances in adult Burkitt lymphoma and leukemia. Curr Opin Oncol 2004; 16: 429–35.

100. Chuang SS, Ye H, Du MQ, et al. Histopathology and immunohistochemistry in distinguishing Burkitt lymphoma from diffuse large B-cell lymphoma with very high proliferation index and with or without a starry-sky pattern: a comparative study with EBER and FISH. Am J Clin Pathol 2007; 128(4): 558–64.

101. Haralambieva E, Boerma EJ, van Imhoff GW, et al. Clinical, immunophenotypic, and genetic analysis

of adult lymphomas with morphologic features of Burkitt lymphoma. Am J Surg Pathol 2005; 29(8): 1086–94.

102. McClure RF, Remstein ED, Macon WR, et al. Adult B-cell lymphomas with Burkitt-like morphology are phenotypically and genotypically heterogeneous with aggressive clinical behavior. Am J Surg Pathol 2005; 29(12): 1652–60.

103. Braziel RM, Arber DA, Slovak ML, et al. The Burkitt-like lymphomas: a Southwest Oncology Group study delineating phenotypic, genotypic, and clinical features. Blood 2001; 97(12): 3713–20.

104. Macpherson N, Lesack D, Klasa R, et al. Small non-cleaved, non-Burkitt's (Burkitt-Like) lymphoma: cytogenetics predict outcome and reflect clinical presentation. J Clin Oncol 1999; 17(5): 1558–67.

105. Traverse-Glehen A, Pittaluga S, Gaulard P, et al. Mediastinal gray zone lymphoma: the missing link between classic Hodgkin's lymphoma and mediastinal large B-cell lymphoma. Am J Surg Pathol 2005; 29(11): 1411–21.

106. Portlock CS, Donnelly GB, Qin J, et al. Adverse prognostic significance of CD20 positive Reed–Sternberg cells in classical Hodgkin's disease. Br J Haematol 2004; 125(6): 701–8.

107. Garcia JF, Mollejo M, Fraga M, et al. Large B-cell lymphoma with Hodgkin's features. Histopathology 2005; 47(1): 101–10.

108. Stein H, Mason DY, Gerdes J, et al. The expression of the Hodgkin's disease associated antigen Ki-1 in reactive and neoplastic lymphoid tissue: evidence that Reed–Sternberg cells and histiocytic malignancies are derived from activated lymphoid cells. Blood 1985; 66: 848–58.

109. Foss HD, Anagnostopoulos I, Araujo I, et al. Anaplastic large-cell lymphomas of T-cell and null-cell phenotype express cytotoxic molecules. Blood 1996; 88(10): 4005–11.

110. Morris SW, Kirstein MN, Valentine MB, et al. Fusion of a kinase gene, ALK, to a nucleolar protein gene, NPM, in non-Hodgkin's lymphoma. Science 1994; 263: 1281–4.

111. Pulford K, Lamant L, Morris SW, et al. Detection of anaplastic lymphoma kinase (ALK) and nucleolar protein nucleophosmin (NPM)-ALK proteins in normal and neoplastic cells with the monoclonal antibody ALK1. Blood 1997; 89(4): 1394–404.

112. Benharroch D, Meguerian-Bedoyan Z, Lamant L, et al. ALK-positive lymphoma: a single disease with a broad spectrum of morphology. Blood 1998; 91(6): 2076–84.

113. Falini B, Pileri S, Zinzani PL, et al. ALK+ lymphoma: clinico-pathological findings and outcome. Blood 1999; 93(8): 2697–706.

114. Brugieres L, Deley MC, Pacquement H, et al. CD30(+) anaplastic large-cell lymphoma in children: analysis of 82 patients enrolled in two consecutive studies of the French Society of Pediatric Oncology. Blood 1998; 92(10): 3591–8.

115. Kinney MC, Collins RD, Greer JP, et al. A small-cell-predominant variant of primary Ki-1 (CD30)+ T-cell lymphoma. Am J Surg Pathol 1993; 17(9): 859–68.

116. Bayle C, Charpentier A, Duchayne E, et al. Leukaemic presentation of small cell variant anaplastic large cell lymphoma: report of four cases. Br J Haematol 1999; 104(4): 680–8.

117. Delsol G, Al Saati T, Gatter KC, et al. Coexpression of epithelial membrane antigen (EMA), Ki-1, and interleukin-2 receptor by anaplastic large cell lymphomas. Diagnostic value in so-called malignant histiocytosis. Am J Pathol 1988; 130(1): 59–70.

118. Chan JK, Buchanan R, Fletcher CD. Sarcomatoid variant of anaplastic large-cell Ki-1 lymphoma. Am J Surg Pathol 1990; 14(10): 983–8.

119. Falini B, Bigerna B, Fizzotti M, et al. ALK expression defines a distinct group of T/null lymphomas ("ALK lymphomas") with a wide morphological spectrum. Am J Pathol 1998; 153(3): 875–86.

120. Pileri SA, Pulford K, Mori S, et al. Frequent expression of the NPM-ALK chimeric fusion protein in anaplastic large-cell lymphoma, lympho-histiocytic type. Am J Pathol 1997; 150(4): 1207–11.

121. Jaffe ES. Post-thymic T-cell lymphomas. In: Surgical Pathology of the Lymph Nodes and Related Organs (Major Problems in Pathology Series, Vol. 16), 2nd edn. Philadelphia: WB Saunders, 1995.

122. Vassallo J, Lamant L, Brugieres L, et al. ALK-positive anaplastic large cell lymphoma mimicking nodular sclerosis Hodgkin's lymphoma: report of 10 cases. Am J Surg Pathol 2006; 30(2): 223–9.

123. Brousset P, Rochaix P, Chittal S, et al. High incidence of Epstein–Barr virus detection in Hodgkin's disease and absence of detection in anaplastic large-cell lymphoma in children. Histopathology 1993; 23(2): 189–91.

124. Stein H, Foss HD, Durkop H, et al. CD30(+) anaplastic large cell lymphoma: a review of its histopathologic, genetic, and clinical features. Blood 2000; 96(12): 3681–95.

125. Hernandez L, Pinyol M, Hernandez S, et al. TRK-fused gene (TFG) is a new partner of ALK in anaplastic large cell lymphoma producing two structurally different TFG-ALK translocations. Blood 1999; 94(9): 3265–8.

126. Lamant L, Dastugue N, Pulford K, Delsol G, Mariame B. A new fusion gene TPM3-ALK in anaplastic large cell lymphoma created by a (1;2)(q25;p23) translocation. Blood 1999; 93(9): 3088–95.

127. Mason DY, Pulford KA, Bischof D. Nucleolar localization of the nucleophosmin-anaplastic lymphoma kinase is not required for malignant transformation. Cancer Res 1998; 58(5): 1057–62.

128. Rosenwald A, Ott G, Pulford K, et al. t(1;2)(q21;p23) and t(2;3)(p23;q21): two novel variant translocations of the t(2;5)(p23;q35) in anaplastic large cell lymphoma. Blood 1999; 94(1): 362–4.

129. Touriol C, Greenland C, Lamant L, et al. Further demonstration of the diversity of chromosomal

changes involving 2p23 in ALK-positive lymphoma: 2 cases expressing ALK kinase fused to CLTCL (clathrin chain polypeptide-like). Blood 2000; 95(10): 3204–7.

130. Wilson MS, Weiss LM, Gatter KC, et al. Malignant histiocytosis. A reassessment of cases previously reported in 1975 based on paraffin section immunophenotyping studies. Cancer 1990; 66(3): 530–6.

131. Wlodarska I, Wolf-Peeters C, Falini B, et al. The cryptic inv(2)(p23q35) defines a new molecular genetic subtype of ALK-positive anaplastic large-cell lymphoma. Blood 1998; 92(8): 2688–95.

132. Trinei M, Lanfrancone L, Campo E, et al. A new variant anaplastic lymphoma kinase (ALK)-fusion protein (ATIC-ALK) in a case of ALK-positive anaplastic large cell lymphoma. Cancer Res 2000; 60(4): 793–8.

133. Cools J, Wlodarska I, Somers R, et al. Identification of novel fusion partners of ALK, the anaplastic lymphoma kinase, in anaplastic large-cell lymphoma and inflammatory myofibroblastic tumor. Genes Chromosomes Cancer 2002; 34(4): 354–62.

134. Meech SJ, McGavran L, Odom LF, et al. Unusual childhood extramedullary hematologic malignancy with natural killer cell properties that contains tropomyosin 4–anaplastic lymphoma kinase gene fusion. Blood 2001; 98(4): 1209–16.

135. Tort F, Pinyol M, Pulford K, et al. Molecular characterization of a new ALK translocation involving moesin (MSN-ALK) in anaplastic large cell lymphoma. Lab Invest 2001; 81(3): 419–26.

136. Piva R, Chiarle R, Manazza AD, et al. Ablation of oncogenic ALK is a viable therapeutic approach for anaplastic large-cell lymphomas. Blood 2006; 107(2): 689–97.

137. Gascoyne RD, Aoun P, Wu D, et al. Prognostic significance of anaplastic lymphoma kinase (ALK) protein expression in adults with anaplastic large cell lymphoma. Blood 1999; 93(11): 3913–21.

138. Shiota M, Nakamura S, Ichinohasama R, et al. Anaplastic large cell lymphomas expressing the novel chimeric protein p80NPM/ALK: a distinct clinicopathologic entity. Blood 1995; 86(5): 1954–60.

139. Liso A, Tiacci E, Binazzi R, et al. Haploidentical peripheral-blood stem-cell transplantation for ALK-positive anaplastic large-cell lymphoma. Lancet Oncol 2004; 5(2): 127–8.

140. Falini B. Anaplastic large cell lymphoma: pathological, molecular and clinical features. Br J Haematol 2001; 114(4): 741–60.

141. Zettl A, Rudiger T, Konrad MA, et al. Genomic profiling of peripheral T-cell lymphoma, unspecified, and anaplastic large T-cell lymphoma delineates novel recurrent chromosomal alterations. Am J Pathol 2004; 164(5): 1837–48.

142. ten Berge RL, de Bruin PC, Oudejans JJ, et al. ALK-negative anaplastic large-cell lymphoma demonstrates similar poor prognosis to peripheral T-cell lymphoma, unspecified. Histopathology 2003; 43(5): 462–9.

143. Song SY, Kim WS, Ko YH, et al. Aggressive natural killer cell leukemia: clinical features and treatment outcome. Haematologica 2002; 87(12): 1343–5.

144. Ruskova A, Thula R, Chan G. Aggressive natural killer-cell leukemia: report of five cases and review of the literature. Leuk Lymphoma 2004; 45(12): 2427–38.

145. Hasserjian RP, Harris NL. NK-cell lymphomas and leukemias: a spectrum of tumors with variable manifestations and immunophenotype. Am J Clin Pathol 2007; 127(6): 860–8.

146. Chan JKC, Sin VC, Wong KF, et al. Nonnasal lymphoma expressing the natural killer cell marker CD56: a clinicopathologic study of 49 cases of an uncommon aggressive neoplasm. Blood 1997; 89: 4501–13.

147. Sun HS, Su IJ, Lin YC, Chen JS, Fang SY. A 2.6 Mb interval on chromosome 6q25.2-q25.3 is commonly deleted in human nasal natural killer/T-cell lymphoma. Br J Haematol 2003; 122: 590–9.

148. Nakashima Y, Tagawa H, Suzuki R, et al. Genome-wide array-based comparative genomic hybridization of natural killer cell lymphoma/leukemia: different genomic alteration patterns of aggressive NK-cell leukemia and extranodal Nk/T-cell lymphoma, nasal type. Genes Chromosomes Cancer 2005; 44(3): 247–55.

149. Ohshima K, Karube K, Hamasaki M, et al. Differential chemokine, chemokine receptor and cytokine expression in Epstein–Barr virus-associated lymphoproliferative diseases. Leukemia Lymphoma 2003; 44: 1367–78.

150. Makishima H, Ito T, Momose K, et al. Chemokine system and tissue infiltration in aggressive NK-cell leukemia. Leuk Res 2007 Sept; 31(9): 1237–45.

151. Teruya-Feldstein J, Setsuda J, Yao X, et al. MIP-1alpha expression in tissues from patients with hemophagocytic syndrome. Lab Invest 1999; 79: 1583–90.

152. Lu D, Lin CN, Chuang SS, Hwang WS, Huang WT. T-cell and NK/T-cell lymphomas in southern Taiwan: a study of 72 cases in a single institute. Leuk Lymphoma 2004; 45(5): 923–8.

153. Kwong YL, Chan AC, Liang R, et al. CD56+ NK lymphomas: clinicopathological features and prognosis. Br J Haematol 1997; 97: 821–9.

154. Suzuki R, Suzumiya J, Nakamura S, et al. NK-cell Tumor Study Group. Aggressive natural killer-cell leukemia revisited: large granular lymphocyte leukemia of cytotoxic NK cells. Leukemia 2004; 18: 763–70.

155. Oshimi K. Progress in understanding and managing natural killer-cell malignancies. Br J Haematol 2007; 139(4): 532–44.

156. Chan JK. Natural killer cell neoplasms. Anat Pathol 1998; 3: 77–145.

157. Siu LL, Chan JK, Kwong YL. Natural killer cell malignancies: clinicopathologic and molecular features. Histol Histopathol 2002; 17: 539–54.

158. Oshimi K, Kawa K, Nakamura S, et al. NK-cell neoplasms in Japan. Hematology 2005; 10: 237–45.

159. Jaffe ES, Chan JK, Su IJ, et al. Report of the Workshop on nasal and related extranodal angiocentric T/natural killer cell lymphomas: definitions, differential diagnosis, and epidemiology. Am J Surg Pathol 1996; 20: 103–11.

160. Chan JK, Yip TT, Tsang WY, et al. Detection of Epstein–Barr viral RNA in malignant lymphomas of the upper aerodigestive tract. Am J Surg Pathol 1994; 18(9): 938–46.

161. Kawamata N, Inagaki N, Mizumura S, et al. Methylation status analysis of cell cycle regulatory genes (p16INK4A, p15INK4B, p21Waf1/Cip1, p27Kip1 and p73) in natural killer cell disorders. Eur J Haematol 2005; 74: 424–9.

162. Cheung MM, Chan JK, Lau WH, et al. Primary non-Hodgkin's lymphoma of the nose and nasopharynx: clinical features, tumor immunophenotype, and treatment outcome in 113 patients. J Clin Oncol 1998; 16(1): 70–7.

163. Aviles A, Neri N, Fernandez R, et al. Nasal NK/T-cell lymphoma with disseminated disease treated with aggressive combined therapy. Med Oncol 2003; 20: 13–17.

164. Savage KJ, Chhanabhai M, Gascoyne RD, Connors JM. Characterization of peripheral T-cell lymphomas in a single North American institution by the WHO classification. Ann Oncol 2004; 15: 1467–75.

MALT lymphoma pathology, initial diagnosis, and post-treatment evaluation

10

Christiane Copie-Bergman and Andrew Wotherspoon

HISTOPATHOLOGICAL FEATURES OF MALT LYMPHOMAS

Mucosa-associated lymphoid tissue (MALT) lymphomas are extranodal marginal zone B-cell lymphomas arising at various sites and account for 7–8% of adults' non-Hodgkin's B-cell lymphomas (NHL).[1] The stomach is the commonest site of involvement (50%), followed by the lung (10%), ocular adnexae (12%), skin (9%), salivary glands (6%), thyroid (4%), and breast (2%).[2] Other sites may rarely be involved, like the liver or the thymus.[3,4] Since the stomach is the most frequent site of involvement, the description of the histopathological features of MALT lymphomas will focus on gastric MALT lymphomas.

Histologically, MALT lymphomas reproduce features of the mucosa-associated lymphoid tissue that is present at the physiological level in the terminal ileum and constitute the Peyer's patches. The latter comprises lymphoid follicles characterized by a germinal center surrounded by the follicular mantle composed of monotonous small lymphoid cells. The follicular mantle is in turn surrounded by the marginal zone composed of memory B cells, plasma cells, and T cells. The epithelium that covers the lymphoid follicles is invaded by memory B cells and forms the lymphoepithelium, which plays an essential role in the immune antigen response.

The diagnosis of MALT lymphoma relies on three characteristic histopathological features reminiscent of Peyer's patches:[5]

- a diffuse (and/or nodular) infiltrate of centrocyte-like (CCL) neoplastic lymphoid cells
- lymphoepithelial lesions (LELs)
- reactive non-neoplastic lymphoid follicles.

Neoplastic cells originate from the marginal zone of reactive lymphoid follicles and spread diffusely to the adjacent lamina propria, surrounding epithelial structures (Figure 10.1). Cytologically, neoplastic cells are characterized by small lymphoid cells with irregular nuclei and scant cytoplasm resembling that of centrocytes, and called therefore 'centrocyte-like' cells (Figure 10.2). Cytological variants may be seen with more regular nuclei similar to small lymphocytes (Figure 10.3) or with abundant clear cytoplasm resembling monocytoid B cells. Neoplastic cells are usually intermingled with scattered transformed blasts. A variable degree of plasma-cell differentiation may be seen, usually beneath the surface epithelium. At the end of the cytological spectrum, MALT lymphomas may be characterized by a predominant plasma cell infiltrate, which may be difficult to differentiate from extramedullary plasmacytoma.

Lymphoepithelial lesions are defined by the infiltration and partial destruction of epithelial structures by neoplastic cells, which form small aggregates within the epithelium. Epithelial cells usually show degenerative changes and acquire an eosinophilic oncocytic aspect (Figure 10.4).

Reactive non-neoplastic lymphoid follicles are an important component of MALT lymphoma.

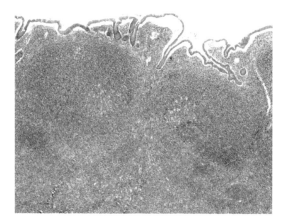

Figure 10.1 MALT lymphoma of the small bowel. The neoplastic cells originate from the marginal zone of reactive non-neoplastic lymphoid follicles and spread diffusely to the adjacent lamina propria (HE ×25).

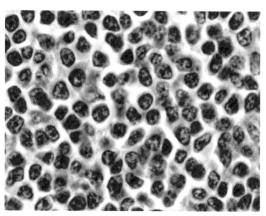

Figure 10.3 Cytological variant of MALT lymphoma: the neoplastic cells present with more regular nuclei and slight plasma cell differentiation (HE ×1000).

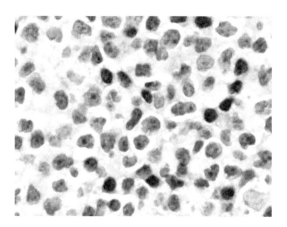

Figure 10.2 Gastric MALT lymphoma: the neoplastic cells are characterized by small lymphocytes with irregular nuclei resembling that of centrocytes and called 'centrocyte-like cells' (CCL) (HE ×1000).

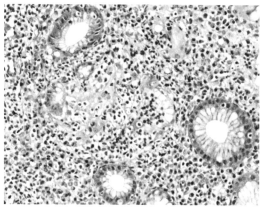

Figure 10.4 Lymphoepithelial lesions (LELs): the epithelial structures are infiltrated and destroyed by CCL neoplastic cells, which form small aggregates within the epithelium. The epithelium shows degenerative changes and acquires an eosinophilic aspect (HE ×200).

They are part of a reactive process that usually precedes the development of MALT lymphoma, and constitute what is called an 'acquired MALT' secondary to inflammation that may be infectious (*Helicobacter pylori* gastritis in the stomach) or autoimmune in nature (Hashimoto's thyroiditis or myoepithelial sialadenitis [MESA] associated with Sjögren's syndrome). Follicular colonization may be seen, and is defined by the invasion of the germinal centers by neoplastic cells.[6]

Neoplastic cells may acquire within the germinal center microenvironment a marked plasma cell differentiation or transform into blasts. Follicular colonization may induce a pure nodular architecture without residual germinal centers and can mimic follicular lymphoma. Follicular colonization with blast transformation restricted to the germinal center may be difficult to differentiate from transformation into high-grade B-cell lymphoma, especially in small gastric biopsies.

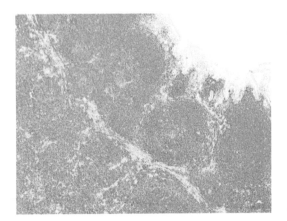

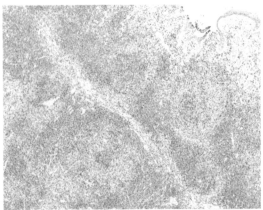

Figure 10.5 Neoplastic lymphoid cells are CD20-positive (CD20 ×25).

Figure 10.6 Neoplastic lymphoid cells are CD5-negative. Numerous CD5+ reactive lymphoid T-cells are observed within the tumor (CD5 ×25).

Although the histological triad described above is helpful for the diagnosis of MALT lymphoma, reactive lymphoid follicles and LELs may be absent in small gastric biopsies. In addition, LELs are not entirely specific of MALT lymphomas and may be seen in reactive conditions and other lymphomatous processes.

MALT lymphoma is usually **multifocal,** and numerous small tumor foci may be seen throughout the gastric mucosa at distance from the main tumor mass.[7,8] Regional lymph nodes are involved in 15–30% of gastric MALT lymphoma.[9] The morphological features are then similar, with a neoplastic lymphoid infiltrate located in the marginal zone of lymphoid follicles which may be colonized. Bone marrow involvement occurs in up to 20% of MALT lymphomas.[10]

Immunohistochemical studies are necessary to confirm the diagnosis of MALT lymphoma. Neoplastic cells display the same immunophenotype as non-neoplastic marginal zone B cells of Peyer's patches and are CD20+ (Figure 10.5), CD79a+, CD5– (Figure 10.6), CD10–, Bcl2+, cyclin D1–, IgM+, IgD–.[11] CD3-positive reactive T cells are usually abundant. Cytokeratin immunostaining is useful to highlight LELs (Figure 10.7). Demonstrating kappa or lambda immunoglobulin light chain restriction helps to differentiate from a reactive lymphoid infiltrate. CD5 and cyclin D1 immunostainings are essential in first intent to exclude mantle cell lymphoma, which is the main differential diagnosis among other

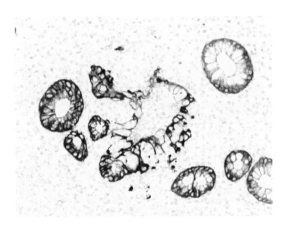

Figure 10.7 Cytokeratin immunostaining highlights LELs (CK ×200).

lymphomatous processes (see below). Careful looking for *H. pylori* infection in gastric biopsies is mandatory using modified Giemsa stain or immunostaining with anti-*H. pylori* antibody.

DIFFERENTIAL DIAGNOSIS OF GASTRIC MALT LYMPHOMA

With other lymphomatous processes

The main differential diagnosis of MALT lymphoma is **mantle cell lymphoma** (MCL). In the gastrointestinal tract, MCL may present as multiple lymphomatous polyposis. Both diseases present a tropism for mucosa and may

Table 10.1 Histological scoring for diagnosis of MALT lymphoma[16]

Grade	Description	Histological features
0	Normal	Scattered plasma cells in lamina propria. No lymphoid follicles
1	Chronic active gastritis	Small clusters of lymphocytes in lamina propria. No lymphoid follicles. No LELs
2	Chronic active gastritis with florid lymphoid follicle formation	Prominent lymphoid follicles with surrounding mantle zone and plasma cells. No LELs
3	Suspicious lymphoid infiltrate in lamina propria, probably reactive	Lymphoid follicles surrounded by small lymphocytes that infiltrate diffusely in lamina propria and occasionally into epithelium
4	Suspicious lymphoid infiltrate in lamina propria, probably lymphoma	Lymphoid follicles surrounded by CCL cells that infiltrate diffusely in lamina propria and into epithelium in small groups
5	Low-grade B-cell lymphoma of MALT	Presence of dense diffuse infiltrate of CCL cells in lamina propria with prominent LELs

CCL, centrocyte-like; LELs, lymphoepithelial lesions.

display very similar histopathological features. MCL is characterized by a diffuse or nodular lymphoid infiltrate composed of small monotonous lymphoid cells, with scant cytoplasm and irregular nuclei. Small residual germinal centers of lymphoid follicles may be seen within the nodules. In the classical form, transformed blasts are usually absent and LELs are not seen. Diagnosis of MCL will rely on histopathological features and the CD20+, **CD5+,** CD10−, Bcl2+, **IgD+, cyclin D1+** immunophenotype of neoplastic cells.[12] Distinguishing these two entities may be difficult in small gastric biopsies, where characteristic histological features of MALT lymphoma (LELs and/or reactive lymphoid follicles) may be absent. In addition, CD5 immunostaining of neoplastic cells may be faint and rare cases of CD5-negative MCL have been reported.[13] MCL is characterized by the t(11;14)(q13;q32) translocation between the immunoglobulin heavy chain *IGH* and the *CYCLIN D1* gene, which is associated with CYCLIN D1 mRNA overexpression and nuclear staining for cyclin D1 demonstrated by immunohistochemistry.[12]

Primary gastrointestinal **follicular lymphoma** (FL) is rare and constitutes 1–3% of gastrointestinal NHL.[14] The small intestine and especially the duodenum is the favored site of involvement. FL may present as small polyps mimicking lymphomatous polyposis or as a diffuse obstructing lesion.[15] Morphologically, FL have a follicular pattern of infiltration and most primary gastrointestinal FL are grade I and composed of predominantly centrocytes. Neoplastic cells are CD20+, CD5−, **CD10+,** Bcl2+. Distinction between MALT lymphoma and FL may be difficult due to follicular colonization, but immunostaining with CD10 is useful to differentiate the two entities. Demonstration of t(14;18)(q32;q21), involving rearrangement of the *BCL2* gene, is characteristic of follicular lymphoma.

With non-lymphomatous process

Distinguishing MALT lymphoma from acquired MALT is difficult, especially in small gastric biopsies. *H. pylori*-**associated chronic follicular gastritis** is characterized by hyperplastic reactive lymphoid follicles with sometimes a poorly defined marginal zone. Lymphoid cells epitheliotropism in gastric glands or crypts surrounding hyperplastic lymphoid follicles may be seen and can be confused with true LELs. Several histological criteria favor *H. pylori*-associated gastritis: the intraepithelial component is usually inconspicuous and located in the proximity of hyperplastic lymphoid follicles; the epithelium does not show degenerative changes and glands are not disintegrated; the lymphoid infiltrate remains well organized and no sheets of CD20+ CCL lymphoid cells are seen in the interfollicular areas or around adjacent epithelial structures.[5]

However, despite these histopathological criteria that may be coupled with immunostaining for CD20 and CD3, some cases remain ambiguous. Wotherspoon et al established a histological scoring system to express the pathologist's confidence of a diagnosis of MALT lymphoma[16] (Table 10.1). This scoring is useful at diagnosis, especially in early or borderline cases of MALT lymphoma that can be confused with *H. pylori*-associated follicular gastritis. Furthermore, a recent study showed that, in difficult cases, Wotherspoon diagnostic criteria combined with detection of monoclonal B-cell populations with a reliable polymerase chain reaction (PCR)-based method (Biomed-2 IgH PCR) for the determination of B-cell clonality helps to resolve most diagnostic problems.[17]

SITE-SPECIFIC DIAGNOSTIC FEATURES (AND PROBLEMS) IN NON-GASTRIC MALT LYMPHOMAS

Extragastric MALT lymphomas of various sites share similar histopathological features, and the diagnosis relies on the three characteristic histological features mentioned previously: a diffuse (and/or nodular) infiltrate of CCL lymphoid cells surrounding reactive nonneoplastic lymphoid follicles and LELs.

MALT lymphoma of the lung results in an interstitial thickening by a nodular lymphoid infiltrate composed of CCL lymphoid cells with a typical marginal zone distribution around reactive lymphoid follicles.[18] Characteristic LELs in the bronchiolar epithelium are usually seen. Coalescing nodules forming a large tumor mass with destruction of the pulmonary parenchyma is usually easy to diagnose. Early lesions without destruction of the pulmonary parenchyma can be difficult to differentiate from follicular bronchiolitis and

lymphoid interstitial pneumonia. In doubtful cases, searching for B-cell monoclonality by immunohistochemistry or molecular analysis will be helpful.

MALT lymphoma of the salivary gland often arises in the setting of MESA associated with Sjögren's syndrome or other autoimmune diseases. MALT lymphoma may be extremely difficult to differentiate from MESA, which recapitulates some of the features of MALT lymphoma, with reactive lymphoid follicles and progressive alteration of salivary gland ducts resulting in epimyoepithelial islands reminiscent of LELs. One of the earliest sign of MALT lymphoma is the occurrence of a clear halo around epimyoepithelial islands characterized by centrocytes and/or monocytoid neoplastic cells.[5] Furthermore, CCL cells expand diffusely around lymphoid follicles and in the interfollicular areas, forming LELs in the adjacent duct epithelium.

MALT lymphoma of the thyroid is very similar to the salivary gland as it usually arises in the setting of an autoimmune condition such as Hashimoto's thyroiditis. The histological features are similar to other MALT lymphomas.[5] Demonstration of B-cell monoclonality will be helpful to differentiate MALT lymphoma of the thyroid and salivary gland from an underlying autoimmune condition.

As in other sites, **MALT lymphoma of the ocular adnexa** can be difficult to differentiate from follicular lymphoid hyperplasia and especially when biopsies are small and subjected to crush artifacts.[5] In these cases, molecular studies are mandatory to demonstrate B-cell monoclonality and to assess a diagnosis of lymphoma.

POST-TREATMENT EVALUATION OF GASTRIC BIOPSIES AFTER ANTIBIOTIC THERAPY

Evaluation of lymphoma response after *H. pylori* eradication relies on the endoscopic features and histopathological assessment of multiple gastric biopsies performed usually every 6 months the first 2 years and then once a year. However, post-treatment evaluation of gastric biopsies remains controversial. Residual lymphoid aggregates in the basal layers of the mucosa in post-treatment gastric biopsies are very common and their reactive or tumoral nature is difficult to establish based on morphological and immunohisto-chemical criteria.

In the natural course of the disease, regression of the neoplastic infiltrate after *H. pylori* eradication is associated with several mucosal changes indicative of an ongoing remission process:

- the diffuse lymphoid infiltrate disappears, usually starting beneath the surface epithelium, and becomes less dense
- a characteristic aspect of an 'empty' lamina propria is seen, which is defined by partial loss of epithelial structures separated by a loose connective tissue with scattered plasma cells but devoid of organized collections of lymphoid cells
- LELs become rare
- subsequently, only small lymphoid aggregates are seen in the basal lamina propria associated with more or less dense fibrosis.

The major difficulty is to interpret these residual lymphoid aggregates, frequently presenting crush artifacts due to the surrounding fibrosis and which cytology is difficult to analyze. Immunostaining is usually not helpful, since these lymphoid aggregates are characterized by numerous reactive T cells and a minority of CD20+ B cells.

Several studies have tried to clarify this issue by using PCR for the immunoglobulin heavy chain *(IGH)* gene.[19] Molecular evidence of monoclonality detected by PCR may help to assess the remission status; however, its usefulness is jeopardized by the possibility of false-negative results and conflicting reports on detectable monoclonality in histologically reactive lesions.[17,19–21] Furthermore, persistent monoclonal disease may be observed in up to 44% of the patients after eradication therapy despite apparent histological remission.[22–26] Whether these monoclonal bands represent active neoplastic cells or resting memory B cells in the gastric mucosa remains to be established. The significance of a persistent malignant clone is still unclear and PCR results should be interpreted only in the context of histology.

More recently, some authors have suggested that molecular monitoring of t(11;18)-positive lymphoma response to therapy (*Hp* eradication and/or chemotherapy) using reverse transcriptase (RT)-PCR for t(11;18)(q21;q21) could be more sensitive then PCR for *IGH*.[27,28] Indeed, ongoing positivity for t(11;18) may be observed in gastric biopsies with complete histological remission and no evidence of *IGH* rearrangement. Further studies of larger series of patients are needed in order to confirm the better sensitivity of RT-PCR for t(11;18) compared to PCR for *IGH* in t(11;18)-associated gastric MALT lymphomas.

However, the clinical relevance of persistent molecular disease, using either PCR for *IGH* or RT-PCR for t(11;18) in patients with otherwise normal gastric mucosa and complete histological remission, is still uncertain. Whether these patients present a higher risk of relapse is not established, and to the best of our knowledge, these patients should be followed up without additional treatment. Therefore, molecular monitoring of lymphoma response to therapy is not recommended in routine practice and should be restricted to patients enrolled in clinical trials where molecular monitoring is under evaluation.

Thus, histological evaluation of follow-up gastric biopsies remains the method of choice for the evaluation of gastric MALT lymphoma response to treatment in addition to endoscopic features. However, variable histological criteria of partial or complete remission have been used among clinical trials. Wotherspoon's histological grading has been used in several trials, although this scoring system was not intended initially to be used for post-treatment evaluation of gastric biopsies. Indeed, many pathologist investigators have found the system difficult to apply and of low interobserver reproducibility.

In order to standardize the histological criteria of gastric MALT lymphoma response to therapy, pathologists from the GELA (Groupe d'Etude des Lymphomes de l'Adulte), together with Dr Wotherspoon, established in 2003 a reliable and reproducible histological

Table 10.2   GELA histological grading system for post-treatment evaluation of gastric MALT lymphoma[29]

Score		Lymphoid infiltrate	LELs	Stromal changes
CR	Complete histological remission	Absent or scattered plasma cells and small lymphoid cells in the LP	Absent	Normal *or* empty LP *and/or* fibrosis
pMRD	Probable minimal residual disease	Aggregates of lymphoid cells or lymphoid nodules in the LP/MM and/or SM	Absent	Empty LP *and/or* fibrosis
rRD	Responding residual disease	Dense, diffuse or nodular, extending around glands in the LP	Focal LEL *or* absent	Focal empty LP *and/or* fibrosis
NC	No change	Dense, diffuse or nodular	Present *or* 'may be absent'	No changes

MM, muscularis mucosa; LP, lamina propria; SM, submucosa; LELs, lymphoepithelial lesions.

grading system (Table 10.2) that aimed to be used by any pathologist and give relevant guidelines to the clinicians.[29] Testing of this scheme in a large number of cases has shown it to be highly reproducible.[30]

This histological grading system of posttreatment gastric biopsies is based only on histological features, independently of immunostaining or molecular studies. Three essential histological diagnostic features are evaluated: the CCL neoplastic cell infiltrate; presence of LELs; and stromal changes. The morphological features observed in post-treatment gastric biopsies are classified in four categories:

- **Complete histological remission** (CR) is defined by the total disappearance of the CCL neoplastic cells and only scattered plasma cells or small lymphoid cells are seen without lymphoid aggregates. Stromal changes characterized by an empty lamina propria and/or loose fibrosis may be seen (Figure 10.8).
- **Probable minimal residual disease** (pMRD) (Figure 10.9) is defined by the persistence of small lymphoid aggregates or lymphoid nodules in the basal lamina propria and/or submucosa associated with stromal changes. LELs are absent. These lymphoid cells do not display characteristic features of CCL and are usually non-suspicious. The meaning of these lymphoid aggregates is still unclear, since in half of these cases, PCR for *IGH* demonstrates

persistence of monoclonal disease. To illustrate this uncertainty, these histological features are classified as 'probable minimal residual disease' (pMRD) but should be considered as a state of remission, since they are not associated with active disease.

- **Responding residual disease** (rRD) (Figure 10.10) is defined by the persistence of a dense nodular or diffuse CCL neoplastic cells infiltrate, extending around glands, but LELs may be absent. Stromal changes is a prominent feature of this state and is indicative of an ongoing remission process.
- **No change** (NC) is defined by the persistence of the CCL neoplastic cells infiltrate, with or without LELs, but no stromal changes are seen.

It is recommended that each follow-up gastric biosy is scored in comparison to the previous gastric biopsy by the same pathologist in order to give the most acurate information to the clinician.

According to this histological scoring system, the recommendations for the clinical management of patients is as follows:

- **CR/pMRD is considered as a state of histological remission** and does not require any additional treatment. Patients should be followed up regularly twice a year for the first 2 years and then once a year with gastroscopy and multiple gastric biopsies.

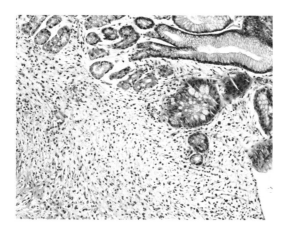

Figure 10.8 'Empty' lamina propria characterized by partial loss of epithelial structures separated by a loose connective tissue with scattered plasma cells but devoid of organized collections of lymphoid cells (HE ×100).

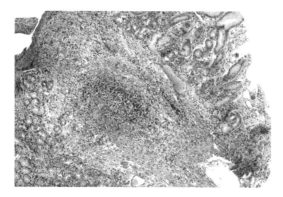

Figure 10.9 Probable minimal residual disease (pMRD): small lymphoid aggregates are observed in the submucosa associated with stromal changes. LELs are absent (HE ×100).

- **rRD is considered as partial remission** of the disease, with histological features indicative of an ongoing remission process. Therefore, additional therapy may be postponed until the next follow-up gastric biopsy (usually 6 months), unless the patient is symptomatic.
- **NC is considered as persistent disease** with no improvement and is indicative of a failure to respond to treatment. In this state, second-line therapy needs to be discussed.

Clinicians must be aware of possible sampling variations between gastroscopies. At

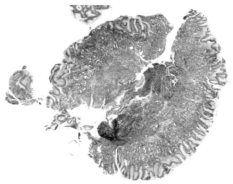

Figure 10.10 Responding residual disease (rRD): persistence of a dense, diffuse CCL neoplastic cells infiltrate in the submucosae with fibrosis (HE ×25).

least two repeated gastroscopies are needed in order to establish a true remission state.

Most patients with *H. pylori*-associated gastric MALT lymphoma stay in remission after eradication. However, relapse may occur in up to 22% of the patients whether associated or not with *H. pylori* reinfection.[31] This relapse may occur several years later and may be focal. Alternatively, the disease may follow a wax and wane evolution, with focal and self-limiting infiltration of the gastric mucosa that may not always require additional treatment.

Long-term endoscopic follow-up of these patients is recommended in order to detect relapse of gastric MALT lymphoma but also to detect preneoplastic modifications of gastric mucosa that may precede the development of gastric cancer. Synchronous occurrence of gastric MALT lymphoma and gastric adenocarcinoma has been reported in several studies.[32,33] Although a rare event, metachronous development of early gastric cancer despite apparent clinical and histological remission of gastric MALT lymphoma has been reported in a few studies, with a mean time of 9.5 years after lymphoma diagnosis in one study.[34–36]

In conclusion, histological evaluation of gastric biopsies remains the method of choice to assess gastric MALT lymphoma response to therapy. The recent development of a simple histological grading system should help pathologists to classify the histopathological features observed in post-treatment gastric biopsies and to give relevant information to the clinicians for the clinical management of the patients. In addition, using this scheme in clinical trials should help to compare the efficacy of different therapeutic approaches in the management of gastric MALT lymphomas resistant to *H. pylori* eradication. Molecular monitoring of lymphoma response is of interest, but is not recommended in routine practice unless its usefulness has been clearly evaluated in large clinical trials.

REFERENCES

1. Anon. A clinical evaluation of the International Lymphoma Study Group classification of non-Hodgkin's lymphoma. The Non-Hodgkin's Lymphoma Classification project. Blood 1997; 89: 3909–18.
2. Thieblemont C, Bastion Y, Berger F, et al. Mucosa-associated lymphoid tissue gastrointestinal and non-gastrointestinal lymphoma behavior: analysis of 108 patients. J Clin Oncol 1997; 15: 1624–30.
3. Issacson PG, Banks PM, Best PV, et al. Primary low-grade hepatic B-cell lymphoma of Mucosa-Associated Lymphoid Tissue. Am J Surg Pathol 1995; 19: 571–5.
4. Ortonne N, Copie-Bergman C, Remy P, et al. Mucosa-associated lymphoid tissue lymphoma of the thymus: a case report with no evidence of MALT1 rearrangement. Virchows Arch 2005; 446: 189–93.
5. Isaacson PG, Norton AJ. Extranodal Lymphomas. Edinburgh: Churchill Livingstone, 1994.
6. Isaacson PG, Wotherspoon AC, Diss T, et al. Follicular colonization in B-cell lymphoma of mucosa-associated lymphoid tissue. Am J Surg Pathol 1991; 15: 819–28.
7. Wotherspoon AC, Doglioni C, Isaacson PG. Low-grade gastric B-cell lymphoma of mucosa-associated lymphoid tissue (MALT): a multifocal disease. Histopathology 1992; 20: 29–34.
8. Du MQ, Diss TC, Dogan A, et al. Clone-specific PCR reveals wide dissemination of gastric MALT lymphoma to the gastric mucosa. J Pathol 2000; 192: 488–93.
9. Levy M, Copie-Bergman C, Traulle C, et al. Conservative treatment of primary gastric low-grade B-cell lymphoma of mucosa-associated lymphoid tissue: predictive factors of response and outcome. Am J Gastroenterol 2002; 97: 292–7.
10. Thieblemont C, Berger F, Dumontet C, et al. Mucosa-associated lymphoid tissue lymphoma is a disseminated disease in one third of 158 patients analyzed. Blood 2000; 95: 802–6.
11. Isaacson PG, Müller-Hermelink HK, Piris MA, et al. Extranodal marginal zone lymphoma of mucosa-associated lymphoid tissue (MALT lymphoma). In: Jaffe ES, Harris NL, Stein H, Vardiman JW, eds. World Health Organization Classification of Tumors. Pathology and Genetics of Tumors of Haematopoietic and Lymphoid Tissues. Lyon, France: IARC Press, 2001.
12. Swerdlow SH, Berger F, Isaacson PG, et al. Mantle cell lymphoma. In: Jaffe ES, Harris NL, Stein H, Vardiman JW, eds. World Health Organization Classification of Tumors. Pathology and Genetics of Tumors of Haematopoietic and Lymphoid Tissues. Lyon, France: IARC Press, 2001.
13. Kaptain S, Zukerberg LR, Ferry JA, et al. BCL1 cyclin D1+ CD5− mantle cell lymphoma. Mod Pathol 1998; 11: 133a.
14. Shia J, Teruya-Feldstein J, Pan D, et al. Primary follicular lymphoma of the gastrointestinal tract: a clinical and pathologic study of 26 cases. Am J Surg Pathol 2002; 26: 216–24.
15. Damaj G, Verkarre V, Delmer A, et al. Primary follicular lymphoma of the gastrointestinal tract: a study of 25 cases and a literature review. Ann Oncol 2003; 14: 623–9.
16. Wotherspoon AC, Doglioni C, Diss TC, et al. Regression of primary low-grade B-cell gastric lymphoma of mucosa-associated lymphoid tissue type after eradication of Helicobacter pylori. Lancet 1993; 342: 575–7.
17. Hummel M, Oeschger S, Barth TFE, et al. Wotherspoon criteria combined with B cell clonality analysis by advanced polymerase chain reaction technology discriminates covert gastric marginal zone lymphoma from chronic gastritis. Gut 2006; 55: 782–7.
18. Kurtin PJ, Myers JL, Adlakha H, et al. Pathologic and clinical features of primary pulmonary extranodal marginal zone B-cell lymphoma of MALT type. Am J Surg Pathol 2001; 25: 997–1008.
19. Savio A, Franzin G, Wotherspoon AC, et al. Diagnosis and posttreatment follow-up of *Helicobacter pylori*-positive gastric lymphoma of mucosa-associated lymphoid tissue: histology, polymerase chain reaction, or both? Blood 1996; 87: 1255–60.
20. Wündisch T, Neubauer A, Stolte M, et al. B-cell monoclonality is associated with lymphoid follicles in gastritis. Am J Surg Pathol 2003; 27: 882–7.
21. de Mascarel A, Dubus P, Belleannee G, et al. Low prevalence of monoclonal B cells in Helicobacter pylori gastritis patients with duodenal ulcer. Hum Pathol 1998; 29: 784–90.
22. Bertoni F, Conconi A, Capella C, et al. Molecular follow-up in gastric mucosa-associated lymphoid tissue lymphomas: early analysis of the LY03 cooperative trial. Blood 2002; 99: 2541–4.
23. Thiede C, Wündisch T, Alpen B, et al. Long-term persistence of monoclonal B cells after cure of *Helicobacter pylori* infection and complete histologic remission in gastric mucosa-associated lymphoid tissue B-cell lymphoma. J Clin Oncol 2001; 19: 1600–9.

24. de Mascarel A, Ruskone-Fourmestraux A, Lavergne-Slove A, et al. Clinical, histological and molecular follow-up of 60 patients with gastric marginal zone lymphoma of mucosa-associated lymphoid tissue. Virchows Arch 2005; 446: 219–24.

25. Wündisch T, Thiede C, Morgner A, et al. Long-term follow-up of gastric MALT lymphoma after *Helicobacter pylori* eradication. J Clin Oncol 2005; 23: 8018–24.

26. Montalban C, Santon A, Redondo C, et al. Long-term persistence of molecular disease after histological remission in low-grade gastric MALT lymphoma treated with H. pylori eradication. Lack of association with translocation t(11; 18): a 10-year updated follow-up of a prospective study. Ann Oncol 2005; 16: 1539–44.

27. Salar A, Bellosillo B, Serrano S, et al. Persistent residual disease in t(11;18)(q21;q21) positive gastric mucosa-associated lymphoid tissue lymphoma treated with chemotherapy or rituximab. J Clin Oncol 2005; 23: 7361–4.

28. Streubel B, Huber D, Wöhrer S, et al. Reverse transcription-PCR for t(11;18)(q21;q21) staging and monitoring in mucosa-associated lymphoid tissue lymphoma. Clin Cancer Res 2006; 12: 6023–8.

29. Copie-Bergman C, Gaulard P, Lavergne-Slove A, et al. Proposal for a new histological grading system for post-treatment evaluation of gastric MALT lymphoma. Gut 2003 ; 52: 1656.

30. Copie-Bergman C, Capella C, Motta T, et al. Validation of the GELA scoring system for evaluating gastric biopsies from patients with MALT lymphoma following eradication of *Helicobacter pylori*. Ann Oncol 2005; 16: v94(Suppl 5; Abstr 194).

31. Raderer M, Streubel B, Woehrer S, et al. High relapse rate in patients with MALT lymphoma warrants lifelong follow-up. Clin Cancer Res 2005; 11: 3349–52.

32. Wotherspoon AC, Isaacson PG. Synchronous adenocarcinoma and low grade B-cell lymphoma of mucosa-associated lymphoid tissue (MALT) of the stomach. Histopathology 1995; 27: 325–31.

33. Goteri G, Ranaldi R, Rezai B, et al. Synchronous mucosa-associated lymphoid tissue lymphoma and adenocarcinoma of the stomach. Am J Surg Pathol 1997; 21: 505–9.

34. Morgner A, Miehlke S, Stolte M, et al. Development of early gastric cancer 4 and 5 years after complete remission of *Helicobacter pylori* associated gastric low grade marginal zone B cell lymphoma of MALT type. World J Gastroenterol 2001; 7: 248–53.

35. Raderer M, Puspok A, Stummvoll G. Early cancer of the stomach arising after successful treatment of gastric MALT lymphoma in patients with autoimmune disease. Scand J Gastroenterol 2003; 38: 294–7.

36. Copie-Bergman C, Locher C, Levy M, et al. Metachronous gastric MALT lymphoma and early gastric cancer: is residual lymphoma a risk factor for the development of gastric carcinoma? Ann Oncol 2005; 16: 1232–6.

PART III

MAIN ENTITIES/LOCATIONS

Primary central nervous system lymphoma

11

Tracy T Batchelor and Andrés JM Ferreri

INCIDENCE AND EPIDEMIOLOGY

Primary central nervous system lymphoma (PCNSL), a rare form of extranodal lymphoma, occurs in the brain, leptomeninges, spinal cord, or eyes; typically, it remains confined to the CNS,[1,2] and accounts for 3.1% of all primary brain tumors.[3] Its incidence increased nearly 3-fold between 1973 and 1984,[4] but, recent data suggest that it may be stabilizing or declining slightly.[5] Congenital or acquired immunodeficiency is the only established risk factor; persons infected with the human immunodeficiency virus (HIV) have a 3600-fold increased risk of developing PCNSL compared with the general population.[6] In HIV-infected patients, a CD4+ count <50 cells/µl and a high peripheral HIV viral load are risk factors for PCNSL development. More than half of patients will have had an acquired immunodeficiency syndrome (AIDS)-defining illness prior to the development of PCNSL, offering additional evidence that immune function must be markedly impaired before this lymphoma arises. AIDS-PCNSL is usually associated with Epstein–Barr virus (EBV);[5] this infection and the *c-myc* translocation result in the development and proliferation of PCNSL. With the advent of highly active antiretroviral therapy (HAART), the incidence of AIDS-related PCNSL has declined.[7]

PATHOLOGY AND BIOLOGY

Diffuse large B-cell lymphoma (DLBCL) is the most common type of PCNSL (90% of cases); the remaining 10% of cases are poorly characterized low-grade lymphomas, Burkitt's lymphomas, and T-cell lymphomas.[8,9] PCNS-DLBCL is a late germinal center or postgerminal center lymphoid neoplasm composed of immunoblasts or centroblasts that have a predilection for blood vessels, resulting in lymphoid clustering around small cerebral vessels (Figure 11.1). Reactive T-cell infiltrates are also present in varying degrees,[10] making it difficult for a pathologist to discriminate between PCNSL and a reactive process. Rare histopathological variants of CNS lymphomas exist; diagnostic, staging, and therapeutic approaches to these malignancies are variable. Mucosa-associated lymphoid tissue (MALT) lymphoma, usually arising in the dura, and immunocytoma are the most common types of indolent CNS lymphomas. These lymphomas have excellent prognosis after local therapy (surgery or radiotherapy). PCNSL of T-cell phenotype is more common in Japan (8% of PCNSL); it should be treated in the same manner as standard PCNSL, with the expectation of similar results, at least in Western countries.[11] Primary CNS anaplastic large-cell lymphoma usually displays a T-cell immunophenotype and the ALK-1 positive histotype, with more frequent meningeal involvement and a better prognosis.[12] Intravascular large B-cell lymphoma is a rare, aggressive, and disseminated malignancy, characterized by large B cells located in the vessel lumen, CNS involvement in 34% of cases, and rapidly progressing multiorgan failure.[13] Anecdotal cases of primary CNS plasmacytoma and Hodgkin lymphoma have been reported. Radiotherapy alone has provided acceptable disease-free survival in both entities.

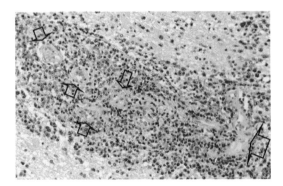

Figure 11.1   Microscopic section from a tumor specimen in a patient with PCNSL (hematoxylin and eosin stain). The tumor cells are pleomorphic, with large nuclei and a coarse chromatin pattern. Tumor cells are clustered around cerebral blood vessels (arrows) in a pattern typical for PCNSL.

Gene expression studies have demonstrated three gene 'signatures' associated with PCNSL: germinal center B-cell, activated B-cell, and type 3 large B-cell lymphomas.[14] Brain lymphoma is distinguished from nodal large B-cell lymphoma by expression of regulators of the unfolded protein response (UPR) signaling pathway, by the oncogenes c-Myc and Pim-1, and by distinct regulators of apoptosis. Interleukin-4 (IL-4) and some associated genes, like XBP-1, a regulator of the UPR, and STAT6, a mediator of IL-4 signaling, are highly expressed by both tumor cells and endothelium in PCNSL.[14]

HIV-related PCNSL is typically EBV-associated large B-cell lymphoma with immunoblastic and more aggressive features.[5] Latent EBV infection induces an activated B-cell state and neoplastic transformation.[15] Expression of several EBV proteins, including LMP1, triggers several oncogenic signaling pathways, probably through BCL6 mutations or c-myc translocations.

CLINICAL FEATURES

In immunocompetent patients, the median age at diagnosis of PCNSL is 60 years, with a male: female ratio of 1.2–1.7.[9,16] In HIV-positive patients, the median age at diagnosis is 31–36 years,[3] with a male:female ratio of 7.38.[7]

Patients with PCNSL typically present with focal neurological deficits (70% of cases), neuropsychiatric symptoms (43%), symptoms of increased intracranial pressure (33%), seizures (14%), and ocular symptoms (4%).[17] Systemic B symptoms are rare.[9] Leptomeningeal involvement, often asymptomatic, occurs in 16–41% of cases.[9] Ocular involvement, generally associated with floaters, blurred vision, diminished visual acuity, and painful red eyes, is detected in ~20% of PCNSL patients at presentation, with both eyes affected in most patients.[18,19] Lymphomatous cells can infiltrate the vitreous humor, retina, and choroid.[18,19] Patients may present with isolated ocular lymphoma; however, in 80–90% of cases, ocular involvement is followed, weeks to months later, by the development of brain lesions.[20–23] Ocular lymphoma may also occur as an isolated site of recurrence after parenchymal PCNSL.

Patients with HIV-related PCNSL are more likely than immunocompetent patients to present with mental status changes or seizures; headache (43%) and ataxia (18%) are frequently reported.[7] The presenting features often span only days to weeks in HIV-positive patients, as opposed to weeks to months in immunocompetent hosts.

DIAGNOSTIC EVALUATION

The International PCNSL Collaborative Group (IPCG) has published guidelines for baseline assessment of PCNSL patients (Table 11.1).[24] The extent of disease evaluation should include a contrast-enhanced brain magnetic resonance imaging (MRI) study, cytological evaluation and flow cytometry of cerebrospinal fluid (CSF) if a lumbar puncture can be safely performed, a complete ophthalmological evaluation, contrast-enhanced CT scans of the chest, abdomen, and pelvis, and a bone marrow biopsy with aspirate.[25,26] Testicular ultrasound examination should also be considered in elderly males, while the role of positron emission tomography (PET) in patients with presumed PCNSL remains to be defined. Conventional lymphoma staging demonstrates the presence of extraneural disease in 4–12% of patients with 'primary' CNS lymphoma.[25,26] The application of molecular diagnostic techniques may increase these percentages. In fact, polymerase chain reaction (PCR) analysis of

Table 11.1 IPCG guidelines for baseline evaluation for clinical trials

Pathology	Clinical	Laboratory	Imaging
Centralized review of pathology	Complete medical and neurological examination	HIV serology Viral BC hepatitis markers	Contrast-enhanced cranial MRI[c]
Immunophenotyping	Dilated eye examination, including slit-lamp evaluation	Serum LDH level	CT of chest, abdomen and pelvis
	Record prognostic factors (age, performance status)	CSF cytology, flow cytometry, IgH PCR Bone marrow biopsy with aspirate	
	Serial evaluation of cognitive function[a]	24 hour urine collection for creatinine clearance[b]	Testicular ultrasound in elderly males

Adapted from Abrey et al.[24]
[a] Mini-mental status examination is used commonly, although improved instruments are being developed.
[b] For patients who will receive HD-MTX (high-dose methotrexate).
[c] Contrast-enhanced cranial CT in patients who have a contraindication for MRI (pacemaker) or who cannot tolerate MRI (claustrophobia).

IgV_H genes detected identical DNA sequences in bone marrow, peripheral blood, and tumor samples in 2 of 24 assessed patients.[27] In one of them, a monoclonal blood product was detectable after 24 months of follow-up despite complete radiographic remission of the brain lymphoma. The clinical relevance, if any, of these observations remains to be elucidated.

Evaluation with slit-lamp examination, indirect ophthalmoscopy, and ophthalmic ultrasonography allows the detection of ocular involvement in 5% of asymptomatic cases. The suspicion of ocular infiltration should be confirmed by vitrectomy and cytological examination of the ocular fluid. Concomitant treatment with steroids may decrease the diagnostic yield of vitrectomy. Routine cytology, immunohistochemistry and/or flow cytometry are useful to characterize cellular phenotype and to confirm the diagnosis.[21] IgV_H gene rearrangement is detected in most cases, and may be useful in confirming the monoclonal nature of the disorder. Intravitreal levels of IL-10 and IL-6 are, probably, adjuncts for B-cell intraocular lymphoma diagnosis.[22,23] A role for human herpes virus 8, EBV, and *Toxoplasma gondii* in the pathogenesis of intraocular lymphoma has been hypothesized.[22]

Neuroimaging

Contrast-enhanced cranial MRI is the best imaging modality for assessing patients with PCNSL; in patients who have a contraindication to MRI, contrast-enhanced cranial CT scans are recommended. In immunocompetent patients with PCNSL, the lesions are often isodense to hyperdense on CT images and isointense to hypointense on T2-weighted MRI, a finding that is attributed to the high cell density and scant cytoplasm of PCNSL lesions (Figure 11.2). On postcontrast CT or MRI there is typically a homogeneous and strong pattern of enhancement in almost all cases.[28] Enhancement along the Virchow–Robin spaces, although not constant, is a highly specific feature of PCNSL. In immunocompetent patients, lesions are solitary in 65% of cases, and located in the hemispheres (38%), thalamus/basal ganglia (16%), corpus callosum (14%), periventricular region (12%), and cerebellum (9%). In HIV-positive patients, lesions are solitary in half of cases, localized to the cerebral cortex (65%), the periventricular region (56%), the basal ganglia (33%), the cerebellum (7%), or to the brainstem (4%), and are often ring-enhancing on MRI.[7] In these patients, toxoplasmosis, abscesses, and progressive multifocal leukoencephalopathy are the main differential diagnoses. Single-photon emission computed tomography (SPECT), PET, and proton MR spectroscopy may distinguish tumor from infectious processes in HIV-positive patients, but are not always definitive. Thus, a brain biopsy is often required for diagnosis, particularly if the patient has rapid neurological deterioration, negative CSF cytology, negative *Toxoplasma*

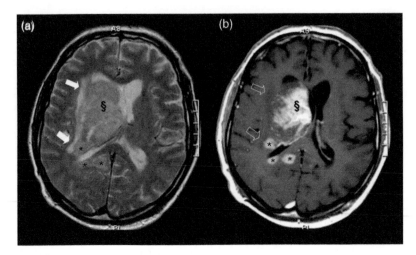

Figure 11.2 Axial MR images of a patient with PCNSL. An axial T2-weighted MR image (A) shows that the right basal ganglia (§) and periventricular (*) lesions are isointense with respect to gray matter; perilesional edema is T2-hyperintense (full arrows). An axial T1-weighted MR image after contrast (B) shows that the lesions enhance intensely. Adjacent edema is T1-hypointense (empty arrows).

serology, radiographic features atypical for toxoplasmosis, and progressing symptoms within the first 2 weeks of antitoxoplasmosis therapy. Surgical biopsy may be avoided in AIDS patients with brain lesions that have both increased thallium uptake on SPECT scanning and a positive CSF for EBV DNA. The combination of these procedures is associated with 100% sensitivity and specificity. SPECT is insufficient as a sole diagnostic modality and may give a false-negative result in lesions <0.6 cm, located near the skull or ependyma, or after steroid therapy.

Cerebrospinal fluid

CSF sampling should be considered in every patient with suspected or confirmed PCNSL; however, increased intracranial pressure may be a relative contraindication to lumbar puncture. CSF evaluation should include cell counts, protein and glucose levels, cytology, flow cytometry, and immunoglobulin heavy-chain gene rearrangement studies. Increases in the white blood cell count and high protein concentrations are often present. Initial CSF cytological studies are positive in approximately 15% of cases.[9,29] CSF cytology may be abnormal, typically showing clumped pleomorphic cells with enlarged nuclei and coarse

chromatin in ~30% of cases.[30] Serial CSF samples result in increased diagnostic sensitivity.

PROGNOSTIC FACTORS

Identification of prognostic factors enables physicians to discuss prognosis with individual patients, may eventually allow the application of risk-adjusted therapeutic strategies, and is critical for prospective study designs. In a review of a large historical PCNSL patient database, the International Extranodal Lymphoma Study Group (IELSG) reported that the following parameters were associated with poor prognosis: age >60 years old; performance status ECOG (Eastern Cooperative Oncology Group) >1; elevated lactate dehydrogenase serum level; high CSF protein concentration; and tumor location within the deep regions of the brain (periventricular regions, basal ganglia, brainstem, and/or cerebellum).[31] Patients with 0–1, 2–3, or 4–5 of these adverse risk factors had 2-year overall survival (OS) rates of 80%, 48%, or 15%, respectively (Figure 11.3).[31] A prognostic model that divided PCNSL patients into three groups according to age and performance status has also been proposed.[32] A prognostic role has also been hypothesized for the expression of the molecular markers STAT6 and BCL-6.[14,33]

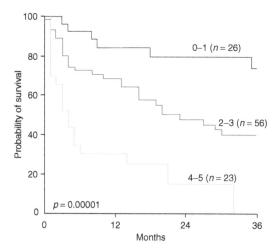

Figure 11.3 Survival distributions for patients grouped according to the IELSG prognostic score:[31] patients with 0–1 (red solid line), 2–3 (blue dotted line), or 4–5 (green dashed line) unfavorable features. Analysis was performed on 105 PCNSL cases in which complete data from all 5 variables were available. The 2-year OS (± standard deviation) were 80 ± 8% for patients with 0–1 unfavorable features, 48% ± 7% for patients with 2–3 unfavorable features, and 15 ± 7% for patients with 4–5 unfavorable features.

TREATMENT

Immunocompetent hosts

Treatment options for immunocompetent patients with newly diagnosed PCNSL include corticosteroids, radiation therapy, and chemotherapy. The IPCG has established guidelines for the assessment of treatment response in patients with PCNSL (Table 11.2).[24] A stereotactic biopsy is indicated for all patients with suspected PCNSL. An attempt to remove as much tumor as possible confers no survival benefit and could result in chemotherapy delay.[34,35] The administration of corticosteroids is associated with significant tumor lysis (radiographic response) in up to 40% of PCNSL patients,[36,37] which seems to be a favorable prognostic marker. However, corticosteroids should be withheld, if possible, prior to biopsy to avoid diagnostic inaccuracy. Moreover, PCNSL patients relapse quickly when treated exclusively with corticosteroids and always require additional therapy.

Radiation

Because of the multifocal nature of PCNSL, radiation has historically been administered to the whole brain. The overall response rate (ORR) in PCNSL patients treated with whole-brain radiation therapy (WBRT) alone (36–40 Gy) is 90%, but response duration is short, with a median OS of 12–18 months.[38,39] A radiation dose–response relationship exists for PCNSL, as dose reduction from 45 Gy to 30 Gy increases relapse risk.[40] Whereas WBRT is effective for the initial control of disease, it produces delayed neurotoxicity, especially in older patients, causing cognitive deficits and diminishing quality of life. For this reason, WBRT is often deferred in PCNSL patients >60 years old in complete remission after primary chemotherapy. Hyperfractionated WBRT delays the onset of, but does not reduce, the frequency of neurotoxicity.[41]

Combined modality therapy

The administration of chemotherapy regimens that are effective for extracranial aggressive lymphomas (i.e. CHOP regimen) produced poor results in PCNSL patients,[42,43] probably because the chemotherapeutic drugs in these regimens (cyclophosphamide, anthracyclines) are associated with limited blood–brain barrier (BBB) penetration.

Methotrexate, when administered at high doses (HD-MTX), is the most effective drug for PCNSL. At doses of 2–8 g/m², cytotoxic CSF levels of MTX are achieved and the need to use intrathecal chemotherapy to treat leptomeningeal spread may be avoided. HD-MTX produces an ORR of 29–88% as monochemotherapy[44,45] and 70–94% as polychemotherapy.[46,47] These chemotherapeutic approaches followed by WBRT are associated with a 2-year OS of 58–72% and 43–73%,[47–52] respectively. An MTX dose of 3 g/m², administered as a 4–6 hour infusion, every 3–4 weeks is recommended, and creatinine clearance and area under the curve (AUC) for MTX seem to predict survival in PCNSL patients treated with HD-MTX.[53]

Several drugs have been added to HD-MTX in an effort to improve outcome. These drugs

Table 11.2 IPCG guidelines for response assessment for clinical trials

Response	Brain imaging	Steroid dose	Eye exam	CSF cytology
Complete response	No enhancing lesion	None	Normal	Negative
Unconfirmed complete response	No enhancing lesion	Any	Normal	Negative
	Minimally enhancing lesion	Any	Minor RPE abnormality	Negative
Partial response	50% decrease in enhancement	N/A	Minor RPE abnormality or normal	Negative
	No enhancing lesion	N/A	Decrease in vitreous cells or retinal infiltrate	Persistent or suspicious
Progressive disease	25% increase in enhancement	N/A	Recurrent or new disease	Recurrent or positive
	Any new lesion			
Stable disease	All scenarios not covered by responses above			

Adapted from Abrey et al.[24]
RPE, retinal pigment epithilium.

were selected based on their capacity to penetrate the BBB and on their demonstrated efficacy against systemic NHL. However, none of these drugs were previously evaluated for efficacy as single agents in patients with relapsed PCNSL. Preliminary results from a few trials in relapsed patients are available with temozolomide, topotecan, rituximab, and the PCV regimen.[54–57] A survival benefit resulting from the addition of HD-cytarabine immediately after HD-MTX[9,58] is being tested in a randomized phase II trial. Although there is no proven benefit of additional drugs, it is likely that an MTX-based polychemotherapy regimen will emerge as the standard therapy for PCNSL.

Chemotherapy alone

Chemotherapy alone has been emphasized to minimize radiation-related neurotoxicity, especially in elderly patients. With this strategy, durable responses are possible, although most patients eventually experience relapse. Treatment with HD-MTX (8 g/m^2) deferring consolidation radiotherapy has been associated with a complete response rate of 52%, a median progression-free survival of 12.8 months, and a median OS of 55.4 months, with mild toxicity.[44] A systemic and intraventicular regimen utilizing a five-drug, HD-MTX-containing combination, without radiotherapy,

has been associated with an ORR of 71%, a median time to progression of 21 months, and a median survival of 50 months.[46] However, this intensive regimen was associated with treatment-related mortality of 9% and Ommaya reservoir infection in 19% of cases. The incidence of adverse events is generally higher in MTX-based polychemotherapy in comparison to MTX monotherapy studies.

Blood–brain barrier disruption

BBB disruption is a strategy aimed at circumventing the BBB in order to deliver higher concentrations of chemotherapeutics to the CNS. BBBD with intra-arterial mannitol + chemotherapy, without WBRT, has been associated with a 75% complete response rate and maintenance of cognitive function in newly diagnosed PCNSL patients.[59] However, BBBD is technically complex and should only be performed in experienced centers.

High-dose chemotherapy and autologous stem cell transplantation

High-dose chemotherapy supported by autologous stem cell transplantation (ASCT) can be used to dose intensify chemotherapy as well as to replace WBRT to avoid treatment-related neurotoxicity. Preliminary results indicate that this strategy is feasible in PCNSL patients

Table 11.3   Studies of high-dose chemotherapy and ASCT in PCNSL

Reference	Therapy line	Number of patients	Induction regimen	Conditioning regimen	CRR (%)	Median follow-up (months)	Survival data	Lethal toxicity
68	2nd	22	araC VP16	thiotepa busulfan CTX	73%	41	3-year EFS: 53%	23%
84	2nd	43	araC VP16	thiotepa busulfan CTX	56	24	mOS: 18 months	14%
60	1st	28	MTX araC	BEAM	18%	27	mEFS: 9 months	0%
85	1st	11	MTX	thiotepa busulfan CTX	82%	22	3-year OS: 61%	18%
61	1st	30	MTX araC thiotepa	thiotepa BCNU + RT	76%	63	5-year OS: 69%	3%
86	1st	25	MTX[a] VP16 BCNU	araC ITX BEAM + RT	64%	25	3-year OS: 55%	6%
87	1st	23	MTX	thiotepa busulfan ± RT	81%	15	mEFS: 17 months	13%

CRR, complete remission rate; MTX, methotrexate; araC, cytarabine; CTX, cyclophosphamide; BEAM, carmustine, etoposide, cytarabine, and melphalan; RT, radiotherapy; BCNU, carmustine; EFS, event-free survival; mEFS, median event-free survival; OS, overall survival; mOS, median overall survival; ITX, ifosfamide.
[a] Intrathecal therapy.

(Table 11.3). The use of HD-MTX-based induction followed by thiotepa-based conditioning seems to be more active than the same induction followed by the BEAM conditioning regimen.[60] The lack of cross-resistance with MTX has been an advantage when this strategy has been used as salvage therapy, but previously irradiated patients had a higher risk of neurotoxicity. In a multicenter trial of 30 patients with newly diagnosed PCNSL under the age of 65 years old,[61] high-dose chemotherapy plus ASCT followed by hyperfractionated WBRT was associated with 65% complete response rate, and a 5-year OS of 87% and 69%, respectively, for patients who received ASCT and for all enrolled patients. The role of this strategy in PCNSL is evolving, and optimal induction and conditioning regimens are being explored.

Intrathecal chemotherapy

The efficacy of intrathecal chemotherapy in PCNSL patients has not been prospectively confirmed. Historical comparisons demonstrated no survival benefit when intrathecal MTX is added to HD-MTX-containing regimens.[9] By giving MTX systemically, the risk of Ommaya placement complications, chemical meningitis, and infection can be avoided. However, as mentioned previously, the intravenous dose must be high enough and administered over a rapid time interval for MTX to penetrate into the CSF and tumor.

Intravitreal chemotherapy

The therapeutic approach to intraocular lymphoma patients is challenging due to the limited knowledge of intraocular drug pharmacokinetics, the limitations in achieving adequate intraocular drug concentrations when administered by the intravenous route,[62] and the high rates of persistent disease in the eyes after conventional therapy. Some protocols using intravitreal injections of MTX, with or without thiotepa, are currently ongoing. A weekly intravitreal injection of 400 µg of MTX/ 0.1 ml, for 4 weeks, and once a month thereafter, has produced encouraging results and low morbidity.[63]

Salvage therapy

Almost all patients with PCNSL will experience tumor relapse or progression and will require salvage therapy. The precise mechanisms that confer treatment resistance in PCNSL are largely unknown. However, promoter methylation of the reduced folate carrier (RFC) gene has been hypothesized as a potential mechanism of MTX resistance in PCNSL patients.[64] The RFC is the predominant transporter of MTX across cell membranes, and deficiencies of this protein have been linked to intrinsic MTX resistance. RFC promoter methylation has been associated with lower response and survival rates in PCNSL patients treated with HD-MTX.[64]

There is no consensus on the best salvage therapy for PCNSL patients, owing to the small number of trials focusing on this issue (Table 11.4). In general, prognosis for patients with relapsed or progressive PCNSL is poor, with a median survival of 4.5 months.[65] For patients who initially responded to an MTX-containing regimen, re-treatment with MTX at the time of relapse may be effective.[66] Activity of some drugs, such as temozolomide[54] and topotecan,[55] has been confirmed in prospective trials, or, like rituximab,[56,67] suggested by retrospective experience (Table 11.4). Some of these agents are gradually being incorporated into trials assessing novel chemotherapy combinations in newly diagnosed PCNSL patients. Salvage high-dose chemotherapy + ASCT has been associated with encouraging results in selected series, which deserves to be confirmed in further studies.[68] Salvage WBRT is effective in PCNSL patients who have failed MTX-based chemotherapy,[69] whereas salvage with stereotactic radiosurgery palliates local symptoms with no effect on tumor spread.[70]

Neurotoxicity

Treatment-related neurotoxicity is more common in elderly patients treated with chemoradiation or radiotherapy and may present as a subcortical dementia with gait ataxia and incontinence. No effective treatment for neurotoxicity exists; CSF shunting may be partially beneficial in a subset of patients. Patients often die from related complications without evidence of recurrent lymphoma. MRI reveals periventricular white matter abnormalities, cortical atrophy, and ventricular enlargement. Pathological studies show demyelination and neuronal loss, gliosis, and white matter rarefaction.[71] Although the pathophysiology of treatment-related neurotoxicity is multifactorial, vascular injury and resultant tissue ischemia is one possible mechanism, while toxicity to neural progenitor cells is another.[71] In one retrospective study,[72] the 5-year cumulative incidence of neurotoxicity was 24% and the use of WBRT was the only predictor. This is in contrast to chemotherapy alone, in which no decline in cognitive function was found in two prospective studies despite evidence of white matter changes on MRI.[73,74]

HIV-related PCNSL

WBRT and HAART are the mainstays of HIV-associated PCNSL treatment. Prior to the introduction of HAART in 1996, a diagnosis of PCNSL was associated with a dismal prognosis (median survival <3 months).[75,76] Since the adoption of HAART, the overall incidence of PCNSL has declined.[77,78] This is probably because fewer patients are reaching such a severe immunocompromised state, reducing the likelihood of latent EBV reactivation in the CNS.

Survival of patients with HIV-associated PCNSL has improved with the advent of HAART, mostly in patients whose viral load dropped after HAART and in those whose CD4 count rose >50 with treatment.[76] The association of HAART with WBRT can prolong survival. These studies, however, are subject to selection bias, since enrolled patients are stable enough to undergo WBRT or tolerate

Table 11.4 Selected salvage therapy trials in PCNSL

Treatment	Number of patients	Responsive patients (%)	OS (months)
WBRT[69]	27	20 (74)	11
Methotrexate[66]	22	20 (91)	62
High-dose chemotherapy + ASCT[68]	22[a]	16 (73)	3-year OS: 64%
Procarbazine, lomustine and vincristine[57]	7	6 (86)	>16
Temozolomide[54]	36	11 (31)	3.5
Temozolomide + rituximab[56]	15	8 (53)	14
Temozolomide + rituximab[67]	7	7 (100)	8
Topotecan[55]	27	9 (33)	8.4
VP-16, ifosfamide, cytarabine[88]	16	6 (38)	1-year OS: 41%
Stereotactic radiosurgery[70]	9 with 17 tumors[b]	13/17 tumors	1-year OS: 58%

[a] Relapsing patients who initially responded to HD-MTX-based chemotherapy.
[b] Seven patients also received chemotherapy.

HAART and may represent a healthier, more compliant subset of subjects.

Chemotherapy has been used in HIV-positive PCNSL patients as well, despite a concern that it will worsen immunosuppression. In 10 HIV-associated PCNSL patients treated with MTX (3 g/m²), the median survival was 290 days.[79] The combination of thiotepa, procarbazine, and MTX was associated with a median survival of 3.5 months overall and 7 months for patients who completed the entire treatment.[80]

Given the association between EBV and HIV-related PCNSL, some studies have examined the effect of EBV-directed therapies on outcome. Preliminary studies have produced promising results with ganciclovir, alone or in combination with zidovudine, interleukin-2 (IL-2), and HAART.[81] IL-2 was used to boost immune reconstitution. Clinical experience with other EBV-specific approaches, like kinase expression up-regulation and lytic induction, is limited and successes are exceptional.[7] It is possible that EBV-related lymphomagenesis could be inhibited by depleting the viral reservoir (i.e. B lymphocytes) in high-risk patients.[82] Rituximab could play a relevant role in this setting.

FUTURE DIRECTIONS

A better understanding of the biology of PCNSL and increasing the fraction of cured patients are critical objectives for future studies. Expanded biospecimen (tumor, blood, CSF) collection and sharing has led to the discovery of specific molecular alterations that may account for some of the unique clinical features of PCNSL and molecular targets for therapeutic exploitation. The IPCG recommendations on extent of disease evaluation and response criteria will be incorporated into prospective PCNSL trials and will enable the generation of historical databases against which new treatments can be compared. Prospective measurement of cognitive function will be a critical endpoint in future trials, mostly those assessing the role of consolidation radiotherapy.[83] International and multidisciplinary collaboration could result in well-designed randomized trials addressing major therapeutic issues, such as the optimal MTX-based chemotherapy, as well as the roles of high-dose chemotherapy with ASCT, intrathecal chemotherapy, and consolidation radiotherapy, in this malignancy.

REFERENCES

1. Batchelor T, Loeffler JS. Primary CNS lymphoma. J Clin Oncol 2006; 24(8): 1281–8.
2. Ferreri AJ, Abrey LE, Blay JY, et al. Summary statement on primary central nervous system lymphomas from the Eighth International Conference on Malignant Lymphoma, Lugano, Switzerland, June 12 to 15, 2002. J Clin Oncol 2003; 21(12): 2407–14.

3. Central Brain Tumor Registry of the United States. Primary brain tumors in the United States 1995–1999. Chicago, III: CBTRUS, 2002–2003.

4. Eby NL, Grufferman S, Flannelly CM, et al. Increasing incidence of primary brain lymphoma in the US. Cancer 1988; 62(11): 2461–5.

5. Kadan-Lottick NS, Skluzacek MC, Gurney JG. Decreasing incidence rates of primary central nervous system lymphoma. Cancer 2002; 95(1): 193–202.

6. Cote TR, Manns A, Hardy CR, Yellin FJ, Hartge P. Epidemiology of brain lymphoma among people with or without acquired immunodeficiency syndrome. AIDS/Cancer Study Group. J Natl Cancer Inst 1996; 88(10): 675–9.

7. Kasamon YL, Ambinder RF. AIDS-related primary central nervous system lymphoma. Hematol Oncol Clin North Am 2005; 19(4): 665–87, vi–vii.

8. Miller DC, Hochberg FH, Harris NL, et al. Pathology with clinical correlations of primary central nervous system non-Hodgkin's lymphoma. The Massachusetts General Hospital experience 1958–1989. Cancer 1994; 74(4): 1383–97.

9. Ferreri AJ, Reni M, Pasini F, et al. A multicenter study of treatment of primary CNS lymphoma. Neurology 2002; 58(10): 1513–20.

10. Ponzoni M, Berger F, Chassagne C, et al. Reactive perivascular T-cell infiltrate predicts survival in primary CNS B-cell lymphomas. Br J Haematol 2007; 138: 316–23.

11. Shenkier TN, Blay JY, O'Neill BP, et al. Primary CNS lymphoma of T-cell origin: a descriptive analysis from the international primary CNS lymphoma collaborative group. J Clin Oncol 2005; 23(10): 2233–9.

12. Ponzoni M, Terreni MR, Ciceri F, et al. Primary brain CD30+ ALK1+ anaplastic large cell lymphoma ('ALKoma'): the first case with a combination of 'not common' variants. Ann Oncol 2002; 13(11): 1827–32.

13. Ferreri AJ, Dognini G, Campo E, et al. Variations in clinical presentation, frequency of hemophagocytosis and clinical behavior of intravascular lymphoma diagnosed in different geographical regions. Haematologica 2007; 92: 486–92.

14. Rubenstein JL, Fridlyand J, Shen A, et al. Gene expression and angiotropism in primary CNS lymphoma. Blood 2006; 107(9): 3716–23.

15. Bashir R, Luka J, Cheloha K, Chamberlain M, Hochberg F. Expression of Epstein–Barr virus proteins in primary CNS lymphoma in AIDS patients. Neurology 1993; 43(11): 2358–62.

16. Fine HA, Mayer RJ. Primary central nervous system lymphoma. Ann Intern Med 1993; 119(11): 1093–104.

17. Bataille B, Delwail V, Menet E, et al. Primary intracerebral malignant lymphoma: report of 248 cases. J Neurosurg 2000; 92(2): 261–6.

18. Peterson K, Gordon KB, Heinemann MH, DeAngelis LM. The clinical spectrum of ocular lymphoma. Cancer 1993; 72(3): 843–9.

19. Akpek EK, Ahmed I, Hochberg FH, et al. Intraocular-central nervous system lymphoma: clinical features, diagnosis, and outcomes. Ophthalmology 1999; 106(9): 1805–10.

20. DeAngelis LM, Yahalom J, Heinemann MH, et al. Primary CNS lymphoma: combined treatment with chemotherapy and radiotherapy. Neurology 1990; 40(1): 80–6.

21. Merle-Beral H, Davi F, Cassoux N, et al. Biological diagnosis of primary intraocular lymphoma. Br J Haematol 2004; 124(4): 469–73.

22. Chan CC. Molecular pathology of primary intraocular lymphoma. Trans Am Ophthalmol Soc 2003; 101: 275–92.

23. Cassoux N, Merle-Beral H, Lehoang P, Herbort C, Chan CC. Interleukin-10 and intraocular-central nervous system lymphoma. Ophthalmology 2001; 108(3): 426–7.

24. Abrey LE, Batchelor TT, Ferreri AJ, et al. Report of an international workshop to standardize baseline evaluation and response criteria for primary CNS lymphoma. J Clin Oncol 2005; 23(22): 5034–43.

25. Ferreri AJ, Reni M, Zoldan MC, Terreni MR, Villa E. Importance of complete staging in non-Hodgkin's lymphoma presenting as a cerebral mass lesion. Cancer 1996; 77(5): 827–33.

26. O'Neill BP, Dinapoli RP, Kurtin PJ, Habermann TM. Occult systemic non-Hodgkin's lymphoma (NHL) in patients initially diagnosed as primary central nervous system lymphoma (PCNSL): how much staging is enough? J Neurooncol 1995; 25(1): 67–71.

27. Jahnke K, Hummel M, Korfel A, et al. Detection of subclinical systemic disease in primary CNS lymphoma by polymerase chain reaction of the rearranged immunoglobulin heavy-chain genes. J Clin Oncol 2006; 24(29): 4754–7.

28. Kuker W, Nagele T, Korfel A, et al. Primary central nervous system lymphomas (PCNSL): MRI features at presentation in 100 patients. J Neurooncol 2005; 72(2): 169–77.

29. Balmaceda C, Gaynor JJ, Sun M, Gluck JT, DeAngelis LM. Leptomeningeal tumor in primary central nervous system lymphoma: recognition, significance, and implications. Ann Neurol 1995; 38(2): 202–9.

30. Fitzsimmons A, Upchurch K, Batchelor T. Clinical features and diagnosis of primary central nervous system lymphoma. Hematol Oncol Clin North Am 2005; 19(4): 689–703, vii.

31. Ferreri AJ, Blay JY, Reni M, et al. Prognostic scoring system for primary CNS lymphomas: the International Extranodal Lymphoma Study Group experience. J Clin Oncol 2003; 21(2): 266–72.

32. Abrey LE, Ben-Porat L, Panageas KS, et al. Primary central nervous system lymphoma: the Memorial Sloan-Kettering Cancer Center prognostic model. J Clin Oncol 2006; 24(36): 5711–15.

33. Braaten KM, Betensky RA, de Leval L, et al. BCL-6 expression predicts improved survival in patients with primary central nervous system lymphoma. Clin Cancer Res 2003; 9(3): 1063–9.

34. Bellinzona M, Roser F, Ostertag H, Gaab RM, Saini M. Surgical removal of primary central nervous system lymphomas (PCNSL) presenting as space occupying lesions: a series of 33 cases. Eur J Surg Oncol 2005; 31(1): 100–5.

35. Reni M, Ferreri AJ, Garancini MP, Villa E. Therapeutic management of primary central nervous system lymphoma in immunocompetent patients: results of a critical review of the literature. Ann Oncol 1997; 8(3): 227–34.

36. DeAngelis LM. Primary CNS lymphoma: treatment with combined chemotherapy and radiotherapy. J Neurooncol 1999; 43(3): 249–57.

37. Mathew BS, Carson KA, Grossman SA. Initial response to glucocorticoids. Cancer 2006; 106(2): 383–7.

38. Nelson DF. Radiotherapy in the treatment of primary central nervous system lymphoma (PCNSL). J Neurooncol 1999; 43(3): 241–7.

39. Shibamoto Y, Ogino H, Hasegawa M, et al. Results of radiation monotherapy for primary central nervous system lymphoma in the 1990s. Int J Radiat Oncol Biol Phys 2005; 62(3): 809–13.

40. Bessell EM, Lopez-Guillermo A, Villa S, et al. Importance of radiotherapy in the outcome of patients with primary CNS lymphoma: an analysis of the CHOD/BVAM regimen followed by two different radiotherapy treatments. J Clin Oncol 2002; 20(1): 231–6.

41. Fisher B, Seiferheld W, Schultz C, et al. Secondary analysis of Radiation Therapy Oncology Group study (RTOG) 9310: an intergroup phase II combined modality treatment of primary central nervous system lymphoma. J Neurooncol 2005; 74(2): 201–5.

42. Mead GM, Bleehen NM, Gregor A, et al. A medical research council randomized trial in patients with primary cerebral non-Hodgkin lymphoma: cerebral radiotherapy with and without cyclophosphamide, doxorubicin, vincristine, and prednisone chemotherapy. Cancer 2000; 89(6): 1359–70.

43. Brada M, Hjiyiannakis D, Hines F, Traish D, Ashley S. Short intensive primary chemotherapy and radiotherapy in sporadic primary CNS lymphoma (PCL). Int J Radiat Oncol Biol Phys 1998; 40(5): 1157–62.

44. Batchelor T, Carson K, O'Neill A, et al. Treatment of primary CNS lymphoma with methotrexate and deferred radiotherapy: a report of NABTT 96–07. J Clin Oncol 2003; 21(6): 1044–9.

45. Herrlinger U, Kuker W, Uhl M, et al. NOA-03 trial of high-dose methotrexate in primary central nervous system lymphoma: final report. Ann Neurol 2005; 57(6): 843–7.

46. Pels H, Schmidt-Wolf IG, Glasmacher A, et al. Primary central nervous system lymphoma: results of a pilot and phase II study of systemic and intraventricular chemotherapy with deferred radiotherapy. J Clin Oncol 2003; 21(24): 4489–95.

47. Abrey LE, Yahalom J, DeAngelis LM. Treatment for primary CNS lymphoma: the next step. J Clin Oncol 2000; 18(17): 3144–50.

48. Ferreri AJ, Dell'Oro S, Foppoli M, et al. MATILDE regimen followed by radiotherapy is an active strategy against primary CNS lymphomas. Neurology 2006; 66(9): 1435–8.

49. Poortmans PM, Kluin-Nelemans HC, Haaxma-Reiche H, et al. High-dose methotrexate-based chemotherapy followed by consolidating radiotherapy in non-AIDS-related primary central nervous system lymphoma: European Organization for Research and Treatment of Cancer Lymphoma Group Phase II Trial 20962. J Clin Oncol 2003; 21(24): 4483–8.

50. DeAngelis LM, Seiferheld W, Schold SC, Fisher B, Schultz CJ. Radiation Therapy Oncology Group Study 93-10. Combination chemotherapy and radiotherapy for primary central nervous system lymphoma: Radiation Therapy Oncology Group Study 93-10. J Clin Oncol 2002; 20(24): 4643–8.

51. Bessell EM, Graus F, Lopez-Guillermo A, et al. CHOD/BVAM regimen plus radiotherapy in patients with primary CNS non-Hodgkin's lymphoma. Int J Radiat Oncol Biol Phys 2001; 50(2): 457–64.

52. Omuro AM, DeAngelis LM, Yahalom J, Abrey LE. Chemoradiotherapy for primary CNS lymphoma: an intent-to-treat analysis with complete follow-up. Neurology 2005; 64(1): 69–74.

53. Ferreri AJ, Guerra E, Regazzi M, et al. Area under the curve of methotrexate and creatinine clearance are outcome-determining factors in primary CNS lymphomas. Br J Cancer 2004; 90(2): 353–8.

54. Reni M, Zaja F, Mason W, et al. Temozolomide as salvage treatment in primary brain lymphomas. Br J Cancer 2007; 96(6): 864–7.

55. Fischer L, Thiel E, Klasen HA, et al. Prospective trial on topotecan salvage therapy in primary CNS lymphoma. Ann Oncol 2006; 17(7): 1141–5.

56. Enting RH, Demopoulos A, DeAngelis LM, Abrey LE. Salvage therapy for primary CNS lymphoma with a combination of rituximab and temozolomide. Neurology 2004; 63(5): 901–3.

57. Herrlinger U, Brugger W, Bamberg M, et al. PCV salvage chemotherapy for recurrent primary CNS lymphoma. Neurology 2000; 54(8): 1707–8.

58. Reni M, Ferreri AJ, Guha-Thakurta N, et al. Clinical relevance of consolidation radiotherapy and other main therapeutic issues in primary central nervous system lymphomas treated with upfront high-dose methotrexate. Int J Radiat Oncol Biol Phys 2001; 51(2): 419–25.

59. Doolittle ND, Miner ME, Hall WA, et al. Safety and efficacy of a multicenter study using intraarterial chemotherapy in conjunction with osmotic opening of the blood-brain barrier for the treatment of patients with malignant brain tumors. Cancer 2000; 88(3): 637–47.

60. Abrey LE, Moskowitz CH, Mason WP, et al. Intensive methotrexate and cytarabine followed by high-dose chemotherapy with autologous stem-cell rescue in patients with newly diagnosed primary CNS lymphoma: an intent-to-treat analysis. J Clin Oncol 2003; 21(22): 4151–6.

61. Illerhaus G, Marks R, Ihorst G, et al. High-dose chemotherapy with autologous stem-cell transplantation and hyperfractionated radiotherapy as first-line treatment of primary CNS lymphoma. J Clin Oncol 2006; 24(24): 3865–70.

62. Batchelor TT, Kolak G, Ciordia R, Foster CS, Henson JW. High-dose methotrexate for intraocular lymphoma. Clin Cancer Res 2003; 9(2): 711–15.

63. Smith JR, Rosenbaum JT, Wilson DJ, et al. Role of intravitreal methotrexate in the management of primary central nervous system lymphoma with ocular involvement. Ophthalmology 2002; 109(9): 1709–16.

64. Ferreri AJ, Dell'Oro S, Capello D, et al. Aberrant methylation in the promoter region of the reduced folate carrier gene is a potential mechanism of resistance to methotrexate in primary central nervous system lymphomas. Br J Haematol 2004; 126(5): 657–64.

65. Reni M, Ferreri AJ, Villa E. Second-line treatment for primary central nervous system lymphoma. Br J Cancer 1999; 79(3–4): 530–4.

66. Plotkin SR, Betensky RA, Hochberg FH, et al. Treatment of relapsed central nervous system lymphoma with high-dose methotrexate. Clin Cancer Res 2004; 10(17): 5643–6.

67. Wong ET, Tishler R, Barron L, Wu JK. Immunochemotherapy with rituximab and temozolomide for central nervous system lymphomas. Cancer 2004; 101(1): 139–45.

68. Soussain C, Hoang-Xuan K, Levy V. Results of intensive chemotherapy followed by hematopoietic stem-cell rescue in 22 patients with refractory or recurrent primary CNS lymphoma or intraocular lymphoma. Bull Cancer 2004; 91(2): 189–92.

69. Nguyen PL, Chakravarti A, Finkelstein DM, et al. Results of whole-brain radiation as salvage of methotrexate failure for immunocompetent patients with primary CNS lymphoma. J Clin Oncol 2005; 23(7): 1507–13.

70. Sakamoto M, Oya N, Mizowaki T, et al. Initial experiences of palliative stereotactic radiosurgery for recurrent brain lymphomas. J Neurooncol 2006; 77(1): 53–8.

71. Lai R, Abrey LE, Rosenblum MK, DeAngelis LM. Treatment-induced leukoencephalopathy in primary CNS lymphoma: a clinical and autopsy study. Neurology 2004; 62(3): 451–6.

72. Correa DD, DeAngelis LM, Shi W, et al. Cognitive functions in survivors of primary central nervous system lymphoma. Neurology 2004; 62(4): 548–55.

73. Neuwelt EA, Guastadisegni PE, Varallyay P, Doolittle ND. Imaging changes and cognitive outcome in primary CNS lymphoma after enhanced chemotherapy delivery. AJNR Am J Neuroradiol 2005; 26(2): 258–65.

74. Fliessbach K, Helmstaedter C, Urbach H, et al. Neuropsychological outcome after chemotherapy for primary CNS lymphoma: a prospective study. Neurology 2005; 64(7): 1184–8.

75. Chamberlain MC, Kormanik PA. AIDS-related central nervous system lymphomas. J Neurooncol 1999; 43(3): 269–76.

76. Hoffmann C, Tabrizian S, Wolf E, et al. Survival of AIDS patients with primary central nervous system lymphoma is dramatically improved by HAART-induced immune recovery. AIDS 2001; 15(16): 2119–27.

77. Chow KU, Mitrou PS, Geduldig K, et al. Changing incidence and survival in patients with AIDS-related non-Hodgkin's lymphomas in the era of highly active antiretroviral therapy (HAART). Leuk Lymphoma 2001; 41(1–2): 105–16.

78. Gates AE, Kaplan LD. AIDS malignancies in the era of highly active antiretroviral therapy. Oncology (Williston Park) 2002; 16(5): 657–65; discussion 665, 668–70.

79. Jacomet C, Girard PM, Lebrette MG, et al. Intravenous methotrexate for primary central nervous system non-Hodgkin's lymphoma in AIDS. AIDS 1997; 11(14): 1725–30.

80. Forsyth PA, Yahalom J, DeAngelis LM. Combined-modality therapy in the treatment of primary central nervous system lymphoma in AIDS. Neurology 1994; 44(8): 1473–9.

81. Raez L, Cabral L, Cai JP, et al. Treatment of AIDS-related primary central nervous system lymphoma with zidovudine, ganciclovir, and interleukin 2. AIDS Res Hum Retroviruses 1999; 15(8): 713–19.

82. Yang J, Tao Q, Flinn IW, et al. Characterization of Epstein–Barr virus-infected B cells in patients with posttransplantation lymphoproliferative disease: disappearance after rituximab therapy does not predict clinical response. Blood 2000; 96(13): 4055–63.

83. Correa D, Maron L, Harder H, et al. Cognitive functions in primary central nervous system lymphoma: literature review and assessment guidelines. Ann Oncol 2007; 18(7): 1145–51.

84. Soussain C, Hoang-Xuan K, Taillander L, et al. Intensive chemotherapy followed by hematopoietic stem cell rescue for refractory or recurrent primary central nervous system (PCNSL) or intra ocular lymphoma (IOL). Results of a Multicentric Phase II Study. Blood 2006; 108(11): abstract #402.

85. Cheng T, Forsyth P, Chaudhry A, et al. High-dose thiotepa, busulfan, cyclophosphamide and ASCT without whole-brain radiotherapy for poor prognosis primary CNS lymphoma. Bone Marrow Transplant 2003; 31(8): 679–85.

86. Colombat P, Lemevel A, Bertrand P, et al. High-dose chemotherapy with autologous stem cell transplantation as first-line therapy for primary CNS lymphoma in patients younger than 60 years: a multicenter phase II study of the GOELAMS group. Bone Marrow Transplant 2006; 38(6): 417–20.

87. Montemurro M, Kiefer T, Schuler F, et al. Primary CNS lymphoma treated with HD-methotrexate, HD-busulfan/thiotepa, autologous stem cell transplantation and response-adapted whole-brain radiotherapy: results of the multicenter OSHO-53 Phase II. Blood 2005; 106(11): abstract #3342.

88. Arellano-Rodrigo E, Lopez-Guillermo A, Bessell EM, et al. Salvage treatment with etoposide (VP-16), ifosfamide and cytarabine (Ara-C) for patients with recurrent primary central nervous system lymphoma. Eur J Haematol 2003; 70(4): 219–24.

Primary testicular lymphoma 12

Umberto Vitolo, Emanuele Zucca and John F Seymour

INCIDENCE AND EPIDEMIOLOGY

Primary testicular lymphoma (PTL) is a rare disease that represents 1–2% of all non-Hodgkin's lymphomas, with an estimated incidence of 0.26 in 100 000 per year. The first case was reported by Malassez in 1877.[1] PTLs account for no more than 5% of all testicular malignancies; however, they are the most frequent testicular cancer in men older than 50 years of age.[2,3] PTL is typically a disease of the elderly: 85% of PTLs are diagnosed in men over 60 years old.[4] Patients with advanced disease have a very adverse prognosis, and also those with stage I–II disease have a high incidence of relapses, leading to a poor outcome overall for patients with PTL.

PTL must be distinguished from systemic lymphomas, which may secondarily involve the testes. Aggressive histological subtypes such as lymphoblastic lymphoma and Burkitt's lymphoma have the highest incidence of secondary testicular involvement, but secondary testicular involvement has been reported with all histological subtypes of lymphoma.

ETIOLOGY AND BIOLOGICAL FEATURES

Although anectodal reports have suggested an association with trauma, chronic orchitis, cryptorchidism, or filiariasis,[5,6] no clear data support these hypotheses. Specific molecular features have been described in PTL such as somatic hypermutation of immunoglobulin heavy-chain gene, indicating a possible antigen-driven stimulation, analogous to what is seen in extranodal marginal zone lymphoma.[7] However, so far no putative antigen has been clearly proven.

The majority of testicular diffuse large B-cell lymphomas (DLBCLs) manifests complete loss of human leukocyte antigen (HLA)-DR and -DQ expression associated with homozygous deletions of the corresponding genes: this loss, also observed in other extranodal lymphomas such as central nervous system (CNS) DLBCL, may help the tumor cells to escape from a cytotoxic T-lymphocyte response.

Associations with certain HLA class II alleles have been reported for several hematological malignancies: testicular DLBCL manifests significantly higher frequencies of *HLA-DRB1*15* and *HLA-DRB1*12* than the controls.[8]

PTL has a rather high incidence of bilateral involvement, and monoclonal lymphoid cells have been shown in contralateral testis even in PTL patients without clinical evidence of disease involvement, suggesting that bilateral testicular involvement is a pattern of a disease of the same origin.[9]

PATHOLOGY

Testicular lymphoma may involve testicle only, but also structures within the scrotum and regional retroperitoneal lymph nodes. Locally, PTL can infiltrate epididymis, spermatic cord, and scrotal skin.[10,11]

The tumor typically involves the body of the testis, with diffuse replacement of testicular parenchyma. However, multiple small nodules and foci of necrosis have also been described.[5,12]

Histologically, >90% of PTLs are DLBCLs (Figure 12.1a,b), but isolated cases of other histological subtypes have been described, such as Burkitt's and Burkitt's-like types in 5–10% of cases, mainly in human immunodeficiency virus-positive (HIV+) patients. Very

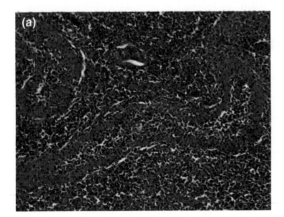 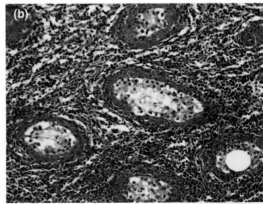

Figure 12.1 Primary diffuse large B-cell lymphoma (DLBCL) of the testis. (a) The edge between interstitial infiltration of large cell lymphoma and still uninvolved parenchyma: in both areas seminiferous tubules show marked hyalinization. H&E, low power. (b) Interstitial infiltration in DLBCL. Hyalinized seminiferous tubules showed maturation arrest of residual germ cells and underwent focal lymphomatous infiltration (lower right). H&E, intermediate power. (By courtesy of D Novero, Pathology University of Turin.)

few cases of T-cell lymphomas have been reported.[12,13] Rarely, cases of PTL of follicular histiotype have been described and, in contrast to the usual age of patients with PTL, they were surprisingly reported in children.[14,15] These cases lacked BCL-2 rearrangement and p53 mutation, along with negativity for the corresponding protein products. In these very rare pediatric cases, the lymphoma seems to lack protection against apoptosis, and this might explain the excellent prognosis in comparison to the most common DLBCL type of PTL. DLBCL can be further subdivided into two major prognostic categories according to different molecular profiling: germinal center B-cell-like type and non-germinal center ('activated') B-cell-like type, with the latter having an inferior prognosis.[16] These profiles may be defined immunohistochemically.[17] Recently, 18 cases of PTL were characterized using the immunohistochemical expression of CD10, BCL-6, and MUM1. Also, the proliferative activity was determined by MIB1 staining.[18] All cases expressed high proliferation activity and 89% belonged to the non-germinal center ('activated') B-cell-like type. Should these findings be confirmed in larger series of patients, they might explain the poor prognosis of PTL.

CLINICAL PRESENTATION

The most common clinical presentation of PTL is a unilateral painless scrotal swelling, rarely with sharp scrotal pain. On physical examination, there is usually a unilateral non-tender firm mass. Hydrocele is observed in 43% of cases, requiring ultrasound of the testis to detect the underlying parenchymal mass. Systemic conventional symptoms such as fever, night sweats, or weight loss are usually present only in advanced stage in 25–41% of patients.[4,19–21] Bilateral testicular involvement may be synchronous at diagnosis or, more frequently, asynchronous during the course of the disease in a portion of cases ranging from 2% to 19%.[4,19–21] Localized stages I and II account for 70–80% of the patients (50–60% stage I and 20–30% stage II). Stage III is very rare (3–5%), whereas the precise incidence of stage IV is not easy to assess because PTL in stage IV is virtually undistinguishable from an advanced-stage systemic lymphoma with testicular involvement.

PTL has a propensity to relapse systemically. Most relapses involve several extranodal sites. Without prophylactic scrotal irradiation, a median rate of 10% contralateral testicular relapse was reported, ranging from 6% to 40%.[20–22] Other frequently involved extranodal sites at relapse were the CNS (6–16%), skin (0–35%), Waldeyer's ring (5%), lung, pleura, and soft tissue.[19,21,23] Overall, the portion of patients showing CNS involvement at diagnosis, 2–16%, is higher than in nodal lymphomas and warrants routine CSF sampling, even in asymptomatic patients.[4,21,23] Involvement of Waldeyer's ring is difficult to explain. This may due to a common embryonic tissue origin, since both the testis and the oropharynx and nasopharynx are derived from the endoderm. Involvement of nodal and extranodal sites may occur either concurrently or subsequently during the course of the disease. These features explain the high rate of relapses in PTL, the majority of them occurring in extranodal sites.

PROGNOSTIC FACTORS

Adverse prognostic factors for PTL reported by some studies were as follows: advanced age, impaired performance status, the presence of systemic symptoms, tumor bulk >9 cm, spermatic cord involvement, an elevated lactate dehydrogenase value, high histological grade, vascular invasion, degree of sclerosis, and advanced stage disease.[5,19,24,25] In the large retrospective study performed by the International Extranodal Lymphoma Study Group (IELSG), clinical features significantly associated with a longer overall survival in multivariate analysis were: low/low-intermediate IPI score, absence of B symptoms, treatment with an anthracycline- containing chemotherapy regimen, and prophylactic scrotal radiotherapy.[21]

DIAGNOSTIC AND STAGING PROCEDURES

For pathological diagnosis, orchiectomy is the method of choice to obtain tissue in preference to fine-needle ultrasound-guided biopsy. Orchiectomy not only provides a better histological definition but also it removes the main tumor mass, allowing a good local tumor control.[26] Moreover, orchiectomy also removes a potential sanctuary site, as the blood–testis barrier makes testis tumors less accessible to systemic chemotherapy.[4]

Ultrasound is the initial investigation of choice. A lymphomatous mass has a sonographic appearance of a focal hypoechoic mass, without a definable capsule or diffuse enlargement and decreased echogenicity of the entire testis, that contrasts with the hyperechoic aspect of normal testis. These findings are not specific for malignant lymphoma. However, hypoechoic striations radiating outward from the center of the testis may be more specific for lymphomatous involvement of the testis because they seem to be due to vascular and lymphatic infiltration by lymphoma cells.[27]

Staging procedures in PTL are similar to those applied in nodal lymphomas, with some specific requirements. A thorough clinical and imaging evaluation, focusing specifically on the CNS, contralateral testis, skin, and Waldeyer's ring, is recommended. Besides the staging work-up usually performed in nodal aggressive lymphoma, additional recommended procedures include cerebrospinal fluid (CSF) examination for malignant cells and ultrasound of contralateral testis. CSF flow cytometry has been recently showed to be more sensitive in the detection of occult CNS disease in aggressive B-cell lymphomas[28] and positron emission tomography (PET) scan may increase accuracy in lymphoma staging.[29] It may be worthwhile to incorporate such new staging procedures into staging work-up of PTL to rule out occult systemic and CNS disease.

PTLs are staged according to Ann Arbor criteria, with few modifications:[30]

- *Stage IE*: involvement of the testis unilateral or bilateral.
- *Stage IIE*: unilateral or bilateral testicular involvement with locoregional lymph nodes (iliac and/or para-aortic).
- *Advanced stage III/IV*: unilateral or bilateral testicular involvement with involvement of distant lymph nodes and/or extranodal sites.

HIV serology should be checked in all cases, as testicular presentations are more frequent in HIV+ patients.

TREATMENT AND OUTCOME

PTLs are very aggressive malignancies with poor prognosis. Five-year survival ranged from 16% to 50%, and median survival has been reported of only 12–24 months according to the different series of patients[3,21,26,31] (Figure 12.2a). Although, very occasionally, long-term survival may be achieved with orchiectomy alone, the majority of the patients treated with surgical excision alone have relapsed within 2 years, suggesting that widespread microscopic disease is present at diagnosis.[32] After surgery alone, most of the patients relapsed, involving regional nodal areas, and leading to the use of pelvic and para-aortic radiotherapy. Radiation therapy on para-aortic or iliac lymph nodes after orchiectomy has been used in stage IE and IIE patients. The results, however, have been disappointing. Despite a high response rate, the overall relapse rate exceeded 70%.[19] PTL is therefore best considered as a systemic malignancy, requiring more than locoregional therapy. Even if PTL is a radiosensitive malignancy, chemotherapy is needed and, apart from the role of radiation to the contralateral testis discussed below, the indications for radiation therapy are limited to patients who are not good candidates for systemic treatment. Testicular lymphoma cells are sensitive to chemotherapy, with most patients achieving apparent remission to their initial therapy, but unfortunately most patients with limited disease still relapse in spite of initial complete remission. The use of anthracycline-based chemotherapy has been associated with a 5-year survival of 30–60% in different series; nevertheless, there appears to be a continuous relapse pattern, with no clear evidence of plateau in the survival curve.[21,33–35] Although it is not possible to individuate the most efficacious chemotherapy regimen, owing to the limited number of patients in the reported series and the lack of randomized trials, doxorubicin-containing regimens have been associated with an improvement in the relapse-free survival compared with orchiectomy ± radiotherapy; however, the advantage on survival time varied greatly among the different series published so far.[21,22,35] In the largest series of patients reported so far by IELSG (373 patents), the outcome of patients was extremely poor, with an actuarial 5-year and 10-year overall survival (OS) of 48% and 27%, respectively, and an actuarial 5-year and 10-year progression-free survival (PFS) of 48% and 33%, respectively.[21] The survival and PFS curves showed no clear evidence of a plateau, suggesting that there may not be the potential for cure of patients affected by primary testicular lymphoma, even for those presenting with localized stage I/II (5-year and 10-year OS in stage I of 58% and 29%, respectively, and stage II of 46% and 29%, respectively).[21] The majority of patients with PTL relapse despite complete response to initial treatment. The pattern of relapse depends on previous primary treatment. When radiation is given to the retroperitoneal lymph nodes, failures are systemic. Very few cases of in-field relapses have been reported. After chemotherapy, both systemic and regional relapses are seen. Most relapses occurred in the first 2 years, but late relapses have also been described.[21,34,36] In most cases, relapses occurred in extranodal sites such as the CNS, skin, lung, pleura, soft tissue, and Waldeyer's ring.[23,37,38] One of the peculiar features of PTL is a contralateral testis relapse occurring in 5–35% of the patients.[19] In the retrospective series of 373 patients reported by IELSG, the commonest sites of relapse were CNS (5-year and 10-year risk of CNS relapse of 20% and 35%, respectively) and contralateral testis (15% at 3 years, 40% at 15 years), occurring in patients not receiving prophylactic scrotal radiotherapy.[21] Prophylactic irradiation of the contralateral testis has been proved to successfully prevent testicular recurrences in some studies. In the IELSG study, prophylactic radiotherapy to contralateral testis significantly reduced the risk of contralateral testis relapse at 3 years and was also associated with better PFS (5-year PFS 36% vs 70%) and OS (5-year OS 38% vs 66%) (Figure 12.2b).[21] These data strongly support the practice that all patients should receive contralateral testis radiotherapy at a dose of 25–30 Gy in 180–200 cGy/day fractions. This approach is feasible with low toxicity also in elderly patients and

(a)

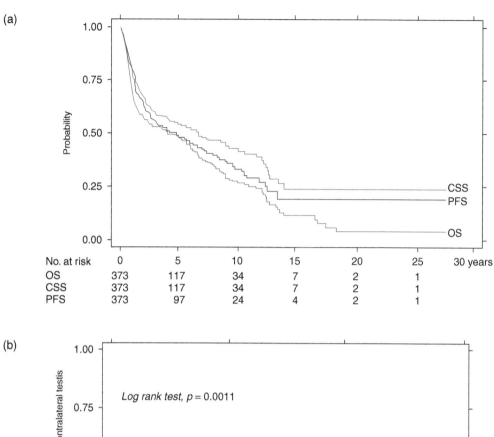

(b)

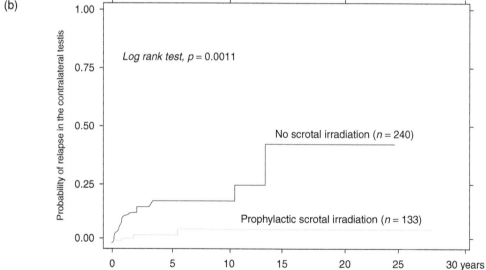

Figure 12.2 IELSG series of 373 patients:[21] (a) Overall survival (OS), cause-specific survival (CSS), and progression-free survival (PFS). (b) Risk of contralateral testis relapse according to scrotal irradiation.

could eliminate the risk of failure at this site. Such treatment is associated with a moderate risk of hypogonadism, and screening of testosterone levels and replacement therapy should be considered in younger or symptomatic patients.

Moreover, CNS relapses are definitely more common than in other aggressive lymphomas and they have been reported up to 30% of the patients within 1–2 years from diagnosis. However, occasionally, late relapses have also been described, sometimes as CNS relapse

(a)

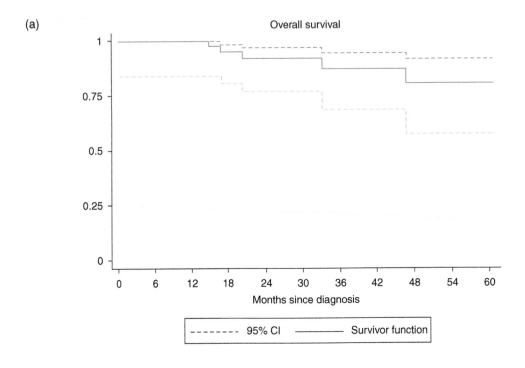

(b)

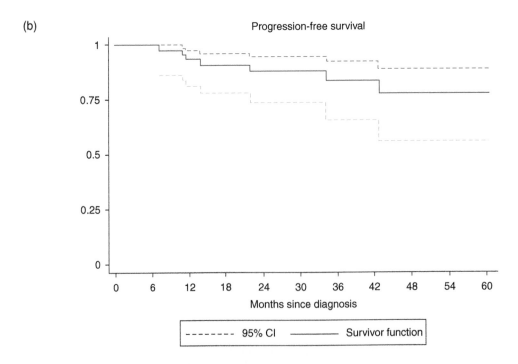

Figure 12.3 IELSG10 study: 49 patients were treated with CHOP + rituximab, intrathecal methotrexate, and prophylactic scrotal radiotherapy and, for stage II patients, locoregional radiotherapy. The 3-year overall survival was 87% (a) and the 3-year progression-free survival was 84% (b).[39]

only.[22,34,38] The high rate of CNS recurrence is troublesome and has led to a recommendation for routine CNS prophylaxis. Although the use of prophylactic intrathecal chemotherapy has been advocated, its value is controversial, because CNS relapses occur more frequently in brain parenchyma than in the meninges and also still occur in patients who had received intrathecal chemotherapy.[21,23] In the IELSG series, an adequate CNS prophylaxis was associated with an improvement in PFS; however, an influence on preventing CNS relapse has not been shown, perhaps because this prophylaxis was delivered to few patients.[21] Perhaps the incorporation of chemotherapy agents that have a better penetration into the CNS, such as high-dose methotrexate, would allow a more effective control of the disease and may prevent CNS recurrence. However, this type of chemotherapy is not easy to administer in elderly patients usually afflicted with PTL. Although all patients with PTL should receive CNS prophylaxis due to the high risk of CNS recurrence, there is little evidence to directly support this commonly adopted strategy and, unfortunately, the best strategy to prevent CNS relapse is still a matter of debate.

As for nodal DLBCL, the addition of rituximab to CHOP chemotherapy may be useful in PTL, as suggested by preliminary data of an IELSG10 study that was recently reported.[39] In this study, 49 patients with stage I-II PTL were treated with 6–8 cycles of CHOP and rituximab and complete prophylaxis with intrathecal methotrexate and scrotal radiotherapy ± locoregional radiotherapy for stage II. The preliminary results suggest an improvement in the outcome, with a 3-year OS and 3-year PFS of 87% and 84%, respectively, no contralateral testis relapses, and a 2.5% actuarial risk of CNS relapse at 3 years (Figure 12.3).

Thus, testicular lymphoma is a unique extranodal presentation of DLBCL. Unlike some other primary extranodal lymphomas, patients with testicular lymphoma appear to have a poor prognosis and they are similar to patients who have primary CNS lymphoma (PCNSL).

Should the results of the IELSG10 study be confirmed with a more mature follow-up in a larger series of patients, a combined treatment of CHOP with rituximab, intrathecal methotrexate, and prophylactic scrotal radiotherapy and, for stage II patients, locoregional radiotherapy, may be regarded as the standard treatment for PTL.

REFERENCES

1. Malassez M. Lymphadenome du testicle. Bull Soc Anta Paris 1877; 52: 176–8.
2. Duncan PR, Checa F, Gowing NF, McElwain TJ, Peckham MJ. Extranodal non-Hodgkin's lymphoma presenting in the testicle: a clinical and pathologic study of 24 cases. Cancer 1980; 45: 1578–84.
3. Zucca E, Roggero E, Bertoni F, Cavalli F. Primary extranodal non-Hodgkin's lymphomas. Part 1: gastrointestinal, cutaneous and genitourinary lymphomas. Ann Oncol 1997; 8: 727–37.
4. Doll DC, Weiss RB. Malignant lymphoma of the testis. Am J Med 1986; 81: 515–24.
5. Sussman EB, Hajdu SI, Lieberman PH, Whitmore WF. Malignant lymphoma of the testis: a clinicopathologic study of 37 cases. J Urol 1977; 118: 1004–7.
6. Talerman A. Primary malignant lymphoma of the testis. J Urol 1977; 118: 783–6.
7. Hyland J, Lasota J, Jasinski M, et al. Molecular pathological analysis of testicular diffuse large cell lymphomas. Hum Pathol 1998; 29: 1231–9.
8. Riemersma SA, Jordanova ES, Haasnoot GW, et al. The relationship between HLA class II polymorphisms and somatic deletions in testicular B cell lymphomas of Dutch patients. Human Immunol 2006; 67: 303–10.
9. Leite KR, Gariocochea B, Srougi M, et al. Monoclonality of asynchronous bilateral lymphoma of the testis. Eur Urol 2000; 38: 774–7.
10. Ahmad M, Khan AH, Mansoor A, et al. Non-Hodgkin's lymphomas with primary manifestation in gonads – a clinicopathological study. JPMA J Pakistan Med Assoc 1994; 44: 86–8.
11. Crellin AM, Hudson BV, Bennett MH, Harland S, Hudson GV. Non-Hodgkin's lymphoma of the testis. Radiother Oncol 1993; 27: 99–106.
12. Ferry JA, Harris NL, Young RH, et al. Malignant lymphoma of the testis, epididymis, and spermatic cord. A clinicopathologic study of 69 cases with immunophenotypic analysis. Am J Surg Pathol 1994; 18: 376–90.
13. Lambrechts AC, Looijenga LH, van't Veer MB, et al. Lymphomas with testicular localisation show a consistent BCL-2 expression without a translocation (14;18): a molecular and immunohistochemical study. Br J Cancer 1995; 71: 73–7.

14. Moertel CL, Watterson J, McCormick SR, Simonton SC. Follicular large cell lymphoma of the testis in a child. Cancer 1995; 75: 1182–6.

15. Pileri SA, Sabattini E, Rosito P, et al. Primary follicular lymphoma of the testis in childhood: an entity with peculiar clinical and molecular characteristics. J Clin Pathol 2002; 55: 684–8.

16. Rosenwald A, Wright G, Chan WC, et al. The use of molecular profiling to predict survival after chemotherapy for diffuse large-B-cell lymphoma. N Engl J Med 2002; 346: 1937–47.

17. Hans CP, Weisenburger DD, Greiner TC, et al. Confirmation of the molecular classification of diffuse large B-cell lymphoma by immunohistochemistry using a tissue microarray. Blood 2004; 103: 275–82.

18. Al-Abbadi MA, Hattab EB, Tarawneh MS, et al. Primary testicular diffuse large B-cell lymphoma belongs to the nongerminal center B-cell like sungroup: a study of 18 cases. Mod Pathol 2006; 19: 1521–7.

19. Shahab N, Doll DC. Testicular lymphoma. Semin Oncol 1999; 26: 259–69.

20. Seymour JF, Solomon B, Wolf MM, et al. Primary large cell non-Hodgkin's lymphoma of the testis: a retrospective analysis of patterns of failure and prognostic factors. Clin Lymphoma 2001; 2: 1–7.

21. Zucca E, Conconi A, Mughal TI, et al. Patterns of outcome and prognostic factors in primary large-cell lymphoma of the testis in a survey by the International Extranodal Lymphoma Study Group J Clin Oncol 2003; 21: 20–7.

22. Tondini C, Ferreri AJ, Siracusano L, et al. Diffuse large-cell lymphoma of the testis. J Clin Oncol 1999; 17: 2854–8.

23. Fonseca R, Habermann TM, Colgan JP, et al. Testicular lymphoma is associated with a high incidence of extranodal recurrence. Cancer 2000; 88: 154–61.

24. Fickers MM, Koudstaal J, van de Weijer FP, Verschueren TA. Malignant lymphoma of the testis. Neth J Med 1991; 39: 92–100.

25. Paladugu RR, Bearman RM, Rappaport H. Malignant lymphoma with primary manifestation in the gonad: a clinicopathologic study of 38 patients. Cancer 1980; 45: 561–71.

26. Salem YH, Miller HC. Lymphoma of genitourinary tract. J Urol 1994; 151: 1162–70.

27. Emura A, Kudo S, Mihara M, et al. Testicular malignant lymphoma; imaging and diagnosis. Radiat Med 1996; 14: 121–6.

28. Hedge U, Filie A, Little RF, et al. High incidence of occult leptomeningeal disease detected by flow cytometry in newly diagnosed aggressive B-cell lymphomas at risk for central nervous system involvement: the role of flow cytometry versus cytology. Blood 2005; 105: 496–502.

29. Spaepen K, Stroobants S, Dupont P, et al. Prognostic value of positron emission tomography (PET) with fluorine-18 fluorodeoxyglucose ([18F]FDG) after first-line chemotherapy in non-Hodgkin's lymphoma: is [18F]FDG-PET a valid alternative to conventional diagnostic methods? J Clin Oncol 2001; 19: 414–19.

30. Carbone PP, Kaplan HS, Musshoff K, Smithers DW, Tubiana M. Report of the Committee on Hodgkin's Disease Staging Classification. Cancer Res 1971; 31: 1860–1.

31. Moller MB, D'Amore F, Christensen BE. Testicular lymphoma: a population-based study of incidence, clinico-pathological correlations and prognosis. Eur J Cancer 1994; 30A: 1760–4.

32. Ciatto S, Cionini L. Malignant lymphoma of the testis. Acta Radiol Oncol Radiat Phys Biol 1979; 18: 572–6.

33. Liang R, Chiu E, Loke SL. An analysis of 12 cases of non-Hodgkin's lymphomas involving the testis [letter]. Ann Oncol 1990; 1: 383.

34. Touroutoglou N, Dimopoulos MA, Younes A, et al. Testicular lymphoma: late relapses and poor outcome despite doxorubicin-based therapy. J Clin Oncol 1995; 13: 1361–7.

35. Connors JM, Klimo P, Voss N, Fairey RN, Jackson S. Testicular lymphoma: improved outcome with early brief chemotherapy. J Clin Oncol 1988; 6: 776–81.

36. Ikeda Y, Nakazawa S, Kudo M. Intracranial malignant lymphoma developing 20 years after total removal of testicular malignant lymphoma – case report. Neurol Med Chir (Tokyo) 1986; 26: 68–70.

37. Zietman AL, Coen JJ, Ferry JA, et al. The management and outcome of stage IAE non Hodgkin's lymphoma of the testis. J Urol 1996; 155: 943–6.

38. Lippuner T, Gospodarowicz M, Pintilie M, et al. Testicular lymphoma, pattern of failure after long-term follow-up. VII International Conference on Malignant Lymphoma, Lugano, Switzerland. Ann Oncol 1999; 10–63 (Suppl 3, Abstr 213).

39. Vitolo U, Zucca E, Martelli M, et al. Primary diffuse large B-cell lymphoma of the testis (PTL): a prospective study of rituximab (R)-CHOP with CNS and contralateral testis prophylaxis. Results of the IELSG 10 study. Blood 2006; 108(11): 208 (Abstr).

Intravascular large B-cell lymphoma 13

Maurilio Ponzoni, Takuhei Murase, Andrés JM Ferreri, and Shigeo Nakamura

INCIDENCE AND EPIDEMIOLOGY

Intravascular large B-cell lymphoma (IVL), or 'angiotropic lymphoma', was earlier regarded, since the original description in 1959 by Pfleger and Tappeiner,[1] as an endothelial neoplasia with vascular dissemination. IVL was recognized as a peculiar form of lymphoid neoplasm only about 22 years ago,[2] and only recently included in lymphoma classifications. IVL is currently defined by the World Health Organization (WHO) classification as an extranodal lymphoma characterized by the presence of neoplastic lymphocytes within the lumina of small vessels.[3]

It is virtually impossible so far to draw incidence figures for IVL: in fact, the main body of literature data is almost exclusively represented by case reports and cumulative reviews, but rare, relatively large series.[4,5] Notwithstanding these difficulties, some clinical features involving presenting symptoms and clinical variants seem to keep IVL diagnosed in Western countries distinct from those IVL reported in Eastern countries, mainly Japan.[6,7]

ETIOLOGY AND BIOLOGICAL FEATURES

Etiological factors in IVL are unknown. The most distinctive property of IVL cells, i.e. their tendency to grow within blood vessel lumina without, if any, substantial extravasation, is a stimulating issue. A few studies that were more or less focused on this topic advanced the hypothesis that neoplastic intravascular B cells may be able to adhere, at least in part, to endothelial cells, but that they seem to lack of some molecules, such as CD29 (β_1 integrin subunit), that are critical for extravasation.[8,9] The

most likely explanation may be that multiple defects are involved in this mechanism: future studies on this topic are therefore warranted.

The relationship with infectious agents has been investigated in few reports. Most of these reports have been written in Japan or other Asian countries, where the Asian variant (i.e. the hemophagocytic syndrome-associated form of the disease, see Clinical presentation section) of IVL occurs most frequently; it appears therefore that, at least in these countries, a link with infectious agent(s) may occur. Apart from an anecdotal evidence associated with *Fasciola* and *Anisakis*,[10] two other agents have been mostly evaluated, i.e. Epstein–Barr virus (EBV) and human T-lymphotropic virus 1 (HTLVI) virus. EBV infection is not frequent in IVL,[11] and usually it accompanies IVL with T-cell[11] or natural killer (NK)-cell[12] phenotype or human immunodeficiency virus (HIV) infection.[13] A single case reports the association of IVL with HTLVI.[14] A few cases have been tested for human herpes virus 8 and resulted negative.[15]

Studies attesting the clonal nature of IVL have been published in the last 20 years. Besides the earlier studies employing the Southern blot technique,[16] the vast majority of clonality studies are carried out with the polymerase chain reaction (PCR) technique,[17] and confirmatory in most cases of gene rearrangement. Five of six cases of IVL evaluated showed somatic hypermutation of the immunoglobulin heavy chain:[18] this feature has been associated with cells that may have experienced a possible transition through the lymph node germinal center. Only one recent report showed t(14;18) rearrangement.[19] Cytogenetic abnormalities in IVL have been seldom investigated and they are not characteristic; in 6 cases, the most frequent defects involved chromosomes 1, 6, and 18.[20] In a recent report, a near-tetraploid karyotype t(11;14)(q13;q32) and chromosome 3q abnormality involving BCL-6 rearrangement were simultaneously present.[21]

PATHOLOGY

Tissue biopsy (i.e. histological examination) is usually mandatory for the diagnosis of IVL; this is due to the lack of a pathognomonic diagnostic immunophenotypic marker for this lymphoma. The demonstration of large cells in the lumina of vessels is the conditio sine qua non for the diagnosis of IVL, but a concomitant minimal extravascular location of neoplastic cells, usually surrounding involved vascular structures, may be seen in occasional cases.[22] Affected vessels range from capillaries to small-to-medium-sized vessels: large arteries and veins are usually spared. In addition, it has been also recognized that IVL involves blood vessels, while lymphatic vessels are usually spared.[22] The degree and growth pattern within blood vessel lumen may vary from case to case or coexist in the same patient. We can basically identify four types of growth pattern in IVL:

- dyscohesive, in which neoplastic lymphocytes are free-floating in the lumen
- cohesive, in which the cells form aggregates completely filling the lumen, sometimes impairing with an easy recognition of the blood vessel structure
- marginating, when lymphomatous cells preferentially adhere to endothelia, without forming neoplastic thrombus
- tumor-associated, when IVL cells preferentially involve vascular structures contained within a tumor and relatively spare vessels contained in the normal surrounding parenchyma.[9]

Classically, the neoplastic cells are large, with high nuclear/cytoplasmic ratio and scant cytoplasm. Nuclear outline is smooth, sometimes with irregular contour in some cases. Nucleolus may single or multiple, and usually readily visible. It appears that IVL cells share intermediate features between centroblasts and immunoblasts. Two exceptions to this rule may occur; in fact, some cases display indented or more irregular nuclear contours, and in some instances cell size may be slightly smaller than the usual one.[22] Recently, a case of IVL with anaplastic morphology has also been described.[23] Most importantly, blood vessel lumen, other than being merely a vehicle, is also a site of active replication for IVL cells; indeed, mitotic features are often easily recognizable within the lymphomatous population. Three anatomical sites show peculiar patterns of involvement. First, renal involvement, other than the classical intravascular location, may preferentially disclose neoplastic cells in glomeruli. In the liver, along with the classic intrasinusoidal distribution, focal, extravascular intraparenchymal spread could be noted. Problematic is sometimes the definition of spleen involvement in IVL. In fact, some cases with splenic localization showed IVL cells within red pulp: the relationship of these occurrences with reported cases of diffuse large B-cell lymphoma with preferential, if not exclusive, red pulp involvement should be clarified.[24] At the present time, it has been proposed to diagnose a splenic involvement by IVL only when an extrasplenic presence of IVL could be detected.[22] Finally, a particular mention should be made of bone marrow involvement. Bone marrow biopsy is usually performed in patients with IVL, because one of the most frequent symptoms is a fever of unknown origin. It should be remembered that the demonstration of lymphoid cells within blood vessel lumen is not exclusive to IVL. Bone marrow intravascular lymphoid cells may be encountered with a variable occurrence in persistent polyclonal B-cell lymphocytosis,[25] hairy cell leukemia, B-cell chronic lymphocytic leukemia, mantle zone lymphoma, splenic marginal zone lymphoma, hepatosplenic gamma-delta lymphoma, and in some cases of secondary[24] or primary[26] bone marrow diffuse large B-cell lymphomas, but these cases also displayed an appreciable extravascular marrow involvement. In these situations, a correct differential diagnosis was made by morphology and immunophenotype in most instances, and was corroborated by clinical findings in the remaining cases. A random tissutal biopsy (for instance gastric biopsy) may disclose another occult site of IVL and facilitate diagnosis.[22] Occasional cases of IVL may occur associated with other non-Hodgkin's lymphoma (NHL); the latter can be of different histotype and are mainly located in the lymph nodes (reviewed in Ponzoni et al.[22]). A recent series of IVL included a significant number of solid NHL with an intravascular component:[27] the relationship between these two lymphomatous populations is presently not entirely clear and therefore specifically addressed studies on this topic are needed. A consistent fraction of IVL diagnosed in Asia (mainly Japan), at a variance with IVL reported in Western countries, is accompanied by morphological signs of hemo/erythrophagocytosis (i.e. phagocytosis by admixed benign-looking histiocytes); this is apparently the only reported morphological difference between Western and Eastern IVL series.[7,28,29] More than 95% of the reported cases invariably display a B-cell phenotype. The most used B-cell marker is CD20, which is often intensely and homogeneously expressed (Figure 13.1); this feature should kept in mind also in view of potential therapeutic implications. Exceptional cases with a B-cell phenotype, CD20-negative cases do exist:[7] in such instances, the most useful B-lineage marker is represented by the CD79a antibody.

Few papers have pursued a more extensive immunophenotypic characterization. For instance, about 20% of a Western series displayed a germinal center phenotype in terms of either of CD10 and bcl-6 immunoreactivity.[30] However, the same authors showed that one-fifth of their IVL were positive for the CD5 molecule, a trend that is even more pronounced in Asian patients (about one-third of cases).[28] Interestingly enough, about 20% of those patients displayed CD5/bcl-6 co-expression.[30]

Taken together, these preliminary data confirm the immunophenotypic heterogeneity of IVL. Much rarer are IVL with T-cell[31] or NK-cell immunophenotype.[12,32] Anecdotal reports describe immunoreactivity of IVL cells for myeloperoxydase[33] or prostatic acid

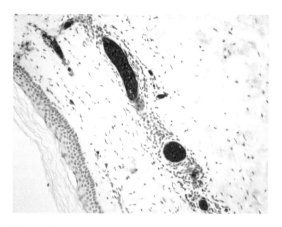

Figure 13.1 Cutaneous blood vessels are filled by large neoplastic cells that are immunoreactive for CD20.

phosphatase;[34] the significance of these latter observations is still obscure.

CLINICAL PRESENTATION

Median age at diagnosis of IVL is 70 years old, but with a wide range (34–90 years old), and with a similar prevalence in males and females. Almost 15% of IVL patients are associated with another malignancy. The median duration of the interval between the diagnosis of these tumors and IVL diagnosis oscillates between 4 and 5 years. In some cases, IVL is diagnosed concomitant to other tumors (see below).

IVL can virtually involve any organ, with a resulting potential proteiform clinical presentation, ranging from monosymptomatic forms, such as fever, pain, or organ-specific local symptoms, to the combination of B symptoms and rapidly progressing manifestations of multiorgan failure. Patients usually present with deterioration in Eastern Cooperative Oncology Group performance status (ECOG-PS score ≥1 in 95% of cases). In the past, a premortem diagnosis was infrequent. More recently, diagnosis is established in vivo in almost 80% of cases, thus reflecting a better awareness of clinical suspicion for IVL among physicians.

The most relevant presenting signs and symptoms are summarized in Table 13.1. More than half of cases complain of systemic symptoms; among these, fever is the most common one (46% of cases). Fever is associated

Table 13.1   Signs and symptoms in IVL patients[4,5]

Systemic symptoms	55%
Fever	46%
Fever + weight loss ± night sweats	23%
Fever + night sweats	3%
Weight loss	10%
Cutaneous lesions	40%
Neurological symptoms	35%
Pain	20%
Fatigue	16%
Urinary symptoms	8%
Gastrointestinal symptoms	5%
Cardiac dysfunction	5%
Edema	5%
Dyspnea	3%

Table 13.2   Involved sites in IVL patients ordered by decreasing frequency[4,5]

Skin	
Single lesion	10%
Multiple lesions	30%
CNS	40%
Bone marrow	32%
Liver	26%
Spleen	26%
Kidney	21%
Endocrine glands	16%
Lung	16%
Prostate	16%
Lymph nodes	11%
Heart	11%
Peripheral blood smear	9%
Gastrointestinal tract	8%
Urinary bladder	8%
Uterus	8%
Gallbladder	3%

with other B symptoms in half of the cases, whereas weight loss alone is present in 10% of cases.

Cutaneous lesions are the dominant presenting feature in 40% of cases (see Table 13.1), but extremely heterogeneous, encompassing painful indurate erythematous eruption, poorly circumscribed violaceous plaques, skin 'peau d'orange', cellulitis, large solitary plaques, painful blue-red palpable nodular discolorations, tumors, ulcerated nodules, small red palpable spots, and erythematous and desquamative plaques. These lesions are commonly situated in the extremities, lower abdomen, and breast region. Cutaneous lesions are single in one-third of cases; they are associated with multiple organ involvement in 30% of cases (Table 13.2). When the disease is exclusively limited to the skin (25% of cases), the cutaneous variant of IVL is diagnosed (see below). Importantly, not every patient with cutaneous involvement carries the cutaneous variant of IVL; in fact, in those patients with cutaneous lesions associated with other symptoms, mostly represented by neurological and B symptoms, standard lymphoma staging procedures are able to disclose additional sites of disease, usually involving the liver, central nervous system (CNS), and bone marrow.

Thirty-five percent of IVL patients present with neurological symptoms at diagnosis. These symptoms include sensory and motor deficits or neuropathies, meningoradiculitis, paresthesias, hyposthenia, aphasia, dysarthria, hemiparesis,

seizures, myoclonus, transient visual loss, vertigo, and impaired cognitive function. IVL limited to the CNS is an extremely rare condition, notwithstanding current standard lymphoma staging results. Neuroimaging discloses CNS involvement only in half of patients with neurological symptoms. There are no pathognomonic neuroradiological findings for IVL; ischemic foci are the most common presentation pattern and therefore vasculitis is the most common differential diagnosis. In spite of possible false-negative results, magnetic resonance imaging (MRI) of the CNS should be routinely included in current staging work-up of IVL. The presence of neoplastic cells in the cerebrospinal fluid (CSF) is rare, and is at a variance with increased CSF protein levels, which is actually much more common.

The most relevant laboratory characteristics of IVL are summarized in Table 13.3. Increased serum lactic dehydrogenase and β_2-microglobulin levels are the most frequent findings. Anemia is the most frequent cytopenia; interestingly enough, leukopenia or thrombocytopenia usually does not occur without anemia. Most cases of thrombocytopenia are associated with bone marrow infiltration and hepatosplenic involvement; patients

Table 13.3 Laboratory findings in patients with IVL in decreased order of frequency[4,5]

High lactic dehydrogenase serum level	86%
High β2-microglobulin serum level	82%
Anemia (<12 g/dl)	63%
Elevated erythrocyte sedimentation rate	43%
Thrombocytopenia (<150000/μl)	29%
Leukopenia (<4000/μl)	24%
Hypoalbuminemia (< 3.6 g/dl)	18%
Monoclonal serum component	14%

with marrow infiltration and without anemia or thrombocytopenia are rare. Patients with hepatic and/or splenic involvement frequently disclose cytopenia. Altered hepatic, renal, or thyroid functional tests are observed in nearly 15% of cases; these function tests are useful tools in the staging of IVL; in fact, altered results are invariably associated with organ involvement by lymphoma cells.

The cutaneous variant

Single or multiple lesions of the skin followed by negative systemic staging are consistent with the recently described cutaneous variant of IVL.[5] The patients with this variant display distinctive clinical characteristics: almost all are females with normal leukocyte and platelet counts, absence of monoclonal gammopathy, ECOG-PS usually ≤1, and a median age significantly lower (59 years old vs 72 years old of usual IVL). Features consistent with lymphoma aggressiveness are less pronounced within this group of patients.

The hemophagocytosis-related variant

In Japanese patients, in contrast to IVL patients in Western countries, IVL has often been associated with hemophagocytic syndrome, bone marrow involvement, fever, hepatosplenomegaly, and thrombocytopenia in 73–100% of cases, whereas CNS and cutaneous involvement are uncommon. Some Japanese authors defined these features as diagnostic for hemophagocytic syndrome-associated IVL[35] (also called Asian variant[7]). Although morphological examination remains the gold standard to

assess hemo/erythrophagocytosis, it has been recently and provisionally accepted that some cases of hemophagocytosis-associated IVL actually lack substantial morphological grounds and therefore are assigned to this category of IVL by virtue of the presence of those clinical findings (i.e. thrombocytopenia, hepatosplenomegaly, and fever), whose combination in the appropriate clinical context is considered diagnostic for hemophagocytic syndrome.[22] On these grounds, it could be therefore interesting to assess whether some IVL with only clinical/laboratory features suggestive for hemophagocytic syndrome and diagnosed in Western countries may fall in the Asian variant.

PROGNOSTIC FACTORS

Patients with cutaneous variant of IVL survive significantly longer than others, independently of the International Prognostic Index (IPI) and all the other prognostic variables investigated.[5] However, therapeutic outcome is remarkably different between patients with single and multiple cutaneous lesions: only patients with single cutaneous lesions are long-term survivors. The favorable clinical behavior of the cutaneous variant of IVL, mainly in cases with a single lesion, may be either explained by the earlier diagnosis of cutaneous lesions or, alternatively, by unknown potential biological and behavioral differences.

STAGING

Ann Arbor stage I_E disease is present in 40% of patients. Most of these cases carry the cutaneous variant or are incidentally diagnosed. Apart from these two exceptions, the limitations of current standard lymphoma staging in IVL patients are highlighted by some cases of death occurring a few weeks later in patients considered as having stage I disease, where the autopsy actually showed a disseminated disease.[5]

Sixty percent of IVL patients have stage IV, and disseminated disease is reported in all autopsied cases. Bone marrow involvement has been reported in one-third of patients, where it is significantly associated with hepatosplenic involvement and pancytopenia.

In exceptional cases, bone marrow is the apparently unique site of disease.

In contrast to most NHL, lymph node involvement is rare (10% of cases), usually located in retroperitoneum; hepatic or splenic infiltration is present in one-third of cases. Simultaneous liver, spleen, and marrow involvement is observed in nearly 20% of IVL in Western countries and more frequently in Japanese series. Peripheral blood smears are positive in only 5–9% of cases and are invariably associated with bone marrow infiltration. However, it has been reported that occasional atypical circulating cells may be observed, or abnormal karyotypes may be detected from peripheral blood leukocytes, thus suggesting that a careful review of peripheral blood films and/or cytogenetic analysis may increase these currently accepted percentages.

Pulmonary IVL is characterized by multifocal disease, leading to dyspnea, air trapping, and severe pulmonary hypertension, with a rapidly aggressive behavior. Endocrine gland involvement is common, with a variable degree of endocrine failure(s) according to the infiltration of one or more related organs. Other frequent sites include the kidney and prostate.

TREATMENT AND OUTCOME

The course of this malignancy is generally rapidly progressive and ultimately fatal, with the exception of some patients who achieve durable remission after chemotherapy and rare cases of untreated long-term survivors. The correct therapeutic assessment in IVL is presently biased by the absence of prospective trials and by the fragmentation of reported data in such rare malignancies. A general rule is that patients with IVL should be considered to have a disseminated disease, and, accordingly, should be treated with combination chemotherapy. A possible exception might be cases with single small cutaneous lesions, which have some probability of cure with a local treatment. The inclusion of anthracycline as part of chemotherapy combinations, due to its 59% response rate, is critical. It should be remembered that response assessment is difficult in IVL patients because

measurable disease (i.e. lymphadenopathy and tumor masses) is usually lacking. Half of patients treated with anthracycline-based chemotherapy experience relapse (median time to treatment failure = 8 months) and die within 18 months from diagnosis, with 3-year event-free survival (EFS) of 27%.

Relapses invariably involve extranodal organs and, in most instances, the primary site of disease; one-third of relapses involves the CNS. Relapses after 5 years of follow-up are rare. In patients treated with anthracycline-based chemotherapy, the 3-year overall survival (OS) is near to 30%; however, long-term survival remains to be defined, since follow-up in reported case series is usually short. The clinical benefit offered by chemotherapy may be contrasted by postsurgical lethal complications or delayed diagnosis. A more intensive combination is needed in cases with CNS involvement, owing to their poor outcome (due to either lymphoma progression or septic complications). Drugs with higher bioavailability in the CNS, such as methotrexate or cytarabine, should be included, mostly in Western patients, where the involvement of these organs is more common.[22] Although experience with rituximab in IVL patients is still limited,[36] the combination of anthracycline-based chemotherapy and rituximab (R-CHOP regimen or similar ones) could have a positive impact on survival in IVL patients.

The use of high-dose chemotherapy supported by autologous stem cell transplantation, an important strategy to intensify treatment against NHL, may theoretically improve current outcomes. However, this strategy appears feasible only in a small proportion of patients with IVL, considering that their median age is 70 years old and PS is usually poor. This strategy therefore deserves to be further investigated mostly in young patients with unfavorable features.

The therapy in cases associated with hemophagocytic syndrome deserves a specific comment. Anthracycline-based chemotherapy produces a 53% complete remission rate and a 2-year OS of 32% in Japanese patients with IVL: these figures do not differ significantly from those reported in IVL patients treated in Western countries.[4]

Radiotherapy may be considered the exclusive treatment for IVL in elderly patients with single cutaneous lesions; outside this context, the role of radiotherapy remains to be determined.

Management of patients with the cutaneous form of IVL remains a matter of debate, considering that some cases show an excellent prognosis even if treated without chemotherapy, whereas others experience early relapse after intensive therapy. Biological studies could help us to stratify patients with the cutaneous form of IVL. With the exception of the cutaneous variant, the classical IVL and the hemophagocytosis-related variant of IVL do not correlate with patient survival.[4,28]

Rare entities sometimes display such peculiar features that detailed studies on their properties may be exported and facilitate a better understanding of much more common diseases. IVL appears therefore one of the best in-vivo candidates for the evaluation of lymphocytic migration, traffic, and invasiveness of lymphoma cells.

REFERENCES

1. Pfleger L, Tappeiner J. On the recognition of systematized endotheliomatosis of the cutaneous blood vessels (reticuloendotheliosis? Hautarzt 1959; 10: 359–63.
2. Sheibani K, Battifora H, Winberg CD, et al. Further evidence that 'malignant angioendotheliomatosis' is an angiotropic large-cell lymphoma. N Engl J Med 1986; 314(15): 943–8.
3. Gatter KC, Warnke RA. Intravascular large B-cell lymphoma. In: Jaffe ES, Harris NL, Stein H, Vardiman J, eds. Tumours of Haematopoietic and Lymphoid Tissues. Lyon: IARC Press, 2001: 177–8.
4. Ferreri AJ, Dognini G, Campo E, et al. Variations in clinical presentation, frequency of hemophagocytosis and clinical behavior of intravascular lymphoma diagnosed in different geographical regions. Haematologica 2007; 92: 486–92.
5. Ferreri AJ, Campo E, Seymour JF, et al. Intravascular lymphoma: clinical presentation, natural history, management and prognostic factors in a series of 38 cases, with special emphasis on the 'cutaneous variant'. Br J Haematol 2004; 127(2): 173–83.
6. Murase T. Asian variant of intravascular large B-cell lymphoma: still a diagnostic enigma? Intern Med 2002; 41(12): 1099–100.
7. Murase T, Nakamura S, Kawauchi K, et al. An Asian variant of intravascular large B-cell lymphoma: clinical, pathological and cytogenetic approaches to

8. diffuse large B-cell lymphoma associated with haemophagocytic syndrome. Br J Haematol 2000; 111(3): 826–34.
8. Ferry JA, Harris NL, Picker LJ, et al. Intravascular lymphomatosis (malignant angioendotheliomatosis). A B-cell neoplasm expressing surface homing receptors. Mod Pathol 1988; 1(6): 444–52.
9. Ponzoni M, Arrigoni G, Gould VE, et al. Lack of CD 29 (beta1 integrin) and CD 54 (ICAM-1) adhesion molecules in intravascular lymphomatosis. Hum Pathol 2000; 31(2): 220–6.
10. Murase T, Tashiro K, Suzuki T, Saito H, Nakamura S. Detection of antibodies to Fasciola and Anisakis in Japanese patients with intravascular lymphomatosis. Blood 1998; 92(6): 2182–3.
11. Au WY, Shek WH, Nicholls J, et al. T-cell intravascular lymphomatosis (angiotropic large cell lymphoma): association with Epstein–Barr viral infection. Histopathology 1997; 31(6): 563–7.
12. Wu H, Said JW, Ames ED, et al. First reported cases of intravascular large cell lymphoma of the NK cell type: clinical, histologic, immunophenotypic, and molecular features. Am J Clin Pathol 2005; 123(4): 603–11.
13. Hsiao CH, Su IJ, Hsieh SW, et al. Epstein–Barr virus-associated intravascular lymphomatosis within Kaposi's sarcoma in an AIDS patient. Am J Surg Pathol 1999; 23(4): 482–7.
14. Shimokawa I, Higami Y, Sakai H, et al. Intravascular malignant lymphomatosis: a case of T-cell lymphoma probably associated with human T-cell lymphotropic virus. Hum Pathol 1991; 22(2): 200–2.
15. Nixon BK, Kussick SJ, Carlon MJ, Rubin BP. Intravascular large B-cell lymphoma involving hemangiomas: an unusual presentation of a rare neoplasm. Mod Pathol 2005; 18(8): 1121–6.
16. Otrakji CL, Voigt W, Amador A, Nadji M, Gregorios JB. Malignant angioendotheliomatosis – a true lymphoma: a case of intravascular malignant lymphomatosis studied by Southern blot hybridization analysis. Hum Pathol 1988; 19(4): 475–8.
17. Sleater JP, Segal GH, Scott MD, Masih AS. Intravascular (angiotropic) large cell lymphoma: determination of monoclonality by polymerase chain reaction on paraffin-embedded tissues. Mod Pathol 1994; 7(5): 593–8.
18. Kanda M, Suzumiya J, Ohshima K, et al. Analysis of the immunoglobulin heavy chain gene variable region of intravascular large B-cell lymphoma. Virchows Arch 2001; 439(4): 540–6.
19. Vieites B, Fraga M, Lopez-Presas E, et al. Detection of t(14;18) translocation in a case of intravascular large B-cell lymphoma: a germinal centre cell origin in a subset of these lymphomas? Histopathology 2005; 46(4): 466–8.
20. Tsukadaira A, Okubo Y, Ogasawara H, et al. Chromosomal aberrations in intravascular lymphomatosis. Am J Clin Oncol 2002; 25(2): 178–81.
21. Rashid R, Johnson RJ, Morris S, et al. Intravascular large B-cell lymphoma associated with a near-tetraploid karyotype, rearrangement of BCL6, and a

t(11;14)(q13;q32). Cancer Genet Cytogenet 2006; 171(2): 101–4.

22. Ponzoni M, Ferreri AJ, Campo E, et al. Definition, diagnosis and management of intravascular large B-cell lymphoma: proposals and perspectives from an international consensus meeting. J Clin Oncol 2007; 25(21): 3168–73.

23. Takahashi E, Kajimoto K, Fukatsu T, et al. Intravascular large T-cell lymphoma: a case report of CD30-positive and ALK-negative anaplastic type with cytotoxic molecule expression. Virchows Arch 2005; 447(6): 1000–6.

24. Morice WG, Rodriguez FJ, Hoyer JD, Kurtin PJ. Diffuse large B-cell lymphoma with distinctive patterns of splenic and bone marrow involvement: clinicopathologic features of two cases. Mod Pathol 2005; 18(4): 495–502.

25. Feugier P, De March AK, Lesesve JF, et al. Intravascular bone marrow accumulation in persistent polyclonal lymphocytosis: a misleading feature for B-cell neoplasm. Mod Pathol 2004; 17(9): 1087–96.

26. Ponzoni M, Li CY. Isolated bone marrow non-Hodgkin's lymphoma: a clinicopathologic study. Mayo Clin Proc 1994; 69(1): 37–43.

27. Sukpanichnant S, Visuthisakchai S. Intravascular lymphomatosis: a study of 20 cases in Thailand and a review of the literature. Clin Lymphoma Myeloma 2006; 6(4): 319–28.

28. Murase T, Yamaguchi M, Suzuki R, et al. Intravascular large B-cell lymphoma (IVLBCL): a clinicopathologic study of 96 cases with special reference to the immunophenotypic heterogeneity of CD5. Blood 2007; 109(2): 478–85.

29. Murase T, Tomita Y, Nakamura S. Clinicopathologic features of intravascular large B-cell lymphoma in Japan: review of the special reference to the Asian variant. Rinsho Ketsueki 2002; 43(1): 5–11.

30. Yegappan S, Coupland R, Arber DA, et al. Angiotropic lymphoma: an immunophenotypically and clinically heterogeneous lymphoma. Mod Pathol 2001; 14(11): 1147–56.

31. Williams G, Foyle A, White D, et al. Intravascular T-cell lymphoma with bowel involvement: case report and literature review. Am J Hematol 2005; 78(3): 207–11.

32. Santucci M, Pimpinelli N, Massi D, et al. Cytotoxic/natural killer cell cutaneous lymphomas. Report of EORTC Cutaneous Lymphoma Task Force Workshop. Cancer 2003; 97(3): 610–27.

33. Conlin PA, Orden MB, Hough TR, Morgan DL. Myeloperoxidase-positive intravascular large B-cell lymphoma. Arch Pathol Lab Med 2001; 125(7): 948–50.

34. Seki K, Miyakoshi S, Lee GH, et al. Prostatic acid phosphatase is a possible tumor marker for intravascular large B-cell lymphoma. Am J Surg Pathol 2004; 28(10): 1384–8.

35. Nakamura S, Murase T, Kinoshita T. Intravascular large B-cell lymphoma: the heterogeneous clinical manifestations of its classical and hemophagocytosis-related forms. Haematologica 2007; 92(4): 434–6.

36. Bazhenova L, Higginbottom P, Mason J. Intravascular lymphoma: a role for single-agent rituximab. Leuk Lymphoma 2006; 47(2): 337–41.

Nasal natural killer/T-cell lymphoma 14

WY Au, Raymond HS Liang, YH Ko, and Won-Seog Kim

INCIDENCE AND EPIDEMIOLOGY

Nasal natural killer (NK)/T-cell lymphoma is a unique type of mature T/NK-cell lymphoma, that is invariably associated with Epstein–Barr virus (EBV), a distinct extranodal homing pattern, and a unique pattern of geographical distribution.[1] The disease is more commonly seen in Oriental Asia (including South East Asia, Southern China, Korea, and Japan) than in the West. It is also well recognized in South America and among Native Americans.[2] The incidence in Southern Asia, the Middle East, and Africa is reported to be low.[3,4] In Oriental countries, it accounts for up to 5% of all cases of lymphoma, and up to 30% of cases of mature T-cell lymphomas (Table 14.1).[5–8]

The relative incidence in Taiwan and Southern Japan is lower, due to dilution by human T-lymphotropic virus 1 (HTLV-1)-related disease.[9] In certain extranodal sites, such as the nasal area,[10] gut,[11] and the skin,[12] it actually represented a significant proportion (5–80%) of all cases of non-Hodgkin's lymphoma (NHL), especially in Orientals[13–16] (Table 14.2). In Europe and North America, the incidence is only 3–5% of the T-cell lymphomas, which in turn contribute to only 5% of all lymphoma cases.[17–19] Since many cases occur in migrants or patients of Oriental and Latin American descent, the true incidence in Caucasians may be even lower. However, the demography and clinical behavior of Caucasian patients, including EBV localization, disease homing, and response to treatment, appeared to be no different from the Oriental cases. In Japan, unique subtypes of EBV-related extranasal NK lineage malignancies – namely, mosquito bite hypersensitivity,[20] cies – namely, mosquito bite hypersensitivity,[20]

hydroa vacciniforme,[21] and chronic active EBV infection (CAEBV) – are reported. The relationship between these subcategories of disease and nasal-type lymphoma is uncertain. Other extranodal EBV negative malignant NK lymphoproliferations (e.g. blastoid NK leukemia, NK lymphocytosis, myeloid-NK leukemia) are unrelated to nasal-type lymphoma and will not be further discussed here.

There is currently no population-based survey of the incidence and epidemiology of nasal NK/T-cell lymphoma. Referral bias may play a part in most retrospective series from tertiary centers (Table 14.3). The reported demography data are, however, remarkably consistent between single institution, multicenter experiences and even international cooperative series. Published series report 20–260 cases, and the mean age of onset is from 40 to 50 years.[22] Very few pediatric cases are reported,[23] whereas elderly patients are common. There is a male predominance, with a male:female ratio ranging from 1.5 to 4. In most series, encompassing both nasal and extranasal disease, nasal cases (including disease in the adjacent upper aerodigestive tract) outnumber extranasal disease by a ratio of 3–8 times (see Table 14.3). There is no significant difference in median age or sex ratio between nasal and extranasal disease. In endemic areas, the incidence of nasal NK/T-cell lymphoma appeared to be relatively stable over time and remained unchanged in migrant populations.[24]

ETIOLOGY

As with most malignant lymphoproliferative diseases, the underlying cause of nasal

Table 14.1   Relative incidences of NK/T-cell lymphoma according to geographic regions

Relative incidence of NK lymphoma	Korea[6]	Canada[17]	Hong Kong[5]	Japan[7]	Worldwide[47]
Percent of all lymphomas	11.8	0.14	6		
Percent of all T-cell lymphomas	32	9	14	24	5–22
Percent of all extranodal lymphomas	Pending	Pending	Pending		

Table 14.2   Extranasal involvement sites of NK/T-cell lymphoma

Relative primary site of extranasal tumor	Lee[36]	Chan[29]	Ng[16]	Oshimi[7]
Skin	7	14	5	15
Gut	10	4	4	1
Testis/soft tissue or muscle	10	5/4	3/2	NA
Liver	4	Classify as stage IV	3	6
Lung	4	NA	NA	3
Orbit	2	NA	NA	NA
Aerodigestive	Classify as nasal	8	7	Classified as nasal
Spleen	Classify as stage IV	4	2	8

NK/T-cell lymphoma is largely unknown. There are, however, certain clues to its possible etiology. One peculiar feature is the invariable association with EBV. In these malignancies, EBV integration occurs directly in the malignant T and NK cells.[25] The consistent association has allowed EBV staining and EBV DNA monitoring in the peripheral blood to serve as diagnostic and prognostic markers.[26] The key to disease etiology probably lies in factors favoring proliferation of EBV-positive T/NK cells. The local EBV activity in the upper aerodigestive tract probably accounts for its unique localization at presentation and relapse. The latency of EBV was reported to be latency II, which is similar to that in nasopharyngeal carcinoma (NPC). There is preliminary evidence suggesting that distinct transforming strains of EBV (strain A with LMP-1 deletion) may favor development of nasal NK/T-cell lymphoma.[27,28] Although EBV integration is probably an early event in nasal lymphoma pathogenesis, the role of the EBV-transforming genes remains uncertain. Furthermore, it is difficult to maintain cell lines of nasal NK/T-cell lymphomas, which unlike NPC cell lines, remains EBV-positive in culture. EBV-negative transformation of nasal

NK/T-cell lymphoma has also never been reported. All these point to the key role of EBV in pathogenesis. The World Health Organization (WHO) classification also recognizes an entity called EBV-negative blastoid NK-cell lymphoma, an unrelated malignant proliferation that is undefined in terms of exact lineage and relationship with other NK and myeloid neoplasms.[29]

The unique racial distribution of nasal NK/T-cell lymphoma suggests a pertinent role for genetic predisposition. This is especially evident in migrant populations, where a relatively higher incidence of nasal NK/T-cell lymphoma persists into the second generation. Furthermore, nasal NK/T-cell lymphoma is seldom reported in Caucasians residing in Oriental areas. The predisposition is likely to be polygenic, and familial cases are very rare.[30] A recent study has shown that patients with nasal NK/T-cell lymphomas have a low frequency of the HLA-A*0201 allele, suggesting the importance of this allele in cytotoxic T-lymphocyte response.[7]

The relative roles of environmental factors in nasal NK/T-cell lymphoma is unknown. One multinational study suggests that risk may be increased with uncontrolled pesticide

Table 14.3   Clinical features and treatment outcomes of nasal NK/T-cell lymphoma

Epidemiology	Lee[22]	Chim[11]	Ng[16]	Oshimi[7]	Bossard[18]	Pagano[19]	Qunitalla	Au[47]
Number of cases	262	67	42	149	48	26	28	136
Year	1991–2004	1980–2002	1997–2003	1994–1998	1987–2003	1997–2004	NA	1990–2002
Country	Korea	Hong Kong	Singapore	Japan	France	Italy	Peru	Worldwide
Nature	Multicenter	Single center	Single center	Multicenter	Multicenter	Multicenter	Single center	Multicenter
Mean age of onset (range)	50 (21–77)	49 (17–84)	44 (27–86)	52 (14–89)	46 (22–79)	50 (20–80)	43 (11–72)	49 (21–89)
Male:female ratio	1.86	3.46 (52 vs 15)	4.26 (81 vs 19)	1.71 (94 vs 55)	1.52 (29 vs 19)	2.7 (19 vs 7)	1.28	2 vs 1
Nasal:extranasal ratio	5.67	Nasal only	2.85	4.73	Nasal only	8.67	Nasal only	2.63
Treatment	Chemo ± RT	CEOP ± RT	RT	Chemo ± RT/BMT	Chemo ± RT/BMT	Chemo ± RT/BMT	NA	85% chemo
Median survival	49% (5 years)	38 months	30 months	6–11 months	49% (5 years)	9 months	NA	6–16 months

RT, radiotherapy; BMT, Bone marrow transplant; CEOP, cyclophosphamide, epirubicin, vincristine, and prednisone.

exposure and drinking, but is reduced in smokers.[31] Despite a high incidence of other EBV-related lymphomas, NK/T-cell lymphoma is seldom reported in immunocompromised patients and among the HIV-infected populations of Asia and Latin America.[32,33] It is also known that local nasal symptoms may persist for years, or even decades, before the subsequent diagnosis of nasal or extranasal disease. Retrospective histological evidence may show long standing dormant EBV-positive malignant NK cells.[34] Hence, it is possible that unknown environmental factors may trigger disease progression in some cases. Rapid progression of nasal NK/T-cell lymphoma had been reported after surgery,[11] and mosquito bite NK reaction is a unique type of malignant NK lymphoproliferation in Japan.

PATHOGENESIS

Nasal NK/T-cell lymphoma cells usually show EBV latency type II phenotype, and express latent viral proteins, including Epstein–Barr nuclear antigen 1 (EBNA-1) and latent membrane protein 1 (LMP-1). LMP-1 up-regulates Th-1 cytokines such as interferon gamma (IFN-γ) and tumor necrosis factor alpha (TNF-α) via TNF receptor-associated factor (TRAF) 2,5/nuclear factor kappaB (NF-κB) signals.[62] DNA microarray analysis also shows up-regulation of many Th-1 type cytokine genes, including inducible (IP-10), IFN-γ, monokine induced by IFN-γ (MIG), and monocyte chemoattractant proteins (MCP)-1, 2, 3, and 4.[63] These cytokines, and especially IP-10 and MIG, are known to enhance NK-cell-mediated cell lysis and the release of granule-derived serine esterases, which explains why the lymphoma cells contain abundant cytotoxic granules such as granzyme B and perforin. As a result, releases of these cytotoxic granules into the cytosol induce prominent cell death of tumor cells, which is a common histological change in NK/T-cell lymphoma.[64–66]

Impairment of apoptotic signaling pathway may provide NK/T-cell lymphoma with a survival advantage. Whereas Fas (APO-1/CD95) and Fas ligand (Fas-L) are frequently expressed in tumor cells, NK/T-cell lymphomas are resistant to Fas-mediated apoptosis. The resistance to Fas-mediated cell death may be explained by mutations of Fas gene, methylation of proapoptotic genes including death-associated protein (DAP) kinase, and overexpression of apoptosis-inhibitory molecules such as c-FLIP (cellular FLICE inhibitory protein).[67–69] Likewise, constitutive activation of NF-κB in NK/T-cell lymphoma may also play a pivotal role in the survival of NK/T-cell lymphoma cells and drug resistance.[70]

Regarding the genetic changes of NK/T-cell lymphoma, no specific cytogenetic abnormality or mutation related to tumorigenesis of NK/T-cell lymphoma has been known. Previous studies using comparative genomic hybridization (CGH) showed frequent deletion of chromosome 1p, 6q, 12q, 13q, 17p, and gain of 2q, 10q, 13q, Xp.[71,72] A recent study using array CGH analysis revealed frequent loss of 6q21-q22.1, 6q22.33-q23.2, 6q25.3, and 6q26-q27, suggesting that the tumor suppressor genes in these regions may be associated with the development of NK/T-cell lymphoma.[73]

PATHOLOGY

Common histological changes of NK/T-cell lymphoma are polymorphous infiltration of small, medium, and large atypical lymphocytes with accompanying inflammatory cells of varying degree. The small to medium-sized tumor cells are often elongated and serpentine. Large tumor cells show vesicular nucleus with prominent nucleoli. The cytoplasm of some tumor cells is clear and abundant. Extensive necrosis of tumor tissue accompanied by numerous apoptotic bodies is common. Angioinvasion or angiocentric infiltration of tumor cells can be observed in 50–60% of cases, but may be absent in a small biopsy. These histological changes are similar, irrespective of site of tumor. In the upper airway, the tumor commonly shows ulceration, with acute inflammatory reaction of the mucosa, which hampers prompt diagnosis in superficial biopsy. Epitheliotropism, characterized by invasion of tumor cells into the epithelium of glands or surface mucosa, can be seen as well as pseudoepitheliomatous hyperplasia of the mucosa. In the soft tissue, tumors

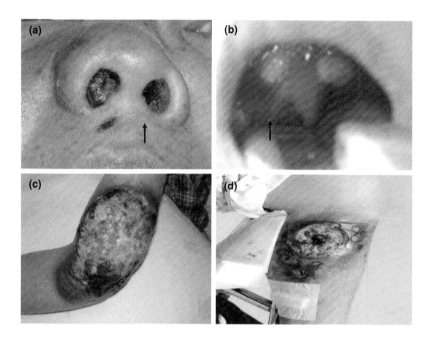

Figure 14.1 (a,b) Nasal NK/ T-cell lymphoma presented as perinasal skin infiltration and palatal ulcer. (c,d) Skin involvement of NK/T-cell lymphoma presented as large non-healing ulceration.

infiltrated in between skeletal muscle cells result in a moth-eaten appearance of each muscle fiber. In fat tissues, tumor cells rim the border of the fat vacuoles. In the skin, the tumor commonly involves the entire cutaneous layer, including the subcutaneous adipose tissue. Some cases involve the lower dermis and subcutaneous adipose tissue, with features of lobular panniculitis simulating subcutaneous panniculitis-like T-cell lymphoma. Extensive necrosis, ulceration of the epidermis, and erythrophagocytic histiocytosis are common. Tumors in the gastrointestinal tract mainly involve the large intestine. Perforation of the bowel wall may occur because of extensive necrosis of tumor tissue.[57,58]

NK/T-cell lymphoma is a tumor of cytotoxic cells of mainly NK lineage, with a minority of T cells. The typical immunophenotype is CD2(+), sCD3(−), cCD3(+), and CD56(+), with expression of cytotoxic molecules such as TIA-1, perforin, and granzyme B. CD56, which is a useful marker to diagnose NK/T-cell lymphoma, may be negative in 10–30% of cases.[16,59,60] Other NK cell markers such as CD16 and CD57 are usually negative. CD30 may be positive in about 30–70% of cases. By definition, EBV is detected by EBER

(EBV-encoded small RNA) in-situ hybridization in virtually all cases. T-cell receptor genes are in the germline in the majority of cases, but 0–27% of cases show clonal T-cell receptor gene rearrangement,[16,59–61] which supports the existence of T-lineage NK/T-cell lymphoma. CD56-negative NK/T-cell lymphomas are similar in histological findings to CD56-positive NK/T-cell lymphoma and show clonal *TCR* gene rearrangement in 30–45% of cases.[16]

CLINICAL PRESENTATION

The histology of NK/T-cell lymphoma is characterized by angioinvasion and necrosis, due to the production of Fas cytokines and cytotoxic granules by the malignant NK cells. Indeed, the previous names for the disease were angiocentric lymphoma and lethal midline granuloma. Hence, the clinical features are mainly dominated by local obstructive and destructive symptoms. Since up to two-thirds of cases occur in the upper aerodigestive tract, symptoms included nasal obstruction, ulcer, hemorrhage, pain, and discharge. Patients may present with nasopharyngeal, or oral or palatal ulcers, that were initially biopsied as carcinoma (Figure 14.1).[35,36] Advanced local

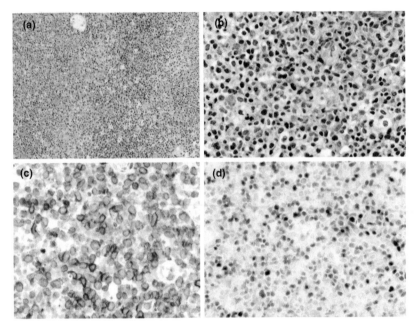

Figure 14.2 (a) NK-HE-lower: nasal NK/T-cell lymphoma. There is extensive necrosis. (b) NK-HE-high: nasal NK/T-cell lymphoma. The tumor is composed of small to medium-sized cells with pale cytoplasm. (c) The neoplastic cells are positive for cytoplasmic CD3e. (d) The neoplastic cells show nuclear labeling for EBV-encoded RNA (EBER).

cases may present as hoarseness of voice or difficulty in swallowing or speech. In some cases, intense local inflammation over an apparent small localized disease mass may be sufficient to cause fever of unknown origin or malignant cachexia. Due to the proximity of the nasal area to the orbit, ophthalmological presentations, such as proptosis, diplopia, or even retinal detachment due to effusion, can occur.[37] These are more commonly due to intense periorbital inflammation than to direct invasion.

Extranasal disease occurs in the skin, gut, soft tissue/testis and occasionally in the ovary, muscle, lung, and adrenals (see Table 14.2).[29] Regional lymph node spread may occur, but isolated nodal disease is uncommon. The clinical presentation of extranodal disease is also dominated by non-healing ulcerative lesions, often accompanied by fever due to necrosis and superinfection (Figure 14.2). Gut perforation and acute abdomen is not uncommon.[11] Hepatosplenic involvement usually accompanies disseminated blood and marrow involvement, and may be impossible to be classified as primary nasal or extranasal. It is notable that in apparently localized cases, occult marrow disease may be discerned by EBER staining. Systemic cases usually present as fulminant multiorgan failure with high lactate dehydrogenase level, fever and acidosis, pancytopenia, and hemophagocytosis. This is sometimes misdiagnosed as severe sepsis or autoimmune diseases. These cases often succumb before treatment and the diagnosis is often made at autopsy.

STAGING OF NK-CELL LYMPHOMA

No specific staging system for NK/T-cell lymphoma has been proposed. Ann Arbor staging has been usually applied for staging. However, the Ann Arbor system is based on the nodal disease with contiguous lymphatic spread. NK-cell lymphoma per se is an extranodal disease and isolated nodal disease is uncommon. Moreover, around 80% of the patients are presented in stage I/II according to the Ann Arbor system.[22] Therefore, the Ann Arbor system itself needs some modification to apply to NK-cell lymphoma.

Recent studies have shown the prognostic importance of local tumor invasiveness and the primary site (upper airway vs extra-upper airway).[36,38–40] The local extent of disease in the nasal region may not be appreciated without radiological evaluation.[41] The use of appropriate

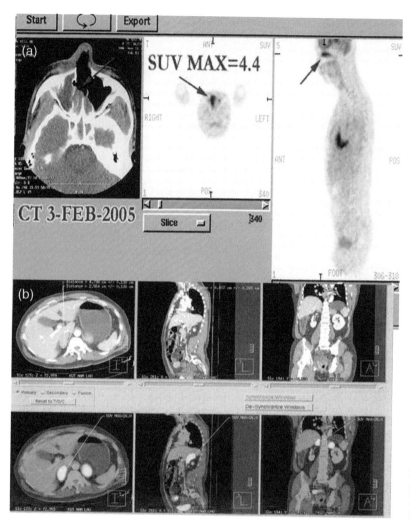

Figure 14.3 (a) CT and PET scans show nasal mass with high SUV. (b) PET scans show adrenal gland metastasis.

computed tomography (CT) reconstruction can show the extent of local invasion, and complete bone erosions are common. Magnetic resonance imaging (MRI) may give a good impression of the extent of soft tissue disease. Both imaging techniques are invaluable to radiotherapy planning. Positron emission tomography (PET) may have an emerging role in staging and disease monitoring, since preliminary experience suggest most lesions are of high standardized uptake value (SUV) (Figure 14.3). For extranasal disease, MRI may be most useful for delineating the extent of involvement in soft tissues, but the imaging appearance is non-diagnostic and must be supplemented by histological biopsy for documentation of

involvement. Although nasal NK/T-cell lymphoma may infiltrate the base of the skull and the orbit, meningeal involvement is not a common finding and there is no consensus for the need for cerebrospinal fluid (CSF) study and intrathecal prophylaxis. There is also the possibility of using circulating EBV DNA titer as a tumor marker,[26] and new staging including these factors should be explored.

PROGNOSTIC FACTORS

Due to the small number of cases, the general poor prognosis of patients, and the heterogeneity of treatment, there are few attempts at deriving prognostic factors for the disease. As in other lymphoma subtypes, the International Prognostic Index (IPI: age/stage/extranodal/lactate dehydrogenase [LDH]/performance status [PS]), initially derived for CHOP (cyclophosphamide, vincristine, prednisone, and doxorubicin)-treated diffuse large B-cell lymphoma, have been adapted for prognostication. However, it is questionable whether the IPI applies to a primarily extranodal T-cell disease.[42] In localized disease, the degree of local invasiveness is more predictive of survival than the complete IPI index.[43] A separate prognostic index for mature T-cell lymphoma applied to a limited subset of NK lymphoma, replacing extranodal site and stage with marrow positivity, has had some success (PIT: age/PS/LDH/bone marrow [BM] +ve).[44] However, it must be noted that T-cell lymphoma itself is histologically and prognostically heterogeneous. There has only been one attempt for an NK-cell lymphoma prognostic index, the result of which eliminates age and PS score and directs more emphasis on disease load (NK/T PI: B symptoms/stage/LDH/lymph node [LN]).[22] Verification by an international collection of nasal NK lymphoma cases have shown that this is the most robust index; the cases are triaged into equally divided prognostic groups, with the highest statistical significance (Figure 14.4).

Additional prognostic factors that may be of significance include anemia, thrombocytopenia, raised C-reactive protein, and histological evidence of more transformed cells and Ki67 positivity. Of note, however, the prognosis of extranasal NK/T-cell lymphoma is so poor that all prognostic scores and factors are clinically and statistically not significant.

TREATMENT

Optimal treatment strategies have not been fully defined yet, because this lymphoma subtype is a rare and relatively newly recognized entity. No prospective randomized clinical trials have been performed. Therefore, current evidence relies mainly on retrospective studies and reports of small series.

Localized disease

Radiotherapy is an important treatment modality for stage I/II nasal NK/T-cell lymphoma. Typically, a total dose of 30–60 Gy is administrated. The overall response rate ranges from 60 to 100%.[42,45–48] Front-line radiotherapy seems to be superior to front-line chemotherapy in disease control and survival,[19,42,46–49] and any forms of inclusion of radiotherapy yielded survival benefit. Although a high rate of response can be achieved through radiotherapy alone, relapses have been reported in 50% of the patients, and long-term survival rate was only 40–60% (Table 14.3).[10,42,45,46] Locoregional failure is the common pattern of failure.[38,45] However, systemic failure occurs in 25–30% of the patients.[38,45,46,48] Therefore, chemotherapy should be part of the treatment.

Front–line chemotherapy gives an average of 20–60% of CR.[42,46,47,50] Like other localized aggressive lymphoma, chemotherapy followed by radiotherapy was widely administrated to treat stage I/II nasal NK/T-cell lymphoma.[46,48,50] Anthracycline-containing chemotherapy treatments, including CHOP or CHOP-like regimens, have been most commonly used.[38,46,50] However, 30–40% of disease progression during the chemotherapy was reported.[46,49,50] Moreover, addition of anthracycline-containing chemotherapy after radiotherapy failed to improve survival.[42,46] Therefore, radiotherapy followed by, or concurrent with, chemotherapy may be the best treatment for localized nasal NK-cell lymphoma, perhaps with non-anthracycline-containing chemotherapy.[51]

Because extranasal NK-cell lymphomas usually present with advanced disease, only very limited data are available about treatment outcome of localized extranasal NK/T-cell lymphoma. Various treatments, including chemotherapy alone, surgery with/without chemotherapy, and radiotherapy with/without chemotherapy, were tried according to the primary site. The treatment outcomes were disappointing and the median survival was only 20 months.[36,39]

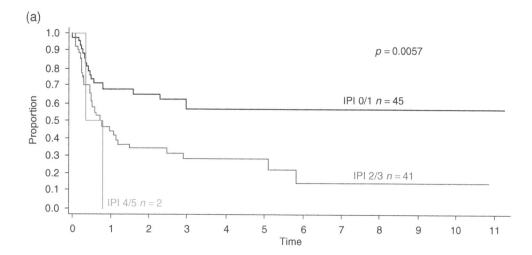

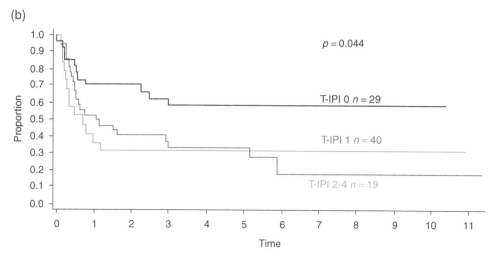

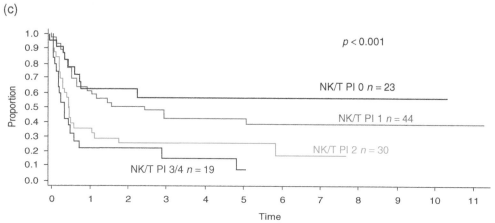

Figure 14.4   Prognostic models. (a) DLCL-B IPI:[74] age/stage/extranodal/LDH/PS. (b) Italian PIT:[41] age/PS/LDH/BM+ve. (c) Korean NK/T PI:[22] B symptoms/stage/LDH/LN.

Advanced-stage disease

Combination chemotherapy is the main treatment for stage III/IV NK/T-cell lymphoma. However, the results were very disappointing. There is no consensus as to the optimal chemotherapy regimen. Anthracycline-containing regimens give less than 20% of response.[36,39] The poor response of anthracycline-containing chemotherapy may be due to high expression of the multidrug resistance (*MDR*) gene.[52] Therefore, the role of non-anthracycline-containing chemotherapy regimens or non-*MDR* targeted agents should be explored.

One of the promising chemotherapeutic agent is L-asparaginase.[40,53] L-asparaginase-based regimens gave 50–60% response rate and around 60% long-term survival for anthracycline-refractory NK/T-cell lymphoma patients.[40,53] Optimal use of L-asparaginase in the first-line treatment should be explored.

Hematopoietic stem cell transplantation

Some reports have demonstrated promising results with auto-HSCT (hematopoietic stem cell transplantation) as salvage treatment. However, most of the nasal NK/T-cell lymphoma patients present with stage I/II or low/low intermediate-risk group by IPI.[22,38] Therefore, only limited data are available to show the role of auto-HSCT in first CR (CR1). For patients transplanted in CR, long-term overall survival was 68–80%.[54–56] These results might appear superior to historical controls, but the patients were highly selected. Moreover, survival benefits were only proved in high-risk patients.[56] Hence, auto-HSCT cannot be used routinely in CR, especially CR1.

Allogeneic-HSCT (allo-HSCT) can be another appealing option: in high-risk patients (including auto-HSCT failures), a 2-year survival of 40% was reported.[40] However, treatment related mortality up to 40–60% can be associated with allo-HSCT.[40,55] The optimal timing and conditioning for allo-HSCT has so far not been explored.

REFERENCES

1. Rudiger T, Weisenburger DD, Anderson JR, et al. Peripheral T-cell lymphoma (excluding anaplastic large-cell lymphoma): results from the Non-Hodgkin's Lymphoma Classification Project. Ann Oncol 2002; 13(1): 140–9.
2. Aviles A, Diaz NR, Neri N, Cleto S, Talavera A. Angiocentric nasal T/natural killer cell lymphoma: a single centre study of prognostic factors in 108 patients. Clin Lab Haematol 2000; 22(4): 215–20.
3. Naresh KN, Agarwal B, Nathwani BN, et al. Use of the World Health Organization (WHO) classification of non-Hodgkin's lymphoma in Mumbai, India: a review of 200 consecutive cases by a panel of five expert hematopathologists. Leuk Lymphoma 2004; 45(8): 1569–77.
4. Nigidie A, Schneider J. Nasal NK/T-cell lymphoma causing diagnostic difficulties. Ethiop Med J 2005; 43(3): 197–201.
5. Au WY, Ma SY, Chim CS, et al. Clinicopathologic features and treatment outcome of mature T-cell and natural killer-cell lymphomas diagnosed according to the World Health Organization classification scheme: a single center experience of 10 years. Ann Oncol 2005; 16(2): 206–14.
6. Kim K, Kim WS, Jung CW, et al. Clinical features of peripheral T-cell lymphomas in 78 patients diagnosed according to the Revised European-American lymphoma (REAL) classification. Eur J Cancer 2002; 38(1): 75–81.
7. Oshimi K, Kawa K, Nakamura S, et al. NK-cell neoplasms in Japan. Hematology 2005; 10(3): 237–45.
8. Tham IW, Lee KM, Yap SP, Loong SL. Outcome of patients with nasal natural killer (NK)/T-cell lymphoma treated with radiotherapy, with or without chemotherapy. Head Neck 2006; 28(2): 126–34.
9. Ohshima K, Liu Q, Koga T, Suzumiya J, Kikuchi M. Classification of cell lineage and anatomical site, and prognosis of extranodal T-cell lymphoma – natural killer cell, cytotoxic T lymphocyte, and non-NK/CTL types. Virchows Arch 2002; 440(4): 425–35.
10. Cheung MM, Chan JK, Lau WH, et al. Primary non-Hodgkin's lymphoma of the nose and nasopharynx: clinical features, tumor immunophenotype, and treatment outcome in 113 patients. J Clin Oncol 1998; 16(1): 70–7.
11. Chim CS, Au WY, Shek TW, et al. Primary CD56 positive lymphomas of the gastrointestinal tract. Cancer 2001; 91(3): 525–33.
12. Bekkenk MW, Jansen PM, Meijer CJ, Willemze R. CD56+ hematological neoplasms presenting in the skin: a retrospective analysis of 23 new cases and 130 cases from the literature. Ann Oncol 2004; 15(7): 1097–108.
13. Mitarnun W, Suwiwat S, Pradutkanchana J. Epstein–Barr virus-associated extranodal non-Hodgkin's lymphoma of the sinonasal tract and

nasopharynx in Thailand. Asian Pac J Cancer Prev 2006; 7(1): 91–4.

14. Kitamura A, Yamashita Y, Hasegawa Y, et al. Primary lymphoma arising in the nasal cavity among Japanese. Histopathology 2005; 47(5): 523–32.

15. Yasukawa K, Kato N, Kodama K, Hamasaka A, Hata H. The spectrum of cutaneous lymphomas in Japan: a study of 62 cases based on the World Health Organization Classification. J Cutan Pathol 2006; 33(7): 487–91.

16. Ng SB, Lai KW, Murugaya S, et al. Nasal-type extranodal natural killer/T-cell lymphomas: a clinicopathologic and genotypic study of 42 cases in Singapore. Mod Pathol 2004; 17(9): 1097–107.

17. Savage KJ, Chhanabhai M, Gascoyne RD, Connors JM. Characterization of peripheral T-cell lymphomas in a single North American institution by the WHO classification. Ann Oncol 2004; 15(10): 1467–75.

18. Bossard C, Belhadj K, Reyes F, et al. Expression of the granzyme B inhibitor PI9 predicts outcome in nasal NK/T-cell lymphoma: results of a Western series of 48 patients treated with first-line polychemotherapy within the Groupe d'Etude des Lymphomes de l'Adulte (GELA) trials. Blood 2006; 31: 31.

19. Pagano L, Gallamini A, Trape G, et al. NK/T-cell lymphomas 'nasal type': an Italian multicentric retrospective survey. Ann Oncol 2006; 17(5): 794–800.

20. Ishihara S, Yabuta R, Tokura Y, Ohshima K, Tagawa S. Hypersensitivity to mosquito bites is not an allergic disease, but an Epstein–Barr virus-associated lymphoproliferative disease. Int J Hematol 2000; 72(2): 223–8.

21. Iwatsuki K, Satoh M, Yamamoto T, et al. Pathogenic link between hydroa vacciniforme and Epstein–Barr virus-associated hematologic disorders. Arch Dermatol 2006; 142(5): 587–95.

22. Lee J, Suh C, Park YH, et al. Extranodal natural killer T-cell lymphoma, nasal-type: a prognostic model from a retrospective multicenter study. J Clin Oncol 2006; 24(4): 612–18.

23. Kim D, Ko Y, Suh Y, et al. Characteristics of Epstein–Barr virus associated childhood non-Hodgkin's lymphoma in the Republic of Korea. Virchows Arch 2005; 447(3): 593–6.

24. Au WY, Gascoyne RD, Klasa RD, et al. Incidence and spectrum of non-Hodgkin lymphoma in Chinese migrants to British Columbia. Br J Haematol 2005; 128(6): 792–6.

25. Chiang AK, Chan AC, Srivastava G, Ho FC. Nasal T/natural killer (NK)-cell lymphomas are derived from Epstein–Barr virus-infected cytotoxic lymphocytes of both NK- and T-cell lineage. Int J Cancer 1997; 73(3): 332–8.

26. Au WY, Pang A, Choy C, Chim CS, Kwong YL. Quantification of circulating Epstein–Barr virus (EBV) DNA in the diagnosis and monitoring of natural killer cell and EBV-positive lymphomas in immunocompetent patients. Blood 2004; 104(1): 243–9.

27. Suzumiya J, Ohshima K, Takeshita M, et al. Nasal lymphomas in Japan: a high prevalence of Epstein–Barr virus type A and deletion within the latent membrane protein gene. Leuk Lymphoma 1999; 35(5–6): 567–78.

28. Kim JE, Kim YA, Jeon YK, et al. Comparative analysis of NK/T-cell lymphoma and peripheral T-cell lymphoma in Korea: clinicopathological correlations and analysis of EBV strain type and 30-bp deletion variant LMP1. Pathol Int 2003; 53(11): 735–43.

29. Chan JK, Sin VC, Wong KF, et al. Nonnasal lymphoma expressing the natural killer cell marker CD56: a clinicopathologic study of 49 cases of an uncommon aggressive neoplasm. Blood 1997; 89(12): 4501–13.

30. Kojya S, Matsumura J, Ting L, et al. Familial nasal NK/T-cell lymphoma and pesticide use. Am J Hematol 2001; 66(2): 145–7.

31. Xu JX, Hoshida Y, Yang WI, et al. Life-style and environmental factors in the development of nasal NK/T-cell lymphoma: a case-control study in East Asia. Int J Cancer 2007; 120(2): 406–10.

32. Oh SC, Choi CW, Kim BS, et al. NK/T-cell lymphoma associated with Epstein–Barr virus in a patient infected with human immunodeficiency virus: an autopsy case. Int J Hematol 2004; 79(5): 480–3.

33. Hoshida Y, Hongyo T, Nakatsuka S, et al. Gene mutations in lymphoproliferative disorders of T and NK/T cell phenotypes developing in renal transplant patients. Lab Invest 2002; 82(3): 257–64.

34. Au W, Kwong Y, Chan A. Scrotal skin ulcer in a patient with a previous tonsillectomy because of natural killer cell lymphoma. Am J Dermatopathol 1998; 20(6): 582–5.

35. Kwong YL, Chan AC, Liang R, et al. CD56+ NK lymphomas: clinicopathological features and prognosis. Br J Haematol 1997; 97(4): 821–9.

36. Lee J, Kim WS, Park YH, et al. Nasal-type NK/T cell lymphoma: clinical features and treatment outcome. Br J Cancer 2005; 92(7): 1226–30.

37. Hon C, Kwok AK, Shek TW, Chim JC, Au WY. Vision-threatening complications of nasal T/NK lymphoma. Am J Ophthalmol 2002; 134(3): 406–10.

38. Au W, Intragumtornchai T, Nakamura S, Armitage JO, Liang R. Clinical and pathological differences between nasal and nasal-type NK/T cell lymphomas: a summary of 136 cases from the International T Cell Lymphoma (ITCL) Project. Blood (ASH Annual Meeting Abstracts): 2006; 108(Abstract 292).

39. Lee J, Park YH, Kim WS, et al. Extranodal nasal type NK/T-cell lymphoma: elucidating clinical prognostic factors for risk-based stratification of therapy. Eur J Cancer 2005; 41(10): 1402–8.

40. Murashige N, Kami M, Kishi Y, et al. Allogeneic haematopoietic stem cell transplantation as a promising treatment for natural killer-cell neoplasms. Br J Haematol 2005; 130(4): 561–7.

41. King AD, Lei KI, Ahuja AT. MRI of neck nodes in non-Hodgkin's lymphoma of the head and neck. Br J Radiol 2004; 77(914): 111–15.

42. Chim CS, Ma SY, Au WY, et al. Primary nasal natural killer cell lymphoma: long-term treatment outcome and relationship with the International Prognostic Index. Blood 2004; 103(1): 216–21.

43. Kim TM, Park YH, Lee SY, et al. Local tumor invasiveness is more predictive of survival than International Prognostic Index in stage I(E)/II(E) extranodal NK/T-cell lymphoma, nasal type. Blood 2005; 106(12): 3785–90.

44. Gallamini A, Stelitano C, Calvi R, et al. Peripheral T-cell lymphoma unspecified (PTCL-U): a new prognostic model from a retrospective multicentric clinical study. Blood 2004; 103(7): 2474–9.

45. Kim GE, Cho JH, Yang WI, et al. Angiocentric lymphoma of the head and neck: patterns of systemic failure after radiation treatment. J Clin Oncol 2000; 18(1): 54–63.

46. Li YX, Yao B, Jin J, et al. Radiotherapy as primary treatment for stage IE and IIE nasal natural killer/T-cell lymphoma. J Clin Oncol 2006; 24(1): 181–9.

47. Ribrag V, Ell Hajj M, Janot F, et al. Early locoregional high-dose radiotherapy is associated with long-term disease control in localized primary angiocentric lymphoma of the nose and nasopharynx. Leukemia 2001; 15(7): 1123–6.

48. You JY, Chi KH, Yang MH, et al. Radiation therapy versus chemotherapy as initial treatment for localized nasal natural killer (NK)/T-cell lymphoma: a single institute survey in Taiwan. Ann Oncol 2004; 15(4): 618–25.

49. Isobe K, Uno T, Tamaru J, et al. Extranodal natural killer/T-cell lymphoma, nasal type: the significance of radiotherapeutic parameters. Cancer 2006; 106(3): 609–15.

50. Kim WS, Song SY, Ahn YC, et al. CHOP followed by involved field radiation: is it optimal for localized nasal natural killer/T-cell lymphoma? Ann Oncol 2001; 12(3): 349–52.

51. Yamaguchi M, Oguchi M, Tobinai K, et al. Phase I/II study of concurrent chemoradiotherapy for newly-diagnosed, localized nasal NK/T-cell lymphoma: results of a phase I portion of JCOG0211-DI. Blood (ASH Annual Meeting Abstracts) 2005; 106(2685).

52. Egashira M, Kawamata N, Sugimoto K, Kaneko T, Oshimi K. P-glycoprotein expression on normal and abnormally expanded natural killer cells and inhibition of P-glycoprotein function by cyclosporin A and its analogue, PSC833. Blood 1999; 93(2): 599–606.

53. Yong W, Zheng W, Zhu J, et al. Midline NK/T-cell lymphoma nasal-type: treatment outcome, the effect of L-asparaginase based regimen, and prognostic factors. Hematol Oncol 2006; 24(1): 28–32.

54. Au WY, Lie AK, Liang R, et al. Autologous stem cell transplantation for nasal NK/T-cell lymphoma: a progress report on its value. Ann Oncol 2003; 14(11): 1673–6.

55. Suzuki R, Suzumiya J, Nakamura S, et al. Hematopoietic stem cell transplantation for natural killer-cell lineage neoplasms. Bone Marrow Transplant 2006; 37(4): 425–31.

56. Kim HJ, Bang SM, Lee J, et al. High-dose chemotherapy with autologous stem cell transplantation in extranodal NK/T-cell lymphoma: a retrospective comparison with non-transplantation cases. Bone Marrow Transplant 2006; 37(9): 819–24.

57. Nakamura S, Katoh E, Koshikawa T, et al. Clinicopathologic study of nasal T/NK-cell lymphoma among the Japanese. Pathol Int 1997; 47(1): 38–53.

58. Ko YH, Cho EY, Kim JE, et al. NK and NK-like T-cell lymphoma in extranasal sites: a comparative clinico-pathological study according to site and EBV status. Histopathology 2004; 44(5): 480–9.

59. Ko YH, Ree HJ, Kim WS, et al. Clinicopathologic and genotypic study of extranodal nasal-type natural killer/T-cell lymphoma and natural killer precursor lymphoma among Koreans. Cancer 2000; 89(10): 2106–16.

60. Gaal K, Sun NC, Hernandez AM, Arber DA. Sinonasal NK/T-cell lymphomas in the United States. Am J Surg Pathol 2000; 24(11): 1511–17.

61. Ohsawa M, Nakatsuka S, Kanno H, et al. Immunophenotypic and genotypic characterization of nasal lymphoma with polymorphic reticulosis morphology. Int J Cancer 1999; 81(6): 865–70.

62. Chuang HC, Lay JD, Hsieh WC, et al. Epstein–Barr virus LMP1 inhibits the expression of SAP gene and upregulates Th1 cytokines in the pathogenesis of hemophagocytic syndrome. Blood 2005; 106(9): 3090–6.

63. Ohshima K, Karube K, Hamasaki M, et al. Differential chemokine, chemokine receptor and cytokine expression in Epstein–Barr virus-associated lymphoproliferative diseases. Leuk Lymphoma 2003; 44(8): 1367–78.

64. Taub DD, Sayers TJ, Carter CR, Ortaldo JR. Alpha and beta chemokines induce NK cell migration and enhance NK-mediated cytolysis. J Immunol 1995; 155(8): 3877–88.

65. Ng CS, Lo ST, Chan JK, Chan WC. CD56+ putative natural killer cell lymphomas: production of cytolytic effectors and related proteins mediating tumor cell apoptosis? Hum Pathol 1997; 28(11): 1276–82.

66. Ko YH, Park S, Jin H, et al. Granzyme B leakage-induced apoptosis is a crucial mechanism of cell death in nasal-type NK/T-cell lymphoma. Lab Invest 2007;

67. Takakuwa T, Dong Z, Nakatsuka S, et al. Frequent mutations of Fas gene in nasal NK/T-cell lymphoma. Oncogene 2002; 21(30): 4702–5.

68. Nakatsuka S, Takakuwa T, Tomita Y, et al. Hypermethylation of death-associated protein (DAP) kinase CpG island is frequent not only in B-cell but also in T- and natural killer (NK)/T-cell malignancies. Cancer Sci 2003; 94(1): 87–91.

69. Jeon YK, Kim H, Park SO, et al. Resistance to Fas-mediated apoptosis is restored by cycloheximide

through the downregulation of cellular FLIPL in NK/T-cell lymphoma. Lab Invest 2005; 85(7): 874–84.

70. Kim K, Ryu K, Ko Y, Park C. Effects of nuclear factor-kappaB inhibitors and its implication on natural killer T-cell lymphoma cells. Br J Haematol 2005; 131(1): 59–66.

71. Siu LL, Wong KF, Chan JK, Kwong YL. Comparative genomic hybridization analysis of natural killer cell lymphoma/leukemia. Recognition of consistent patterns of genetic alterations. Am J Pathol 1999; 155(5): 1419–25.

72. Ko YH, Choi KE, Han JH, Kim JM, Ree HJ. Comparative genomic hybridization study of nasal-type NK/T-cell lymphoma. Cytometry 2001; 46(2): 85–91.

73. Nakashima Y, Tagawa H, Suzuki R, et al. Genome-wide array-based comparative genomic hybridization of natural killer cell lymphoma/leukemia: different genomic alteration patterns of aggressive NK-cell leukemia and extranodal NK/T-cell lymphoma, nasal type. Genes Chromosomes Cancer 2005; 44(3): 247–55.

74. Shipp et al. A predictive model for aggressive non-Hodgkin's lymphoma. N Engl J Med 1993; 329(14): 987–94.

Primary breast lymphoma

15

Giovanni Martinelli and Gail Ryan

INTRODUCTION

Primary malignant lymphoma of the breast is a rare entity, representing less than 0.5% of all malignant breast tumors and less than 1% of all malignant lymphomas.[1,2] The criteria for primary breast lymphoma were defined by Wiseman and Liao in their original article published in 1972:

- a technically adequate specimen for pathological evaluation
- mammary tissue and lymphomatous infiltrate must be in close association
- no evidence of concurrent systemic lymphoma or previous extramammary lymphoma (the presence of ipsilateral axillary node involvement is considered acceptable).[3]

The published literature on breast lymphomas documents several hundred cases identified over a 30-year period, mostly in small single institution series including both primary and secondary involvement of the breast by lymphoma, and using varying classification systems.[4–8] This has made it difficult to define the exact nature of the condition, and to draw accurate conclusions on the incidence of different histological subtypes, prognostic factors, and outcomes. However, a recent large multi-institutional retrospective series,[9] and a prospective study,[10] in association with literature reviews, have made the picture much clearer, and provide valuable insights into the nature and management of the group of diseases included in the general classification of primary breast lymphoma.

The etiology of primary breast lymphoma remains uncertain, with no specific predisposing factors identified. A complex biological and hormonal relationship between the breast and the lymphoma is suggested by the occurrence of bilateral presentations of primary breast lymphoma, and the presence of estrogen and/or progesterone receptors in some breast lymphomas,[11] but the nature of this relationship is currently unclear.

The clinical presentation of breast lymphoma is almost always as a palpable rubbery mass in the breast, which is not fixed to the chest wall or to overlying skin. It is generally painless, is often large at the time of diagnosis, and is commonly rapidly growing.[1,2,12] However, the clinical features, while suggestive, are not sufficiently specific to distinguish primary breast lymphoma from other breast tumors.

Diagnostic procedures for primary breast lymphomas include radiological examination (mammography, ultrasound, magnetic resonance imaging [MRI]),[13,14] radioisotope imaging (gallium scan, positron emission tomography [PET] scan),[15,16] fine needle aspiration cytology,[17] and histopathological biopsy. Mammography and ultrasound are performed in the majority of patients, but although they have a high degree of sensitivity (~90% positivity) in detecting lymphomatous masses in the breast, their specificity is relatively low, and they are unable to distinguish reliably between breast lymphoma and other breast tumors.[18,19] MRI of the breast may have greater specificity; however, the lack of large comparative studies makes this procedure unsuitable for routine use.[20–22] Both gallium and 18-fluorodeoxyglucose (FDG)-PET scans are positive in a high percentage of patients with primary breast lymphoma, but specificity is once again a limitation, so they are most useful in response evaluation, particularly in the setting of a residual mass.[15,16] Fine needle aspiration cytology is positive for lymphoma in around two-thirds of cases,[9] but subclassification may be inaccurate or impossible,[17] and basing treatment decisions on cytology alone is therefore inappropriate. Thus, the most important diagnostic procedure is excisional biopsy. Once the diagnosis of lymphoma is confirmed or suspected on conventional histological grounds, additional immunohistochemistry and accurate subtyping of the tumor is critical for planning subsequent local or systemic treatments.

Almost all reported primary breast lymphomas are of B-cell origin, with diffuse large B-cell histology – World Health Organization (WHO)/Revised European–American Classification of Lymphoid Neoplasms (REAL) – accounting for approximately 70–80% of all primary breast lymphomas. Less frequent are Burkitt's lymphoma, follicular lymphoma, and marginal zone (mucosa-associated lymphoid tissue [MALT]) lymphoma.[2,4,5,9] In the large retrospective series compiled by Ryan et al on behalf of the International Extranodal Lymphoma Study Group (IELSG), more than 300 cases of primary breast lymphoma were evaluated. In this series, 73% were of diffuse large B-cell histology, 13% were follicular lymphomas, 9% marginal zone lymphomas (M, 2% Burkitt's lymphoma, 2% other B-cell lymphomas, and only 1% were of T-cell origin.[9]

PRIMARY DIFFUSE LARGE B-CELL LYMPHOMA OF THE BREAST

Diffuse large B-cell lymphoma (DLBCL) of the breast is predominantly a disease of older patients, with a median age at diagnosis of 64 years old. Many series report a slightly higher rate of occurrence in the right breast compared with the left, of uncertain significance. The incidence of bilateral involvement at the time of initial diagnosis is ~5%. The median tumor diameter at diagnosis is 4 cm, and nodal involvement is present in 25–30% of patients.

Eastern Cooperative Oncology Group (ECOG) performance status is 0 or 1 in almost all patients. B symptoms are uncommon, being present in less than 5% of patients at diagnosis, with lactate dehydrogenase (LDH) being raised in ~25%.

Variable treatment approaches have been used in the past, the variability mostly reflecting different treatment eras. There appears to be no advantage to mastectomy, as compared to conservative surgery (excision biopsy/wide local excision).[9] Data from both the IELSG series[9] and the prospective study of Aviles et al[10] showed the best results to be achieved by conservative surgery, followed by the combination of at least three cycles of an anthracycline-based chemotherapy regimen (usually CHOP [cyclophosphamide, vincristine, prednisone, and doxorubicin]) and radiotherapy to at least the involved breast. With this approach, results similar to those achieved in the ECOG[23] and Southwest Oncology Group (SWOG)[24] studies of early-stage, predominantly nodal, DLBCL were achieved, with actuarial 5- and 10-year progression-free survivals of ~65% and 60%, and 5- and 10-year overall survivals of ~75% and 65% (Figures 15.1 and 15.2).

Patterns of relapse seen in almost all studies of primary DLBCL of the breast are distinctly different from those seen in patients presenting with a nodal DLBCL. Relapses in breast, central nervous system (CNS), and other extranodal sites are much more frequent than nodal relapses. Interestingly, the sites of relapse in the two major DLBCL primary breast lymphoma studies were different. Breast was the major site of relapse in the IELSG series[9] (16% of first relapses, with one-third occurring in the initially involved breast, and two-thirds in the contralateral breast), whereas in the Aviles series[10] the CNS was the major site of relapse. The reason for this difference is not immediately clear, but may relate to the competing risks of breast and CNS relapse in this disease entity. The IELSG data suggested that chemotherapy reduced the risk of contralateral breast relapse and, as the average number of anthracycline cycles was 4 in this series, as compared to the 6 cycles used in the Aviles study, a higher rate of breast relapse might be expected. Conversely,

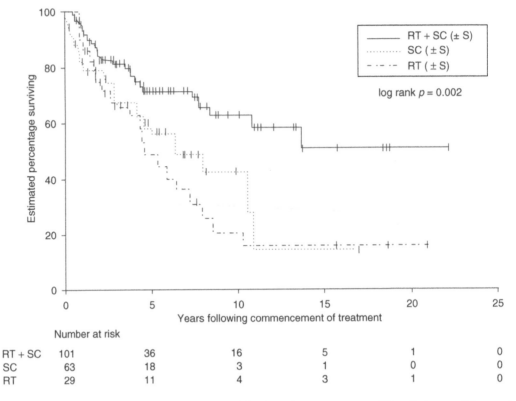

Figure 15.1 Overall survival of patients with DLBCL of the breast by treatment type. RT, radiotherapy; SC, systemic chemotherapy; S, surgery.

superior breast control achieved in the Aviles study may then have resulted in CNS becoming the major site of relapse.

Currently, the role of CNS prophylaxis has not been resolved, and further study is required to confirm whether or not it is of benefit. It may be that, with the combination of optimal chemotherapy and radiotherapy, CNS prophylaxis is not necessary. Similarly, the theoretical benefit of contralateral breast radiation in reducing the risk of contralateral breast relapse, and thus improving outcomes generally, as suggested by IELSG data,[9] may be reduced or negated by optimal chemotherapy.

Survival following relapse is generally poor, irrespective of second-line therapy, with median survival of only 12 months post-relapse (Figure 15.3).

Patients with bilateral presentation appear to have a significantly worse prognosis than those presenting with unilateral disease, with

actuarial 3-year progression-free and overall survivals of only 36% and 46%, respectively, in the IELSG series.[9] Although the numbers are small, and evidence-based recommendations thus impossible to make, there appears to be a strong case for intensive chemotherapy, bilateral breast radiotherapy, and CNS prophylaxis.

Other potential prognostic factors for DLBCL of the breast have been examined in multivariate analysis. In the IELSG series,[9] International Prognostic Index (IPI) and the use of anthracycline were significantly associated with improved progression-free survival (p = 0.01 and 0.001, respectively), and for overall survival IPI, use of anthracycline and radiotherapy were all significantly associated with improvement (p <0.001, 0.02, and 0.03, respectively). Other factors not found to be significant included primary tumor size, nodal involvement, treatment era, and number of cycles of anthracycline chemotherapy.

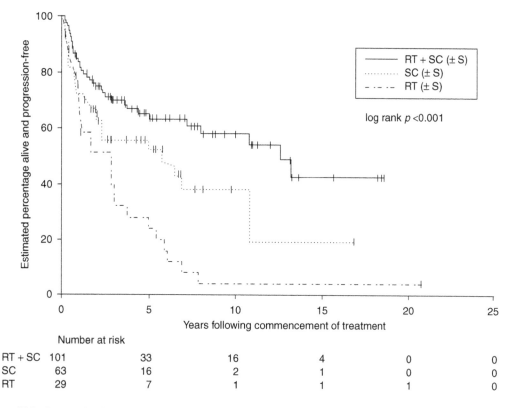

Figure 15.2 Progression-free survival of patients with DLBCL of the breast by treatment type.

Although patients with DLBCL of the breast treated with CHOP chemotherapy and local radiotherapy achieve outcomes similar to those of the SWOG and ECOG studies, these latter results are considerably inferior to those recently reported in landmark studies of DLBCL,[25,26] in which rituximab, a chimeric monoclonal antibody against the CD20 B-cell antigen, has been added to standard chemotherapy protocols ± radiotherapy. Although these studies included very few patients with primary breast DLBCL, it is likely that similar improvements in progression-free and overall survival will accrue from its use in this scenario. A recent retrospective analysis examined the outcome of DLBCL according to site of origin, and found that whether the presentation was extranodal or nodal did not influence outcome; other clinical and biological factors such as IPI and immunophenotypic characteristics (e.g. BCL2, BCL6, MUM1, CD10) appear to be more significant in determining prognosis;

however, in this study all the extranodal lymphomas originating outside the gastrointestinal tract or the Waldeyer's ring were grouped together, thus limiting the possibility of proper evaluation of the clinical characteristics and the prognostic role of each particular primary site.[27] The addition of rituximab to anthracycline-based chemotherapy and radiotherapy is therefore recommended for primary DLBCL.

Whether the improvement in outcomes as a result of the use of rituximab will result in changes to other recommendations, e.g. the need for radiotherapy or CNS prophylaxis, will only be resolved through well-conducted prospective studies.

PRIMARY FOLLICULAR AND MARGINAL ZONE (MALT) LYMPHOMA OF THE BREAST

Approximately 25% of all primary breast lymphomas are of 'low-grade' histology.[28] The

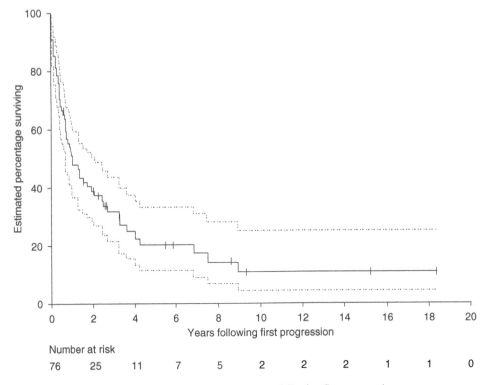

Figure 15.3   Overall survival of patients with DLBCL of the breast following first progression.

follicular subtype seems to be the more common histology, accounting for approximately 10–15% of all low-grade breast lymphomas. The true incidence of MALT lymphoma of the breast is uncertain, with the incidence in different series ranging from 0 to 40%.[4,29] This wide range of results is likely to relate to the relatively recent characterization of this entity of malignant lymphoma,[30] and the lack of standardized procedures for its diagnosis used in most of these retrospective studies.[2,4,29] However, a reasonable estimate of the incidence of marginal zone lymphoma (MALT) in retrospective series of primary breast lymphoma is 8–10%.

Clinical presentation and investigation of the 'low-grade' variants is similar to that of primary DLBCL of the breast, although follicular lymphomas tend to occur at a later age, with a median age at diagnosis around 10 years older. Occasionally, there are cases of follicular/ MALT lymphoma presenting with involvement of the breast and other extranodal or nodal sites, and in these cases the site of origin can be difficult to determine, even with complete staging.

'Low-grade' primary breast lymphomas appear to have similar clinical behavior to lymphomas of similar histology and stage presenting in other extranodal or nodal sites: i.e. breast presentation does not appear to be an adverse prognostic factor. In general, conservative surgery followed by radiotherapy is the recommended treatment for localized follicular/ MALT lymphoma of the breast.

OTHER SUBTYPES OF PRIMARY BREAST LYMPHOMA

Other subtypes are so uncommon that no specific features or treatment recommendations can be given. Treatment appropriate to that histological subtype presenting elsewhere in the body is appropriate in this situation.

REFERENCES

1. Abbondanzo SL, Seidman JD, Lefkowitz M, et al. Primary diffuse large B-cell lymphoma of the breast. A clinicopathologic study of 31 cases. Pathol Res Pract 1996; 192(1): 37–43.

2. Giardini R, Piccolo C, Rilke F. Primary non-Hodgkin's lymphomas of the female breast. Cancer 1992; 69(3): 725–35.

3. Wiseman C, Liao KT. Primary lymphoma of the breast. Cancer 1972; 29: 1705–12.

4. Kuper-Hommel MJ, Snijder S, Janssen-Heijnen ML, et al. Treatment and survival of 38 female breast lymphomas: a population-based study with clinical and pathological review. Ann Hematol 2003; 82(7): 397–404.

5. Vignot S, Ledoussal V, Nodiot P, et al. Non-Hodgkin's lymphoma of the breast: a report of 19 cases and a review of the literature. Clin Lymphoma 2005; 6(1): 37–42.

6. Lyons JA, Myles J, Pohlman B, et al. Treatment and progress of primary breast lymphoma: a review of 13 cases. Am J Clin Oncol 2000; 23: 334–6.

7. Wong WW, Schild SF, Halyard MY, et al. Primary non-Hodgkin lymphoma of the breast: the Mayo Clinic experience. J Surg Oncol 2002; 23: 334–6.

8. Ryan GF, Roos DR, Seymour JF. Primary non-Hodgkin's lymphoma of the breast: retrospective analysis of prognosis and patterns of failure in two Australian centers. Clin Lymphoma Myeloma 2006; 6: 337–41.

9. Ryan G, Martinelli G, Kuper-Hommel M, et al. Primary diffuse large B-cell lymphoma of the breast: prognostic factors and outcomes of a study by the International Extranodal Lymphoma Study Group. Ann Oncol 2008; 19(2): 233–41.

10. Aviles A, Delgado S, Nambo MJ, et al. Primary breast lymphoma: results of a controlled clinical trial. Oncology 2005; 69: 256–60.

11. Hugh JC, Jackson FI, Hanson JP, et al. Primary breast lymphoma: an immunohistologic study of 20 new cases. Cancer 1990; 66: 2602.

12. Bobrow LG, Richards MA, Haperfield LC, et al. Breast lymphomas: a clinical pathologic review. Hum Pathol 1982; 24: 274.

13. Liberman L, Giess CS, Dershaw DD, et al. Non Hodgkin lymphoma of the breast: imaging characteristics and correlation with histopathologic findings. Radiology 1994; 192: 157–60.

14. Liberman L, Mason G, Morris EA, et al. Does size matter? Positive predictive value of MRI-detected breast lesions as a function of lesion size. AJR Am J Roentgenol 2006; 186: 426–30.

15. Gasparini M, Bombardieri E, Castellani M, et al. Gallium-67 scintigraphy evaluation of therapy in non-Hodgkin's lymphoma. J Nucl Med 1998; 39: 1586–90.

16. Delbeke D. Oncological applications of FDG PET imaging: brain tumors, colorectal cancer lymphoma and melanoma. J Nucl Med 1999; 40: 591–603.

17. Levine PH, Zamuco R, Yee HT. Role of fine-needle aspiration cytology in breast lymphoma. Diagn Cytopathol 2004; 30(5): 332–40.

18. Jackson FI, Lalani ZH. Breast lymphoma: radiologic imaging and clinical appearances. Can Assoc Radiol J 1991; 42(1): 48–54.

19. Kiresi DA, Kivrak AS, Ecirli S, et al. Secondary breast, pancreatic, and renal involvement with non-Hodgkin's lymphoma. Imaging findings. Breast 2006; 15: 106–10.

20. Demirkazik FB. MR imaging features of breast lymphoma. Eur J Radiol 2002; 42(1): 62–4.

21. Morrow M, Freedman G, Darnell A, et al. A clinical oncology perspective on the use of breast MR. Magn Reson Imaging Clin N Am 2006; 14(3): 363–78.

22. Morrow M, Freedman G, Darnell A, et al. Primary lymphoma of the breast: MR imaging features. A case report. J Magn Res Imaging 1999; 17: 199–202.

23. Horning SG, Weller E, Kim K, et al. Chemotherapy with or without radiotherapy in limited stage diffuse aggressive non-Hodgkin's lymphoma: Eastern Cooperative Oncology Group Study 1484. J Clin Oncol 2004; 22: 3032–8.

24. Miller T, Dahlberg S, Cassady J, et al. Chemotherapy alone compared with chemotherapy plus radiotherapy for localized intermediate- and high-grade non-Hodgkin's lymphoma. N Engl J Med 1998; 339: 21–6.

25. Pfreundschuh M, Trumper L, Osterborg A, et al. CHOP-like chemotherapy plus rituximab versus CHOP-like chemotherapy alone in young patients with good-prognosis diffuse large B-cell lymphoma: a randomised controlled trial by the MabThera International Trial (MInT) Group. Lancet Oncol 2006; 7: 379–91.

26. Feugier P, Van Hoof A, Sebban C, et al. Long-term results of the R-CHOP study in the treatment of elderly patients with diffuse large B-cell lymphoma: a study by the Groupe d'Etude des Lymphomes de l'Adulte. J Clin Oncol 2005; 23(18): 4117–26.

27. Lopez-Guillermo A, Colomo L, Jimenez M, et al. Diffuse large B-cell lymphoma: clinical and biological characterization and outcome according to nodal or extranodal primary origin. J Clin Oncol 2005; 23: 2797–804.

28. Mattia AR, Ferri JA, Harris NL. Breast lymphoma. A B-cell spectrum including low-grade B-cell lymphoma of mucosa associated lymphoid tissue. Am J Surg Pathol 1993; 17: 574–89.

29. Thiebelmant C, Bastion Y, Bergen F, et al. Mucosa associated lymphoid tissue gastrointestinal and non-gastrointestinal lymphoma behaviour: analysis of 108 patients. J Clin Oncol 1997; 15: 1624–30.

30. Isaacson P, Wright DH. Malignant lymphoma of mucosal associated lymphoid tissue. A distinctive type of B-cell lymphoma. Cancer 1983; 52: 1410–16.

Bone lymphoma

16

David Christie and Julie Vose

INCIDENCE AND EPIDEMIOLOGY

Primary bone lymphoma (PBL) is a rare non-Hodgkin's lymphoma (NHL) that has been described in many small and a few large retrospective reports.[1,2] The International Extranodal Lymphoma Study Group (IELSG) recently collected data on 499 cases in their IELSG-14 retrospective study.[1] Unless otherwise indicated, the data described in this chapter relate to the results of this study, which is larger than any other modern series.

The first identified cases are commonly attributed to Oberling, who described in 1928[3] a tumor consistent with primary bone lymphoma using the methods available and named it reticulum cell sarcoma (RCS). Since then, there have been refinements in the diagnosis, perhaps further lowering the incidence by excluding cases of Ewing's sarcoma. Although the exact incidence is difficult to define, the relative incidence of PBL has been described in a variety of ways: e.g. as the proportion of all malignant primary bone tumors, varying between 3% and 7%.[4–9] It has also been described as a proportion of all extranodal lymphomas, usually around 5%.[4,6,7,10–14] In Australasia, the term osteolymphoma was proposed[6,7] to overcome difficulties in literature searching, although it is yet to gain acceptance.

PBL has been reported in association with some specific conditions, including the human immunodeficiency virus (HIV),[15,16] sarcoidosis,[17] Gaucher disease,[18,19] hereditary exostoses,[20] Paget's disease,[2,21] osteomyelitis,[2] and following some specific treatments including hip replacements,[22,23] CLL (chronic lymphocytic leukemia) after cladribine chemotherapy,[24] and renal transplants.[25] None of these are consistent enough to suggest a true association or predisposition towards the development of the condition.

ETIOLOGY AND BIOLOGICAL FEATURES

The distribution of PBL sites in the skeleton reflects the distribution of bone marrow. Bone marrow makes up around 20% of the weight of the skeleton generally, and its distribution is different to the other components of bone such as cancellous bone or trabecular bone, as it concentrates in the axial skeleton and proximal parts of the long bones.[26] Although NHL may diffusely affect bone marrow, in PBL the disease is concentrated into specific infiltrative bone lesions. These occur most often in the diaphysis; involvement of the metaphysis and epiphysis probably reflect progressive disease.[27] There are indications that a homing mechanism may be active, as the initial presentation of PBL may involve multiple bony sites in the relative absence of soft tissue disease.[7] Also, recurrences tend to occur primarily in bone rather than in soft tissues. However, the reason for this remains unknown and the difficulties in distinguishing true PBL from secondary involvement of bone by soft tissue lymphoma masses remains problematic. The reason for bone marrow to develop into PBL is unknown and no distinctive biological or molecular features are established. A role for osteoclast activating factors such as macrophage inflammatory protein 1 alpha (MIP1-α) has been proposed.[28,29]

PATHOLOGY

To obtain sufficient material for classification, a surgical biopsy is usually required. However, the risk of pathological fracture following biopsy is significant and potentially disabling, so biopsies should be limited in size to around 2 mm. Morphologically, there are some unique problems in the diagnosis of PBL, including the presence of fibrosis (either delicate reticulum fibrosis, bands, or dense hyalinized fibrosis), inflammation, and some specific diagnostic traps (including sarcoma-like spindle cells and carcinoma-like clustering).[2] Crush artifacts are common in biopsy specimens[4] and fine needle aspirates (FNAs) may yield low numbers of recognizable diagnostic cells.[30] Some bony sites, such as the skull base, can be particularly difficult to biopsy[31] and falsely negative biopsy results have led to delayed diagnosis.[32]

Morphologically, most reports describe cells that are large and consistent with follicle center or centroblastic cell type.[2,33,34] Additionally, some large multilobated cells are reported in around half the cases. Nuclear cleavage is common.

In studies that report immunophenotyping,[4,35,36] high proportions of cells with positive staining for LCA (CD45), B1 (CD20), B2 (CD21) have been noted. Monotypic IgG, IgH, and HLA-DR have been noted, and clonality has been confirmed between initial and progressed tumors.[36] T-cell markers are usually negative but small T cells (CD3+) are often present. Molecular heterogeneity is common, but expression of BCL-2, BCL-6, and strong p53 protein expression have been noted when sought in around half of the cases tested.

Most reported series predate modern NHL classification systems, but the more recent reports classify the majority of their cases as diffuse large B-cell NHL. Evidence of germinal center derivation has been noted in at least 50% of cases.[37] A variety of other types from previous classification systems are often included in each series, including poorly differentiated lymphocytic lymphoma, but no other type is predominant.

Several cases of T-cell PBL have been reported,[8,38,39] most of which are anaplastic large cell lymphoma. Positivity for CD30, for the t(2;5)(p23;q35) translocation, and anaplastic lymphoma kinase immunoreactivity[8,38] were noted, and the cases were treated with combination chemotherapy and radiotherapy with varying degrees of success. The IELSG-14 series contains a small number of T-cell tumors and the IELSG will shortly issue a report relating to these. In the meantime, the data are too sparse to conclude that there are any features to distinguish these T-cell PBL from other PBL or other T-cell lymphomas. Hodgkin's disease rarely presents in bone, but the nodular sclerosing subtype has been recorded.[40,41]

CLINICAL AND RADIOGRAPHIC PRESENTATION

Although PBL can occur in children,[14] most reports describe adults with a mean age of 45–60 years old[2,42] and a wide age range (15–99 years old). In older papers, prior to immunohistochemistry, the mean age was lower, at 35–45 years old, perhaps indicating the inclusion of other histological types.[11,27,43] There is usually a slight predominance of males (55–60%). The majority of patients in the reported series have ECOG (Eastern Cooperative Oncology Group) performance status of 0–1, although the tumor itself can affect performance, particularly if it occurs in weight-bearing bones. No racial or geographic predominance has been demonstrated.

In early disease the most common bone described as affected is the femur.[2] Most papers group individual bones rather than specifying each bone separately: e.g. the vertebrae are grouped as the spine, and the limb bones are often reported together as long bones. Every bone in the body is a potential site for PBL and many case reports describe cases in specific bones, such as bones of the thumb,[12] the feet,[5] and the jaws.[25,44]

The commonest presenting feature is pain (80–95%), swelling is present in 30–40%, and 15–20% present with a pathological fracture.

Spinal cord compression was noted in 14% of patients in a recent larger series.[45] B symptoms are relatively uncommon, at 5–15%. Lactate dehydrogenase (LDH) levels may be elevated in around 30% of patients. A modified IPI (International Prognostic Index) scoring system can be applied to PBL, and patients are often well spread across the prognostic categories. The majority of patients present with unifocal disease. However, it is possible to get multifocal disease both within a single bone (monostotic disease) and in different bones (polyostotic disease). In the case of multifocal, monostotic disease, it can be difficult to distinguish between disease that has permeated the bone extensively and continuously, and those with multiple, discontinuous lesions. In around 20% of patients, soft tissue disease may also be present, most commonly in the form of regional nodes, although other nodes and other soft tissues can be affected. Median tumor sizes are 5–10 cm, but vary widely from 1 to 30 cm. Extraosseous extension is present in around 50% of cases and can make it difficult to be certain that the disease has arisen in bone rather than adjacent lymph nodes. An example is presented in Figure 16.1, in which a patient presented with pain above the hip, and films revealed a tumor mass in the right ilium. Although the tumor mass predominantly affected areas where pelvic lymph nodes might be expected to give rise to nodal masses, the presence of widespread bony disease in other areas indicated that the tumor was likely to be exhibiting a tendency to occur in bone.

The typical plain film appearances were noted as early as 1971.[27] In that series, all 47 were lytic (see Figure 16.1a), and just under half were also blastic. The cortex shows a mixture of permeative, moth-eaten, or destructive patterns. Pathological fractures may be detected Nearly all periostei showed reactive changes, but only occasionally was there onion skin layering, breach of the periosteum, or the sunburst appearance. These latter features are known to occur in sarcomatous bone lesions, but have not been reported in PBL. In the series by Shoji, those with more aggressive changes had a poorer prognosis.

Computed tomography (CT) scanning may demonstrate the boundaries of any extraosseous extension (see Figure 16.1b), as well as indicating cortical breakthrough by the tumor.[46] Osteolysis, osteosclerosis, and fragments of bone sequestra may be apparent.[47] Magnetic resonance imaging (MRI) scanning may reveal the extent of disease in more detail, particularly by identifying cortical changes such as linear channels of cortical destruction, as well as intratumoral fibrosis, replacement of trabecular bone and bone marrow by tumor.[48,49] Abnormal signal intensity areas are visible on both T1- and T2-weighted images with contrast enhancement.

Bone lesions usually result in increased uptake on technetium 99 scanning (see Figure 16.1d), whereas functional imaging (previously gallium scanning, now PET [positron emission tomography] scanning) usually reveals associated soft tissue disease. Combined use of these modalities was suggested in 1981.[50] Isotope bone scanning has the advantage of including the whole skeleton, whereas functional imaging may show the presence or absence of soft tissue disease. PET scanning can be expected to take over functional imaging from gallium scanning, although it is performed in different ways at different centers and usually does not fully cover the limbs, as demonstrated in Figure 16.1c. Therefore, need for isotope bone scanning remains.

PROGNOSTIC FACTORS

Prior to the recent IELSG-14 study,[1] no consistent prognostic factors were noted. The only study large enough to assess factors in detail was the study by Ostrowski et al.[2] In that series, significantly worse survival rates were noted for patients with multifocal disease, advanced disease, disease site (mandible and maxilla worst), presentation prior to 1960, and age >50 years old. The use of chemotherapy ($n=19$) was associated with worse survival, although the difference was not statistically significant and was presumably a reflection of more advanced disease. Other studies have reported significant associations on multivariate analysis between better outcomes and younger age,[37,42,51] IPI score,[45] the dose of radiotherapy,[42] the use of multimodality therapy,[51] and the use of rituximab.[45]

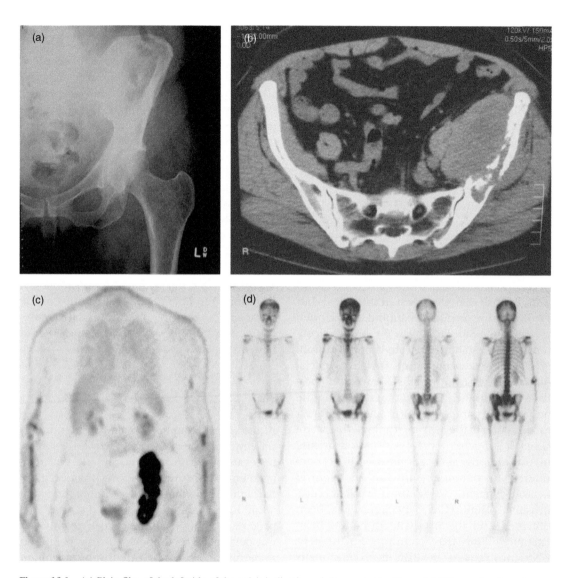

Figure 16.1 (a) Plain film of the left side of the pelvis indicating a lytic area in the ilium. (b) CT scan showing a tumor mass involving the left ilium and with extensive extraosseous extension. (c) FDG PET scan indicating dense uptake in the left ilium, but also in other bones, including bones of the arms. (d) Technetium 99 bone scan showing widespread bony disease, beyond that indicated by the PET scan.

The IELSG-14 study has revealed significantly better results with age <60 years old, ECOG performance status <2, normal LDH, combined modality therapy, higher radiation dose, and more than three cycles of chemotherapy.

DIAGNOSTIC CRITERIA AND STAGING PROCEDURES

No established criteria for the diagnosis of PBL exist, although several authors have made proposals. Whereas there is general agreement that cases with solitary lymphoma that appears to arise in bone should be included, regardless of histological type, there is disagreement over the inclusion of cases with multifocal or soft tissue disease. Some clinicians have considered multifocal disease to warrant classifying the patients as stage IV,[51] while others have considered stage II to be more appropriate.[2] Some clinicians have excluded cases with soft tissue disease,[27,42] whereas others have included it if it is apparent within 6 months before or after the appearance of the bone lesion,[2,43,52] or if it is limited to extraosseous extension[53] or to regional draining nodes.[52,54] The opinion of the authors is that the criteria should include patients with the particular biological feature of a predisposition of the lymphoma to originate in bone. Therefore, cases would be included if they represent a single focus of bony disease, multiple foci of bony disease, or predominantly bony disease that exceeds in volume any associated soft tissue disease. Although regional nodes have been described, the disease is primarily blood-borne, so that the regional location or other anatomical aspects of any associated soft tissue should be irrelevant. Disease that has arisen in soft tissues but involved bone secondarily should be excluded and should be identifiable if the tumor is centered in an established node group location, eroding an adjacent bony surface. Special difficulties arise in specific anatomical locations – e.g. in the case of tumors affecting the bones of the paranasal region – as it is difficult to distinguish these from tumors that arise from the mucosal surfaces. Tumors arising in parameningeal locations should be considered to potentially involve the central nervous system (CNS) until a clear cerebrospinal fluid (CSF) specimen has been obtained and the overlying dura has been examined by MRI scanning. Fortunately, CNS involvement by PBL is exceptionally rare. In many cases a subjective judgment will be required about whether a case should be categorized as PBL or lymphoma secondarily affecting bone; isotope bone scanning should be performed in such a case to exclude widespread bony disease. Fortunately, the influence of such a decision on management and outcome is unlikely to be significant. Tumors should be biopsied, limiting the size of the biopsy to avoid pathological fractures, and the specimens should be tested with immunohistochemistry for B-cell lineage, particularly CD20.

Staging in PBL should include plain films, CT or MRI of the primary tumor, CT scanning of the neck, chest, abdomen, and pelvis, isotope bone scanning, and either gallium or PET scanning. Blood tests should include a complete blood count, biochemistry including alkaline phosphatase, lactate dehydrogenase, erythrocyte sedimentation rate, C-reactive protein, β_2-microglobulin, and protein electrophoresis. CSF aspiration and cytology should be performed for tumors in parameningeal locations. Until a more suitable staging system is available, staging should be performed using the Ann Arbor system, and taking care to limit the diagnosis of stage IV to those with diffuse involvement of bone marrow beyond any focus of bony disease detectable by imaging. An IPI score can be assigned in the usual way, except that the primary tumor should not be considered to contribute any points to the score in the category of extranodal disease, but any additional extranodal sites would be scored.

TREATMENT AND OUTCOME

After diagnosis, an immediate consideration is stability, and internal fixation may be required, necessitating orthopedic involvement in management. There are few reports describing the particular difficulties involved in obtaining fixation in this setting, but expedition of the process is required so that cancer treatment is not delayed.[9] The tendency for the condition to permeate bone more extensively than might be obvious should be taken into account by extending the prosthetic devices used over greater distance and into healthy bone. The opportunity should be taken to gather additional biopsy material at the time of operation and to complete the staging investigations while recovering from surgery.

Apart from fixation, the role of surgery is limited. While the excision of weight-bearing bones has been recommended, it is not usually required. Amputation for local control has been performed in previous series, but no clear indications for it exist. Excision biopsy should be avoided, as biopsies should be kept to a limited size in order to preserve bone strength. In at least one series,[55] the use of surgery in a large proportion of the cases has been associated with a relatively poor result.

Although the first reports of PBL described the use of radiotherapy alone, and although local control rates were reasonably high, long-term survival was limited by distant failure. No modern series has recommended treatment by radiotherapy alone.

A historical treatment called Coley's toxin appeared in several papers. It is a mixture of toxins derived from *Streptococcus pyogenes* and *Serratia marcescens* injected intratumorally and intravenously. Some long remissions were recorded,[27,43,56–58] particularly in those patients who became febrile and had longer courses (>6 weeks). The dose was adjusted according to the febrile response. In 1971, a series was published[27] of 47 primary cases in which 21 patients receiving the toxin in addition to radiotherapy had a 5-year survival of 17.6%, compared with 38% among those treated by radiotherapy alone, and therefore the toxin was not considered effective thereafter.

Since then, combined treatment (radiotherapy and chemotherapy) was reported and found to produce higher rates of distant control and survival in several studies and most patients reported in the last 20 years have received combined treatment.[1,45,51] Although combined modality treatment is usually agreed as appropriate by experts, wide variation in the specific aspects of the treatments were noted when a case of PBL was circulated for comment.[59]

The mostly commonly reported sequence of treatments has been chemotherapy first, followed by radiotherapy. Regarding the chemotherapy, the most commonly used type of chemotherapy has been conventional CHOP chemotherapy – cyclophosphamide, Adriamycin (doxorubicin), vincristine, and prednisone – with a medina of six cycles. Rituximab should be routinely added (R-CHOP).[45] Its use should be restricted to those with CD20-positive immunohistochemistry. The doses and scheduling are done in combination with chemotherapy, as for nodal lymphoma. The use of intrathecal methotrexate treatment should be considered for patients that have positive CSF cytology or MRI evidence of dural involvement from a parameningeal tumor. Other types of chemotherapy would be appropriate for other histological subtypes, as they would be in the setting of nodal disease.

Regarding radiotherapy, a recent survey[59] of radiotherapy experts has suggested that the majority favored whole bone treatment, with a dose of 38–40 Gy. In previous reports, doses of 36–45 Gy in 1.8–2.0 Gy fractions have usually been prescribed. The volume to be enclosed varies widely with the disease site and should take into account the exposure of sensitive organs such as adjacent lung or kidney. However, in general, it is possible to treat the whole of an affected bone to that dose while keeping the risk of late effects on bone at negligible levels. Neither whole bone treatment nor treatment of regional graining nodes has been shown to be beneficial; however, whole bone treatment overcomes the difficulty in discerning the border of a permeative lesion in an affected bone. In cases where the use of whole bone treatment appears risky due to exposure of adjacent organs, wide margins (3–5 cm) around prechemotherapy tumor margins within bone should still be achievable. Margins around the soft tissue or extraosseous borders can be further restricted to 1–2 cm around postchemotherapy volumes, as the distinction between normal and abnormal tissue is not so problematic.

The role of radiotherapy in patients with multifocal disease is unknown, although it would be reasonable to add a lighter radiation dose (say 30 Gy) to areas of initially bulky tumor if these were limited to two or three sites. Although radiotherapy alone has been proposed for small lesions of the mandible,[60] the results of treatment for PBL in this site have not always been highly successful,[2,44] and combined modality treatment should still be considered.

Responses to treatment are difficult to assess, as there can be persisting activity for many years on isotope bone scans and architectural distortion on plain films. Persisting changes on isotope bone scanning and other imaging modalities in the absence of disease prevent the designation of complete response using the recently revised response criteria.[61] The designation of response is usually made upon resolution of any symptoms, particularly pain, signs such as swelling, and resolution of soft tissue disease as discernible on CT, MRI, or PET scanning. The conclusion of complete response is supported if there is evidence of bone healing on plain films and if there are no other signs of progressive disease during the follow-up period. Follow-up MRI scans may show replacement of intraosseous tumor and adjacent bone marrow with fatty marrow and sclerosis. Functional imaging (gallium or PET scanning) has been considered more useful than bone scanning in the assessment of response to treatment.[62,63] The limitations of PET scanning for bone and bone marrow disease are acknowledged in the recent consensus statement[64] on the use of PET scanning in the assessment of response, including false-positive findings due to marrow hyperplasia and false-negative findings relating to the resolution of the equipment, the technique, and the variability of fluorodeoxyglucose (FDG) avidity among histological subtypes. The description of response rates in reports about the success of treatment for this condition should be considered with caution.

Local control and survival rates

High rates of local control (around 80%) have been reported for many years, including historical series treated with radiotherapy alone.[34] Rates of 5-year overall survival have gradually increased from around 50% to around 75%, as the proportion of patients receiving combined modality treatment has increased.[7]

Toxicity

The toxicities related to CHOP chemotherapy and moderate doses of radiotherapy have been well reported elsewhere, but in the case of PBL there is a special form of toxicity, which is pathological fracture. Such fractures can occur in the absence of local recurrence and can lead to persisting non-union, with subsequent disability if occurring in a bone of the

lower limb. Contributing factors may include architectural disturbance due to previous tumor, pathological fractures prior to treatment, osteonecrosis due to radiotherapy, the use of steroids in association with CHOP chemotherapy, and the existence of other medical conditions such as osteomyelitis following surgery, Paget's disease and osteoporosis, particularly among patients who are older and female. The frequency of late pathological fracture is unknown, but attention was drawn to it by two studies[53,65] reporting a total of 11 patients with pathological fractures. In these patients there was a high incidence of high radiation doses (>50 Gy), large fraction size, and local recurrence was present at the fracture site in some of the cases. Treatment regimens should therefore include orthopedic fixation of fractures prior to treatment where indicated, limitation of the use of corticosteroids, limited radiation doses and fraction sizes, and monitoring of patients for signs of subsequent pain or disability. Amputations have been reported in the absence of local failure as a way of dealing with painful non-healing fractures. However, such drastic measures like these are likely to be avoidable if the preventive measures described herein are adopted. Second malignancies after treatment for PBL are usually limited to incidental skin cancers and are otherwise rarely reported.[7]

Future studies of PBL are likely to include prospective studies aimed at defining the roles of PET scanning in staging and response assessment, the addition of monoclonal antibody treatments, and detailed molecular biology studies aimed at clarifying the mechanisms of homing.

REFERENCES

1. Christie D, Gracias E, Mary Gospodarowicz M, et al. Patterns of outcome and prognostic factors in primary bone lymphoma (osteolymphoma): a survey of 499 cases by the International Extranodal Lymphoma Study Group. Haematologica 2007; 92 (S1): abstract 0863.
2. Ostrowski M, Unni KK, Banks P, et al. Malignant lymphoma of bone. Cancer 1986; 58: 2646–55.
3. Oberling C. Les reticulosarcomes et les reticuloendothliosarcomes de la moelle osseuse (Sarcomes d'Ewing). Bull Assn Francais Etudes Cancer 1928; 17: 259–96.

4. Pettit CK, Zuckerburg LR, Gray MH, et al. Primary lymphoma of bone. A B-cell neoplasm with a high frequency of multilobated cells. Am Surg J Pathol 1990; 14(4): 329–34.

5. Singh DP, Dhillon MS, Kumar R, Sharma SC, Radotra BD. Primary lymphoma of the bones of the foot: management of two cases. Foot Ankle 1991; 11(5): 314–16.

6. Christie D, Cahill SP, Barton M. Primary bone lymphoma (osteolymphoma). Australas Radiol 1996; 40: 319–23.

7. Christie DRH, Barton MB, Bryant G, et al. Osteolymphoma (primary bone lymphoma): an Australian review of 70 cases. Aust NZ J Med 1999; 29: 214–19.

8. Lones MA, Sanger W, Perkins SL, Mediros LJ. Anaplastic large cell lymphoma arising in bone: report of a case of monomorphic variant with the t(2;5)(p23;q35) translocation. Arch Pathol Lab Med 2000; 124(9): 1339–43.

8. Lones MA, Perkins SL, Sposto R, et al. Non-Hodgkins' lymphoma arising in bone in children and adolescents is associated with an excellent outcome: a Children's Cancer Group report. J Clin Oncol 2002; 20(9): 2293–301.

9. Gabel GT, Sim FH, Beabout JW, Haberman TH, Wold LE. Non-Hodgkin's lymphoma of bone. Orthopedics 1989; 12(8): 1139–42.

10. Zucca E, Roggero E, Bertoni F, Conconi A, Cavalli F. Primary extranodal non-Hodgkin's lymphomas. Part 2 Head and neck, central nervous system and other less common sites. Ann Oncol 1999; 10: 1023–33.

11. Susnerwala SS, Dinshaw KA, Pande S, et al. Primary lyphoma of bone: experience of 39 cases at the Tata Memorial Hospital, India. J Surg Oncol 1990; 44(4): 229–33.

12. Davies AN, Salisbury JR, Dobbs HJ. Primary bone lymphoma: report of an unusual case with a review of the literature. Clin Oncol 1994; 6: 411–12.

13. Parvinen LM, Jereb B, Nisce L. Primary non-Hodgkin's lymphoma ('reticulum cell sarcoma') of bone in adults. Acta Radiol Oncol 1983; 22(6): 449–54.

14. Loeffler JS, Tarbell NJ, Kozakewich H, Cassody R, Weinstein HJ. Primary lymphoma of bone in children: analysis of treatment results with adriamycin, prednisone, Oncovin (APO), and local radiation therapy. J Clin Oncol 1986; 4(4): 496–501.

15. Thurner MM, Rieger A, Kleibl-Popov C, Schindler E. Malignant lymphoma of the cranial vault in an HIV-positive patient: imaging findings. Eur Radiol 2001; 11(8): 1506–9.

16. Sipsas NV, Kontas A, Panayiotkopoulos, et al. Extranodal non-Hodgkin lymphoma presenting as a soft tissue mass in the proximal femur in a HIV+ patient. Leuk Lymphoma 2002; 43(12): 2405–7.

17. Kobayashi H, Kato Y, Hakamada M, et al. Malignant lymphoma of the bone associated with systemic sarcoidosis. Intern Med 2001; 40(5): 435–8.

18. Bohm P, Kunz W, Horny HP, Einsele H. Adult Gaucher disease in association with primary malignant bone tumors. Cancer 2001; 91(3): 457–62.

19. Manz M, Riessen R, Poll L, et al. High grade lymphoma mimicking bone crisis in Gaucher's disease. Br J Haematol 2001; 113(1): 191–3.

20. Neben K, Werner M, Bernd L, et al. A man with hereditary exostoses and high grade non-Hodgkin's lymphoma of the bone. Ann Hematol 2001; 80(11): 682–4.

21. Stephens GC, Lennington WJ, Schwartz HS. Primary lymphoma and Paget's disease of the femur. Am J Clin Pathol 1994; 101(6): 783–6.

22. Syed AA, Agarwal M, Fenelon G, Toner M. Osseous malignant non-Hodgkin's B-cell lymphoma associated with total hip replacement. Leuk Lymphoma 2002; 43(11): 2213–16.

23. Ito H, Shimizu A. Malignant lymphoma at the site of a total hip replacement. Orthopedics 1999; 22(1): 82–4.

24. Robak T, Kasznicki M, Bartkowiak J, et al. Richter's syndrome following cladirabine therapy for chronic lymphocytic leukemia first manifested as pathological fracture of the femur. Leuk Lymphoma 2001; 42(4): 789–96.

25. Maxymiw WG, Wood RE, Lee L. Primary multifocal non-Hodgkin's lymphoma of the jaws presenting as periodontal disease in a renal transplant patient. Int J Oral Maxillofac Surg 1991; 20: 69–70.

26. International Commission on Radiological Protection (ICRP). Report 23. Report of the task group on reference man. London: Pergamon, 1975; reprinted 1994.

27. Shoji H, Miller TR. Primary reticulum cell sarcoma of bone – significance of clinical features upon the prognosis. Cancer 1971; 28(5): 1234–44.

28. Hicks D, Gokan T, O'Keefe RJ, et al. Primary lymphoma of bone. Correlation of magnetic resonance imaging features with cytokine production by tumour cells. Cancer 1995; 75: 973–80.

29. Matsuhashi Y, Tasaka T, Uehara E, et al. Diffuse large B-cell lymphoma presenting with hypercalcemia and multiple osteolysis. Leuk Lymphoma 2004; 45(2): 397–400.

30. Htwe WM, Lucas DR, Bedrossian CWM, Ryan JR. Fine-needle aspirate of primary lymphoma of bone. Diagn Cytopathol 1996; 15: 421–6.

31. Amara H, Elomri H, Cherni N, et al. [Primary lymphoma of bone: imaging features]. J Radiol 2002; 83(1): 55–8. [in French]

32. Theodorou DJ, Theodorou SJ, Sartorius DJ, Haghighi P, Resnick D. Delayed diagnosis of primary non-Hodgkin's lymhoma of the sacrum. Clin Imaging 2000; 24(3): 169–73.

33. Bacci G, Jaffe N, Emiliani E, et al. Therapy for non-Hodgkin's lymphoma of bone and a comparison of results with Ewing's sarcoma. Cancer 1986; 57: 1468–72.

34. Dosoretz DE, Raymond AK, Murphy GF, et al. Primary lymphoma of bone. The relationship of morphological diversity to clinical behaviour. Cancer 1982; 50: 1009–14.

35. Huebner-Chan D, Fernandes B, Yang G, Lim MS. An immunophenotypic and molecular study of primary large B-cell lymphoma of bone. Mod Pathol 2001; 14(10): 1000–7.

36. Chang ST, Chuang SS, Wang YH. Polyostotic primary bone lymphoma with progression in the skeleton: identical clonal origin of the initial and progressed tumours and a late relapse by VDJ rearrangement analysis. Leuk Lymphoma 2006; 47(6): 1144–8.

37. Zinzani PL, Carillo G, Ascani S, et al. Primary bone lymphoma: experience with 52 patients. Haematologica 2003; 88: 280–5.

38. Biasotti S, Fondelli P, Garaventa A. Anaplastic large cell lymphoma of the parietal bone. Br J Haematol 2002; 117: 258.

39. Ali R, Ozkalamkas F, Ozcelik T, et al. Primary non-Hodgkin's T-cell lymphoma of bone. Leuk Lymphoma 2004; 45(8): 1719–20.

40. Pilo G, Casula P. Uncommon sites in initial involvement of Hodgkin's disease. Presented at the Lugano International Conference on Malignant Lymphoma, 2002. Abstract 395.

41. Mlczoch L, Attarbaschi A, Dworzak M, Gadner H, Mann G. Alopecia areata and multifocal bone involvement in a young adult with Hodgkin's disease. Leuk Lymphoma 2005; 46(4): 623–7.

42. Fairbanks RK, Bonner JA, Inwards CY, et al. Treatment of stage IE primary lymphoma of bone. Int J Radiat Oncol Biol Phys 1993; 28: 363–72.

43. Coley BL, Higinbotham NL, Groesbeck HP. Primary reticulum-cell sarcoma of bone. Radiology 1959; 55(5): 641–57.

44. Rosado MF, Morgensztern D, Peleg M, Lossus IS. Primary diffuse large cell lymphoma of the mandible. Leuk Lymphoma 2004; 45(5): 1049–53.

45. Ramadan KM, Shenkier T, Sehn LH, Gascoyne RD, Connors JM. A clinicopathological retrospective study of 131 patients with primary bone lymphoma: a population-based study of successively treated cohorts from the British Columbia Cancer Agency. Ann Oncol 2007; 18: 129–35.

46. Phillips, Kattapuram, Dosoretz, et al. Primary lymphoma of bone: relationship of radiographic appearance and prognosis. Diagn Radiol 1982; 144(2): 285–90.

47. Mulligan ME, Kransdorf MJ. Sequestra in primary lymphoma of bone: prevalence and radiologic features. AJR Am J Roentgenol 1993; 160: 1245–8.

48. Stiglbauer R, Augustin I, Kramer J, et al. MRI in the diagnosis of primary lymphoma of bone: correlation with histopathology. J Comput Assist Tomogr 1992; 16(2): 248–53.

49. Hicks DG, Gokan T, O'Keefe, et al. Primary lymphoma of bone. Correlation of magnetic resonance imaging features with cytokine production by tumour cells. Cancer 1995; 75: 973–80.

50. Sweet DL, Mass D, Simon MA, Shapiro CM. Histiocytic lymphoma (reticulum cell sarcoma) of bone. JBJS 1981; 63(1): 79–84.

51. Beal K, Alen L, Yahalom J. Primary bone lymphoma: treatment results and prognostic factors with long term follow-up in 82 patients. Cancer 2006; 106(12): 2652–6.

52. Desai S, Jambhekar NA, Soman CS, Advani SH. Primary lymphoma of bone: a clinicopathological study of 25 cases reported over 10 years. J Surg Oncol 1991; 46: 265–9.

53. Stokes SH, Walz BJ. Pathological fracture after radiation therapy for primary non-Hodgkin's malignant lymphoma of bone. Int J Radiat Oncol Biol Phys 1983; 9: 1153–9.

54. Rathmel AJ, Gospdarowicz MK, Sutcliffe SB, Clark RM. Localised lymphoma of bone: prognostic factors and treatment recommendations. Br J Cancer 1992; 66: 603–6.

55. Bayrakei K, Yildiz Y, Saglik Y, et al. Primary lymphoma of bones. Int Orthop 2001; 25(2): 123–6.

56. Francis KC, Higinbotham NL, Coley BL. Primary reticulum cell sarcoma of bone; report of 44 cases. Surg Gynecol Obstet 1954; 92(2): 142–6.

57. McCormack LJ, Ivins JC, Dahlin DC, Johnson EW. Primary reticulum-cell sarcoma of bone. Cancer 1952; 5(6): 1182–92.

58. Miller TR, Nicholson JT. End results in reticulum cell sarcoma of bone treated by bacterial toxin therapy alone or combined with surgery and/or radiotherapy (47 cases) or with concurrent infection (5 cases). Cancer 1971; 27(3): 524–47.

59. Tsang RW, Gospodarowicz MK, O'Sullivan B. Staging and management of localised non-Hodgkin's lymphomas: variation among experts in radiation oncology. Int J Radiat Oncol Biol Phys 2002; 52(4): 747–56.

60. Barbieri, Camelli S, Mauro F, et al. Primary non-Hodgkin's lymphoma of the bone: treatment and analysis of prognostic factors for stage I and II. Int J Radiat Oncol Biol Phys 59(3): 760–4.

61. Cheson BD, Pfistner B, Juweid ME, et al. The International Harmonization Project on Lymphoma. Revised response criteria for malignant lymphoma. J Clin Oncol 2007; 25(5): 579–86.

62. Israel O, Mekel M, Bar-Shalom, R, et al. Bone lymphoma: Ga67 scintigraphy and CT for prediction of outcome after treatment. J Nucl Med 2002; 43(10): 1295–303.

63. Moon TY, Kim EE, Kim YC, et al. Comparison of nuclear bone and gallium scanning in the therapeutic evaluation of bone lymphoma. Clin Nucl Med 1995; 20(8): 721–4.

64. Juweid ME, Stroobants S, Hoekstra OS, et al; Imaging Subcommittee of International Harmonization Project in Lymphoma. Use of positron emission tomography for response assessment of lymphoma: consensus of the Imaging Subcommittee of International Harmonization Project in Lymphoma. J Clin Oncol 2007; 25(5): 571–8.

65. Lucraft HH. Primary lymphoma of bone: a review of 13 cases emphasising orthopaedic problems. Clin Oncol 1991; 3: 265–9.

Lung lymphoma

17

Stefano A Pileri, V Poletti, C Campidelli, PL Zinzani,
and Maurizio Martelli

DEFINITION, INCIDENCE, AND EPIDEMIOLOGY

The lung can be involved in a variety of malignant lymphomas, either primarily or in the course of a systemic disease. Primary lung lymphomas comprise all the clonal lymphoid processes involving mainly the lung parenchyma and/or large airways without extension to the extrapulmonary sites at the diagnosis or during the 3 months after the diagnosis; hilar or mediastinal lymph nodes may be enlarged but the neoplastic burden is more evident in the lung tissue.[1]

In this chapter, the authors focus on tumors that present in the lung or whose behaviour is largely affected by pulmonary involvement. These lymphomas are a heterogeneous group and include a spectrum of conditions ranging from indolent to aggressive disease.[1-3]

The most common type of primary pulmonary lymphoma is the extranodal marginal zone B-cell lymphoma of MALT (mucosa-associated lymphoma tissue) type, which arises from bronchus-associated lymphoid tissue (BALT).[1] It represents approximately 70–90% of all primary lung lymphomas, 10% of all MALT lymphomas, 3–4% of extranodal non-Hodgkin's lymphoma (NHL), and 0.5–1% of primary pulmonary malignancies.[3,4] Diffuse large B-cell lymphomas (DLBCL) make up 10% of cases of primary pulmonary lymphomas.[1] T-cell lymphomas and Hodgkin's disease rarely occur primarily in the lungs.[1,5]

An association of primary lung lymphomas with collagen vascular diseases, mainly Sjögren's syndrome, and with immunodeficiency disorders such as common variable immunodeficiency and human immunodeficiency virus (HIV) infection

has been reported.[6] Among the Epstein–Barr virus (EBV)-associated lymphoproliferative diseases that can be induced by primary or acquired immunosuppression, a particular condition, the lymphomatoid granulomatosis, a rare systemic angiodestructive EBV-associated lymphoproliferative disease, is usually characterized by prominent pulmonary involvement.[7] The EBV-associated post-transplant lymphoproliferative disorders can also affect the lungs.[8]

ETIOLOGY, BIOLOGICAL FEATURES, AND HISTOPATHOLOGY

Almost every type of malignant lymphoma listed in the World Health Organization (WHO) classification[8] can develop in the lungs (Figure 17.1). The same tumors can, however, affect other extranodal sites and/or lymph nodes. This is the reason why the classification adopted a pathobiological rationale for disease entity definition instead of a topographic one. In addition, when dealing with lung lymphoid proliferations, one should take into consideration neoplasms affecting the pleura as well as conditions that, although included in the lymphoma classification, may have different biological potential. The main categories of lymphoid proliferations that can affect the lung are summarized in Table 17.1.

PULMONARY MARGINAL ZONE B-CELL LYMPHOMA (BALT LYMPHOMA)

This tumor is felt to derive from the BALT.[9-11] It can be preceded by an infection or autoimmune disease or be concomitant with an

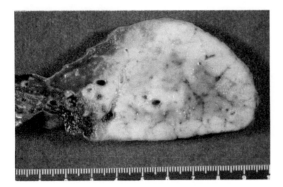

Figure 17.1   Macroscopic view of a marginal zone lymphoma of the lung infiltrating the upper right lobe.

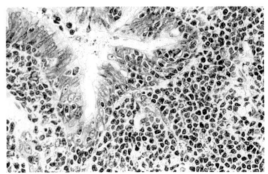

Figure 17.2   Marginal zone lymphoma of the lung showing prevalent lymphoplasmacytic cytology and infiltrating the bronchial wall (Giemsa, ×250).

Table 17.1   Main histological types of lymphoma observed at the lung level

Peripheral B-cell lymphoma
Extranodal marginal zone lymphoma of MALT type
Extramedullary plasmacytoma
Follicular lymphoma
Diffuse large B-cell lymphoma, including intravascular lymphoma, primary effusion lymphoma, pyothorax-associated lymphoma, lymphomatoid granulomatosis grade III, and other forms occurring in immunocompromised patients (e.g. post-transplant)

B-cell proliferation of uncertain malignant potential
Lymphomatoid granulomatosis, grade I and II
Post-transplant lymphoproliferative disorders, polymorphic

Peripheral T-cell lymphoma

Hodgkin's lymphoma

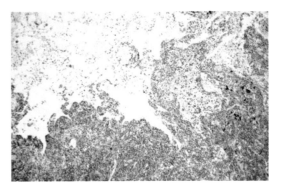

Figure 17.3   Low-power view of the same case: the tumor diffusely substitutes the normal lung parenchyma (Giemsa, ×40).

immunodeficiency.[12–15] All these events would favor a reactive lymphoid proliferation within which a pathological clone does emerge due to the accumulation of genetic damage and altered immunological surveillance. In a proportion of cases, however, a predisposing condition is not recorded.

On morphological grounds, BALT lymphoma is characterized by the proliferation of small neoplastic cells (Figure 17.2) that can display centrocyte-like, lymphoplasmacytic-like or B-monocytoid profile.[8] One component usually predominates over the others, although they may be variably admixed. Neoplastic cells do usually grow diffusely[8] (Figure 17.3).

However, they tend to colonize pre-existing germinal centers (thus producing a vague nodularity), and form characteristic lymphoepithelial lesions that are highlighted by cytokeratin immunostaining[8] (Figure 17.4a). Notably, the tumor can display prominent plasma cell differentiation that at times obscures the small cell component[8] (Figure 17.5). The latter can be easily picked up by an anti-CD20 antibody: in this respect, one should remember that the in-vivo administration of rituximab may be of limited efficacy under these circumstances, the plasma cell component remaining unaffected by the therapy.[16] At least some of the primary pulmonary plasmacytomas of the past would today be classified as marginal zone lymphomas with prominent plasma cell differentiation.[17] This variety of the tumor can be more

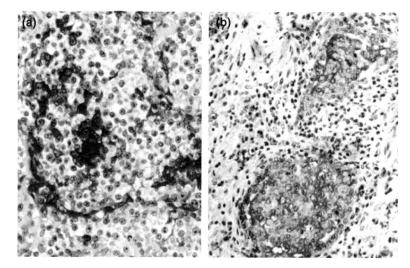

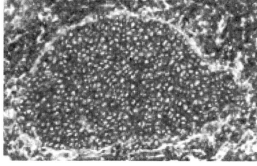

Figure 17.4 Marginal zone lymphoma of the lung. (a) Remnants of alveolar structures infiltrated by the lymphomatous growth evidenced by an anticytokeratin antibody (alkaline phosphatase antialkaline phosphatase complexes [APAAP] technique; Gill's hematoxylin counterstain; ×250); (b) Neoplastic cells stain for the IRTA-1 molecule (APAAP technique; Gill's hematoxylin counterstain; ×250).

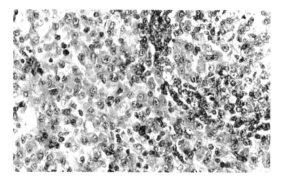

Figure 17.5 Marginal zone lymphoma of the lung with prominent plasma cell differentiation (Giemsa, ×500).

Figure 17.6 Marginal zone lymphoma of the lung: lymphomatous cells strongly express CD20 (APAAP technique; Gill's hematoxylin counterstain; ×400).

easily associated with paraproteinemia, amyloidosis, storage of immunoglobulin (Ig) crystals by foamy macrophages, and deposition of Ig heavy and/or light chains.[18–20] Finally, clusters or increased amounts (>10%) of blasts can be seen at times.[21] As there is no consensus on their meaning, they should only be quoted in the report, along with increased proliferation rate (Ki-67 marking) and expression of p53 in more than 5% of the neoplastic cells, in order to see in prospective studies whether or not these findings herald progression to DLBCL.[21] Notably, the association of marginal zone lymphoma and DLBCL in the same specimen does not necessarily imply that the latter ensues from the former:[21] such a conclusion can be drawn only on the basis of the demonstration

of the clonal relationship between the two populations.[21] Some exceptional examples of association between BALT lymphoma and classic Hodgkin's lymphoma (cHL) have also been described.[22]

At immunohistochemistry, neoplastic cells express B-cell markers (CD19, CD20, CD79a, and PAX-5/BSAP) (Figure 17.6) and show monotypic Ig light-chain restriction.[21] With the exception of cases with pronounced plasma cell differentiation, the demonstration of the latter may be problematic, being more often confined to the perinuclear spaces, and its visualization requires a very sensitive detection method.[21] Recently, it has been shown that lymphomatous elements do carry, at least in part, the *IRTA-1* gene product that represents the first specific

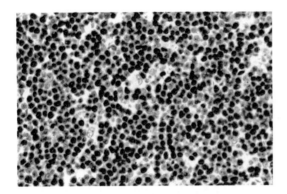

Figure 17.7 Marginal zone lymphoma of the lung: expression of Bcl-10 in a case carrying t(11;18) (EnVision+ method; Gill's hematoxylin counterstain; ×400).

histogenetic marker proposed in the literature[23] (Figure 17.4b). In addition, they can express MUM1/IRF4, depending on their degree of plasma cell differentiation.[21] The staining for CD5, CD10, Bcl-6, and cyclin D1 usually turns out negative.[21] The Ki-67/Mib-1 marking is below 10% on average. Remnants of follicular dendritic cells are evidenced by antibodies against CD21, CD23, and CD35.[21] Bcl-2 is variably expressed, although the stain never reaches the same intensity as observed in follicular lymphoma.[21]

Molecular biology shows IgV_H gene clonal rearrangements with a high load of somatic mutations.[21] The latter are usually stable, but can become ongoing in case of follicular colonization.[21] Fluorescent in-situ hybridization (FISH) and/or polymerase chain reaction (PCR) analysis reveals the occurrence of t(11;18)(q21;q21) with formation of the *MALT1–API2* fusion gene in 25–40% of cases.[24–26] This is generally associated with (1) the absence of any underlying autoimmune disease, (2) normal serum lactate dehydrogenase (LDH), (3) 'typical' histology without marked plasmacytic differentiation or an increased number of large cells, and (4) aberrant nuclear Bcl-10 expression (Figure 17.7) that, however, is not limited to t(11;18), being observed also in t(1;14)(p22;q32) and t(14;18)(q32;q21) (see later), as all these abnormalities imply direct or indirect up-regulation of the corresponding gene and nuclear factor kappaB (NF-κB) pathway activation.[27] Trisomy 3 can concur in some instances. In about 10% of cases, a t(14;18)

with *IgH–MALT1* fusion is encountered, at times in conjunction with trisomy 3 and 12.[25] Interestingly, t(11;18) and t(14;18) seem to be mutually exclusive. The detection of aneuploidy occurs in 35–40% of patients, with trisomy 3 and 18 being the most common aberrations.[26] Finally, the detection of t(1;14) is rare in BALT lymphoma.[24] Besides chromosomal abnormalities, molecular analysis shows *p16* gene methylation in about 60% cases of BALT lymphomas.[28] The gene is similarly methylated in DLBCL cases (55%). Statistical analysis indicates that the *p16* gene methylation status does not correlate with *API2–MALT1* fusion or any of the clinicopathological factors, including serum LDH, clinical stage, and increased large cells. This suggests that *p16* methylation is not associated with tumor progression, but may be an early event in MALT lymphomagenesis that might be maintained through the progression of the tumor. Extramedullary plasmacytoma has anecdotally been reported to occur in the lung.[29] As mentioned above, it is likely that most cases of the past do actually represent examples of BALT lymphoma with extreme plasma cell differentiation.

PULMONARY DIFFUSE LARGE B-CELL LYMPHOMA

DLBCL can affect the lung, either primarily or secondarily. Among the latter, one should note the involvement per continuum or at the time of relapse by a primary mediastinal large B-cell lymphoma (PMBL) that frequently evokes fibrotic reaction with compartmentalization[8,30] (Figure 17.8). Neoplastic cells show a high load of stable somatic mutations that is consistent with a late germinal center cell derivation, as is the phenotypic profile that shows co-expression of Bcl-6 and MUM1/IRF4.[30] Interestingly, in most if not all cases, they carry CD30 (Figure 17.8) (in the absence of CD15), CD45, MAL protein, HLA-DR, BOB.1, Oct.2, and PU.1, but lack Ig production.[30] Gene expression profiling studies have revealed that PMBL share a signature that largely overlaps the one of cHL.[31,32] Thus, it is not surprising that a gray zone exists between the two forms.[33]

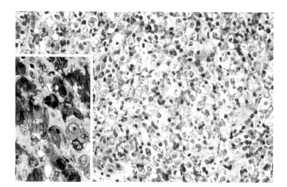

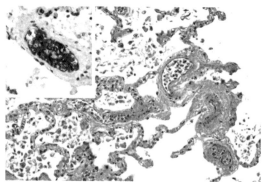

Figure 17.8 Lung parenchyma infiltrated by primary mediastinal large B-cell lymphoma (Giemsa, ×250). Inset, neoplastic cells express CD30 (APAAP technique; Gill's hematoxylin counterstain; ×600).

Figure 17.9 Pulmonary involvement by intravascular B-cell lymphoma: please note the presence of large neoplastic cells within the vessel lumina (hematoxylin and eosin; ×250). Inset: lymphomatous elements are highlighted by an anti-CD79a antibody (APAAP technique; Gill's hematoxylin counterstain; ×400).

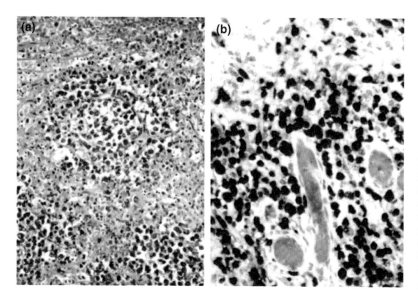

Figure 17.10 EBV-related large B-cell lymphoma: (a) neoplastic cells show prominent angiocentricity and angioinvasiveness, producing extensive necrosis (hematoxylin and eosin; ×250); (b) EBNA2 expression (APAAP technique; Gill's hematoxylin counterstain; ×400).

Primary DLBCL of the lung may belong to one of the usual clinicopathological subtypes or correspond to a rare variant, such as intravascular lymphoma or an EBV-related form, also termed grade III lymphomatoid granulomatosis (LYG).[8] The former can also affect organs other than the lung (e.g. central nervous system [CNS], bone marrow, skin, liver, kidney, and spleen), although the pulmonary involvement may represent one of the main clinical manifestations: tumoral cells are confined within small to medium-sized vessels (Figure 17.9) and express an activated B-cell-like (ABC) phenotype and – in 20% of cases – CD5.[8,34–36] The process has a very aggressive clinical course that may be worsened by an associated hemophagocytic syndrome.[36] The so-called LYG grade III corresponds to an EBV-driven DLBCL (Figure 17.10) (more often a T-cell-rich B-cell lymphoma with a huge amount of reactive cytotoxic T lymphocytes), which displays prominent angiocentricity and angioinvasiveness producing infarct-like necrosis (Figure 17.10).[8,37,38] The latter is due

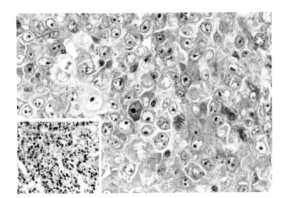

Figure 17.11 Pyothorax-associated lymphoma: neoplastic cells display immunoblastic/plasmablastic morphology (Giemsa, ×600). Inset: EBV integration at in-situ hybridization (×150).

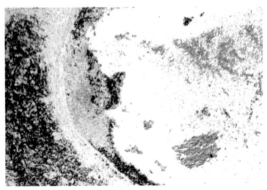

Figure 17.12 Primary effusion lymphoma showing strong expression of the HHV8-related latent nuclear antigen (APAAP technique; Gill's hematoxylin counterstain; ×100).

to both vascular occlusion by the lymphoid infiltrate and fibrinoid necrosis of blood vessels mediated by EBV-induced chemokines. The process, which can actually involve several organs, was originally described by Liebow et al in the lung as being characterized by vanishing nodules.[39] Interestingly, it may be related to varying degrees of immunosuppression, including acquired immunodeficiency syndrome (AIDS) or antigraft therapy in organ-transplant recipients.[40,41] In the WHO classification, the term LYG is applied to a spectrum of lesions carrying different histological atypia and clinical aggressiveness that correlate with the proportion of large atypical B cells. A histopathological grading system was proposed on the basis of the proportion of large cells.[8] These are rare or absent in grade I lesions, occasionally seen in grade II, and numerous in grade III LYG.[8] Only grade III LYG is considered a frank lymphoma, grade I being usually polyclonal and grade II oligoclonal.[8]

Within the context of primary DLBCLs of the lung, one should also consider the so-called primary effusion lymphoma (PEL) and pyothorax-associated lymphoma (PAL).[8] Both involve the pleura more than the lung parenchyma, are associated with conditions predisposing systemic or local decreased immunosurveillance, and are characterized by a very aggressive clinical course. The former usually occurs in AIDS patients, although it can also be observed in transplanted individuals or in elderly males

living in suburban areas.[8,42] Lymphoma cells display immunoblastic or plasmablastic morphology (Figure 17.11), aberrant phenotype (CD45+, CD30+/−, CD38+/−, CD138+/−, and conventional B-cell markers, including Ig), and regular integration of human herpes virus 8 (HHV8) (Figure 17.12) with frequent EBV co-infection.[8,43–46] The latter is demonstrated by EBER (EBV-encoded RNA) in-situ hybridization (ISH), the search for latent membrane protein-1 (LMP-1) turning out negative.[8] Neoplastic elements induce high levels of interleukins IL-6 and IL-10 in the pleural fluid and reveal monoclonal IgV_H gene rearrangement with a high load of stable somatic mutations.[43–46] PAL develops in the thoracic wall of patients affected by long-standing pyothorax resulting from lung tuberculosis.[8,47–50] It usually shows a diffuse large cell morphology and constantly contains EBV genome (Figure 17.12). The tumor is composed of large B lymphocytes at the differentiation stage of the late/postgerminal center, as suggested by the expression of Bcl-6 and MUM1/IRF4 and by molecular studies.[51] Occasionally, examples of T-cell PAL quoted in the literature[52] are a matter of debate and probably should be differently classified.

Rarely, other types of lymphoma may be encountered in the lung, including follicular lymphoma with or without marginal zone differentiation,[53] ALK-positive anaplastic large cell lymphoma (Figure 17.13),[54] cHL (which may also represent diffusion from an adjacent

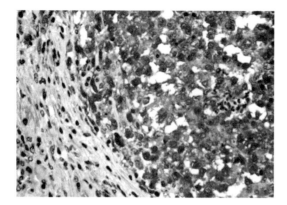

Figure 17.13 Lung infiltration by an ALK+ anaplastic large cell lymphoma (APAAP technique; Gill's hematoxylin counterstain; ×500).

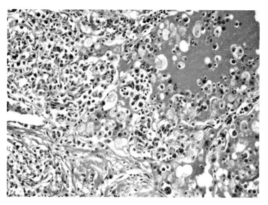

Figure 17.15 Partial involvement of the lung parenchyma by a peripheral T-cell lymphoma (hematoxylin and eosin; ×250).

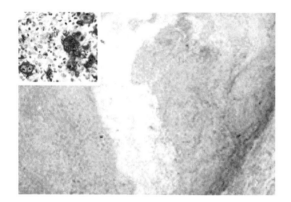

Figure 17.14 Primary classical Hodgkin's lymphoma of the lung, producing extensive necrosis (Giemsa, ×40). Inset: Hodgkin and Reed–Sternberg cells strongly express CD30 (APAAP technique; Gill's hematoxylin counterstain; ×400).

mediastinal mass, more often of the nodular sclerosing type)[55] (Figure 17.14), and peripheral T-cell lymphoma (PTCL)[56] (Figure 17.15). They show the morphological and phenotypical characteristics observed at other anatomical sites. Notably, examples of PTCL of the nasal type have been reported in the literature.[56] These generally occur in immunocompromised patients and are characterized by a pleomorphic neoplastic infiltrate showing EBV integration and an angiocentric and angiodestructive growth pattern with ensuing extensive necrosis.[8] This tumor should not be confused with EBV-related DLBCL. In this respect, phenotypical analysis plays a fundamental role: in fact, lymphomatous elements

express CD56, CD2, cytoplasmic CD3, cytotoxic molecules, and Fas/Fas ligand.[8] Molecular biology is of limited value by showing germ-like configuration of the genes encoding for both IgV$_H$ and T-cell receptor, as expected in a tumor supposed to be derived from natural killer(NK)/T cells.[8]

CLINICAL, DIAGNOSTIC, AND STAGING PROCEDURES

Many patients with primary pulmonary lymphoma of BALT type are asymptomatic, and the disease is discovered incidentally on a chest radiograph done for other purposes: rarely chronic cough, dyspnea, hemoptysis, chest pain, or constitutional symptoms have been described.[1] Patients tend to be in their fifth, sixth, or seventh decades, with a slight male preponderance. Chest X-ray films demonstrate solitary nodule or infiltrates in a minority of cases (<10%) multiple nodules or a diffuse alveolar or interstitial infiltrate is seen. The computed tomography (CT) scan of BALT consists of a solitary nodule of poorly defined focal opacity or a localized area of consolidation with an air bronchogram (Figure 17.16). This appearance is related to the proliferation of the tumor cells within the interstitium such that the alveolar air spaces are obliterated, thereby simulating parenchymal consolidation. Because the bronchi tend to be unaffected, an air bronchogram is common. Ground-glass attenuation is also seen.

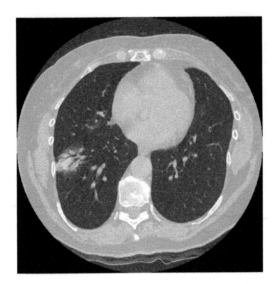

Figure 17.16   High-resolution CT scan of the thorax: an area of alveolar opacification with the bronchogram sign evident in the right lower lobe: low-grade B-cell lymphoma – MALT type – primary in the lung.

Furthermore, CT of the thorax may clarify the hilar or mediastinal lymph node enlargement.[57,58] Recently, [^{18}F] fluorodeoxyglucose positron emission tomography [^{18}FDG-PET] has been shown to be a useful tool in order to stage, restage, or monitor disease in patients with extranodal MALT lymphoma also in the lungs.[59] Bronchoscopy may show mucosal 'inflammatory changes' in more than 10% of patients and bronchial biopsies may document lymphomatous infiltration in about 15–20% of cases.[60] Different surgical procedures may be used to obtain diagnostic tissue. Endoscopic bronchial or transbronchial biopsy is the most frequently used technique. Open lung biopsy or video-assisted thoracoscopic surgery can be chosen if tissue from endoscopic biopsy is not sufficient. Serum lactate dehydrogenase (LDH) may be increased and β_2-microglobulin level is significantly more elevated in disseminated disease; a monoclonal peak of serum protein is present in about 40% of cases. A multifocal involvement outside the lungs may be documented in more than 40% of cases.[61]

TREATMENT AND OUTCOME

For most patients, the course is indolent and these lymphomas may remain confined to the lung for long periods. This indolent behavior can explain why many pulmonary MALT lymphoma cases were previously describe as 'pseudolymphoma'. The estimated 5-year overall survival (OS) is about 80%, but the risk of relapse seems to be constant, with an estimated incidence of 35% at 5 years. Relapses may occur in the same pulmonary localization, but also in other mucosal and non-mucosal sites. Therapy for primary pulmonary lymphomas of MALT type is still debated mainly because the reported series are small and heterogeneous or quite old.[60,62-66]

Thoracic surgery may be part of the diagnostic approach; however, early studies suggested that radical operation could be considered the definitive therapeutic act. Ferraro et al[67] operated on 48 patients for primary pulmonary non-Hodgkin's lymphoma, of which MALT type were 35 (73%) and non-MALT type were 13 (27%). A complete resection was obtained in 19 cases (40%). In patients with MALT-type lymphoma, the OS at 1, 5, and 10 years were 91%, 68%, and 53%, respectively. These data need to be weighed taking into account the fact that this lymphoma is an indolent disease, usually with a long natural course; it is a multifocal disease, in which a radical resection is not easy to reach. Furthermore, lung surgery is not without risks: thoracic pain and lung function impairment are observed in about 10–15% of cases. Radiotherapy alone, with a total dose of 30–35 Gy in 15–20 fractions (3–4 weeks), although shown to guarantee a high failure-free rate in MALT lymphomas of the thyroid, did not demonstrate the same results in primary pulmonary lymphomas of MALT type. This may be explained by considering the lungs as mobile organs.[68] Chemotherapy with anthracyclines or combined modality therapy, mainly with a CHOP (cyclophosphamide, doxorubicin, vincristine, prednisone) regimen, was associated with a 10-year lymphoma-specific survival of 72% in a study on 50 patients.[66] In this study no survival differences were seen between subjects with low-grade MALT lymphoma and patients in which MALT lymphoma was associated with areas of large B-cell lymphoma. Zinzani et al[69] reported a series in which 20 patients received either fludarabine/mitoxantrone (FM) or CVP (cyclophosphamide, vincristine, prednisone). Twenty patients were treated with the FM regimen and 11 patients were treated with the CVP regimen. The recurrence-free survival rate was almost 100% at 60 months. Recently Conconi et al reported that rituximab as single agent is safe, with significant activity in untreated or relapsed BALT lymphoma patients. However, the role of rituximab in BALT lymphoma, as in other extranodal MALT lymphoma, is now well explored in prospective randomized trials.[70–72] A few short series or single case reports using cladribine, oxaliplatinum, and low-dose thalidomide[73–76] have recently been reported with encouraging results.

In conclusion, surgical resection can be performed in patients with localized disease, whenever a wedge resection or middle right lobe and lingula excision are possible. The standard first-line therapy should include chlorambucil/cyclophosphamide monotherapy or CHOP–CHOP-like containing regimens. Radiotherapy has to be reserved for patients with a solitary, small lesion in a poorly mobile site and in patients not suitable for surgery. Rituximab alone or in combination therapy can be administered only within approved clinical trials.

OTHER B-CELL PRIMARY LUNG LYMPHOMAS

Rare cases of lymphocytic lymphoma follicular and DLBCL without low-grade MALT lymphoma are described in different series and make up 10% of cases of primary pulmonary lymphomas.[1] They present as nodules or masses, frequently escavated, with cough, dyspnea, hemoptysis, and often with systemic symptoms (fever, malaise). Clinical behavior, prognosis, and treatment outcome of these lymphomas is scanty but should parallel that for lymphomas arising at other sites. A proportion of cases show association of large B-cell lymphomas with a typical low–grade pulmonary MALT lymphoma (nearly 50% of primary high-grade lymphoma).[62,66] These cases are clinically indistinguishable from other low-grade cases without a large cell component and should be distinguished from other, more aggressive, large cell lymphomas affecting the lung (either primary or secondary) such as DLBCL occurring in immunocompromised patients, either for HIV infection or for immunosuppressive treatment for solid organ transplantation. Pulmonary acquired HIV-related lymphoma are rare (<10% of HIV-related NHL) and mostly appear as multiple nodular opacities on CT scan.

Primary pulmonary DLBCL require a multiagent anthracycline-based chemotherapy regimen combined with rituximab, as for the nodal counterpart. Despite such therapy, systemic progression is common, and relapse-free survival rates are calculated at about 50–60%.

As mentioned before, a peculiar type of DLBCL is grade III lymphomatoid granulomatosis. LYG was first described in the late 1960s.[39] This condition often presents with signs and symptoms that suggest infection. Characteristic CT features include peribronchovascular distribution of nodules, coarse irregular opacities, small thin-walled cysts, and conglomerating small nodules. Formation of large masses and occlusion of vessels also occur (Figure 17.17).[77] Although some reports have described spontaneous regression without any therapy,[78] progression from grade I-II to a frank aggressive lymphoma (grade III) occurs very frequently and prognosis is usually quite poor, with a mortality rate between 53% and 63%.[1,79,80] Contemporary involvement of the CNS, kidneys, or skin is not unusual.[79] Treatment options include corticosteroids, antiviral therapy, interferon-α, chemotherapy, and, more recently, anti CD-20 monoclonal antibodies and autologous hematopoietic stem cell transplantation.[80–82]

PERIPHERAL T-CELL LYMPHOMAS INVOLVING THE LUNG

Different types of extranodal T/NK-cell lymphomas, as defined by the WHO classification, can primarily occur in the lungs, but, due to their rarity, only anecdotal descriptions of their features are available. Nasal T/NK-cell

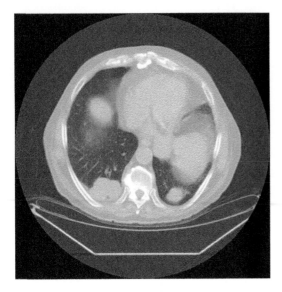

Figure 17.17 CT scan of the thorax. Bilateral basal nodule infiltration. On clinical grounds, one should note that this variety of the tumor can be more easily associated with paraproteinemia, amyloidosis, or deposition of heavy and/or light chains.

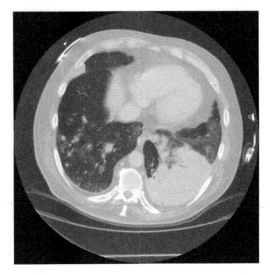

Figure 17.18 CT scan of the thorax showing an alveolar opacification in the left lower lobe, nodules with 'halo sign' in the right lower lobe, and bilateral areas of ground-glass attenuation: NK/T-cell lymphoma, nasal type, primary in the lung.

lymphomas, when occurring in the lung, can present many similarities with LYG, including angioinvasion, expression of EBV infection, necrosis, immune disturbances, and a rich T-cell infiltrate exhibiting cytotoxic immunophenotype. The occurrence of EBV marker expression is heterogeneous in other pulmonary T-cell lymphomas.[83-86]

Pulmonary localization is observed in nearly 10% of cases of T-cell lymphomas. Analogous to nodal peripheral T-cell lymphoma, they have a poor prognosis, with 50% mortality at 2 years, even when intensive combined modality treatments are applied.

PRIMARY HODGKIN'S LYMPHOMA OF THE LUNG

Primary pulmonary Hodgkin's lymphoma is a rare, but distinct, disease, to be distinguished from secondary lung involvement by nodal Hodgkin's disease. Usually localized in the upper lobes, it can present as a solitary mass or with multinodular lesions,[87-89] rarely as an endobronchial tumor.[90] The involvement of mediastinal lymph nodes must be excluded to define the lymphoma as truly primary. The

differential diagnosis includes many lung diseases, and a surgical biopsy is needed. Various modifications can be observed in the parenchyma adjacent to the neoplastic nodules, including focal organizing pneumonia, endoalveolar accumulation of macrophages, and interstitial lymphoid infiltration. The same staging procedures and therapeutic programs of the classic nodal presentation should be employed.

ACKNOWLEDGMENTS

The authors thank Bologna AIL (Bologna, Italy) and Fondazione della Banca del Monte e di Ravenna (Bologna, Italy) for economic support given to our research projects on the topics presented in this chapter.

REFERENCES

1. Chilosi M, Poletti V, Zinzani PL. Lymphoproliferative lung disorders. Semin Respir Crit Care Med 2005; 26: 490–501.
2. Li G, Hansmann ML, Zwingers T, et al. Primary lymphomas of the lung: morphological, immunohistochemical and clinical features. Histopathology 1990; 16: 519–31.

3. Cadranel J, Wislez M, Antoine M. Primary pulmonary lymphoma. Eur Respir J 2002; 20: 750–62.
4. Thieblemont C, Berger F, Dumontet C, et al. Mucosa-associated lymphoid tissue lymphoma is a disseminated disease in one third of 158 patients analyzed. Blood 2000; 95(3): 802–6.
5. Chetty R, Slavin JL, O'Leary JJ, Ansari NA, Gatter KC. Primary Hodgkin's disease of the lung. Pathology 1995; 27: 111–14.
6. Nansen IA, Prakash UBS, Colby TV. Pulmonary lymphoma in Sjögren's syndrome. Mayo Clin Proc 1989; 64: 920–31.
7. Nicholson AG, Wotherspoon AC, Diss TC, et al. Lymphomatoid granulomatosis: evidence that some cases represent Epstein–Barr virus-associated B-cell lymphoma. Histopathology 1996; 29: 317–24.
8. Jaffe ES, Harris NL, Stein H, Vardiman JW. Tumours of haematopoietic and lymphoid tissue. In: Jaffe ES, Harris NL, Stein H, Vardiman JW, eds. Pathology & Genetics. Lyon: IRAC Press, 2001.
9. Isaacson PG. Gastric MALT lymphoma: from concept to cure. Ann Oncol 1999; 10: 637–45.
10. Farinha P, Gascoyne RD. Molecular pathogenesis of mucosa-associated lymphoid tissue lymphoma. J Clin Oncol 2005; 23: 6370–8.
11. Gaur S, Trayner E, Aish L, Weinstein R. Bronchus-associated lymphoid tissue lymphoma arising in a patient with bronchiectasis and chronic Mycobacterium avium infection. Am J Hematol 2004; 77: 22–5.
12. Papiris SA, Kalomedis I, Malagari K, et al. Extranodal marginal zone B-cell lymphoma of the lung in Sjögren's syndrome patients: reappraisal of clinical, radiological, and pathology findings. Respir Med 2007; 101: 84–92.
13. Aghamohammadi A, Parvaneh N, Tirgari F, et al. Lymphoma of mucosa-associated lymphoid tissue in common variable immunodeficiency. Leuk Lymphoma 2006; 47: 343–6.
14. Okamoto M, Inaba T, Uchida R, et al. Human immunodeficiency virus (HIV)-negative, API-MALT1 fusion-negative bronchus-associated lymphoid tissue (BALT) lymphoma in a young male. Leuk Lymphoma 2004; 45: 2165–8.
15. Woehrer S, Streubel B, Chott A, et al. Transformation of MALT lymphoma to pure plasma cell histology following treatment with the anti-CD20 antibody rituximab. Leuk Lymphoma 2005; 46: 1645–9.
16. Niitsu N, Kohri M, Hayama M, et al. Primary pulmonary plasmacytoma involving bilateral lungs and marked hypergammaglobulinemia: differentiation from extranodal marginal zone B-cell lymphoma of mucosa-associated lymphoid tissue. Leuk Res 2005; 29: 1361–4.
17. Sakamaki Y, Yoon HE, Oda N, et al. Pulmonary lymphoma of mucosa-associated lymphoid tissue type followed as a long-standing indeterminate lesion in immunoglobulin M-type paraproteinemia. Jpn J Thorac Cardiovasc Surg 2006; 54: 293–6.
18. Papla B, Rudnicka L. Primary amyloid tumors of the lungs – six cases. Pol J Pathol 2005; 56: 197–202.
19. Fairweather PM, Williamson R, Tsikleas G. Pulmonary extranodal marginal zone lymphoma with massive crystal storing histiocytosis. Am J Surg Pathol 2006; 30: 262–7.
20. Pileri SA, Zinzani PL, Went Ph, Pileri A Jr, Bendandi M. Indolent lymphomas: the pathologist's view point. Ann Oncol 2004; 15: 12–18.
21. Zettl A, Rudiger T, Marx A, Muller-Hermelink HK, Ott G. Composite marginal zone B-cell lymphoma and classical Hodgkin's lymphoma: a clinicopathological study of 12 cases. Histopathology 2005; 46: 217–28.
22. Falini B, Tiacci E, Pucciarini A, et al. Expression of the IRTA1 receptor identifies intraepithelial and subepithelial marginal zone B cells of the mucosa-associated lymphoid tissue (MALT). Blood 2003; 102: 3684–92.
23. Bertoni F, Zucca E. Delving deeper into MALT lymphoma biology. J Clin Invest 2006; 116: 22–6.
24. Okabe M, Inagaki H, Ohshima K, et al. API2-MALT1 fusion defines a distinctive clinicopathologic subtype in pulmonary extranodal marginal zone B-cell lymphoma of mucosa-associated lymphoid tissue. Am J Pathol 2003; 162: 1113–22.
25. Streubel B, Simonitsch-Klupp I, Mullauer L, et al. Variable frequencies of MALT lymphoma-associated genetic aberrations in MALT lymphomas of different sites. Leukemia 2004; 18: 1722–6.
26. Remstein ED, Kurtin PJ, Einerson RR, et al. Primary pulmonary MALT lymphomas show frequent and heterogeneous cytogenetic abnormalities, including aneuploidy and translocations involving API2 and MALT1 and IGH and MALT1. Leukemia 2004; 18: 156–60.
27. Takino H, Okabe M, Ohshima K, et al. p16/NK4a gene methylation is a frequent finding in pulmonary MALT lymphomas at diagnosis. Mod Pathol 2005; 18: 1187–92.
28. Edelstein E, Gal AA, Mann KP, et al. Primary solitary endobronchial plasmacytoma. Ann Thorac Surg 2004; 78: 1448–9.
29. Pileri SA, Gaidano G, Zinzani PL, et al. Primary mediastinal B-cell lymphoma (PMBL): high frequency of Bcl-6 mutations and consistent expression of the transcription factors OCT-2, BOB. 1, and PU. 1 in the absence of immunoglobulins. A co-operative study of the international Extranodal Lymphoma Study Group. Am J Pathol 2003; 162: 243–53.
30. Rosenwald A, Wright G, Leroy K, et al. Molecular diagnosis of primary mediastinal B cell lymphoma identifies a clinically favourable subgroup of diffuse large B cell lymphoma related to Hodgkin lymphoma. J Exp Med 2003; 198: 851–862.
31. Savae KJ, Monti S, Kutok JL, et al. The molecular signature of mediastinal large B-cell lymphoma differs from that of other diffuse large B-cell lymphomas and shares features with classical Hodgkin lymphoma. Blood 2003; 102: 3872–9.

32. Traverse-Glehen A, Pittaluga S, Gaulard P, et al. Mediastinal grey zone lymphoma: the missing link between classic Hodgkin's lymphoma and mediastinal large B-cell lymphoma. Am J Surg Pathol 2005; 29: 1411–21.

33. Murase T, Nakamura S, Kawauchi K, et al. An Asian variant of intravascular large B-cell lymphoma: clinical, pathological and cytogenetic approaches to diffuse large B-cell lymphoma associated with haemophagocytic syndrome. Br J Haematol 2000; 111: 826–34.

34. Ferreri AJM, Campo E, Seymour JF, et al. Intravascular lymphoma: clinical presentation, natural history, management and prognostic factors in a series of 38 cases, with special emphasis on the 'cutaneous variant'. Br J Haematol 2004; 127: 173–83.

35. Ponzoni M, Ferreri AJM, Campo E, et al. Definition, diagnosis and management of intravascular large B-cell lymphoma: proposals and perspectives from an international consensus meeting. J Clin Oncol 2007; 25: 3168–73.

36. Percik R, Serr J, Segal G, et al. Lymphomatoid granulomatosis: a diagnostic challenge. Isr Med Assoc J 2005; 7: 198–9.

37. Katzenstein AL, Peiper SC. Detection of Epstein–Barr virus genomes in lymphomatoid granulomatosis: analysis of 29 cases by the polymerase chain reaction technique. Mod Pathol 1990; 3: 435–41.

38. Liebow AA, Carrington CR, Friedman PJ. Lymphomatoid granulomatosis. Hum Pathol 1972; 3: 457–558.

39. Corti M, Villafane MF, Trione N, et al. Primary pulmonary AIDS-related lymphoma. Rev Med Trop Sao Paulo 2005; 47: 231–4.

40. Saxena A, Dyker KM, Angel S, et al. Posttransplant diffuse large B-cell lymphoma of 'lymphomatoid granulomatosis' type. Virchows Arch 2002; 441: 622–8.

41. Carbone A, Gloghini A. AIDS-related lymphomas: from pathogenesis to pathology. Br J Haematol 2005; 130: 662–70.

42. Carbone A, Gloghini A, Larocca LM, et al. Expression profile of MUM1/IRF4, BCL-6, and CD138/syndecan-1 defines novel histogenetic subsets of human immunodeficiency virus-related lymphomas. Blood 2001; 97: 744–51.

43. Carbone A, Gloghini A, Vaccher E, et al. Kaposi's sarcoma-associated herpesvirus/human herpesvirus type 8-positive solid lymphomas: a tissue-based variant of primary effusion lymphoma. J Mol Diagn 2005; 7: 17–27.

44. Klein U, Gloghini A, Gaidano G, et al. Gene expression profile analysis of AIDS-related primary effusion lymphoma (PEL) suggests a plasmablastic derivation and identifies PEL-specific transcripts. Blood 2003; 101: 4115–21.

45. Chadburn A, Hyjek E, Mathew S, et al. KSHV-positive solid lymphomas represent an extra-cavitary variant of primary effusion lymphoma. Am J Surg Pathol 2004; 28: 1401–16.

46. Ascani S, Piccioli M, Poggi S, et al. Pyothorax-associated lymphoma: description of the first two cases detected in Italy. Ann Oncol 1997; 8: 1133–8.

47. Nakatsuka S, Yao M, Hoshida Y, et al. Pyothorax-associated lymphoma: a review of 106 cases. J Clin Oncol 2002; 20: 4255–60.

48. Aozasa K, Takakuwa T, Nakatsuka S. Pyothorax-associated lymphoma: a lymphoma developing in chronic inflammation. Adv Anat Pathol 2005; 12: 324–31.

49. Aozasa K. Pyothorax-associated lymphoma. J Clin Exp Hematop 2006; 46: 5–10.

50. Nishiu M, Tomita Y, Nakatsuka S, et al. Distinct pattern of gene expression in pyothorax-associated lymphoma (PAL), a lymphoma developing in long-standing inflammation. Cancer Sci 2004; 95: 828–34.

51. Hashizume T, Aozasa K, Tomita Y, Matsushita K: Pyothorax-associated T-cell lymphoma: a case report. Jpn J Clin Oncol 2003; 33: 145–7.

52. Yegappan S, Schnitzer B, Hsi ED. Follicular lymphoma with marginal zone differentiation: microdissection demonstrates the t(14;18) in both the follicular and marginal zone components. Mod Pathol 2001; 14: 191–6.

53. Siordia-Reyes AG, Fernan-Cano F, Rodriguez-Velasco A. [ALK-1 positive anaplastic large cell lymphoma of the lung. Report of a pediatric case]. Gac Med Mex 2005; 141: 531–4. [in Spanish]

54. Rodriguez J, Tirabosco R, Pizzolitto S, et al. Hodgkin lymphoma presenting with exclusive or preponderant pulmonary involvement: a clinicopathologic study of 5 new cases. Ann Diagn Pathol 2006; 10: 83–8.

55. Lee BH, Kim SY, Kim MY, et al. CT of nasal-type T/NK cell lymphoma in the lung. J Thorac Imaging 2006; 21: 37–9.

56. King LJ, Padley SP, Wotherspoon AC, Nischolson AG. Pulmonary MALT lymphoma: imaging findings in 24 cases. Eur Radiol 2000; 10: 1932–8.

57. Do KH, Lee JS, Seo JB, et al. Pulmonary parenchymal involvement of low-grade lymphoproliferative disorders. J Comput Assist Tomogr 2005; 825: 1–7.

58. Alinari L, Castellucci P, Elstrom R, et al. ^{18}F-FDG PET in mucosa-associated lymphoid tissue (MALT) lymphoma. Leuk Lymphoma 2006; 47: 2096–101.

59. Cordier JF, Fouque D, Laville F, et al. Primary pulmonary lymphomas. A clinical study of 70 cases in non immuno-compromised patients. Chest 1993; 103: 201–8.

60. Raderer M, Wohrer S, Streubel B, et al. Assessment of disease dissemination in gastric compared with extragastric mucosa-associated lymphoid tissue lymphoma using extensive staging: a single-center experience. J Clin Oncol 2006; 24: 3136–41.

61. Li G, Hansmann ML, Zwingers T, et al. Primary lymphomas of the lung: morphological, immunohistochemical and clinical features. Histopathology 1990; 16: 519–53.

62. Ahmed S, Kussick SJ, Siddiqui AK, et al. Bronchial-associated lymphoid tissue lymphoma: a clinical

study of a rare disease. Eur J Cancer 2004; 40: 1320–6.

63. Zinzani PL, Tani M, Gabriele A, et al. Extranodal marginal zone B-cell lymphoma of MALT-type of the lung: single experience with 12 patients. Leuk Lymphoma 2003; 44: 821–4.

64. Zucca E, Conconi A, Pedrinis E, et al. Nongastric marginal zone B-cell lymphoma of mucosa-associated lymphoid tissue. Blood 2003; 101: 2489–95.

65. Kurtin PJ, Myers JL, Adlakha H, et al. Pathologic and clinical features of primary pulmonary extranodal marginal zone B-cell lymphoma of MALT type. Am J Surg Pathol 2001; 25: 997–1008.

66. Ferraro P, Trastek VF, Adlakha H, et al. Primary non-Hodgkin's lymphoma of the lung. Ann Thorac Surg 2000; 69: 993–7.

67. Tsang RW, Gospodarowicz MK, Pintilie M, et al. Localized mucosa-associated lymphoid tissue lymphoma treated with radiation therapy has excellent clinical outcome. J Clin Oncol 2003; 21: 4157–64.

68. Zinzani PL, Stefoni V, Musuraca G, et al. Fludarabine-containing chemotherapy as frontline treatment of nongastrointestinal mucosa-associated lymphoid tissue lymphoma. Cancer 2004; 100: 2190–4.

69. Conconi A, Martinelli G, Thieblemont C, et al. Clinical activity of rituximab in extranodal marginal zone B-cell lymphoma of MALT type. Blood 2003; 102: 2741–5.

70. Raderer M, Jager G, Brugger S, et al. Rituximab for treatment of advanced extranodal marginal zone B cell lymphoma of the mucosa-associated lymphoid tissue lymphoma. Oncology 2003; 65: 306–10.

71. Chong FA, Svoboda J, Cherian S, et al. Regression of pulmonary MALT lymphoma after treatment with rituximab. Leuk Lymphoma 2005; 46: 1383–6.

72. Jager G, Neumeister P, Ouehenberger F, et al. Prolonged clinical remission in patients with extranodal marginal zone B-cell lymphoma of the mucosa-associated lymphoid tissue type treated with cladribine: 6 year follow-up of a phase II trial. Ann Oncol 2006; 11: 1722–3.

73. Jager G, Neumeister P, Brezinschek R, et al. Treatment of extranodal marginal zone B-cell lymphoma of mucosa-associated lymphoid tissue type with cladribine: a phase II study. J Clin Oncol 2002; 20: 3872–7.

74. Raderer M, Wohrer S, Bartsch R, et al. Phase II study of oxaliplatin for treatment of patients with mucosa-associated lymphoid tissue lymphoma. J Clin Oncol 2005; 23: 8442–6.

75. Kees M, Raderer M, Metz-Schimmerl S, et al. Very good partial response in a patient with MALT-lymphoma of the lung after treatment with low-dose thalidomide. Leuk Lymphoma 2005; 46: 1379–82.

76. Lee JS, Tuder R, Lynch DA. Lymphomatoid granulomatosis: radiologic features and pathologic correlations. AJR Am J Roentgenol 2000; 175: 1335–9.

77. Wu SM, Min Y, Ostrzega N, Clements PJ, Wong AL. Lymphomatoid granulomatosis: a rare mimicker of vasculitis. J Rheumatol 2005; 32: 2242–5.

78. MaconWR, Williams ME, Greer JP, et al. Natural killer-like T-cell lymphomas: aggressive lymphomas of T-cell large granular lymphocytes. Blood 1996; 87: 1474–83.

79. Katzenstein AL, Carrington CB, Liebow AA. Lymphomatoid granulomatosis: a clinicopathologic study of 152 cases. Cancer 1979; 43: 360–73.

80. Wilson WH, Kingma DW, Raffeld M, Wittes RE, Jaffe ES. Association of lymphomatoid granulomatosis with Epstein–Barr viral infection of B lymphocytes and response to interferon-alpha 2b. Blood 1996; 87: 4531–7

81. Jordan K, Grothey A, Grothe W, et al. Successful treatment of mediastinal lymphomatoid granulomatosis with rituximab monotherapy. Eur J Haematol 2005; 74: 263–6.

82. Johnston A, Coyle L, Nevell D. Prolonged remission of refractory lymphomatoid granulomatosis after autologous hemopoietic stem cell transplantation with post-transplantation maintenance interferon. Leuk Lymphoma 2006; 47: 323–8. .

83. de Bruin PC, Jiwa M, Oudejans JJ, et al. Presence of Epstein–Barr virus in extranodal T-cell lymphoma: differences in relation to site. Blood 1994; 83: 1612–18.

84. Karakus S, Yalcin S, Guler N, Coplu L, Ayhan A. Angiocentric T-cell lymphoma of the lung mimicking metastatic carcinoma: case report. J Exp Clin Res 1998; 17: 371–3.

85. Maerjima S, Kitano K, Ichikawa S, et al. T-cell non-Hodgkin's lymphoma of the lung. Intern Med 1993; 32: 403–7.

86. Beltran Beltran S, de Tomas Labar MF, Ferreras Fernadez P, et al. [Primary Ki-1 positive anaplastic large cell non Hodgkin's lymphoma of the lung. A case study and review of the literature]. An Med Interna 2001; 18. 587–90. [in spanish]

87. Radin AI. Primary pulmonary Hodgkin's disease. Cancer 1990; 65: 550–63.

88. Chetty R, Slavin JI, O'Leary JJ, Ansari NA, Gatter KC. Primary Hodgkin's disease of the lung. Pathology 1995; 27: 111–14.

89. Catterall JR, Mc Cabe RE, Brooks RG, Remington JS. Open lung biopsy in patients with Hodgkin's diasease and pulmonary infiltrates. Am Rev Respir Dis 1989; 139: 1274–9.

90. Kiani B, Magro CM, Ross P. Endobronchial presentation of Hodgkin lymphoma: a review of the literature. Ann Thorac Surg 2003; 76: 967–72.

Primary mediastinal (thymic) large B-cell lymphoma

18

Kerry J Savage and Philippe Gaulard

INTRODUCTION

Since its first description in the early 1980s, primary mediastinal (thymic) large B-cell lymphoma (PMBCL) has been recognized as an distinct subtype of diffuse large B-cell lymphoma (DLBCL) in the REAL (Revised European–American Classification of Lymphoid Neoplastics) classification in 1994 and more recently included in the WHO (World Health Organization) classification,[1] based on unique clinical, pathological, and genetic features. PMBCL is defined pathologically by a diffuse proliferation of large cells thought to derive from thymic B cells and often compartmentalized by fine bands of sclerosis. It primarily occurs in young, adult females with primary involvement of the mediastinum and is often associated with locally invasive behavior. Recent microarray studies have shown a unique gene signature, distinct from other DLBCL, but with striking similarities to that of classical Hodgkin's lymphoma (cHL).[2,3]

INCIDENCE AND EPIDEMIOLOGY

PMBCL accounts for 5–10% of adult diffuse large cell lymphoma[4-6] and occurs mainly in young adults, with a median age of approximately 35 years old and a female predominance (ratio F:M, 2:1) (Table 18.1).

HISTOPATHOLOGY

PMBCL has distinct morphological and phenotypic features. PMBCL typically shows a diffuse growth pattern: tumor cells are large or medium to large B cells with abundant pale cytoplasm. PMBCL is commonly associated with fibrosis, which tends to compartmentalize the tumor[4-8] (Figures 18.1a,b). As a result, PMBCL can mimic a carcinoma or thymoma. PMBCL can exhibit a wide morphological/ cytological spectrum, with variable size and shape of the neoplastic cells observed among cases. In some tumors, lymphoma cells have multilobated nuclei which may resemble Hodgkin's Reed–Sternberg cells. The diagnosis may be difficult, particularly when biopsies are small or obscured by the presence of sclerosis, necrosis, and/or cellular crush artifacts. In such cases, immunohistochemistry is required to definitively establish the B-cell origin of the tumor and to support that a case represents a PMBCL. Remnants of thymic epithelial structures may be observed, particularly on large biopsies or surgical specimen, which are often better highlighted using cytokeratin staining.

IMMUNOPHENOTYPE

PMBCL tumors demonstrate the leukocyte common antigen (CD45) as well as B-cell lineage antigens such as CD19, CD20, and CD22 (Figure 18.1c). However, unlike other B-cell lymphomas, they often lack surface or cytoplasmic immunoglobulin (Ig),[4,8,9] despite expression of the Ig co-receptor, CD79a (see Table 18.1). This discordant expression of components of the B-cell receptor (BCR) is characteristic of PMBCL.[9] It does not appear to be due to a lack of functional Ig gene rearrangements or to a defect in the transcription factors

Table 18.1   Comparison of the clinical and pathological features of diffuse large B-cell lymphoma (DLBCL), primary mediastinal large B-cell lymphoma (PMBCL), and nodular sclerosis classical Hodgkin's lymphoma (NScHL)

Features	DLBCL	PMBCL	NScHL
Female:male ratio	1:1	2:1	1:1
Median age	55	35	28
Stage I–II	30	70–80%	55%
Mediastinal presentation	20%	All	80%
Extranodal sites	Common	Uncommon	Uncommon
Bone marrow	10–15%	2%	3%
Spleen	20%	5%	10%
Elevated LDH	50%	70–80%	Rare
B symptoms	50%	50%	40%
Bulky disease (≥10 cm)	10–15%	70–80%	54%
Relapse past 2 years	2% per year	Rare	Rare
Morphology	Sheets of large cells with variable aspects	Sheets of large cells Clear cells No inflammatory polymorphous infiltrate	Lacunar Hodgkin Reed–Sternberg cells Inflammatory polymorphous infiltrate
Sclerosis	Absent or rare	70–100% (alveolar, fine bands)	100% (large bands), annular
CD45	Positive	Positive	Negative
CD30	Variable (anaplastic variant)	Positive weak (70–85%)	Positive
CD15	Negative	Negative	Positive (75–85%)
CD20	Positive	Positive	Negative or heterogeneous (40%)
CD79a	Positive	Positive	Usually negative
Pax-5	Positive	Positive	Weak positive
Mum-1	Variable (Non-GC type)	Positive	Positive
Immunoglobulin	Positive	Usually negative	Negative
BOB.1	Positive	Positive	Frequently negative
OCT-2	Positive	Positive	Frequently negative
MAL expression	<10%	60–70%	<20%
TRAF1 expression	12%	60–70%	Most cases (84%)
Nuclear cRel	18%	60–70%	Most cases (92%)
BCL6 rearrangements	30%	Usually absent	Absent
BCL2 rearrangements	20%	Absent	Absent
Gains/amp 9p	Absent	70%	33%
Gains/amp 2p (Rel, BCL11A)	15% (> in GCB)	50%	25%
SOCS1 mutations/deletions	?Unknown	45%	42%

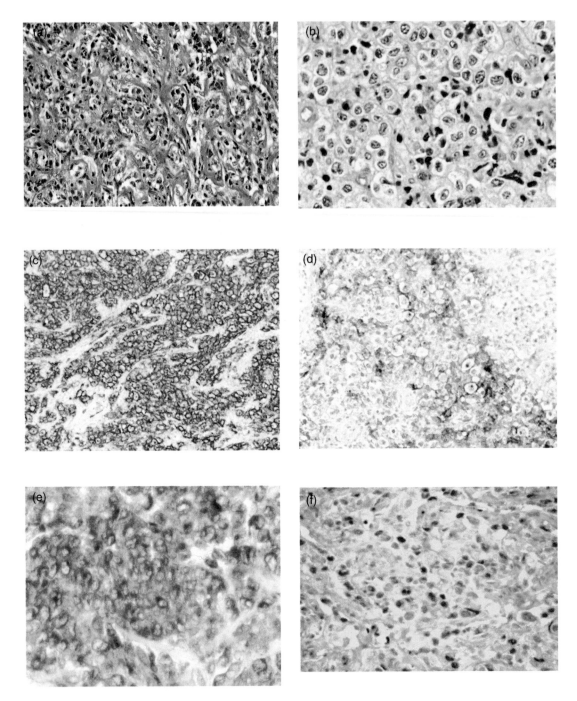

Figure 18.1   Primary mediastinal B-cell lymphoma. (a) H&E staining, illustrating the fibrotic bands without annular distribution compartmentalizing the tumor cells. (b) In another case, the clear cytoplasm of the neoplastic large cells is shown. (c) Tumor cells express CD20 at their membrane. (d) CD23 (note, the more heterogeneous membrane and dot-like staining). (e) Tumor cells also show strong cytoplasmic staining for MAL antigen. (f) Most PMBCL exhibit the presence of phosphorylated STAT6 protein in the nuclei of neoplastic cells.

BOB.1, OCT-2, and PU.1[8] (see Table 18.1). Recent studies suggest that the absence of Ig may be the result of down-regulation of the intronic heavy-chain enhancer[10] or post-transcriptional blockage.[11] Despite some controversies, PMBCL tumors are CD10-negative in the majority of cases, whereas most cases have a MUM1/IRF4+ phenotype with variable BCL6 expression.[8,12] Tumor cells are CD21-negative, but can be CD23-positive in up to 80% of cases[13] (Figure 18.1d). Expression of MAL antigen, a lipid raft component, is another unique characteristic feature of PMBCL, that is not found in other DLBCL[14,15] (Figure 18.1e). CD30 is often present but is usually weak and heterogeneous, in comparison to Hodgkin's lymphoma.[8,16] However, CD15 is absent. Lack of HLA class I and/or class II molecules has been reported.[17,18]

CELL OF ORIGIN

It is postulated that PMBCL derives from the small subset of thymic B cells with asteroid shape located around the Hassall's corpuscles in the medullary thymus which share with PMBCL a CD10−, CD21−, CD23+/−, CD35+/− phenotype[19] and express AID.[20] The clinical presentation within the anterior mediastinum and the identification of normal thymic medullary B cells that express MAL supports this hypothesis.[15]

DIAGNOSTIC CRITERIA

As discussed above, PMBCL can be difficult to distinguish from both nodular sclerosis-HL (Hodgkin's lymphoma) and 'classical' DLBCL associated with secondary mediastinal invasion. The similarities between nodular sclerosis classical Hodgkin's lymphoma (NScHL) may explain the occurrence of cases of mediastinal gray zone lymphomes (MZGL) that combine morphological and phenotypic features of both nodular sclerosis-HL and PMBCL, and can be a diagnostic challenge to pathologists.[4,24] The distinct characteristic morphological features of PMBCL, such as clear cell proliferation and sclerosis, may be difficult to evaluate on small biopsies, and there is a lack of definitive diagnostic criteria that can be routinely applied. In the absence of such criteria, the diagnosis in such cases should be based on the distinctive phenotype of PMBCL, i.e. usually CD15−, but positive for CD45, CD20, CD79a, and transcription factors PU.1, OCT-2, and the co-activator BOB.1. Expression of CD30 (weak), CD23, and BCL6 can also aid in the diagnosis of PMBCL. The presence of MAL antigen may be helpful, although the antibody is not commercially available (Figures 18.1c–e). Another consideration in the differential diagnosis is 'classical' DLBCL associated with secondary mediastinal invasion which most likely originates from mediastinal lymph nodes; however, in contrast to PMBCL, extrathoracic disease is typically present at diagnosis and tumor sclerosis is absent. More recently, the presence of both TRAF1 and nuclear cREL has been shown to be highly specific for the diagnosis of PMBCL, compared to other DLBCLs.[22] Nuclear phosphorylated STAT6 may also aid in differentiating PMBCL from the morphologically similar DLBCL[23] (Figure 18.1f). These and other markers that can reliably and reproducibly differentiate PMBCL will also facilitate future study comparisons.

GENETICS

PMBCL has distinct biological features. Molecular studies of PMBCL can show discrepant results, which may reflect the heterogeneity of the cases studied in the absence of strict diagnostic criteria for PMBCL. However, several studies indicate that PMBCL usually lacks alterations observed in other DLBCLs, such as rearrangements of the BCL2 and BCL6 genes[24] (see Table 18.1). Although most cases carry a high Ig mutational burden, they lack ongoing mutational activity[25] despite constitutive expression of AID.[26] Mutations of the BCL6 gene are also common.[8] Abnormalities in c-myc, p16INK4A, and p53 have also been reported.[27] Together with the frequent CD10–/bcl–6+/MUM1+ phenotype, these studies may suggest that PMBCL originates from a postgerminal center B cell, although a derivation from another B-cell subset which acquired this mutational activity without transit through the germinal center (GC) cannot be excluded.

Comparative genomic hybridization (CGH) studies, have shown that PMBCL is characterized by distinctive chromosomal aberrations, including recurrent chromosomal gains in 9p23-24 in approximately 70% of cases, in addition to gains in chromosome 2p15 (~50%), Xp11.4-21 (33%), Xq24-26 (33%), 7q22 (32%), 9q34 (32%), and 12q31 (30%).[28–31] This genomic profile is unique among DLBCL. The biological significance of these alterations is not fully understood. However, candidate genes include REL and BCL11A, at chromosome 2p, which are amplified in a proportion of PMBCL, leading to frequent nuclear accumulation of their respective proteins.[22,32,33] At chromosome 9p, amplification of JAK2 – a gene which is involved in cytokine-dependent signal transduction – has been demonstrated in a proportion of cases.[23,28,34] Despite amplification at the genetic level, JAK2 does not appear to be overexpressed at the RNA level in many cases, and increased JAK2 activity has rather been associated with mutations in the suppressor of cytokine signaling (SOCS1) gene.[34] The PMBCL cell lines MEDB-1 and Karpas 1106 have biallelic mutations and deletions in SOCS1, respectively, both resulting in constitutive activation of the JAK–STAT pathway. Mutations or deletions in SOCS1 have also been recently found in 45% of PMBCL primary tumors (see Table 18.1) and more recently cHL cell lines as well as in laser microdissected Reed–Sternberg cells of 40% of cHL primary tumors, supporting that this oncogenic pathway is prominent in both tumors.[34–36] The amplicon on chromosome 9p also includes PDL1 and PDL2, which encode members of the B7 family and are ligands for the PD-1 receptor on T-cells; however, the pathogenic significance in PMBCL is unknown.

More recently, detailed analysis of chromosomal aberrations using tiling-resolution array CGH has revealed that chromosomal losses are also frequently encountered in PMBCL, most commonly, 1p13.1-p13.2 (42%), in addition to 3p, 4q, 6q, 7p, and 17p losses.[31] The functional significance is not yet known; however, given the similar frequency of losses compared to gains of DNA, they are likely to play an important role in disease pathogenesis.

PMBCL has a characteristic gene signature that is distinct from other DLBCL and shares features with classical Hodgkin's lymphoma. Two recent molecular profiling studies have shown that PMBCL has a unique transcriptional signature, distinct from that of other types non-mediastinal DLBCL – i.e. germinal-center (GC) B cells or activated-B (ABC) DLBCL[2,3] (Figures 18.2a and 18.2b). This transcriptional signature defines a distinct clinical entity that affects young patients who have a mediastinal tumor, with preferential locoregional extension and a relatively good outcome, and distinguishes these tumors from DLBCL associated with secondary mediastinal invasion.[3]

Although PMBCL is considered a subtype of DLBCL, it has long been appreciated that it shares several notable overlapping clinical and pathological features with NScHL[21,37] (see Table 18.1). Both occur most often in young adults who present with a prominent mediastinal mass but lack extrathoracic disease. Pathologically, sclerosis is present in both tumors, and Reed–Sternberg-like cells can be seen in PMBCL. Further, the Hodgkin's Reed–Sternberg cells (HRS) are also typified by the absence of Ig. Classical Hodgkin's lymphoma also harbor gains in chromosome 2p and 9p and, in addition, SOCS1 mutations have also recently been found, resulting in activation of the JAK–STAT pathway, supporting that this pathway may be critical in both tumors.[34–37] MAL is differentially expressed in PMBCL compared with DLBCL, but is found in some cases of NScHL[3,15] and may be associated with a worse prognosis.[38] In addition to these striking clinical, immunological, and molecular similarities, there have been reported cases of composite or sequential NScHL and PMBCL in addition to (MZGL), as previously described, with features between NScHL and PMBCL.[21] In cases of sequential lymphoma, IgH rearrangements of a similar size have been found, confirming a common origin.[21] These observations support that a close biological relationship exists between PMBCL and NSCHL, whereby MGZL represents the 'missing link' between these entities.[21]

Despite these similarities, there are still important differences between PMBCL and NScHL. Unlike HRS cells, PMBCL tumor cells retain several B-cell differentiation markers and, histologically, they appear more similar to other DLBCLs. The brisk inflammatory background seen in cHL is not usually seen in PMBCL. In addition, PMBCL has not been shown to be associated with EBV.

Overall, the above observations support that PMBCL may be pathogenetically related to cHL. Evidence of an overlapping relationship is further supported by the above gene expression profiling studies that demonstrated that the molecular signature of PMBCL is not only distinct from that of DLBCL but also has a striking resemblance to the expression profile of HRS cell lines (see Figures 18.2).[2,3] The signature is characterized by high expression of

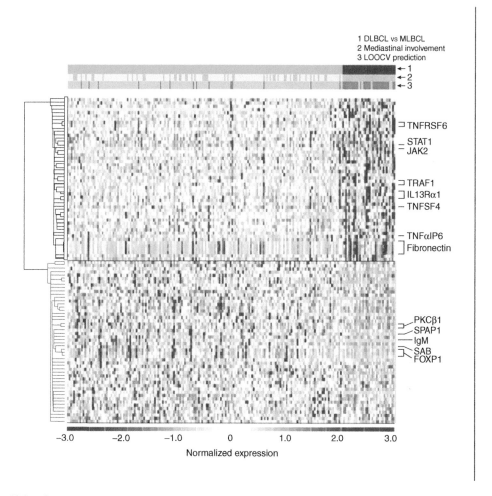

Figure 18.2a Comparative gene expression profiles of DLBCL and MLBCL (or PMBCL). At the top, the actual clinical/pathological diagnosis of DLBCL vs MLBCL (green vs red), presence or absence of mediastinal disease (pink vs light green), and molecular prediction of DLBCL vs MLBCL (green vs red) are compared. Genes are clustered using hierarchical clustering. Expression profiles of 176 DLBCLs are on the left; profiles of the 34 MLBCLs are on the right. Note: red = high relative expression, blue = low expression. Column = sample, row = gene. (© American Society of Hematology; adapted and used with permission.)

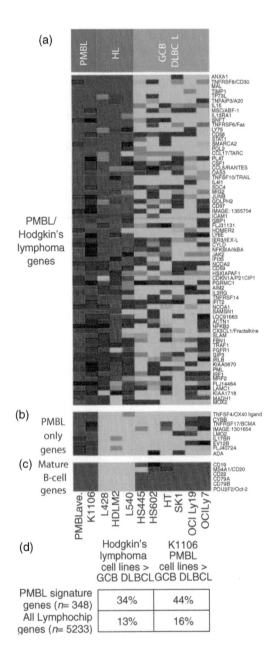

Figure 18.2b Relationship of PMBL to Hodgkin's lymphoma. Relative gene expression is shown in primary PMBLs (average of all biopsy samples), the PMBL cell line K1106, three Hodgkin's lymphoma (HL) cell lines, and six GCB DLBCL cell lines, according to the color scale shown in (a) PMBL signature genes that are also expressed at high levels in Hodgkin's lymphoma cell lines compared with GCB DLBCL cell lines. (b) PMBL signature genes not expressed in Hodgkin's lymphoma cell lines. (c) Mature B-cell markers expressed in PMBL and GCB DLBCL but not in Hodgkin's lymphoma. (d) Enrichment within the set of PMBL signature genes of genes highly expressed in Hodgkin's lymphoma cell lines or in the K1106 PMBL cell line relative to GCB DLBCL cell lines. (Reproduced from the *Journal of Experimental Medicine*; © and permission of the Rockafeller University Press.)

genes involved in cytokine and interleukin IL-4/IL-13 signaling (including *IL-13R alpha1, JAK2, TARC, IL-4-1/FIG1, RANTES*), many of which have been identified in HRS cells or cHL cell lines.[39] IL-4-1/FIG1 and MAL, which had previously been shown to be differentially expressed in PMBCL, were also identified.[14,40] Co-stimulatory molecules of the B7 family (*CD80, CD86, and PDL-2*) were highly expressed in PMBCL[2,3] and are evident in HRS cells. Both

PMBCL and cHL exhibit sclerosis, highlighting the importance of the extracellular matrix. Consistent with this, PMBCL demonstrated high levels of expression of the adhesion molecule CD58/LFA3, CD11b/integrinαM, and additional components of the extracellular matrix (*fibronectin, metalloproteinases*).[2,3]

Tumor necrosis factor (TNF) superfamily signaling pathway members were also identified (including *CD30, Fas/CD95, TRAF1*), all prominent in HRS cells. The nuclear factor kappa B (NF-κB) has been shown to promote HRS cell survival and, similarly, nuclear localization of c-REL, consistent with activation, is seen in the majority of cases of PMBCL.[2,22] Furthermore, increased expression of downstream targets of NF-κB is also seen in PMBCL, supporting that this pathway may be critical in disease pathogenesis.[2,41]

In addition to evidence of activation of NF-κB, it has been further shown that PMBCL activates the JAK–STAT signaling pathways,[23,34] with phosphorylated STAT6 detected in the nuclei of PMBCL, being also found in cHL[23,36,42] (Figure 18.1f). As outlined above, activation of the JAK–STAT signaling pathway seems to be frequently related to mutations in SOCS1.[34–36]

CLINICAL PRESENTATION

PMBCL typically occurs in young adult females (ratio F:M, 2:1; median age 35 years old) (see Table 18.1) who present with an anterior mediastinal mass and associated respiratory symptoms. Superior vena caval syndrome can occur with facial swelling, dyspnea, headache, neck vein distention, and, occasionally, thrombosis. Most patients have bulky, stage I or II disease and B symptoms at diagnosis. Intrathoracic extension into the lung, chest wall, pericardial, and pleural spaces is common (see Table 18.1). Extrathoracic disease, including bone marrow involvement, at presentation is rare. Furthermore, spread to peripheral lymph nodes is infrequent, although localized extension to the supraclavicular nodes can occur. Although the lactate dehydrogenase (LDH) is commonly elevated, the β$_2$-microglobulin level is usually normal, probably related to the low level of human leukocyte antigen (HLA) class I expression in the lymphoma cells. At relapse, disease in unusual extranodal sites such as the liver, kidneys, ovaries, and central nervous system (CNS) can occur.[37]

DIAGNOSTIC AND STAGING PROCEDURES

Staging of PMBCL is the same as that routinely used for DLBCL and the Ann Arbor

staging is applied. It includes a comprehensive history and physical examination, baseline laboratory parameters, including a complete blood count (CBC) and LDH, and computed tomography (CT). Despite infrequent bone marrow involvement, bone marrow aspirate and biopsy should be performed in all patients. Typically, an anterior mediastinotomy or a minithoracotomy is necessary for a tissue diagnosis. Positron emission tomography (PET) scanning is optional at staging but may be useful in monitoring response to therapy.[43]

PROGNOSTIC FACTORS

The International Prognostic Index (IPI) was originally developed in diffuse large cell lymphoma prior to the recognition of PMBCL. Thus, although there may have been cases of PMBCL included in this analysis, they were not evaluated as a separate group. Subsequent studies evaluating the IPI or the aaIPI (age-adjusted) have been discrepant in PMBCL.[44–47] This may in part reflect differences between studies assigning patients as stage IV or stage 2E if multiple but contiguous extranodal sites are involved. In the few studies that have found the index useful, it has been the IPI that was applied, suggesting that it is primarily age that drives the poor prognosis. Even if the aaIPI is used, which eliminates the number of extranodal sites as a risk factor, most patients will have an elevated LDH, again reducing its discrimatory power.[46] Other factors in individual studies that have been found to have a prognostic relevance include pleural and/or pericardial effusion and poor performance status.[47,49]

Recent gene expression studies support that low expression of major histocompatibility class (MHC) II gene correlates with poor outcome,[50] which may reflect decreased immunosurveillance.

TREATMENT AND OUTCOME

Five-year overall survival rates of PMBCL have varied widely in retrospective series in the literature (46–93%) (Table 18.2).[6,44–49,51–57] These broad differences may reflect diagnostic

Table 18.2 Selected PMBCL treatment and survival studies in the last 10 years

Reference	No. of Patients	Mediastinal radiation	Chemotherapy regimen (n)	PFS/EFS (%)	OS (%)	Comment
Savage[47]	153	Before 1998 variable / After 1998 routine	All / MACOPB/VACOPB (47)[a] / CHOP/CHOP-like (63) / CHOPR (18)	69	75 / 87 / 71 / 82 $p = 0.048$	Type of treatment not significant in MVA ($p = 0.09$) / Addition of radiation did not improve PFS or OS / PMBCL had more favorable PFS and OS compared to DLBCL
Hamlin[46]	141	No (23%)	All / CHOP/CHOP-like (intensive)[b] / NHL-15 / ASCT	50 / 34 / 60 $p < 0.001$ / 60	66 / 51 / 84 $p < 0.001$ / 78	Type of chemo (NHL-15/ASCT vs CHOP/CHOP-like) improved EFS/OS in MVA / Minority of patients treated with CHOP/CHOP-like and NHL-15 received RT
Todeschini[45]	138	Yes / Yes (If CR or CRu)	CHOP (43) / MACOPB/VACOPB (95)	39.5 / 76 / $p < 0.001$		Type of chemo (MACOPB/VACOPB) improved OS in MVA / RT improved EFS in pts in CR
Zinzani[44]	426	Yes (80%)	All / CHOP (105) / MACOPB (204) /VACOPB (34) or ProMACE CytaBOM (39) / High-dose sequential (27) or ASCT (17)	62 (10 y) / 35 / 67 / 78 $p = 0$	65 (10 y) / 44 / 71 / 77 $p = 0$	Type of chemotherapy (intensive vs CHOP) improved OS but not PFS in MVA
Nguyen[55]	40	Yes (85%)	CHOP(12)[c] / CHOP-like (intensified) (13) / Doxorubicin/salvage-type (14)	67 (5 y)	72 (5 y)	
Bieri[53]	27	No (41%)	CHOP (11)[d] / CHOP-like (intensified) (12) / CVP (4 elderly)	44 (5 y)	55 (5 y)	Type of chemotherapy ('Intensive' vs CHOP) improved PFS in MVA / RT improved PFS in MVA but no RT group may also include induction failures
Zinzani[52]	50	Yes (94%)	MACOPB	82 (8 y)	93 (8 y)	
Abou Ellela[56]	43	Not reported	CHOP-like regimens[e]	38 (5 y)	46 (5 y)	Similar outcome vs 'non-mediastinal' / Heterogeneous treatment – some with non-anthracycline regimens
Martelli[57]	37	Yes (89%) / No	MACOPB / F-MACHOP	91 (2 y) / 60 (2 y) / $p < 0.02$	93 / 70 / $p = $ ns	
Lazzarino[49]	106	Yes (77%)	CHOP (36) / MACOPB/VACOPB (29) / CHOP-like intensive (41)[f]	N/A	52 (3 y)	No difference in relapse rate whether patients received RT or not

(Continued)

Table 18.2 (Continued)

Reference	No. of Patients	Mediastinal radiation	Chemotherapy regimen (n)	PFS/EFS (%)	OS (%)	Comment
Cazals-Hatem[6]	141	No	Intensive regimens[g] Group 1 (14) Group 2 (104) Group 3 (23) Treatments were not compared	61 (2 y) – 59 58	66 100 60 69	Similar outcome vs 'non-mediastinal' DLBCL Only 1 patient received RT Treatment regimens were not formally compared
Zinzani[54]	22	Yes (100%)	MACOPB F-MACHOP	86 (2 y)		

PFS, progression-free survival; EFS, event-free survival; OS, overall survival; MVA multicheriate analysis; RT radiotherapy

[a] Three treatment groups[47]
1. CHOP or CHOP-like (ACOP12, ECV (CHOP ×4 then high-dose etoposide, cyclophosphamide, vincristine))
2. MACOPB/VACOPB
3. CHOPR

[b] Three treatment groups[46]
1. Includes CHOP and CHOP-like (CHOP-bleomycin, ProMACE-CytaBom, MACOPB). Only 10 patients received radiotherapy
2. NHL-15 – dose-dense sequential chemotherapy with GCSF support. Only 5 patients received radiotherapy
3. TBI and upfront transplant – this patient group were from a trial comparing ASCT to MACOPB for patients with bulky disease or LDH > 2.5 times ULN – All received TBI and a boost to site of initial bulk

[c] Three treatment groups[55]
1. CHOP
2. CHOP-like intensive (CHOP-Bleo; CHOP-Bleo/OPEN (vincristine, prednisone, etoposide, mitroxantrone))
3. ASHAP (doxorubicin, methylprednisone, AraC, cisplatin)/MBACOS (methotrexate, bleomycin, doxorubicin, cyclophosphamide, vincristine, methylprednisolone) and MINE (Mesna, ifosfamide, mitroxantrone, etoposide)

[d] Three treatment groups[53]
1. CHOP
2. Third generation CHOP-like intensive (doxorubicin D1/8, cyclophosphamide D1/D8, vincristine D1/D8, methotrexate alternating q 22 days with etoposide, AraC, bleomycin, procarbazine
3. CVP (elderly)

[e] Four treatment groups[56]
1. Cyclophosphamide, doxorubicin, vincristine, procarbazine, prednisone, bleomycin
2. Cyclophosphamide, doxorubicin, vincristine, procarbazine, dexamethasone, bleomycin
3. Cyclophosphamide, mitoxantrone, vincristine, procarbazine, prednisone
4. Cyclophosphamide, mitoxantrone, vincristine, prednisone

[f] Three treatment groups[49]
1. CHOP
2. MACOPB or VACOPB
3. CHOP-like intensive (CH2OP(11) (doxorubicin repeated day 2); CHOEP(10); hCHOP(high-dose cyclophosphamide)/IVEP (ifosfamide, vindesine, etoposide, prednisone) or CHOP/VIM (etoposide, ifosfamide, methotrexate, prednisone) (13)

[g] Three treatment groups[6]
No poor prognostic factors and <70
1. ACVBP vs mBACOD
   Adverse prognostic factors and <55 years old
2. ACVBP vs NCVBP (N = mitoxatrone) – patients achieving CR randomized condolidation chemotherapy
   LNH-84 vs intensive consolidation with CBV + autologous stem cell transplant
   Adverse prognostic factors and >55 years old
   Adverse prognostic factor = Bulky disease ≥10 cm, bone marrow or CNS involvement, 2 extranodal sites, PS ≥ 2
3. LNH-84 vs VIM3

imprecision, since they rely solely on typical clinicopathological features, with no single biological marker to reliably identify PMBCL. A distinct molecular signature does differentiate PMBCL from DLBCL, as described above;[2,3] however, application in routine practice remains difficult and the newer markers described above are also not uniformly applied. As a result of this diagnostic uncertainty, some reports have probably included cases of DLBCL with secondary mediastinal involvement, complicating study comparison. This discrepancy is highlighted in earlier studies where a more aggressive course was observed,[49,51] with cure rates comparable to DLBCL despite the younger of age of presentation. In contrast, more recent analyses have demonstrated outcome patterns at least equivalent or superior to DLBCL[6,44,45,47,52] (see Table 18.2 and Figures 18.3a and 18.3b). Furthermore, using a refined molecular definition of PMBCL through gene expression profiling, a more favorable survival is seen,[3] suggesting that it does have a natural history that is different from DLBCL. This is further highlighted by the clear plateau seen in the progression-free survival curve of PMBCL, with rare relapses (other than CNS) seen

beyond 2 years[47] (see Figure 18.3a). This is in distinct comparison to DLBCL, where the rate of late relapse is estimated at approximately 2% per year, a proportion of which represent low-grade follicular lymphoma (see Figure 18.1b).

The optimal type of chemotherapy and role of consolidative radiotherapy in the management of PMBCL is unknown. Treatments at various study centers have been extremely heterogeneous with respect to the choice of chemotherapy regimen and whether radiotherapy was utilized in the primary therapy (see Table 18.2). In several retrospective analyses, there is emerging evidence that dose-intensified therapy such as MACOPB (methotrexate, Adriamycin [doxorubicin], cyclophosphamide, vincristine, prednisone, bleomycin) or (etoposide, Adriamycin [doxorubicin], cyclophosphamide, vincristine, prednisone, bleomycin) VACOPB may be superior to CHOP (cyclophosphamide, doxorubicin, vincristine, prednisone) chemotherapy[44,45] (see Table 18.2). In retrospective or phase II studies, the reported overall survival is lower with CHOP (40–71%) than for MACOPB/VACOPB (71–93%) (see Table 18.2). Since the large prospective Southwest Oncology Group (SWOG) study comparing CHOP to second- and third-generation regimens (including

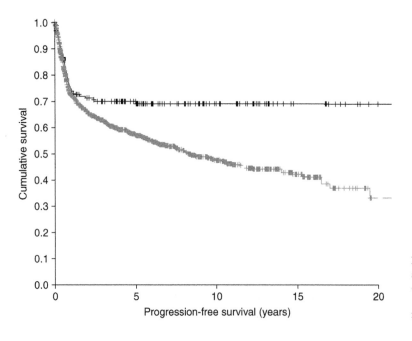

Figure 18.3a Progression-free survival of PMBCL (black) compared with DLBCL (gray). (Adapted with permission from Savage et al.[47])

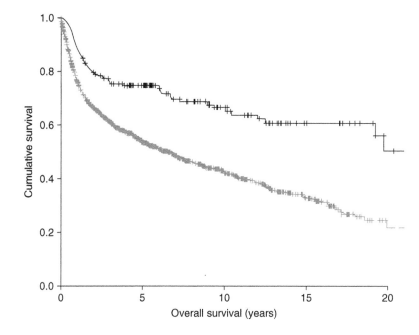

Figure 18.3b Overall survival of PMBCL (black) compared with DLBCL (gray). (Adapted with permission from Savage et al.[47])

MACOPB) in the treatment of aggressive non-Hodgkin's lymphoma was performed prior to the recognition of PMBCL as a separate clinical entity, it is unknown whether these intensive regimens are superior to CHOP in a randomized trial.[58] The Memorial-Sloan-Kettering recently reported a retrospective series comparing 'CHOP-like' chemotherapy, which included second- and third-generation regimens, to an even more intensified regimen, NHL-15 (dose-dense sequential induction with doxorubicin followed by cyclophosphamide with GCSF support) (see Table 18.2) and found that NHL-15 was associated with a more favorable outcome in multivariate analysis (see Table 18.2).[46] Interestingly, a comparison of CHOP with second- and third-generation regimens demonstrated similar clinical outcomes. However, the number of patients receiving specific regimens was too small for individual comparisons. In addition, there may be an inherent selection bias of patients chosen to be treated with more intensive regimens such as NHL-15.

Some researchers support using autologous stem cell transplant (ASCT) in the primary treatment of PMBCL, with one small report of 15 patients with high-intermediate or high-risk disease achieving a disease-free survival (DFS) of 93% after a median follow-up of 35 months with transplant.[59] However, all but 2 patients were in a complete response (CR) or a partial response (PR) prior to transplant, with induction therapy consisting of VACOPB, and due to the high frequency of residual masses in this disease, many of the PR patients by imaging may be in a pathological CR; thus, the true impact of consolidative ASCT is unknown.

Further complicating the evaluation of the effectiveness of dose-dense and dose-intensive regimens is that these studies were undertaken in the 'pre-rituximab' era. The addition of rituximab to CHOP chemotherapy has been shown in multiple studies to improve cure rates in DLBCL over CHOP alone.[60–62] The value of adding rituximab to CHOP (R-CHOP) in PMBCL is unknown; however, it is likely that the same magnitude of benefit seen in DLBCL will be observed, and this may negate any benefit of dose intensity. This effect has already been reported in comparisons of CHOP with CHOEP (cyclophosphamide, doxorubicin, etoposide, vincristine, prednisone) in young good-prognosis aggressive lymphoma patients, the majority of which were DLBCL (NHL-B1).[62] In this pre-rituximab treatment era, patients treated with CHOEP had an improved event-free survival (EFS) over CHOP alone. However, with the addition of rituximab, this benefit was no longer apparent, suggesting that rituximab may be the 'equalizer' of treatment regimens.[63] The utility of more intensive chemotherapy regimens in the treatment of PMBCL can only be evaluated in a well-designed randomized clinical trial that includes the addition of rituximab to each treatment arm. Until such studies are available, it is reasonable to consider R-CHOP as the standard treatment in PMBCL, akin to the current practice in DLBCL.

Consolidative radiotherapy in the treatment of PMBCL

A major challenge in the management of PMBCL is the evaluation of a residual mass following chemotherapy, and whether it represents active lymphoma. There is poor correlation between the size of a residual mass on CT and the risk of relapse.[64,65] In many instances, the residual density represents fibrotic tissue rather than active lymphoma, similar to the problem encountered in bulky mediastinal NScHL.[64] Consolidative mediastinal radiotherapy is often delivered; however, it is unclear whether this impacts on relapse or cure rates. There is an inherent concern of long-term toxicities of mediastinal radiotherapy, including increased risk of cardiovascular disease and secondary malignancies, particularly given the young population at risk,[66] similar to treatment considerations in NScHL. Although some studies have supported that radiotherapy improves EFS[44,45,53] (see Table 18.1), other analyses have demonstrated that chemotherapy alone is effective in many cases,[6,46,47,67] suggesting that radiotherapy is not mandatory in all patients. A recent analysis evaluating the impact on progression-free survival, with a policy recommending routine radiotherapy following primary chemotherapy, failed to demonstrate a benefit.[47] The retrospective nature of such analyses, including definitions of response rates, is problematic, and randomized studies addressing this question are lacking. Improved identification of patients who may benefit from the addition of radiotherapy is needed.

Gallium (^{67}Ga) scintigraphy has been used to detect persistent viable tumor in patients with a residual mass after therapy.[64] [^{18}F]-FDG (fluorodeoxyglucose) PET is superior to ^{67}Ga for the detection of residual disease.[68] Numerous studies have confirmed the value of PET scanning for response assessment in DLBCL at the conclusion of front-line therapy. A meta-analysis performed recently reports a pooled sensitivity of 72% and specificity of 100%, the former reflecting the limitations of PET in the detection of minimal residual disease.[69] In comparison, the sensitivity and specificity in Hodgkin's lymphoma is 84% and 90%, respectively; thus, false-positive results are more common. However, there is no literature available on the sensitivity and specificity of PET scanning in patients with bulky disease, or specifically in PMBCL.

Future studies are needed that evaluate the utility of [^{18}F]-FDG PET to select patients with PMBCL who may benefit from consolidative radiotherapy and, alternatively, identify those cases where it can be safely withheld without compromising cure rates, with the goal of reducing secondary long-term complications.

Salvage therapy

Treatment failures in PMBCL tend to occur within the first 6–12 months after therapy completion, with recurrences uncommon beyond 2 years.[44,47] Typically, such patients are given a salvage regimen and, if chemosensitivity is demonstrated, high-dose chemotherapy (HDC) and ASCT is performed. One difficulty in interpreting the literature of outcomes in relapsed/refractory PMBCL is that the majority of studies report only on those patients who are able to receive transplant as opposed to those in whom transplant is intended but who fail to respond to salvage chemotherapy. Limited data suggest that PMBCL patients may be less likely than DLBCL patients to respond to salvage chemotherapy and proceed to ASCT; however, in those patients who can be transplanted, outcomes appear to be similar[70] or superior.[71] There is little information regarding the utility of transplant of patients with refractory PMBCL.

One study in refractory patients suggested that survival was superior to relapsed patients;[61] however, other studies have found that they may less frequently respond to salvage chemotherapy,[47,49] with a lower likelihood of survival compared to patients with relapsed disease.[46] In summary, HDC and ASCT should be offered to patients with relapsed or refractory PMBCL, if chemosensitivity is demonstrated to a salvage regimen, similar to the practice in DLBCL.

REFERENCES

1. Jaffe ES, Harris NL, Stein H, Vardiman J, eds. World Health Organization Classification of Tumours. Pathology and Genetics of Tumors of Haematopoietic and Lymphoid Ttissues. Lyon: IARC Press, 2001.
2. Savage KJ, Monti S, Kutok JL, et al. The molecular signature of mediastinal large B-cell lymphoma differs from that of other diffuse large B-cell lymphomas and shares features with Hodgkin lymphoma. Blood 2003; 102: 3871–9.
3. Rosenwald A, Wright G, Leroy K, et al. Molecular diagnosis of primary mediastinal B cell lymphoma identifies a clinically favorable subgroup of diffuse large B cell lymphoma related to Hodgkin lymphoma. J Exp Med 2003; 198(6): 851–62.
4. Banks PM, Warnke RA. Mediastinal (thymic) large B-cell lymphoma. In: Jaffe ES, Harris NL, Stein H, Vardiman JW, eds. World Health Organization Classification of Tumors: Pathology and Genetics of Tumors of Hematopoetic and Lymphoid Tissues. Lyon: IARC Press, 2001: 175–8.
5. Barth T, Leithäuser F, Joos S, Benz M, Möller P. Mediastinal (thymic) large B-cell lymphoma: where do we stand? Lancet Oncol 2002; 3: 229–34.
6. Cazals-Hatem D, Lepage E, Brice P, et al. Primary mediastinal large B-cell lymphoma: a clinicopathologic study of 141 cases compared with 916 non-mediastinal large B-cell lymphomas – A GELA ("Groupe d'Etude des Lymphomes de l'Adulte") study. Am J Surg Pathol 1996; 20: 877–88.
7. Paulli M, Strater J, Gianelli U, et al. Mediastinal B-cell lymphoma: a study of its histomorphologic spectrum based on 109 cases. Hum Pathol 1999; 30: 178–87.
8. Pileri SA, Gaidano G, Zinzani PL, et al. On behalf of the International Extranodal Lymphoma Study Group (IELSG). Primary mediastinal B-cell lymphoma (PMBL): high frequency of BCL-6 mutations and consistent expression of the transcription factors oct-2, BOB.1 and PU-1 in the absence of immunoglobulins. Am J Pathol 2003; 162: 243–53.
9. Kanavaros P, Gaulard P, Charlotte F, et al. Discordant expression of immunoglobulin and its associated molecule mb-1/CD79a is frequently found in mediastinal large B cell lymphomas. Am J Pathol 1995; 146: 735–41.
10. Ritz O, Leithäuser F, Hasel C, et al. Downregulation of internal enhancer activity contributes to abnormally low immunoglobulin expression in the MedB-1 mediastinal B-cell lymphoma cell line. J Pathol 2005; 205: 336–48.
11. Loddenkemper C, Anagnostopoulos I, Hummel M, et al. Differential Emu enhancer activity and expression of BOB.1/OBF.1, Oct2, PU.1, and immunoglobulin in reactive B-cell populations, B-cell non-Hodgkin lymphomas, and Hodgkin lymphomas. J Pathol 2004; 202: 60–9.
12. de Leval L, Ferry JA, Falini B, Shipp M, Harris NL. Expression of bcl-6 and CD10 in primary mediastinal large B-cell lymphoma: evidence for derivation from germinal center B cells? Am J Surg Pathol 2001; 25: 1277–82.
13. Calaminici M, Piper K, Lee AM, Norton A. CD23 expression in mediastinal large B-cell lymphoma. Histopathology 2004; 45: 619–24.
14. Copie-Bergman C, Gaulard P, Maouche-Chrétien L, et al. The MAL gene is expressed in primary mediastinal large B-cell lymphoma. Blood 1999; 94: 3567–75.
15. Copie-Bergman C, Plonquet A, Alonso M, et al. MAL expression in lymphoid cells: further evidence for MAL as a distinct molecular marker of primary mediastinal large B-cell lymphomas. Mod Pathol 2002; 15: 1172–80.
16. Higgins JP, Warnke RA. CD30 expression is common in mediastinal large B-cell lymphoma. Am J Clin Pathol 1999; 112: 241–7.
17. Möller P, Moldenhauer G, Momburg F, et al. Mediastinal lymphoma of clear cell type is a tumor corresponding to terminal steps of B cell differentiation. Blood 1987; 69: 1087–95.
18. Momburg F, Herrmann B, Moldenaheru G, Möller P. B-cell lymphomas of high-grade malignancy frequently lack HLA-Dr, DP, and DQ antigens and the associated invariant chain. Int J Cancer 1997; 40: 598–601.
19. Isaacson PG, Norton AJ, Addis BJ. The human thymus contains a novel population of B lymphocytes. Lancet 1987; 2: 1488–91.
20. Moldenhauer G, Popov SW, Wotschke B, et al. AID expression identifies interfollicular large B cells as putative precursors of mature B-cell malignancies. Blood 2006; 107: 2470–3.
21. Traverse-Glehen A, Pittaluga S, Gaulard P, et al. Mediastinal gray zone lymphoma: the missing link between classic Hodgkin's lymphoma and mediastinal large B-cell lymphoma. Am J Surg Pathol 2005; 29: 1411–21.
22. Rodig SJ, Savage KJ, LaCasce AS, et al. Expression of TRAF1 and nuclear c-Rel distinguishes primary mediastinal large cell lymphoma from other types of diffuse large B-cell lymphoma. Am J Surg Pathol 2007; 31: 106–12.
23. Guiter C, Dusanter-Fourt I, Copie-Bergman C, et al. Constitutive STAT6 activation in primary mediastinal large B-cell lymphoma. Blood 2004; 104: 543–9.

24. Tsang P, Cesarman E, Chadburn A, Liu YF, Knowles DM. Molecular characterization of primary mediastinal B cell lymphoma. Am J Pathol 1996; 148: 2017–25.

25. Laithäuser F, Bäuerle M, Huynh MQ, Möller P. Isotype-switched immunoglobulin genes with a high load of somatic hypermutation and lack of ongoing mutational activity are prevalent in mediastinal B-cell lymphoma. Blood 2001; 98: 2762–70.

26. Popov SW, Moldenhauer G, Wotschke B, et al. Target sequence accessibility limits activation-induced cytidine deaminase activity in primary mediastinal B-cell lymphoma. Cancer Res 2007; 67: 6555–64.

27. Scarpa A, Moore PS, Rigaud G, et al. Molecular features of primary mediastinal B-cell lymphoma: involvement of p16^{INK4A}, p53 and c-myc. Br J Haematol 1999; 107: 106–13.

28. Joos S, Otano-Joos M, Ziegler S, et al. Primary mediatinal (thymic) B-cell lymphoma is characterized by gains of chromosomal material including 9p and amplification of the REL gene. Blood 1996; 87: 1571–8.

29. Bentz M, Barth TFE, Brüderlein S, et al. Gain of chromosome arm 9p is characteristic of primary mediastinal B-cell lymphoma (MBL): comprehensive molecular cytogenetic analysis and presentation of a novel MBL cell line. Genes Chromosomes Cancer 2001; 30: 393–401.

30. Wessendorf S, Barth TFE, Viardot A, et al. Further delineation of chromosomal consensus regions in primary mediastinal B-cell lymphomas – an analysis of 37 tumor samples using high resolution genomic profiling (array-CGH). Leukemia 2007; 21: 2463–9.

31. Kimm LR, deLeeuw RJ, Savage KJ, et al. Frequent occurrence of deletions in primary mediastinal B-cell lymphoma. Genes Chromosomes Cancer 2007; 46: 1090–7.

32. Weniger MA, Pulford K, Gesk S, et al. Gains of the proto-oncogene BCL11A and nuclear accumulation of BCL11AXL protein are frequent in primary mediastinal B-cell lymphoma. Leukemia 2006; 20: 1880–2.

33. Weniger MA, Gesk S, Ehrlich S, et al. Gains of REL in primary mediastinal B-cell lymphoma coincide with nuclear accumulation of Rel protein. Genes Chromosomes Cancer 2007; 46: 406–15.

34. Melzner I, Bucur AJ, Brüderlein S, et al. Biallelic mutation of SOCS-1 impairs JAK2 degradation and sustains phosphor-JAK2 action in MedB-1 mediastinal lymphoma line. Blood 2005; 105: 2535–42.

35. Melzner I, Weniger MA, Bucur AJ, et al. Biallelic deletion within 16p13.13 including SOCS-1 in Karpas1106P mediastinal B-cell lymphoma line is associated with delayed degradation of JAK2 protein. Int J Cancer 2006; 118: 1941–4.

36. Weniger MA, Melzner I, Menz CK, et al. Mutations of the tumor suppressor gene SOCS-1 in classical Hodgkin lymphoma are frequent and associated with nuclear phospho-STAT5 accumulation. Oncogene 2006; 25: 2679–84.

37. Savage KJ. Primary mediastinal large B-cell lymphoma. Oncologist 2006; 11: 488–95.

38. Hsi ED, Sup SJ, Alemany C, et al. MAL is expressed in a subset of Hodgkin lymphoma and identifies a population of patients with poor prognosis. Am J Clin Pathol 2006; 125: 776–82.

39. Maggio E, van den Berg A, Diepstra A, et al. Chemokines, cytokines and their receptors in Hodgkin's lymphoma cell lines and tissues. Ann Oncol 2002; 13(Suppl 1): 52–6.

40. Copie-Bergman C, Boulland ML, Dehoulle C, et al. Interleukin 4-induced gene 1 is activated in primary mediastinal large B-cell lymphoma. Blood 2003; 101: 2756–61.

41. Feuerhake F, Kutok JL, Monti S, et al. NFkappaB activity, function, and target-gene signatures in primary mediastinal large B-cell lymphoma and diffuse large B-cell lymphoma subtypes. Blood 2005; 106: 1392–9.

42. Skinnider BF, Elia AJ, Gascoyne RD, et al. Signal transducer and activator of transcription 6 is frequently activated in Hodgkin and Reed–Sternberg cells of Hodgkin lymphoma. Blood 2002; 99: 618–26.

43. Cheson BD, Pfistner B, Juweid ME, et al. Revised response criteria for malignant lymphoma. J Clin Oncol 2007; 25: 579–86.

44. Zinzani PL, Martelli M, Bertini M, et al. Induction chemotherapy strategies for primary mediastinal large B-cell lymphoma with sclerosis: a retrospective multinational study on 426 previously untreated patients. Haematologica 2002; 87: 1258–64.

45. Todeschini G, Secchi S, Morra E, et al. Primary mediastinal large B-cell lymphoma (PMLBCL): long-term results from a retrospective multicentre Italian experience in 138 patients treated with CHOP or MACOP-B/VACOP-B. Br J Cancer 2004; 90: 372–6.

46. Hamlin PA, Portlock CS, Straus DJ, et al. Primary mediastinal large B-cell lymphoma: optimal therapy and prognostic factor analysis in 141 consecutive patients treated at Memorial Sloan Kettering from 1980 to 1999. Br J Haematol 2005; 130: 691–9.

47. Savage KJ, Al-Rajhi N, Voss N, et al. Favorable outcome of primary mediastinal large B-cell lymphoma in a single institution: the British Columbia experience. Ann Oncol 2006; 17: 123–30.

48. van Besien K, Kelta M, Bahaguna P. Primary mediastinal B-cell lymphoma: a review of pathology and management. J Clin Oncol 2001; 19: 1855–64.

49. Lazzarino M, Orlandi E, Paulli M, et al. Treatment outcome and prognostic factors for primary mediastinal (thymic) B-cell lymphoma: a multicenter study of 106 patients. J Clin Oncol 1997; 15: 1646–53.

50. Roberts RA, Wright G, Rosenwald AR, et al. Loss of major histocompatibility class II gene and protein expression in primary mediastinal large B-cell lymphoma is highly coordinated and related to poor patient survival. Blood 2006; 108: 311–18.

51. Todeschini G, Ambrosetti A, Meneghini V, et al. Mediastinal large-B-cell lymphoma with sclerosis: a clinical study of 21 patients. J Clin Oncol 1990; 8: 804–8.

52. Zinzani PL, Martelli M, Magagnoli M, et al. Treatment and clinical management of primary mediastinal large B-cell lymphoma with sclerosis: MACOP-B regimen and mediastinal radiotherapy monitored by (67)Gallium scan in 50 patients. Blood 1999; 94: 3289–93.

53. Bieri S, Roggero E, Zucca E, et al. Primary mediastinal large B-cell lymphoma (PMLCL): the need for prospective controlled clinical trials. Leuk Lymphoma 1999; 35: 139–46.

54. Zinzani PL, Bendandi M, Frezza G, et al. Primary mediastinal B-cell lymphoma with sclerosis: clinical and therapeutic evaluation of 22 patients. Leuk Lymphoma 1996; 21: 311–16.

55. Nguyen LN, Ha CS, Hess M, et al. The outcome of combined-modality treatments for stage I and II primary large B-cell lymphoma of the mediastinum. Int J Radiat Oncol Biol Phys 2000; 47: 1281–5.

56. Abou-Elella AA, Weisenburger DD, Vose JM, et al. Primary mediastinal large B-cell lymphoma: a clinicopathologic study of 43 patients from the Nebraska Lymphoma Study Group. J Clin Oncol 1999; 17: 784–90.

57. Martelli MP, Martelli M, Pescarmona E, et al. MACOP-B and involved field radiation therapy is an effective therapy for primary mediastinal large B-cell lymphoma with sclerosis. Ann Oncol 1998; 9: 1027–9.

58. Fisher RI, Gaynor ER, Dahlberg S, et al. Comparison of a standard regimen (CHOP) with three intensive chemotherapy regimens for advanced non-Hodgkin's lymphoma. N Engl J Med 1993; 328: 1002–6.

59. Cairoli R, Grillo G, Tedeschi A, et al. Efficacy of an early intensification treatment integrating chemotherapy, autologous stem cell transplantation and radiotherapy for poor risk primary mediastinal large B cell lymphoma with sclerosis. Bone Marrow Transplant 2002; 29: 473–7.

60. Coiffier B, Lepage E, Briere J, et al. CHOP chemotherapy plus rituximab compared with CHOP alone in elderly patients with diffuse large-B-cell lymphoma. N Engl J Med 2002; 346: 235–42.

61. Sehn LH, Antin JH, Shulman LN, et al. Primary diffuse large B-cell lymphoma of the mediastinum: outcome following high-dose chemotherapy and autologous hematopoietic cell transplantation. Blood 1998; 91: 717–23.

62. Pfreundschuh M, Trumper L, Kloess M, et al. Two-weekly or 3-weekly CHOP chemotherapy with or without etoposide for the treatment of young patients with good-prognosis (normal LDH) aggressive

lymphomas: results of the NHL-B1 trial of the DSHNHL. Blood 2004; 104: 626–33.

63. Pfreundschuh M, Ho A, Wolf E, et al. Treatment results of CHOP-21, CHOEP-21, MACOP-B and PMITCEBO with and without rituximab in young good-prognosis patients with aggressive lymphomas: rituximab as an 'equalizer' in the MInT (MABTHERA International Trial Group) study. J Clin Oncol 2005; 23(Suppl): 567s (abstract 6529).

64. Canellos GP. Residual mass in lymphoma may not be residual disease. J Clin Oncol 1988; 6: 931–3.

65. Jerusalem G, Beguin Y, Fassotte MF, et al. Whole-body positron emission tomography using 18F-fluorodeoxyglucose for posttreatment evaluation in Hodgkin's disease and non-Hodgkin's lymphoma has higher diagnostic and prognostic value than classical computed tomography scan imaging. Blood 1999; 94: 429–33.

66. Aleman BM, van den Belt-Dusebout AW, Klokman WJ, et al. Long-term cause-specific mortality of patients treated for Hodgkin's disease. J Clin Oncol 2003; 21: 3431–9.

67. Dunleavy K, Pittaluga S, Janik J, et al. Primary mediastinal large B-cell lymphoma (PMBL) outcome is signficantly improved by the addition of rituximab to dose adjusted (DA)-EPOCH and overcomes the need for radiation. Blood 2005; 106(11): 929a.

68. Kostakoglu L, Goldsmith SJ. Fluorine-18 fluorodeoxyglucose positron emission tomography in the staging and follow-up of lymphoma: is it time to shift gears? Eur J Nucl Med 2000; 27: 1564–78.

69. Zijlstra JM, Lindauer-van der Werf G, Hoekstra OS, et al. 18F-fluoro-deoxyglucose positron emission tomography for post-treatment evaluation of malignant lymphoma: a systematic review. Haematologica 2006; 91: 522–9.

70. Kuruvilla J, Nagy T, Pintilie M, Keating A, Crump M. Outcomes of salvage chemotherapy and autologous stem cell transplantation for relapsed or refractory primary mediastinal large B-cell lymphoma (PMLCL) are inferior to diffuse large B-cell lymphoma. Blood 2005; 106(11): 2085a.

71. Popat U, Przepiork D, Champlin R, et al. High-dose chemotherapy for relapsed and refractory diffuse large B-cell lymphoma: mediastinal localization predicts for a favorable outcome. J Clin Oncol 1998; 16: 63–9.

72. Paulli M, Sträter J, Gianelli U, et al. Mediastinal B-cell lymphoma: a study of its histomorphologic spectrum based on 109 cases. Hum Pathol 1999; 30(2): 178–87.

MALT-type lymphoma of the orbit and ocular adnexae

19

Andrés JM Ferreri, John Radford, Claudio Doglioni, and Maurilio Ponzoni

INCIDENCE AND EPIDEMIOLOGY

Non-Hodgkin's lymphomas constitute one-half of all orbital malignancies.[1] Five to 15% of all extranodal lymphomas arise in the ocular adnexae (conjunctiva, lachrymal gland, orbital fat, eyelid, and lachrymal sac).[2] Marginal zone B-cell lymphoma of mucosa-associated lymphoid tissue (MALT) is the most common lymphoma category arising in these anatomical structures (Ocular Adnexal MALT Lymphoma; OAML).[3] The rapidly increasing incidence of OAML is not correlated to changes in classification schemes, since a comparable increase has not been observed at other extranodal sites associated with a similar incidence of MALT lymphoma,[4] and calls for further studies to identify environmental and genetic risk factors, including the potential role of infectious agents.[4] The recently reported association between chlamydial infection and OAML[5] offers new pathogenic insights that have led to the development of innovative antimicrobial therapies.

ETIOLOGY AND BIOLOGICAL FEATURES

Molecular features and cytogenetics

As for other MALT lymphomas, polymerase chain reaction (PCR) analysis of immunoglobulin heavy-chain gene rearrangement shows a clonal B-cell population in 55% of OAML[3] and somatic hypermutations in two-thirds of these cases.[6] In particular, the V_H3 family is expressed in nearly half of cases, followed by V_H4 (23%), which shows a biased usage when compared to adult peripheral blood B lymphocytes.[6] The most frequently involved germline genes are DP-8, DP-10, DP-53, DP-63, DP-49, DP-54, and DP-47,[3,6] which are commonly implicated in the assembly of autoantibodies. Ongoing mutations have been described in OAML; their frequency is lower than that reported in gastrointestinal MALT lymphomas, but it is higher in cases with follicular dendritic cell networks, which supports a potential role of microenvironmental stimuli.[7] Taken together, these molecular features support the view that OAML represent a clonal expansion of postgerminal center memory B cells, where, in two-thirds of cases, antigen selection may have occurred.[6]

The overall frequency of MALT lymphoma-associated chromosomal translocations in OAML is low (Table 19.1). t(11;18)(q21;q21)/API2-MALT1, t(1;14)(p22;q32)/IgH-BCL10, and t(14;18)(q32;q21)/IgH-MALT1 are nearly exclusively found in MALT lymphomas and their oncogenic products share the ability to enhance the activation of nuclear factor kappa B (NF-κB).[17] t(3;14)(p14;q32)/IgH-FOXP1 has been detected in different types of B-cell lymphomas,[13,16] and the molecular mechanism of FOXP1-mediated lymphomagenesis remains to be investigated. The clinical significance of these chromosomal translocations in OAML remains to be investigated. In particular, as reported for gastric MALT lymphomas,[18] the potential correlation between these translocations and the response of OAML to antibiotic treatment[19] deserves to be investigated in future trials.

Table 19.1   Chromosomal abnormalities in OAML

Features	Genes involved	Organs	Frequency in OAML	References
t(11;18)(q21;q21)	API2, MALT1	Lung (40%) Stomach (25%)	0–10%	8–12
t(1;14)(p22;q32)	IgH, BCL10	Lung (9%) Stomach (4%)	0%	10, 11
t(14;18)(q32;q21)	IgH, MALT1	Skin (14%) Salivary gland (5%)	7–11%[a]	11, 12
t(3;14)(p14;q32)	IgH, FOXP1	Thyroid (50%) Skin (10%)	0%[b]	13
Trisomy 3	–		38–62%	8, 10 12, 14
Trisomy 18	–		14–47%	8, 10 12, 14

IgV_H = variable region of immunoglobulin heavy chain.

[a] t(14;18) was found in 3 out of 8 analyzed cases of OAML in the original study.[15]

[b] t(3;14) was originally reported in 4 out of 20 cases of OAML,[16] whereas more recent studies showed that this translocation is absent in OAML.

There are only limited cytogenetic data in OAML (see Table 19.1). Both conventional karyotyping and interphase fluorescent in-situ hybridization (FISH)-based cytogenetic analyses demonstrate that aneuploidy, particularly trisomy 3 and 18, occur frequently in OAML,[8,10,12,14] and their role as predictors of multifocal disease should be investigated.[20] OAML with trisomy 18 seems to have distinct clinical features: it involves the conjunctiva, in young females, and shows a higher recurrence rate.[12] Analysis of chromosomal imbalances in 10 cases of OAML using comparative genomic hybridization (CGH) showed recurrent chromosomal gains at 6p21 and 9q33-qter, in addition to trisomy 3, 12, and 18.[21] It will be interesting to survey the genomic gains and losses of OAML to determine whether these MALT lymphomas are also characterized by a conserved pattern of chromosomal gains, and how these genomic alterations correlate with causation and treatment response.

Pathogenesis

OAML shares several clinicopathological features with other MALT lymphomas. It arises in tissues normally devoid of innate immunoreactive cells,[22] often develops on a background of preexisting chronic inflammation (i.e. conjunctivitis),[7] and shows an indolent clinical course. The presence of a preexisting inflammatory background seems to be of pathogenic relevance for MALT lymphomas, underlying the possible role of infection and autoimmune conditions. Somatic immunoglobulin ongoing mutations detected in OAML are consistent with a process driven by chronic antigenic stimulation. Moreover, the biased usage of V_H genes, frequently rearranged in autoantibodies production[23] and often overrepresented in B-cell malignancies,[24] further supports the occurrence of an antigen selection process during OAML development. A pathogenic model of antigen-driven lymphoproliferation similar to that reported for *Helicobacter pylori* (*Hp*)-associated gastric MALT lymphoma may be applied to OAML. In line with this hypothesis, the DNA of *Chlamydia psittaci (Cp)*, an obligate intracellular pathogen, has been detected in 80% of OAML patients, and immunohistochemical data identified cells of the monocyte/macrophage system as likely carriers of the infection.[5]

Chlamydia are responsible for a wide spectrum of human diseases,[25] cause persistent infections,[26] inhibit apoptosis of infected cells, and have complex immunomodulatory effects that may play a role in tumorigenesis.[25,27] *Cp* is the etiological agent of psittacosis, a human infection caused by exposure to infected birds and household animals.[25] Half of OAML patients report close contact with household animals,[5] and *Chlamydia* are also etiologically linked to chronic follicular or 'inclusion' conjunctivitis.[28]

In OAML patients, *Cp* establishes a persistent systemic infection, as demonstrated by the detection of the bacterial DNA in PBMC (peripheral blood mononuclear cells) of patients with *Cp*-positive lymphoma,[5] which is favored by molecular mimicry, a phenomenon by which antigens derived from microorganisms are able to induce immune reactions, cross-reacting with host self-antigens.[29] The expression of antigenic motifs shared with the host allows the persistence of microbial pathogens, since the immune system is usually tolerant towards autoantigens. It remains to be defined whether, similarly to *Hp*,[30] *Chlamydia* may also provide antigens, like heat shock proteins,[31] which may act as 'molecular mimickers' capable of triggering both humoral and cell-mediated immune responses that at least partially cross-react against the human protein counterpart and other related self-antigens. This phenomenon may contribute to break local tolerance, leading to chronic stimulation by antigens that cannot be successfully eliminated by the host and that may ultimately favor the onset of OAML.[32,33]

The prevalence of *Cp* infection in OAML patients varies among the different series so far published (Table 19.2), and geographical variations have also been reported.[37] Available evidence seems to rule out the possible involvement of other infectious agents commonly associated with chronic eye diseases, such as *Chlamydia trachomatis*, herpes simplex virus 1 and 2, and adenovirus 8 and 19,[5,37] whereas *Chlamydia pneumoniae* DNA was detected sporadically in a few cases of OAML[45] (R Dolcetti, unpublished results). Hepatitis C virus (HCV) seropositivity has been detected in 13–36% of OAML patients.[46,47] Although the role of HCV in the development of OAML

remains to be elucidated, this infection seems to be associated with more disseminated and aggressive lymphoma.[46]

The study of putative mechanism(s) regulating lymphocytes homing to the ocular adnexa constitutes an interesting issue in the genesis of these neoplasms. Data are preliminary and involve the absence of expression of the $\alpha_4\beta_7$ integrin, a crucial regulator of lymphocyte trafficking, and its ligand, mucosal addressin cell adhesion molecule 1 (MAdCAM-1),[48] and the expression of the chemoattractant cytokine CXCL13 on neoplastic lymphocytes.[49]

PATHOLOGY

Every non-Hodgkin's lymphoma subtype can arise in the ocular adnexae (Table 19.3), and surgical biopsy for histopathological diagnosis is mandatory. MALT-type lymphoma is the most common category arising at this site, varying from 50–78% of all ocular adnexal lymphomas in Western countries to 80–90% in Japan and Korea.[3] The orbital region lacks both resident lymphoid tissue and lymphatic drainage, and it is controversial whether MALT is present in normal human conjunctiva.[6] MALT lymphomas arising in these sites may therefore derive from MALT acquired following chronic inflamma-tory or autoimmune disorders.[22] Many ocular adnexal neoplasms previously classified as 'pseudolymphomas' or 'benign lymphoid hyperplasia' may actually contain clonal B-cell expansions[50] and are, presumably, B-cell lymphomas. In different studies, a variable number of cases were diagnosed as 'lymphoma, not otherwise specified', mostly because of the scarcity of diagnostic tissue; the majority of the entities hereby described, however, fall into the 'low-grade lymphoma' category.

OAML displays the well-described histopathology of most MALT lymphomas, comprising a triad of features: neoplastic cells (i.e. centrocytic-like, monocytoid, or small lymphocytes), reactive germinal centers, and epithelium. With respect to other MALT lymphomas, peculiar features for OAML include a frequent absence of epithelium,[51] presence of Dutcher bodies (22% of cases), rarity of follicular colonization,[7] and a

Table 19.2   Prevalence of *Chlamydia psittaci* infection in OAML

Geographical area	No.	Cp+	% Cp+ (95% CI)[a]	Reference
Austria	2	2	100 (16–100)[a]	34
Cuba	19	2	10 (1–33)	35
France	6	0	0 (0–46)[a]	36
Germany	19	9	47 (24–71)	37
Hungary	2	1	50 (22–61)	19
Italy	24	21	87 (68–97)	5
Italy	15	2	13 (2–40)	37
Japan	18	0	0 (0–19)[a]	38
Japan	12	0	0 (0–26)[a]	39
South Korea	30	23	77 (58–90)	40
Southern China	37	4	11 (3–25)	37
The Netherlands	19	0	0 (0–18)[a]	41
The Netherlands	21	6	29 (11–52)	37
United Kingdom	33	4	12 (3–28)	37
USA, East Coast	17	6	35 (14–62)	37
USA, Florida	46	0	0 (0–8)[a]	42
USA, North-East	7	0	0 (0–41)[a]	43

No., number of analyzed patients; *Cp+*, number of *C. psittaci*-positive cases; % *Cp+*, percentage of *C. psittaci*-positive cases.

[a] Binomial exact 95% confidence intervals (95% CI) were calculated; the one-sided, 97.5% CI is given when the percent of positive cases is either 0 or 100.

Modified from Zucca and Bertoni.[44]

Table 19.3   Prevalence of different lymphoma histotypes arising in the ocular adnexae

Histotype	Percentage
Marginal zone B-cell lymphoma	52–64
Follicular lymphomas	10–23
Diffuse large B-cell lymphoma	8–17
Mantle cell lymphoma	4–7
Plasmacytoma	5–6
Chronic lymphocytic leukemia	2–4
Lymphoma, not otherwise specified	1–5
Lymphoplasmacytic lymphoma	1–2

Rare forms:
  Lymphoblastic lymphoma
  Peripheral T-cell lymphomas
  Extranodal NK/T-cell lymphomas
  Hodgkin's lymphoma
	<1

more pronounced degree of plasmacellular differentiation (40% of cases).[52]

OAML displays the classical immunophenotype of MALT lymphoma (CD20+, CD79a+, usually IgM+ with light-chain restriction, PAX5+, bcl-2+, TCL1+, CD11c+/−, CD43+/−, CD21+/−, CD35+/−, and IgD−, CD3−, CD5−, CD10−, CD23−, cyclin D1−, bcl-6−, MUM1− cells). A few exceptions do occur, with 3–10% of cases CD5+.[51,53] Cases with plasmacellular differentiated tumor cells exhibit an aberrant immune profile for plasma cell-related antigens when compared with normal plasma cells,[52] a feature that may be useful in distinguishing from a reactive process.[52] The cell cycle-related molecule profile of OAML comprises p16+, p21−, pRB−, p53− immunophenotype;[53] in addition, these neoplasms display deregulation of apoptotic machinery.[54] Almost two-thirds of OAML exhibit strong immunohistochemical positivity for bcl-10 in both the nucleus and the cytoplasm.[55]

CLINICAL FEATURES

Clinical presentation

Lymphomas can infiltrate any orbital and ocular adnexal tissue, and the clinical picture depends on the structures involved (Table 19.4). Usually, there is a slowly growing, painless mass that displaces rather than infiltrates the normal structures, causing an eyelid lump, ptosis or proptosis, the latter eventually causing limitation of movement of the eye and diplopia. The classic presentation of conjunctival lymphoma is the fleshy 'salmon red patch' (Figure 19.1). Presenting symptoms in patients with intraorbital lymphoma are variable (see Table 19.4). In cases of rapidly growing tumors, visual acuity and field defects or choroidal folds can be observed, and a few cases of OAML infiltrating the eye with devastating consequences have been reported.

Neuroimaging

Neuroimaging techniques are fundamental for differential diagnosis, staging, and definition of therapeutic response (precise volumetric measurement) in patients with OAML. At neuroimaging examination, OAML usually present as well-defined lesions, mostly placed in the superior-lateral quadrant of the orbit, often surrounding and displacing extraocular muscles, without signs of ocular infiltration (Figure 19.2). On basal computed tomography (CT) images, OAML appears homogeneously iso- or slightly hyperdense compared to extraocular muscles. OAML contrast enhancement is homogeneous and its intensity is comparable to that of lachrymal glands and extraocular muscles. Magnetic resonance imaging (MRI) shows a great potential in differentiating OAML from other orbital expansive lesions. Location, margins, and the distinctive T2- and diffusion-weighted imaging (DWI) signal intensities allow OAML identification and

Table 19.4 Clinical features of OAML

Median age (range)	65 (29–87) years old
Males (%)	30%
ECOG-PS >1	0
Sites of disease:	
Conjunctiva involvement	25%
Involvement of lachrymal gland or orbit	75%
Bilateral orbit involvement	10–15%
Extraorbital disease:	
Regional lymphadenopathies	5%
Extranodal disease	10–15%
Symptoms and signs:	
'Salmon red patch' appearance	25%
Swollen conjunctiva	20%
Exophthalmos	27%
Palpable mass	19%
Eyelid ptosis	6%
Diplopia	2%
Eyelid nodule	2%
Visual acuity and field defects	<1%
Others: orbital edema, epiphora, impaired ocular motility	5%
Systemic symptoms	0%
Elevated LDH serum levels	0%
Median interval clinical onset–diagnosis (range)	6 (1–135) months
Autoimmune disorders	
Thyrotoxicosis	5%
Sjögren's syndrome	10%
Gastric *Helicobacter pylori* infection	35%
Hepatitis C virus infection	13%
Prolonged contact with household animals	45%
History of chronic conjunctivitis	42%

ECOG-PS, Eastern Cooperative Oncology Group performance status; LDH, lactate dehydrogenase.

characterization. Similarly to lymphomas at other sites, OAML presents high DWI signal and low apparent diffusion coefficient (ADC) values due to the high cellularity and high nucleus-to-cytoplasm ratio. Preliminary data suggest that the ADC of OAML is lower than that of all orbital

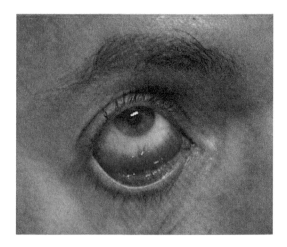

Figure 19.1 An example of classic presentation of conjunctival MALT lymphoma, with 'salmon red patch' appearance and swollen conjunctiva. (Kindly provided by Carlo De Conciliis, Ophthalmology Unit, Ospedale San Giuseppe, Milan, Italy).

normal structures and expansive lesions, and thus may be useful for differential diagnosis. Furthermore, DWI is helpful in establishing involvement or persistence of disease in the lachrymal gland, where both signal intensity and contrast enhancement do not allow unambiguous differentiation between normal and pathological tissue.

CLINICAL BEHAVIOR AND PROGNOSTIC FACTORS

OAML shows a better prognosis compared to other lymphoma subtypes arising in the ocular adnexae.[56,57] Most OAML patients display good prognostic indicators like limited disease, good performance status, and absence of systemic symptoms, and if adequately treated, these patients have a favorable outcome.[42,58] Some anecdotal cases of spontaneous tumor remission have been reported, mostly in Japanese patients with conjunctival MALT lymphoma,[59] but the incidence of this phenomenon remains to be defined. Presenting symptoms often demand immediate treatment. Local control rates vary according to the

therapy used, with an overall 5-year relapse-free survival of ~65%. Some patients experience multiple relapses, usually involving the contralateral orbit and distant extranodal organs. Systemic dissemination occurs in 5–10% of cases overall, but is rare in patients with conjunctival lymphoma. Less than 5% of OAML patients die of lymphoma, with a 5-year cause-specific survival of ~100%.[57,60]

Reliable prognostic factors remain to be defined. Nodal involvement (<5% of cases), systemic symptoms (1%), increased lactate dehydrogenase serum levels (1%), and non-conjunctival sites have been proposed as negative predictors of outcome.[42,60,61] Some of these parameters predict transformation to large cell lymphoma, which has been reported in 1–3% of cases.[58,62] Some histopathological and immunophenotypic parameters useful as predictors of outcome are summarized in Table 19.5.

STAGING PROCEDURES

More than 75% of OAML presents with a single lesion (stage I_E). With conventional lymphoma staging procedures, regional lymphadenopathies are detected in <5% of cases (stage II_E), and extraorbital disease, mostly in other extranodal organs, is observed in 10–15% of cases (stage IV), rarely in patients with conjunctival lymphoma.[5,42,56,57,60,61] Conversely, the use of more extensive and invasive staging showed that 38% of OAML patients have at least one concomitant, extraorbital site of disease at diagnosis.[20] The usefulness of extended staging in OAML remains a matter of debate. On the one hand, the definition of stage I disease is important because these patients are usually treated with radiotherapy alone. On the other hand, even if patients with stage I disease have significantly better relapse-free survival in comparison to those with advanced disease, no difference in cause-specific survival between these subgroups has been reported.[20,57] Our recommendation is that OAML patients should be assessed with conventional lymphoma staging procedures, but, in the absence of symptoms suggestive of gastrointestinal involvement, an extensive work-up is unnecessary.[20]

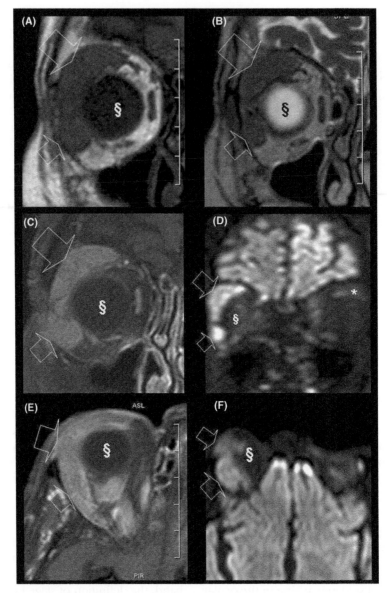

Figure 19.2   Magnetic resonance imaging (MRI) of OAML. Coronal basal T1-weighted (w) image (**A**), coronal T2-w (**B**), coronal and axial postgadolinium T1-w (**C–E**), coronal and axial diffusion-weighted imaging (DWI) image (**D–F**), obtained with a *b value* of 700 mm²/s. Coronal scans display only right orbit, whereas axial scans display both orbits. The OAML (arrows) is located in the superior-lateral quadrant of the right orbit and involves both intra- and extraconal structures. It surrounds the superior pole of the left ocular globe (§), the lateral rectus, and the superior extraocular muscles (EOM). The right lachrymal gland is infiltrated. On T1-w image (**A**), the OAML signal is comparable to that of EOM. On the T2-w image (**B**), OAML presents the same signal intensity of cerebral gray matter and is slightly hyperintense to EOM. Usually, T1 and T2 signal intensities within the lesion are homogeneous. OAML contrast enhancement is uniform and its conspicuity is comparable to that observed in lachrymal glands and EOM. Using parallel imaging technique it is now possible to obtain DWI images of the orbit with reasonable scan times and without the occurrence of significant susceptibility artifacts (**D–F**). DWI is an MRI-based technique that evaluates the rate of microscopic water diffusion in tissues and represents a useful technique for characterizing lymphomas of the central nervous system, the neck, and the orbits. On DWI images, OAML appears hyperintense compared to all other orbital structures. DWI is also helpful in establishing involvement of the lachrymal gland, where both signal intensity and contrast enhancement do not allow unambiguous differentiation between normal and pathological tissue. Please compare the DWI signal intensity of the affected right lachrymal gland and the normal left one (*).

Table 19.5 Histopathological parameters with proposed prognostic value

Parameters	Observation	References
MIB-1 rate >20%	Advanced stage and poor outcome	51, 53
Higher proliferation rate, overexpression of cyclin A, cyclin E, survivin, and bcl-XL	High-grade transformation	54
Increased blast cells, immunoreactivity for p53, bcl-6, pRB, MUM1, and MIB1	Poor prognosis	53
Increased bcl-6+ blast cells	High risk of local recurrence and disseminated disease	53
CD5 immunoreactivity	Stage >I	51
CD43 expression	Adverse prognosis	63
bcl-10 nuclear expression	Conflicting results	54, 55

TREATMENT AND OUTCOME

Current therapeutic knowledge in OAML results from a limited number of small, and variably treated, retrospective series, which included different lymphoma categories, diagnosed before the World Health Organization (WHO) classification era. Surgical resection, radiotherapy, and alkylating agent-based chemotherapy are the standard approaches for OAML patients, whereas bacteria-eradicating antibiotic therapy, anti-CD20 therapy, and intralesional interferon represent experimental strategies. Therapeutic decision making is usually driven by several variables related to the patient (age, performance status, comorbidity, concomitant infections useful as therapeutic targets), the lymphoma itself (stage, site of disease, symptoms, and histological and molecular features), and the risk of treatment-related toxicity. Efficacy and the kinetics of response are two important parameters for therapeutic choice, mostly in 'less indolent' lymphomas that could affect the ocular function.

Surgical resection

Surgical resection is a necessary diagnostic step and, in selected cases, a part of the therapeutic approach to OAML. Efforts to completely resect lymphomatous lesions should be avoided in OAML patients, considering that an aggressive approach could be associated with a high risk of complications, especially in the area of the lachrymal gland and in the deeper orbit, and the fact that the extent of surgical resection does not influence survival.[58] 'Watch and wait' strategies after surgical resection or biopsy in patients with stage I disease produce similar results to those reported with immediate radiotherapy, with a 10-year overall survival of 94%.[58] A watch and wait strategy could be safely proposed for elderly patients or patients with severe comorbidity and those with completely resected lesions and/or indolent and asymptomatic disease.

Radiotherapy

Radiotherapy is the most extensively studied treatment in OAML patients. However, only a few series have been focused on OAML treated exclusively with radiotherapy.[57,60,64,65] A universally accepted radiation schedule for OAML patients does not exist. Recently reported studies suggest an electron beam irradiation (4–12 MeV) of the entire conjunctiva in patients with conjunctival lymphomas and 4–9 mV photon beam irradiation of the entire orbit in intraorbital lymphomas, with a dose of 25–30 Gy in 10–15 fractions (minimal target dose >25 Gy).[60,64,65] A single anterior field or a wedge pair of anterior fields have been used in most series. Brachytherapy can provide local control in conjunctival lymphomas, but the risk of complications and marginal relapses is unacceptably high.[66]

Most irradiated patients with stage I OAML achieve a slow and gradual objective response.[60,64] In-field relapses are rare, and seem to be related to low radiation doses[65] or to the use of lens shielding.[60] The relapse rate at 4 years is 20–25%, with most involving the contralateral orbit (half of relapses) and distant extranodal organs.[57,64,65]

Radiotherapy is usually well tolerated.[60,64] The most common toxicities of grade ≥ 2 are cataract (38% of cases), retinal disorders (17%), xerophthalmia (17%), and glaucoma (2%)[64] and patients should be made aware of these before starting treatment. Toxicity is more common with doses >36 Gy.[64]

Chemotherapy

Only a small proportion of OAML patients in reported series have been treated with chemotherapy alone. The largest experience is with chlorambucil, which has been well-tolerated and associated with a 100% overall response rate (79% complete remission rate), and a 5-year relapse-free survival of 60% in patients with stage I OAML.[62] Relapses mostly involved extraorbital tissues, with rare cases (3%) of high-grade transformation.[62] Chlorambucil could be proposed, especially for OAML patients who experience relapse in previously irradiated areas, or with disseminated or bilateral disease and in the case of radiotherapy inaccessibility. The use of other drugs (fludarabine,[67] cladribine,[68] and oxaliplatin[69]) deserves more caution. These drugs have significant toxicity,[68] and evidence of their efficacy comes from a few prospective trials in unselected MALT lymphomas that have included a small number of OAML patients. The use of upfront anthracycline-based chemotherapy does not improve outcome in comparison with chlorambucil alone.[2]

Bacteria-eradicating therapy

A role for Hp in sustaining the growth also of non-gastric MALT lymphomas has been hypothesized. However, reported evidence shows that concomitant gastric Hp infection is irrelevant to the presentation and course of OAML, and that Hp-eradicating antibiotic therapy is inactive against these lymphomas.[70] Conversely, Cp eradication with doxycycline, a tetracycline derivative largely used in the treatment of psittacosis, appears to be effective.[71] In a multicenter phase II trial,[19] 11 patients with Cp-positive OAML and 16 with Cp-negative OAML have been treated with doxycycline and a 48% overall response rate (ORR) obtained (median follow-up = 14 months). Lymphoma regression was usually slow, and has been observed in both Cp-positive and Cp-negative patients (ORR = 64% vs 38%; $p = 0.25$), with a 2-year failure-free survival of 66%. This trial confirmed that doxycycline is a cheap, safe, and active therapy for Cp-positive OAML, and a valid alternative even in patients with multiple failures, involving previously irradiated areas or regional lymphadenopathies.[19] This latter feature is distinctive from gastric MALT lymphomas, where the detection of nodal disease is considered as a negative response predictor.[72]

Intriguingly, one-third of patients with $Chlamydia$-negative OAML experienced tumor regression after doxycycline treatment.[19,71] These observations could be due to methodological pitfalls, but could also be explained by the involvement of other doxycycline-responsive bacteria and, if so, suggest that doxycycline could be used in most OAML patients, independently of the diagnosis of Cp infection. However, smaller studies where OAML patients received doxycycline without a molecular assessment for chlamydial infection have led to conflicting results.[73,74] Antibiotic therapy therefore remains an experimental strategy that should be always preceded by chlamydial infection assessment, until wider experience becomes available.

Other therapies

As for other indolent lymphomas,[75] the efficacy of antiviral therapy with interferon and ribavirin in HCV-positive patients with OAML should be investigated. Even if active in MALT lymphomas,[76] rituximab has been only anecdotally used in OAML patients.[76–78] Preliminary data suggest that response duration is short in OAML and that relapse rate is clearly higher than those reported for gastric MALT lymphoma.[78] This drug could be used to obtain transient symptomatic benefit in OAML patients for whom other treatments are contraindicated.[77,78] Intralesional injection of interferon alpha is a relatively simple and quick procedure that has been successfully used for conjunctival lymphomas.[79,80] Side effects consist of local hemorrhage, chemosis, and minor systemic effects.[79,80] However, its efficacy remains to be defined, considering that follow-up of reported cases is short and that unsuccessfully treated patients may not have been reported.

ACKNOWLEDGMENTS

The authors are thankful to Riccardo Dolcetti (Immunovirology and Biotherapy Unit, Department of Pre-Clinical and Epidemiological Research, Centro di Riferimento Oncologico, Aviano, Italy), Ming-Qing Du (Division of Molecular Histopathology, Department of Pathology, University of Cambridge, Addenbrooke's Hospital, Cambridge, UK) and Letterio S Politi (Neuroradiology Unit, San Raffaele Scientific Institute, Milan, Italy) for their sustained scientific collaboration. We appreciate the helpful suggestions of Antonio Giordano Resti (Ophthalmology Unit, San Raffaele Scientific Institute, Milan, Italy), Carlo De Conciliis (Ophthalmology Unit, Ospedale San Giuseppe, Milan, Italy), and Francesco Bertoni (Oncology Institute of Southern Switzerland, Osp. San Giovanni, Bellinzona, Switzerland).

REFERENCES

1. Margo CE, Mulla ZD. Malignant tumors of the orbit. Analysis of the Florida Cancer Registry. Ophthalmology 1998; 105(1): 185–90.
2. Sasai K, Yamabe H, Dodo Y, et al. Non-Hodgkin's lymphoma of the ocular adnexa. Acta Oncol 2001; 40(4): 485–90.
3. Mannami T, Yoshino T, Oshima K, et al. Clinical, histopathological, and immunogenetic analysis of ocular adnexal lymphoproliferative disorders: characterization of malt lymphoma and reactive lymphoid hyperplasia. Mod Pathol 2001; 14(7): 641–9.
4. Moslehi R, Devesa SS, Schairer C, Fraumeni JF Jr. Rapidly increasing incidence of ocular non-Hodgkin lymphoma. J Natl Cancer Inst 2006; 98(13): 936–9.
5. Ferreri AJ, Guidoboni M, Ponzoni M, et al. Evidence for an association between Chlamydia psittaci and ocular adnexal lymphomas. J Natl Cancer Inst 2004; 96(8): 586–94.
6. Coupland SE, Foss HD, Anagnostopoulos I, Hummel M, Stein H. Immunoglobulin VH gene expression among extranodal marginal zone B-cell lymphomas of the ocular adnexa. Invest Ophthalmol Vis Sci 1999; 40(3): 555–62.
7. Hara Y, Nakamura N, Kuze T, et al. Immunoglobulin heavy chain gene analysis of ocular adnexal extranodal marginal zone B-cell lymphoma. Invest Ophthalmol Vis Sci 2001; 42(11): 2450–7.
8. Remstein ED, Kurtin PJ, James CD, et al. Mucosa-associated lymphoid tissue lymphomas with t(11;18)(q21;q21) and mucosa-associated lymphoid tissue lymphomas with aneuploidy develop along different pathogenetic pathways. Am J Pathol 2002; 161(1): 63–71.
9. Murga Penas EM, Hinz K, Roser K, et al. Translocations t(11;18)(q21;q21) and t(14;18)(q32;q21) are the main chromosomal abnormalities involving MLT/MALT1 in MALT lymphomas. Leukemia 2003; 17(11): 2225–9.
10. Streubel B, Simonitsch-Klupp I, Mullauer L, et al. Variable frequencies of MALT lymphoma-associated genetic aberrations in MALT lymphomas of different sites. Leukemia 2004; 18(10): 1722–6.
11. Ye H, Gong L, Liu H, et al. MALT lymphoma with t(14;18)(q32;q21)/IGH-MALT1 is characterized by strong cytoplasmic MALT1 and BCL10 expression. J Pathol 2005; 205(3): 293–301.
12. Tanimoto K, Sekiguchi N, Yokota Y, et al. Fluorescence in situ hybridization (FISH) analysis of primary ocular adnexal MALT lymphoma. BMC Cancer 2006; 6: 249.
13. Haralambieva E, Adam P, Ventura R, et al. Genetic rearrangement of FOXP1 is predominantly detected in a subset of diffuse large B-cell lymphomas with extranodal presentation. Leukemia 2006; 20(7): 1300–3.
14. Ott G, Katzenberger T, Greiner A, et al. The t(11;18)(q21;q21) chromosome translocation is a frequent and specific aberration in low-grade but not high-grade malignant non-Hodgkin's lymphomas of the mucosa-associated lymphoid tissue (MALT-) type. Cancer Res 1997; 57(18): 3944–8.
15. Streubel B, Lamprecht A, Dierlamm J, et al. T(14;18)(q32;q21) involving IGH and MALT1 is a frequent chromosomal aberration in MALT lymphoma. Blood 2003; 101(6): 2335–9.
16. Streubel B, Vinatzer U, Lamprecht A, Raderer M, Chott A. T(3;14)(p14.1;q32) involving IGH and FOXP1 is a novel recurrent chromosomal aberration in MALT lymphoma. Leukemia 2005; 19(4): 652–8.
17. Isaacson PG, Du MQ. MALT lymphoma: from morphology to molecules. Nat Rev Cancer 2004; 4(8): 644–53.
18. Liu H, Ye H, Ruskone-Fourmestraux A, et al. T(11;18) is a marker for all stage gastric MALT lymphomas that will not respond to H. pylori eradication. Gastroenterology 2002; 122(5): 1286–94.

19. Ferreri AJ, Ponzoni M, Guidoboni M, et al. Bacteria-eradicating therapy with doxycycline in ocular adnexal MALT lymphoma: a multicenter prospective trial. J Natl Cancer Inst 2006; 98(19): 1375–82.

20. Raderer M, Wohrer S, Streubel B, et al. Assessment of disease dissemination in gastric compared with extragastric mucosa-associated lymphoid tissue lymphoma using extensive staging: a single-center experience. J Clin Oncol 2006; 24(19): 3136–41.

21. Matteucci C, Galieni P, Leoncini L, et al. Typical genomic imbalances in primary MALT lymphoma of the orbit. J Pathol 2003; 200(5): 656–60.

22. Du MQ, Isaccson PG. Gastric MALT lymphoma: from aetiology to treatment. Lancet Oncol 2002; 3(2): 97–104.

23. Pascual V, Capra JD. VH4-21, a human VH gene segment overrepresented in the autoimmune repertoire. Arthritis Rheum 1992; 35(1): 11–18.

24. Bahler DW, Campbell MJ, Hart S, et al. Ig VH gene expression among human follicular lymphomas. Blood 1991; 78(6): 1561–8.

25. Byrne GI, Ojcius DM. Chlamydia and apoptosis: life and death decisions of an intracellular pathogen. Nat Rev Microbiol 2004; 2(10): 802–8.

26. Smith JS, Munoz N, Herrero R, et al. Evidence for Chlamydia trachomatis as a human papillomavirus cofactor in the etiology of invasive cervical cancer in Brazil and the Philippines. J Infect Dis 2002; 185(3): 324–31.

27. Miyairi I, Byrne GI. Chlamydia and programmed cell death. Curr Opin Microbiol 2006; 9(1): 102–8.

28. Yeung L, Tsao YP, Chen PY, et al. Combination of adult inclusion conjunctivitis and mucosa-associated lymphoid tissue (MALT) lymphoma in a young adult. Cornea 2004; 23(1): 71–5.

29. Oldstone MB. Molecular mimicry and immune-mediated diseases. FASEB J 1998; 12(13): 1255–65.

30. Negrini R, Savio A, Poiesi C, et al. Antigenic mimicry between Helicobacter pylori and gastric mucosa in the pathogenesis of body atrophic gastritis. Gastroenterology 1996; 111(3): 655–65.

31. Lamb DJ, El-Sankary W, Ferns GA. Molecular mimicry in atherosclerosis: a role for heat shock proteins in immunisation. Atherosclerosis 2003; 167(2): 177–85.

32. Ishii E, Yokota K, Sugiyama T, et al. Immunoglobulin G1 antibody response to Helicobacter pylori heat shock protein 60 is closely associated with low-grade gastric mucosa-associated lymphoid tissue lymphoma. Clin Diagn Lab Immunol 2001; 8(6): 1056–9.

33. Yamasaki R, Yokota K, Okada H, et al. Immune response in Helicobacter pylori-induced low-grade gastric-mucosa-associated lymphoid tissue (MALT) lymphoma. J Med Microbiol 2004; 53(Pt 1): 21–9.

34. Aigelsreiter A, Stelzl E, Deutsch A, et al. Association between Chlamydia psittaci infection and extranodal marginal zone B-cell lymphoma of mucosa associated lymphoid tissue (MALT)-lymphomas. Proc Annu Meet Am Soc Clin Oncol 2006; 24(18S): 7568.

35. Gracia E, Frosch L, Mazzucchelli L, et al. Low prevalence of Chlamydia psittaci in ocular adnexal lymphomas from Cuban patients. Leuk Lymphoma 2007; 48(1): 104–8.

36. De Cremoux P, Subtil A, Ferreri AJ, et al. Low prevalence of Chlamydia psittaci infection in French patients with ocular adnexal lymphomas. J Natl Cancer Inst 2006; 98(5): 365–6.

37. Chanudet E, Zhou Y, Bacon CM, et al. Chlamydia psittaci is variably associated with ocular adnexal MALT lymphoma in different geographical regions. J Pathol 2006; 209(3): 344–51.

38. Daibata M, Nemoto Y, Togitani K, et al. Absence of Chlamydia psittaci in ocular adnexal lymphoma from Japanese patients. Br J Haematol 2006; 132(5): 651–2.

39. Liu YC, Ohyashiki JH, Ito Y, et al. Chlamydia psittaci in ocular adnexal lymphoma: Japanese experience. Leuk Res 2006; 30(12): 1587–9.

40. You C, Ryu M, Huh J, et al. Ocular adnexal lymphoma is highly associated with Chlamydia psittaci. Cancer Res Treatment 2005; 37(4 (Suppl 2)).

41. Mulder MM, Heddema ER, Pannekoek Y, et al. No evidence for an association of ocular adnexal lymphoma with Chlamydia psittaci in a cohort of patients from the Netherlands. Leuk Res 2006; 30(10): 1305–7.

42. Rosado MF, Byrne JG, Ding F, et al. Ocular adnexal lymphoma: a clinicopathological study of a large cohort of patients with no evidence for an association with Chlamydia psittaci. Blood 2005; 107(2): 467–72.

43. Vargas RL, Fallone E, Felgar RE, et al. Is there an association between ocular adnexal lymphoma and infection with Chlamydia psittaci? The University of Rochester experience. Leuk Res 2006; 30(5): 547–51.

44. Zucca E, Bertoni F. Chlamydia or not Chlamydia, that is the question: which is the microorganism associated with MALT lymphomas of the ocular adnexa? J Natl Cancer Inst 2006; 98(19): 1348–9.

45. Shen D, Yuen HK, Galita DA, Chan NR, Chan CC. Detection of Chlamydia pneumoniae in a bilateral orbital mucosa-associated lymphoid tissue lymphoma. Am J Ophthalmol 2006; 141(6): 1162–3.

46. Ferreri AJ, Viale E, Guidoboni M, et al. Clinical implications of hepatitis C virus infection in MALT-type lymphoma of the ocular adnexa. Ann Oncol 2006; 17(5): 769–72.

47. Arcaini L, Burcheri S, Rossi A, et al. Prevalence of HCV infection in nongastric marginal zone B-cell lymphoma of MALT. Ann Oncol 2007; 18(2): 346–50.

48. Liu YX, Yoshino T, Ohara N, et al. Loss of expression of alpha4beta7 integrin and L-selectin is associated with high-grade progression of low-grade MALT lymphoma. Mod Pathol 2001; 14(8): 798–805.

49. Falkenhagen KM, Braziel RM, Fraunfelder FW, Smith JR. B-Cells in ocular adnexal lymphoproliferative lesions express B-cell attracting chemokine 1 (CXCL13). Am J Ophthalmol 2005; 140(2): 335–7.

50. Neri A, Jakobiec FA, Pelicci PG, Dalla-Favera R, Knowles DM. Immunoglobulin and T cell receptor beta chain gene rearrangement analysis of ocular adnexal lymphoid neoplasms: clinical and biologic implications. Blood 1987; 70(5): 1519–29.

51. Coupland SE, Krause L, Delecluse HJ, et al. Lymphoproliferative lesions of the ocular adnexa. Analysis of 112 cases. Ophthalmology 1998; 105(8): 1430–41.

52. Coupland SE, Damato B. Lymphomas involving the eye and the ocular adnexa. Curr Opin Ophthalmol 2006; 17(6): 523–31.

53. Coupland SE, Hellmich M, Auw-Haedrich C, Lee WR, Stein H. Prognostic value of cell-cycle markers in ocular adnexal lymphoma: an assessment of 230 cases. Graefes Arch Clin Exp Ophthalmol 2004; 242(2): 130–45.

54. Franco R, Camacho FI, Caleo A, et al. Nuclear bcl10 expression characterizes a group of ocular adnexa MALT lymphomas with shorter failure-free survival. Mod Pathol 2006; 19(8): 1055–67.

55. Adachi A, Tamaru JI, Kaneko K, et al. No evidence of a correlation between BCL10 expression and API2-MALT1 gene rearrangement in ocular adnexal MALT lymphoma. Pathol Int 2004; 54(1): 16–25.

56. Jenkins C, Rose GE, Bunce C, et al. Histological features of ocular adnexal lymphoma (REAL classification) and their association with patient morbidity and survival. Br J Ophthalmol 2000; 84(8): 907–13.

57. Fung CY, Tarbell NJ, Lucarelli MJ, et al. Ocular adnexal lymphoma: clinical behavior of distinct World Health Organization classification subtypes. Int J Radiat Oncol Biol Phys 2003; 57(5): 1382–91.

58. Tanimoto K, Kaneko A, Suzuki S, et al. Long-term follow-up results of no initial therapy for ocular adnexal MALT lymphoma. Ann Oncol 2006; 17(1): 135–40.

59. Matsuo T, Yoshino T. Long-term follow-up results of observation or radiation for conjunctival malignant lymphoma. Ophthalmology 2004; 111(6): 1233–7.

60. Uno T, Isobe K, Shikama N, et al. Radiotherapy for extranodal, marginal zone, B-cell lymphoma of mucosa-associated lymphoid tissue originating in the ocular adnexa: a multiinstitutional, retrospective review of 50 patients. Cancer 2003; 98(4): 865–71.

61. Martinet S, Ozsahin M, Belkacemi Y, et al. Outcome and prognostic factors in orbital lymphoma: a Rare Cancer Network study on 90 consecutive patients treated with radiotherapy. Int J Radiat Oncol Biol Phys 2003; 55(4): 892–8.

62. Ben Simon GJ, Cheung N, McKelvie P, Fox R, McNab AA. Oral chlorambucil for extranodal, marginal zone, B-cell lymphoma of mucosa-associated lymphoid tissue of the orbit. Ophthalmology 2006; 113(7): 1209–13.

63. Nola M, Lukenda A, Bollmann M, et al. Outcome and prognostic factors in ocular adnexal lymphoma. Croat Med J 2004; 45(3): 328–32.

64. Ejima Y, Sasaki R, Okamoto Y, et al. Ocular adnexal mucosa-associated lymphoid tissue lymphoma treated with radiotherapy. Radiother Oncol 2006; 78(1): 6–9.

65. Tsang RW, Gospodarowicz MK, Pintilie M, et al. Localized mucosa-associated lymphoid tissue lymphoma treated with radiation therapy has excellent clinical outcome. J Clin Oncol 2003; 21(22): 4157–64.

66. Regueiro CA, Valcarcel FJ, Romero J, de la Torre A. Treatment of conjunctival lymphomas by beta-ray brachytherapy using a strontium-90-yttrium-90 applicator. Clin Oncol (R Coll Radiol) 2002; 14(6): 459–63.

67. Zinzani PL, Stefoni V, Musuraca G, et al. Fludarabine-containing chemotherapy as frontline treatment of nongastrointestinal mucosa-associated lymphoid tissue lymphoma. Cancer 2004; 100(10): 2190–4.

68. Jager G, Neumeister P, Quehenberger F, et al. Prolonged clinical remission in patients with extranodal marginal zone B-cell lymphoma of the mucosa-associated lymphoid tissue type treated with cladribine: 6 year follow-up of a phase II trial. Ann Oncol 2006; 17(11): 1722–3.

69. Raderer M, Wohrer S, Bartsch R, et al. Phase II study of oxaliplatin for treatment of patients with mucosa-associated lymphoid tissue lymphoma. J Clin Oncol 2005; 23(33): 8442–6.

70. Ferreri AJ, Ponzoni M, Viale E, et al. Association between *Helicobacter pylori* infection and MALT-type lymphoma of the ocular adnexa: clinical and therapeutic implications. Hematol Oncol 2006; 24(1): 33–7.

71. Ferreri AJ, Ponzoni M, Guidoboni M, et al. Regression of ocular adnexal lymphoma after *Chlamydia psittaci*-eradicating antibiotic therapy. J Clin Oncol 2005; 23(22): 5067–73.

72. Ruskone-Fourmestraux A, Lavergne A, Aegerter PH, et al. Predictive factors for regression of gastric MALT lymphoma after anti-*Helicobacter pylori* treatment. Gut 2001; 48(3): 297–303.

73. Abramson DH, Rollins I, Coleman M. Periocular mucosa-associated lymphoid/low grade lymphomas: treatment with antibiotics. Am J Ophthalmol 2005; 140(4): 729–30.

74. Grunberger B, Hauff W, Lukas J, et al. 'Blind' antibiotic treatment targeting *Chlamydia* is not effective in patients with MALT lymphoma of the ocular adnexa. Ann Oncol 2006; 17(3): 484–7.

75. Vallisa D, Bernuzzi P, Arcaini L, et al. Role of anti-hepatitis C virus (HCV) treatment in HCV-related, low-grade, B-cell, non-Hodgkin's lymphoma: a multicenter Italian experience. J Clin Oncol 2005; 23(3): 468–73.

76. Conconi A, Martinelli G, Thieblemont C, et al. Clinical activity of rituximab in extranodal marginal zone B-cell lymphoma of MALT type. Blood 2003; 102(8): 2741–5.

77. Nuckel H, Meller D, Steuhl KP, Duhrsen U. Anti-CD20 monoclonal antibody therapy in relapsed MALT lymphoma of the conjunctiva. Eur J Haematol 2004; 73(4): 258–62.

78. Ferreri AJ, Ponzoni M, Martinelli G, et al. Rituximab in patients with mucosal-associated lymphoid tissue-type lymphoma of the ocular adnexa. Haematologica 2005; 90(11): 1578–9.

79. Lachapelle KR, Rathee R, Kratky V, Dexter DF. Treatment of conjunctival mucosa-associated lymphoid tissue lymphoma with intralesional injection of interferon alfa-2b. Arch Ophthalmol 2000; 118(2): 284–5.

80. Blasi MA, Gherlinzoni F, Calvisi G, et al. Local chemotherapy with interferon-alpha for conjunctival mucosa-associated lymphoid tissue lymphoma: a preliminary report. Ophthalmology 2001; 108(3): 559–62.

20

Primary splenic marginal zone lymphomas and other non-MALT marginal zone lymphomas

Catherine Thieblemont and Miguel A Piris

DEFINITION

Splenic marginal zone lymphoma (SMZL) is considered as a distinct entity among non-Hodgkin's lymphomas (NHL), after the proposal as a provisional entity in the Revised European–American Classification of Lymphoid Neoplasms (REAL) classification,[1] and the subsequent recognition as a distinct entity in the World Health Organization (WHO) classification.[2] MZLs represent a group of lymphomas whose cells originate from B lymphocytes normally present in a distinct anatomical location, the so-called 'marginal zone' (MZ) of secondary lymphoid follicles. These cells are anatomically located in spleen and mucosa-associated lymphoid tissue (MALT), although they have been recognized also in lymph nodes draining mucosa.

According to the sites involved and characteristic molecular findings, the International Lymphoma Study Group individualized three distinct subtypes of MZL:

- extranodal MZL of MALT type
- splenic MZL (with or without villous lymphocytes)
- nodal MZL (with or without monocytoid B cells).[1–3]

Despite this progress in the classification of MZL, patients with generalized disease at diagnosis are not easily ascribed to precise diagnostic groups (Figure 20.1). Their relative rarity, as well as the difficulties in distinguishing these lymphomas from other low-grade lymphoma subtypes are crucial issues in conducting epidemiological surveys and in describing the clinical features and outcomes of these lymphomes. This chapter examines current data on the epidemiology, clinical features, staging, and treatment of these lymphomas.

EPIDEMIOLOGY AND THE ROLE OF HEPATITIS C VIRUS

In adults, MZLs account for 5–17% of all NHL, depending on the series. MALT lymphoma is the most frequent of MZL subtypes, representing 50–70% of MZL and 7–8% of NHL. Splenic and nodal MZLs represent 20% and 10% of MZL, respectively, and account for less than 2% of NHL.[4,5] The median age of occurrence for SMZL is 65 years old,[6,7] although younger patients can develop an SMZL (upto 22 years old).[8] Increasing evidence indicates that MZLs in extranodal localizations can be associated with a chronic antigenic stimulation, either of endogenous type due to autoantibodies, or of exogenous type due to microbial pathogens, inducing an accumulation of lymphoid tissues in the typical sites of involvement for each lymphoma entity: i.e. in the mucosae of organs that contain no native lymphoid tissues for MALT lymphomas; in the spleen for SMZL; and in the lymph nodes for nodal MZL.

Since 1994, numerous epidemiological studies have found a correlation between NHL and hepatitis C virus (HCV) infection. Several genotypes of HCV have been identified, and

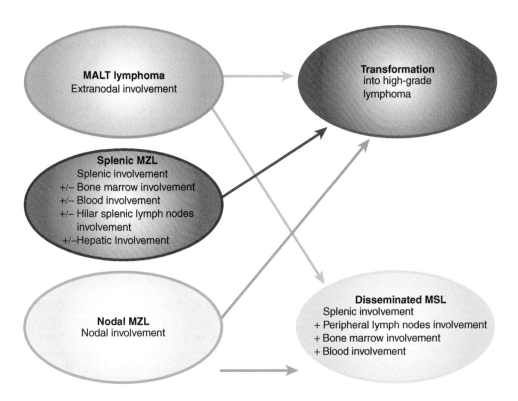

Figure 20.1   Clinical description of the different MZL entities.
Marginal zone lymphomas – SMZL, MZL-MALT, and nodal MZL – at diagnosis have specific clinicopathological features. In the course of the follow-up, the tumors may progress to large cell lymphomas, or disseminate; cytogenetic, phenotypic, and clinical studies are required to reveal the tumor origin.

classified in 9 groups and 30 subgroups (1a, 1b, 1c …). Reported genotypes differ according to country, as well as modalities and period of infection. For instance, the genotype 1 is the most frequent in France, followed by genotypes 2 and 3. In a given patient, changes in the genomic viral population occur because of mutations in hypervariable regions that may result in a failure of the immune system and, consequently, may favor the maintenance of a chronic viral infection. Thereby, 50–80% of HCV-infected patients develop a chronic infection. Most of epidemiological studies on the association between HCV and NHL have been conducted in Italy. They have found a prevalence of HCV infection, ranging from 10–40% in NHL patients, as compared with 1–7% in a control population, consisting mainly of low-grade, B-cell NHL with frequent extranodal localizations,

especially hepatosplenic. The association with HCV seems to be highly correlated in cases of lymphoplasmacytic lymphoma/immunocytoma, SMZL and other nodal or extranodal MZLs.[9,10] In the setting of SMZL the presence of HCV is of major relevance, due to the possible therapeutic implications.[11,12] Interestingly, a subset of SMZL, denominated as tropical splenic lymphoma, and characterized by splenomegaly and circulating naive CD5-negative villous B lymphocytes, has been described in malaria-endemic areas, which supports the role of infectious agents in the pathogenesis of SMZL.

PHYSIOPATHOLOGY

In the spleen, the SMZL is characterized by a micronodular expansion of small B lymphocytes inside the white pulp, associated with variable degree of involvement of the splenic red pulp (Figure 20.2a). The precursor cell is a B cell, presumably derived from a memory B cell from the marginal zone of a secondary follicle.

Marginal zone

The marginal zone is located around lymphoid follicles of secondary lymphoid organs, including lymph nodes, spleen, and extranodal mucosa-associated lymphoid tissue (MALT), such as Peyer's patches of small intestine. The marginal zone is mainly developed in spleen and MALT, whereas it is rarely identifiable in lymph nodes.[13] Marginal zone B lymphocytes are involved in the T-cell-independent antigenic response (quite the reverse of the B-lymphocyte antigenic response of germinal centers, which is a T-cell-dependent antigenic response). Marginal zone B lymphocytes are memory B cells derived from the differentiation of a centrocyte; they have a high-affinity B receptor (BCR). These cells gather in the marginal zone, circulate in blood, and survive several months or even years, ready to display a fast response in case of reintroduction of the same antigen. These memory B cells are remarkable for their speed at evolving towards plasmocytes, yielding antibodies when faced with a new antigenic contact. They differentiate in plasmocytes, diffuse in a few hours to the red pulp, stay inside, and secrete immunoglobulins (Ig) directly in the blood flow, providing a rapid humoral response directed against bacteremia. This bulky response is achieved in less than 48 hours, whereas the germinal center pathway takes at least 6 days to produce antibodies. Marginal zone memory B lymphocytes provide a fast T-cell-independent immune response, and play a key and decisive role in the instant eradication of an IgM-specific bacteremia. Antigens recognized by marginal zone B cells are mainly polysaccharidic antigens of bacterial capsules.[14]

Postgerminal origin

The SMZL is a marginal zone memory B cell, claimed in most cases to have a postgerminal origin, as demonstrated by the study of somatic mutations in Ig heavy-chain variable (Ig-VH) region genes.[15] However, a limited degree of heterogeneity in the mutational profile among SMZL has been recently described, one-third of the cases being non-mutated.[16,17] These lymphomas exhibit a low frequency of somatic mutations, concerning the oncogenes *bcl-6, PAX5, PIM1, RHO-H*[18] findings that suggest a particular differentiation pathway, possibly without transit through the germinal center.[16,17] Interestingly, a bias in the use of VH1.2 has been found in these cases, suggesting the antigen selection of some SMZLs.[16]

Role of the B-cell receptor and chronic antigenic stimulation

Survival and selection of B cells depend on the BCR, even when they are mature and quiescent. This survival signal is delivered either independently, or is secondary to an antigenic stimulation (pre-BCR). In NHL, the BCR signal is also mandatory for B cells' survival, as demonstrated by the absence of BCR-negative variants in NHL and the occurrence of somatic hypermutations of the lymphoma B-cell B receptor.

The SMZL pathogenesis may be associated with a chronic antigenic stimulation.[19] A clear relationship has been highlighted between HCV infection and SMZL with or without villous lymphocytes.[9,10] The E2 glycoprotein of HCV could interact with CD81 in the B cells, and could be responsible for an activation of B cells through BCR signal, leading to their increased proliferation (see Figure 20.2).[19] In murine models, MZLs have been described following a chronic stimulation by HCV, and have been associated with mutations of *FAS, AP12/ML*, and *p53*.[20] A special form of splenic NHL related to HCV has been correlated with the presence of cryoglobulin.[21] A decrease in lymphoproliferation following antiviral treatments reinforces the data pointing towards a contribution of a chronic antigenic stimulation to the physiopathological process of HCV-related MZL.[11,12]

CLINICAL PRESENTATION

The hallmark of the clinical presentation is usually a massive splenomegaly. Small splenic

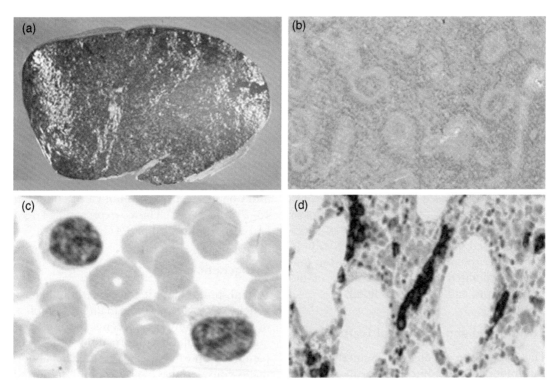

Figure 20.2   Main features of the SMZL at the spleen, bone marrow, and peripheral blood.

hilar lymph nodes are frequently involved. The involvement of peripheral lymph nodes (see Figure 20.1), an infrequent phenomenon in SMZL, is generally associated with a poorer outcome.[22]

Clinically, patients with SMZL complain of asthenia and/or pain of the left hypochondrium. Sometimes, patients take medical advice because of an abnormal blood cell count, especially anemia and/or thrombocytopenia, which are more related to splenic sequestration than to bone marrow infiltration. In these conditions, a splenomegaly is detectable at clinical examination. The general status is generally preserved with a WHO performance status <2 in 85% of cases.[23] General symptoms (fever, weight loss, night sweats) are unusual. The median age is 65 years old. This clinical presentation is associated with bone marrow and blood involvement in more than 90% of patients.[23,24] The serum lactate dehydrogenase (LDH) level is usually normal in SMZL, whereas the β_2-microglobulin

level is increased. A considerable proportion of patients (10–40% of cases) have a serum monoclonal paraprotein (M-component), mainly of the μ (IgM).[4,7,25–27] Autoimmune phenomena are described in 10–15% of patients, including autoiummune hemolytic anemia, immune thrombocytopenia, cold agglutinin, circulating anticoagulant (lupic or cardiolipidic), acquired von Willebrandt's disease, and angioedema due to acquired deficit in C1-esterase inhibitor. In these patients presenting with a combination of autoimmune phenomena and SMZL, the morphological aspect of the tumor consistently shows plasmacytic differentiation.

Few differences in the clinical presentation between patients with leukemic and nonleukemic forms of the disease have been found, except a significantly older age and an absence of immune disorders in the cases with leukemic presentation, formerly denominated as SLVL.[7, 23] The median age at diagnosis for SMZL patients with villous cells on the peripheral blood is 75 years old, as compared with 63 years old for the non-leukemic forms. Thus, clinically, it does not seem crucial to distinguish these two entities, which can be considered as a leukemic phase of SMZL. HCV-associated SMZLs are indistinguishable from typical SMZLs, except for the presence of HCV viral replication, and coexistence of a liver disease.[11]

DIAGNOSIS

The diagnosis is based on the study of peripheral blood lymphocytes, bone marrow biopsies or, when appropriate, on the study of surgically removed spleens. Most cases of SMZL do not require splenectomy for the diagnosis that can be accurately based on the study of the bone marrow and peripheral blood.

Histological and cytological features

Histology of the spleen shows a micronodular infiltration of the white pulp, with marginal zone differentiation and a variable degree of red pulp involvement. Typically, the marginal zone is occupied by a polymorphic population of B cells, including small cells, marginal cells, and scattered immunoblasts. With some frequency, there is plasmacytoid differentiation, both in the marginal zone and the in colonized germinal centers. Likewise, the blood infiltration is pleomorphic, showing small lymphocytes, centrocyte-type lymphocytes, and villous lymphocytes. A variable degree of blood infiltration by villous lymphocytes is a frequent finding in this tumor. In the bone marrow, the involvement can be paratrabecular, nodular, or diffuse. Intrasinusoidal infiltration is highly typical of SMZL.

Immunophenotypic data

SMZL B cells are characterized by the expression of the antigenic markers pan-B CD19, CD20, CD22, and CD79b.[2,28] The expression of other markers (CD5, FMC7, CD22 or CD79b, CD23, surface Ig expression), integrated into the Matutes international score,[29] can be helpful for a differential diagnosis between chronic lymphocytic leukemia (CLL) or other small B-cell lymphomas. This scoring system is based on the presence or absence of the most typical CLL immunophenotype markers (CD5+, CD23+, FMC7−, and weak expression of surface Ig and CD22).[29] According to the study of Matutes et al, 87% of CLL present with a 4–5 score, whereas SMZL is generally <3. Classically, the immunophenotypic analysis of tumoral cells shows CD19+, CD20+, CD5−, CD10−, CD23−, CD43+/−, FMC7 +/−. CD103−, bcl-2+, and cyclin D_1 cells. On the other hand, the expression of CD5 is found in 15–20% of cases.[6] The co-expression of IgM and IgD SIg is typical of SMZL.

Cytogenetic data

Several studies have demonstrated the heterogeneity of caryotypic abnormalities. Complete or partial trisomy 3 represents the most frequent cytogenetic abnormalities (85% of patients) reported in SMZL.[30-34] The abnormality considered as typical of SMZL, reported in 40% of cases, consists of deletion or translocation of chromosome 7q32.[34,35] No tumor suppressor genes have been found in this region, and there are good reasons to think that the deletion of a cluster of miRNAs located in this region could contribute to the deregulation of some of the key oncogenes in this disorder, such as TCL1. More rare translocations involving CDK6 and cyclin D_3 with IgH have been identified in small subsets of cases.[36]

Other chromosomal abnormalities reported at diagnosis include trisomy 18, trisomy 12, 17q isochrome, 13q14 deletion, and structural abnormalities of chromosome 1.[29,30,32-34,36-40] A translocation t(11;14)(q13;q32), combined with a rearrangement of bcl-1 and/or the expression of cyclin D_1, was described as present in 15% of cases diagnosed as SLVL, but these cases could represent a subset of splenic lymphoma with intermediate features between mantle cell lymphoma (MCL) and SMZL.[41-43] None of the above-mentioned cytogenetic abnormalities, with the exception of the 7q32 deletion, is considered typical of SMZL, but they may be helpful for the diagnosis. Contrary to other MZLs, translocations involving the MALT1 gene are not found in SMZL.

Mutational status of the immunoglobulin variable heavy-chain genes

The process of somatic hypermutations of Ig-VH genes is a crucial mechanism, diversifying the B cells' repertoire. Initial analyses of the mutational status of the Ig-VH genes showed the presence of somatic hypermutations in most cases, suggesting that the precursor cell of MZL was a memory B cell of postgerminal origin.[15] However, more recent studies have found an absence of somatic mutations in one-third of the cases studied, with biased use of the VH1.2 gene, which supports a relative degree of molecular heterogeneity of MZL and the existence of a clonal selection.[16,17]

Gene expression profiling: the molecular signature of SMZL

SMZLs have a specific transcriptional profile compared with other lymphomas, especially small B-cell lymphomas, such as follicular lymphomas, lymphocytic lymphomas, and MCLs.[44,45] This specific molecular signature includes genes involved in the signaling cascade of the AKT1 pathway,[45] but also the BCR signaling pathway, tumor necrosis factor (TNF), and nuclear factor kappa B (NF-κB) targets.[44] To date, gene expression analysis is not routinely available and cannot be applied in the routine diagnosis.

DIFFERENTIAL DIAGNOSIS

The association of bone marrow involvement and splenomegaly, with or without monoclonal IgM, is not exclusive for SMZL. This clinical presentation may be observed also for CLL and some NHL, such as MCL or lymphoplasmacytic lymphoma (LPL). The diagnosis often requires the integration of clinical, histological, and immunophenotypic data. Cytology, as well as expression of CD5 and CD23, with a low CD79b, enables differentiation between SMZL and CLL. The differential diagnosis between SMZL and MCL is facilitated by the cytology, expression of CD5 and CD43, overexpression of cyclin D_1 and loss of p27, even if borderline cases need a detailed study and

data integration. The presence of t11;14 is exceptional, if present at all, on SMZL bona fide cases.[40,42,43]

Diffuse large B-cell lymphoma, when involving the spleen, is usually characterized by one or several large nodules and very rarely involves the bone marrow.

Follicular lymphoma may show a pattern of splenic infiltration quite similar to that seen on SMZL, even with marginal zone differentiation, although the expression of BCL6, CD10, or the presence of t14;18, are useful for the diagnosis.[1–4]

Differential diagnosis with LPL/ Waldenström's macroglobulinemia (WM) may have a special difficulty.[2] These LPLs share numerous joint characteristics with SMZL with plasmacytoid differentiation.[1,2,22,46,47] including the clinical presentation.[2] Immunophenotypic and cytogenetic analyses may be helpful for the diagnosis. A high expression of CD22, and a more frequent presence of 7q21 deletion could be in favor of SMZL, whereas the presence of a 6q deletion is more in favor of LPL.[48] However, it remains difficult to distinguish between separate entities and morphological variants of a same entity. In this setting, prospective clinical trials could be warranted to evaluate the patient's outcome.

PROGNOSTIC FACTORS AND SURVIVAL

The median overall survival ranges between 5 and 10 years, but in case of aggressive disease, which is the case in roughly one-third of patients, median survival does not reach 4 years.[7,23,25,27,49] Treatment is indicated in case of symptomatic splenomegaly, cytopenia, or general symptoms.[23,49] Prognostic factors have been identified. The Italian Intergroup of Lymphomas (IIL) have developed a prognostic model in 309 patients based on three factors – hemoglobin level <12 g/dl, LDH level greater than normal, and albumin level <3.5 g/dl – leading to a prognostic index.[50] This index has allowed separation of patients into three groups, displaying different 5-year survival rates: 88% in the low-risk group (no risk factor); 73% in the intermediate-risk group (one risk factor); and 50% in the high-risk group (more than one factor).[50] In this analysis, the International Prognostic Index (IPI) was found to predict survival, although the multivariate analysis selected the three indicated parameters.[50] Other biological prognostic factors have been described, such as expression of CD38, unmutated Ig-VH gene status, and expression of NF-κB-activated genes by using gene expression analysis.[44]

A histological transformation into large cell lymphoma remains uncommon, occurring in only 10–20% of patients. The transformation sets in a median time, ranging from 12 to 85 months.[52] This situation is associated with the appearance of general symptoms, increase in LDH level, and disseminated lymphoma involvement. After histological progression, the median survival time was shortened to 26 months.[7]

TREATMENT

A treatment is required only in symptomatic patients with painful splenomegaly, associated or not with cytopenia due to hypersplenism. Asymptomatic patients may be followed by clinical examinations and laboratory tests. The absence of treatment does not influence the course of disease, and these patients often have a stable disease for at least 10 years.[7,53]

When a treatment is indicated, because of the occurrence of clinical signs, the recommended first-line therapy is splenectomy.[7,25,26,49,53,54] The benefit consists of an improvement of performance status in a few months, and a correction of anemia, thrombocytopenia, and neutropenia within 6 months after splenectomy. This improvement is maintained for years with a free-of-treatment period lasting 8 years in median.[7] Thereby, patients are considered to achieve a partial response with a persisting bone marrow and blood lymphocytosis.

Is there a place for chemotherapy in the management of MZL? Adjuvant chemotherapy to splenectomy provides an increased remission rate without modifying relapse-free and overall survival.[23] Chemotherapy may be proposed to patients with contraindications to surgery, to elderly patients, or to those who have progressed after surgery. Regimens are based on alkylating agents (chlorambucil, cyclophosphamide), purine analogues (fludarabine), and monoclonal antibody (rituximab) single agent or combined with cytotoxics.[10,55–57] A retrospective study of the MD Anderson have reported 88% of response in patients treated with rituximab single agent, 83% in those receiving rituximab + chemotherapy, and 55% in those receiving chemotherapy alone with 3-year survival rates of 95%, 100%, and 55%, respectively.[58] The use of rituximab single agent gave a normalization of splenic size in 92% of patients, and then could be considered as a good therapeutic option for elderly patients and for patients who could not undergo splenectomy. When the MZL is associated with an active HCV infection, the first-line therapy is based on the control of viral infection using interferon-α with or without ribavirin.[11]

CONCLUSIONS

SMZLs represent a distinct entity among NHLs with definite clinical criteria. The clinical presentation shows a splenic involvement with bone marrow and blood infiltration, associated with a lymph node involvement of the splenic hilum, but usually without peripheral lymph node involvement. No differences in the clinical presentation are clearly detectable between cases denominated in the past as SLVL and the classical form of the disease. Various immune phenomena (hemolytic anemia, immune thrombocytopenia, acquired coagulation disorders, etc), and a monoclonal serum paraproteinemia, IgM type, may be associated to SMZL. Splenectomy is an efficient therapy, improving performance status and reducing hypersplenism. The achievement of a complete response is not considered as a necessary step to extend long-term survival and preserve the quality of life. The association with an active HCV infection is possible, requiring antiviral treatment that often results in regression of the splenic lymphoma.

REFERENCES

1. Harris NL, Jaffe ES, Stein H, et al. A revised European–American Classification of lymphoid neoplasms. A proposal from the International Lymphoma Study Group. Blood 1994; 84: 1361–92.
2. Jaffe ES, Harris NL, Stein H, Vardiman J. World Health Organization Classification of Tumours: Pathology and Genetics of Tumours of Haematopoietic and Lymphoid Tissues. Lyon, France: IARC Press, 2001.
3. Isaacson P, Wright D. Malignant lymphoma of mucosa-associated lymphoid tissue. A distinctive type of B-cell lymphoma. Cancer 1983; 52: 1410–16.
4. Berger F. The different entities and diagnostic problems. Educational Program of the European Hematology Association meeting. Birmingham 2000: 5.
5. Nathwani B, Anderson J, Armitage J, et al. Marginal zone B-cell lymphoma: a clinical comparison of nodal and mucosa-associated lymphoid tissue types. Non-Hodgkin's Lymphoma Classification Project. J Clin Oncol 1999; 17: 2486–92.
6. Oscier D, Owen R, Johnson S. Splenic marginal zone lymphoma. Blood Rev 2005; 19: 39–51.
7. Thieblemont C, Felman P, Berger F, et al. Treatment of splenic marginal zone B-cell lymphoma: an analysis of 81 patients. Clin Lymphoma 2002; 3: 41–7.
8. Depowski PL, Dunn H, Purdy S, Ross JS, Nazeer T. Splenic marginal zone lymphoma: a case report and review of the literature. Arch Pathol Lab Med 2002; 126: 214–16.
9. Arcaini L, Burcheri S, Rossi A, et al. Prevalence of HCV infection in nongastric marginal zone B-cell lymphoma of MALT. Ann Oncol 2007; 18: 346–50.
10. Arcaini L, Paulli M, Boveri E, et al. Splenic and nodal marginal zone lymphomas are indolent disorders at high hepatitis C virus seroprevalence with distinct presenting features but similar morphologic and phenotypic profiles. Cancer 2004; 100: 107–15.
11. Hermine O, Lefrere F, Bronowicki J, et al. Regression of splenic lymphoma with villous lymphocytes after treatment of hepatitis C virus infection. N Engl J Med 2002; 11: 89–94.
12. Kelaidi C, Rollot F, Park S, et al. Response to antiviral treatment in hepatitis C virus-associated marginal zone lymphomas. Leukemia 2004; 18: 1711–16.
13. Cyster JG. B cells on the front line. Nat Immunol 2000; 1: 9–10.
14. Weller S, Reynaud CA, Weill JC. Vaccination against encapsulated bacteria in humans: paradoxes. Trends Immunol 2005; 26: 85–9.
15. Zhu DL, Oscier DG, Stevenson FK. Splenic lymphoma with villous lymphocytes involves B cells with extensively mutated Ig heavy chain variable region genes. Blood 1995; 85: 1603–7.
16. Algara P, Mateo MS, Sanchez-Beato M, et al. Analysis of the IgV(H) somatic mutations in splenic marginal zone lymphoma defines a group of unmutated cases with frequent 7q deletion and adverse clinical course. Blood 2002; 99: 1299–304.
17. Traverse-Glehen A, Davi F, Ben Simon E, et al. Analysis of VH genes in marginal zone lymphoma reveals marked heterogeneity between splenic and nodal tumors and suggests the existence of clonal selection. Haematologica 2005; 90: 470–8.
18. Traverse-Glehen A, Verney A, Baseggio L, et al. Analysis of IgVH, BCL6, PIM, RHO/TTF and PAX5 mutational status in splenic and nodal marginal B cell lymphoma suggest a particular B cell origin. Blood 2005; 106: 51a (abstract 162).
19. Suarez F, Lortholary O, Hermine O, Lecuit M. Infection-associated lymphomas derived from marginal zone B cells: a model of antigen-driven lymphoproliferation. Blood 2006; 107: 3034–44.
20. Morse HC, Kearney JF, Isaacson PG, et al. Cells of the marginal zone – origins, function and neoplasia. Leuk Res 2001; 25: 169–78.
21. Saadoun D, Boyer O, Trebeden-Negre H, et al. Predominance of type 1 (Th1) cytokine production in the liver of patients with HCV-associated mixed cryoglobulinemia vasculitis. J Hepatol 2004; 41: 1031–7.
22. Berger F, Felman P, Thieblemont C, et al. Non-MALT marginal zone B-cell lymphomas: a description of clinical presentation and outcome in 124 patients. Blood 2000; 95: 1950–6.
23. Thieblemont C, Felman P, Callet-Bauchu E, et al. Splenic marginal-zone lymphoma: a distinct clinical and pathological entity. Lancet Oncol 2003; 4: 95–103.
24. Franco V, Florena A, Stella M, et al. Splenectomy influences bone marrow infiltration in patients with splenic marginal zone cell lymphoma with or without villous lymphocytes. Cancer 2001; 91: 294–301.
25. Chacon J, Mollejo M, Munoz E, et al. Splenic marginal zone lymphoma: clinical characteristics and prognostic factors in a series of 60 patients. Blood 2002; 100: 1648–54.
26. Troussard X, Valensi F, Duchayne E, et al. Splenic lymphoma with villous lymphocytes: clinical presentation, biology and prognostic factors in a series of 100 patients. Groupe Francais d'Hematologie Cellulaire (GFHC). Br J Haematol 1996; 93: 731–6.
27. Parry-Jones N, Matutes E, Gruszka-Westwood AM, et al. Prognostic features of splenic lymphoma with villous lymphocytes: a report on 129 patients. Br J Haematol 2003; 120: 759–64.
28. Matutes E, Morilla R, Owusu-Ankomah K, Houlihan A, Catovsky D. The immunophenotype of splenic lymphoma with villous lymphocytes and its relevance to the differential diagnosis with other B-cell disorders. Blood 1994; 83: 1558–62.
29. Matutes E, Owusu-Ankomah K, Morilla R, et al. The immunological profile of B-cell disorders and proposal of a scoring system for the diagnosis of CLL. Leukemia 1994; 8(10): 1640–5.
30. Dierlamm J, Pittaluga S, Wlodarska I, et al. Marginal zone B-cell lymphomas of different sites share similar cytogenetic and morphologic features. Blood 1996; 87: 229–307.

31. Gruszka-Westwood AM, Matutes E, Coignet LJA, Wotherspoon A, Catovsky D. The incidence of trisomy 3 in splenic lymphoma with villous lymphocytes: a study by FISH. Br J Haematol 1999; 104: 600–4.

32. Hernandez JN, Garcia JL, Gutierrez NC, et al. Novel genomic imbalances in B-cell splenic marginal zone lymphomas revealed by comparative genomic hybridization and cytogenetics. Am J Pathol 2001; 158: 1843–50.

33. Sole F, Woessner S, Florensa L, et al. Frequent involvement of chromosomes 1, 3, 7 and 8 in splenic marginal zone B-cell lymphoma. Br J Haematol 1997; 98: 446–9.

34. Wotherspoon A, Doglioni C, Isaacson P. Low-grade gastric B-cell lymphoma of mucosa-associated lymphoid tissue (MALT): a multifocal disease. Histopathology 1992; 20: 29–34.

35. Andersen CL, Gruszka-Westwood A, Atkinson S, et al. Recurrent genomic imbalances in B-cell splenic marginal-zone lymphoma revealed by comparative genomic hybridization. Cancer Genet Cytogenet 2005; 156: 122–8.

36. Mateo M, Mollejo M, Villuendas R, et al. 7q31–32 allelic loss is a frequent finding in splenic marginal zone lymphoma. Am J Pathol 1999; 154: 1583–9.

37. Corcoran M, Mould S, Orchard J, et al. Dysregulation of cyclin dependent kinase 6 expression in splenic marginal zone lymphoma through chromosome 7q translocations. Oncogene 1999; 18: 6271–7.

38. Callet-Bauchu E, Baseggio L, Felman P, et al. Cytogenetic analysis delineates a spectrum of chromosomal changes that can distinguish non-MALT marginal zone B-cell lymphomas among mature B-cell entities: a description of 103 cases. Leukemia 2005; 19: 1818–23.

39. Dierlamm J, Michaux L, Wlodarska I, et al. Trisomy 3 in marginal zone B-cell lymphoma: a study based on cytogenetic analysis and fluorescence in situ hybridization. Br J Haematol 1996; 93: 242–9.

40. Gruszka-Westwood AM, Hamoudi RA, Matutes E, Tuset E, Catovsky D. p53 abnormalities in splenic lymphoma with villous lymphocytes. Blood 2001; 97: 3552–8.

41. Troussard X, Mauvieux L, Radfordweiss I, et al. Genetic analysis of splenic lymphoma with villous lymphocytes: a Groupe Français d'Hématologie Cellulaire (GFHC) study. Br J Haematol 1998; 101: 712–21.

42. Cuneo A, Bardi A, Wlodarska I, et al. A novel recurrent translocation t(11;14)(p11;q32) in splenic marginal zone B cell lymphoma. Leukemia 2001; 15: 1262–7.

43. Jadayel D, Matutes E, Dyer M, et al. Splenic lymphoma with villous lymphocytes: analysis of bcl-1 rearrangements and expression of the cyclin D1 gene. Blood 1994; 83: 3664–71.

44. Oscier DG, Matutes E, Gardiner A, et al. Cytogenetic studies in splenic lymphoma with villous lymphocytes. Br J Haematol 1993; 85: 487–91.

45. Ruiz-Ballesteros E, Mollejo M, Rodriguez A, et al. Splenic marginal zone lymphoma: proposal of new diagnostic and prognostic markers identified after

46. Thieblemont C, Nasser V, Felman P, et al. Small lymphocytic lymphoma, marginal zone B-cell lymphoma, and mantle cell lymphoma exhibit distinct gene-expression profiles allowing molecular diagnosis. Blood 2004; 103: 2727–37.

47. Owen RG, Treon SP, Al-Katib A, et al. Clinicopathological definition of Waldenström's macroglobulinemia: consensus panel recommendations from the Second International Workshop on Waldenström's Macroglobulinemia. Semin Oncol 2003; 30: 110–15.

48. Lin P, Bueso-Ramos C, Wilson CS, Mansoor A, Medeiros LJ. Waldenström macroglobulinemia involving extramedullary sites: morphologic and immunophenotypic findings in 44 patients. Am J Surg Pathol 2003; 27: 1104–13.

49. Ocio EM, Hernandez JM, Mateo G, et al. Immunophenotypic and cytogenetic comparison of Waldenström's macroglobulinemia with splenic marginal zone lymphoma. Clin Lymphoma 2005; 5: 241–5.

50. Bertoni F, Zucca E. State-of-the-art therapeutics: marginal-zone lymphoma. J Clin Oncol 2005; 23: 6415–20.

51. Arcaini L, Lazzarino M, Colombo N, et al. Splenic marginal zone lymphoma: a prognostic model for clinical use. Blood 2006; 107: 4643–9.

52. Thieblemont C, Chettab K, Felman P, et al. Identification and validation of seven genes, as potential markers, for the differential diagnosis of small B cell lymphomas (small lymphocytic lymphoma, marginal zone B cell lymphoma, and mantle cell lymphoma) by cDNA macroarrays analysis. Leukemia 2002; 16(11): 2326–9.

53. Camacho FI, Mollejo M, Mateo MS, et al. Progression to large B cell lymphoma in splenic marginal zone lymphoma – a description of a series of 12 cases. Am J Surg Pathol 2001; 25: 1268–76.

54. Catovsky D, Matutes E. Splenic lymphoma with circulating villous lymphocytes/splenic marginal-zone lymphoma. Semin Hematol 1999; 36: 148–54.

55. Mulligan SP, Matutes E, Dearden C, Catovsky D. Splenic lymphoma with villous lymphocytes. Natural history and response to therapy in 50 cases. Br J Haematol 1991; 78: 206–9.

56. Bolam S, Orchard J, Oscier D. Fludarabine is effective in the treatment of splenic lymphoma with villous lymphocytes. Br J Haematol 1997; 99 :158–61.

57. Lefrere F, Hermine O, Belanger C, et al. Fludarabine: an effective treatment in patients with splenic lymphoma with villous lymphocytes. Leukemia 2000; 14: 573–5.

58. Paydas S, Yavuz S, Disel U, Sahin B, Ergin M. Successful rituximab therapy for hemolytic anemia associated with relapsed splenic marginal zone lymphoma with leukemic phase. Leuk Lymphoma 2003; 44: 2165–6.

59. Tsimberidou AM, Catovsky D, Schlette E, et al. Outcomes in patients with splenic marginal zone lymphoma and marginal zone lymphoma treated with rituximab with or without chemotherapy or chemotherapy alone. Cancer 2006; 107: 125–35.

tissue and cDNA microarray analysis. Blood 2005; 106: 1831–8.

Gastrointestinal tract lymphomas

21

Andreas Neubauer and Emanuele Zucca

EPIDEMIOLOGY AND CLASSIFICATION

The gastrointestinal (GI) tract is the most frequent extranodal localization, representing 30–40% of extranodal lymphomas[1-3] and from 4 to 20% of all non-Hodgkin's lymphoma (NHL) cases.[4,5]

In Western countries, the most common location is the stomach (approximately 50–60%), followed by the small intestine (30%), and the large intestine (around 10%). Esophagus localization is very rare. These proportions can differ geographically; small intestinal lymphomas are more common in the Middle East (Table 21.1). In the stomach, NHL represents the second most frequent tumor, following adenocarcinoma.[6]

GI tract lymphomas encompass a number of distinct clinicopathological entities which can be defined according to the World Health Organization (WHO) classification.[7] (Table 21.2) The most common histological subtype in localized GI presentations is diffuse large B-cell lymphoma (DLBCL), which is present in approximately 60% of the gastric and 70% of the intestinal cases. Lymphomas of the mucosa-associated lymphoid tissue (MALT) represent about 35–40% of primary gastric lymphoma cases but less than 10% of the intestinal ones.[8] In recent outpatient series, the percentage of MALT lymphomas with regard to gastric lymphomas may be somewhat higher and reach up to 70% (T Wündisch and M Stolte, pers comm). A Japanese survey also reported that the proportion of patients with low-grade GI lymphoma vs aggressive histologies have increased (from about 40% to 60%) during the past decades.[9] Follicular lymphomas are very rare in the stomach but have been reported in up to 17% of intestinal cases. The other histological subtypes, including T-cell lymphomas, Burkitt's lymphoma, and mantle cell lymphomas (which in the GI tract often present as a multiple lymphomatous polyposis), are much less common and taken together constitute <5% of the cases.[8,10]

The incidence of gastrointestinal lymphoma may have increased over the past decades.[9,11-13] This may be due to a true increase, but more efficient case registration and improved diagnostic tools may have also played a role. An epidemiological study carried out in comparable demographic areas in the UK and northern Italy showed a higher incidence of gastric NHL in the northeastern regions of Italy (13.2 × 10^5/year vs $1 × 10^5$/year). This suggests the existence of geographical variations, perhaps correlated to the rate of chronic gastritis caused by *Helicobacter pylori* (HP) in the regions under examination.[12] Less consistent epidemiological information is available on intestinal than on gastric NHL. Numerous studies have reported on the significant association between celiac disease and the otherwise uncommon enteropathy-type (or enteropathy-associated) T-cell lymphoma (ETL). Patients with celiac disease have an increased risk of developing ETL, as they have an increased risk of developing adenocarcinoma of the upper gastrointestinal tract, including esophageal cancer.[14] Aberrant clonal intraepithelial T-cell populations can be found in patients with refractory celiac sprue[15,16] and some authors have even hypothesized that adult-onset celiac disease can itself be a form of lymphoma.[17,18] More recent large epidemiological studies have confirmed the association (relative risk ≃3) of celiac disease with ETL, and possibly with lymphoma types other than ETL, even though the

Table 21.1   Frequency of lymphomas at different gastrointestinal sites in different series

Author	Country	Total GI tract cases	Stomach	Intestine (small and large)	Small bowel	Colon and rectum
Dragosics[106]	Austria	133	79%	21%[a]	10%	6%
Shenkier[8]	Canada	176	48%	52%	–	–
d'Amore[96]	Denmark	139	63%	37%	–	–
Koch[10]	Germany	371	75%	22%[a]	9%	–
Liang[107]	Hong Kong	425	56%	–	31%	12%
Tondini[67]	Italy	135	73%	27%[a]	15%	9%
Nakamura[9]	Japan	455	75%	25%[b]		
Amer[108]	Saudi Arabia	185	51%	49%	–	–
Zucca[97]	Switzerland	103	68%	–	24%	7%
Otter[2]	The Netherlands	96	56%	44%[c]	13%	16%
Isikdogan[109]	Turkey	145	43%	–	50%	7%
Morton[95]	UK	175	45%	54%[a]	33%	15%
List[110]	USA	87	60%	–	26%	14%

[a] Including cases (approx. 3–6.5% of all cases) with multifocal gastrointestinal involvement.
[b] Including cases (approx. 4% of all cases) with concomitant gastric and intestinal involvement.
[c] Mesenterial localization was considered as primary intestinal and cases with multifocal GI tract involvement were also included.

Table 21.2   Distribution of the main histological types in 393 patients with localized gastric lymphoma enrolled in a large German clinical trial performed mainly in referral hospitals[59]

Histological type (REAL classification criteria)	Frequency
Diffuse, large B-cell lymphoma	59%
with MALT component	14%
without MALT component	45%
Marginal zone lymphoma of the MALT	38%
Mantle cell lymphoma	1%
Follicular lymphoma	0.5%
Peripheral T-cell lymphomas	1.5%

risk seems lower than previously thought.[14,19–22] However, frequently, the diagnosis of celiac disease is not made before ETL is diagnosed.

DIAGNOSIS AND STAGING PROCEDURES

Regardless of histological type, the presenting symptoms are generally due to the local lesion (abdominal pain, dyspepsia, nausea and vomiting, anorexia, obstruction, hemorrhage). Fever and night sweats are uncommon and are often associated with a T-cell phenotype and/or intestinal localization, e.g. in Burkitt's lymphoma.[4]

Compared to nodal lymphomas, fewer patients with gastric lymphoma present with bone marrow involvement or elevated lactate dehydrogenase (LDH) levels.[23] The percentage of marrow involvement in gastrointestinal MALT lymphomas may be underestimated by clinical means such as changes in blood counts, and occurs in about 15% of patients referred to large centers.[24] Weight loss, however, is common, but usually as a consequence of the localization of the primary lymphoma rather than a constitutional B symptom.[25] Gastrointestinal bleeding may occur at presentation in 20–30% of patients, whereas gastric occlusion and perforation are quite uncommon.[10,26–29]

There is no consensus concerning classification and staging of GI NHL. An international workshop was held in Lugano in 1993 to discuss the problems of evaluating patients with GI tract lymphoma, which proposed a modification – known as 'Lugano staging' – to the Blackledge's staging system.[30] However, this was not generally accepted, and the best 'staging' for GI lymphoma remains controversial with a variety of staging systems still in clinical use.[30–32]

Table 21.3 Remission rate and time needed to document the histological remission of the lymphoma after anti-*Helicobacter* therapy for stage I gastric MALT lymphoma

Author	No. of patients	Staging procedures	Percent CR	Months to CR	No. of relapses
Pinotti[111]	45	CT	67	3–18	2
Neubauer[112]	50	CT± EUS	80	1–9	5
Nobre-Leitao[113]	17	CT+ EUS	100	1–12	1
Steinbach[40]	23	CT± EUS	56	3–45	0
Montalban[114]	19	CT± EUS	95	2–19	0
Ruskone-Formestraux[41]	24	CT+ EUS	79	2–18	2
Bertoni[83]	189	CT	56	3–24	15

CR, complete response; CT, computed tomography; EUS, endoscopic ultrasound.

Until recently, when surgery was the main therapy for GI lymphomas, it was also considered as the correct diagnostic work-up since it provided adequate tumor specimens for histological diagnosis. However, sufficient material for diagnosis is now obtained in the vast majority of cases by endoscopic biopsy. Surgery for diagnostic purposes, at least in gastric lymphomas, is not needed anymore. Imaging techniques have also improved significantly and, in the past decade, the introduction of endoscopic ultrasonography has been proven to be useful in assessing the depth of the stomach wall infiltration and the presence of perigastric lymph nodes and in identifying patients at high risk of bleeding and/or perforation.[33–38] In MALT lymphomas, deep infiltration of the gastric wall is associated with a greater risk of lymph nodal positivity and a smaller chance of response to antibiotics only.[39–41]

In general, a computed tomography (CT) scan of the chest and abdomen is recommended in all GI lymphomas to exclude systemic, lymph nodal involvement and/or extension to the adjacent structures. The usefulness of a positron emission tomography (PET) scan has been documented only for DLBCLs but is controversial for MALT lymphomas, which are frequently reported as PET-negative due to their often limited tumor volume and indolent behavior.[42,43] In addition, since normal gastric mucosa also sometimes shows [18F]-fluorodeoxyglucose (FDG) uptake, specificity is rather low. Nevertheless, recent studies suggest that many gastric MALT lymphomas with known active disease may have positive FDG uptake.[44,45] An ear, nose, and throat (ENT) examination is also often recommended in gastric lymphomas in order to exclude concomitant involvement of Waldeyer's ring, occasionally associated with a gastric presentation.[46]

CLINICAL MANAGEMENT

For gastric lymphomas, until 10 years ago surgery employing partial or total gastrectomy was the main therapy with curative intention.[47,48] In some series, surgery was combined with postoperative radiotherapy (RT) and/or chemotherapy. A retrospective review of the Danish Lymphoma Study Group found that patients with gastric lymphoma who received irradiation as part of their therapy had a reduced risk of relapse.[4] The benefit of low dose (20–25 Gy) postoperative RT in patients with stage IA and IIA gastric lymphoma was also shown in the series from the Princess Margaret Hospital in Toronto, which reported an 86% 10-year relapse-free survival.[49–51] Other clinicians have shown good results in patients with complete resection of tumor followed by chemotherapy alone or combined modality therapy.[52] It has been shown by several studies that chemotherapy alone or chemotherapy followed by RT may produce similar results, and that gastrectomy is thus redundant.[53–56] Taal and colleagues reported a a 5-year relapse-free survival of 85% in stage I and 58% in stage II patients treated with chemotherapy and RT or RT alone, without prior tumor resection.[57,58] In a recent large German study, 393 patients with localized primary gastric lymphoma were treated with RT and/or chemotherapy only or additional surgery. The survival rate at 42 months for those treated with surgery was 86% compared with 91% for those without surgery.[59]

Hence, the need for surgery for diagnostic purposes has disappeared, at least for the gastric tumors, and the assumption of an increased risk of perforation and bleeding associated with front-line chemotherapy, for which 'debulking surgery' was carried out preventively, has not been confirmed in any modern series. Indeed, the presence of a bulky mass is sometimes itself an obstacle to surgical intervention, and surgery does not necessarily prevent these complications, as episodes of bleeding or perforation have also been reported to occur despite surgical resection. On the contrary, several studies have reported a high degree of postsurgical complications that resulted in a delay in the start of chemotherapy[55,56,59–62] and surgical resection has been replaced by conservative therapeutic approaches for gastric lymphomas.[10,28,59,63–66] For primary intestinal lymphoma, however, there are no studies clearly demonstrating that surgery is unnecessary.

Albeit the scarcity of randomized studies comparing surgery alone with the addition of adjuvant chemotherapy and/or RT, combined modality treatment is nowadays considered the procedure of choice for patients with primary intestinal lymphoma.[67–69] It is noteworthy that with such an approach in the large series of the Istituto Nazionale dei Tumori in Milan,[67] primary gastric and intestinal lymphomas appear to have similar outcomes if they are comparable with respect to histology and prognostic index, while, in the past, the prognosis for the intestinal localization was considered to be generally worse.[4] Recently retrospective studies have proposed modifications of the International Prognostic Index (IPI) to effectively identify subsets of patients with primary GI DLBCL with significantly different outcomes.[70–73] Optimal treatment of GI lymphomas depends mainly on the histological type, but also on the site and the stage of the disease. The different situations will therefore be discussed separately.

Primary diffuse large B-cell lymphoma of the stomach

DLBCL represents the most common histological type among GI lymphomas, when patients in large referral centers are investigated. Patients with locally advanced or disseminated aggressive GI lymphomas appear to behave in the same manner as other advanced lymphomas, with comparable histology and prognostic factors.[54] Therefore, treatment of disseminated DLBCL is today based on chemotherapy combined with rituximab. In general, the same guidelines followed for nodal DLBCL can also be applied to GI lymphomas with aggressive histologies. These guidelines suggest – for localized stages – a front-line chemoimmunotherapy with 3–4 cycles of standard CHOP-rituximab (CHOP-R) followed by 'involved-field' RT. RT toxicity can be reduced by using conformational techniques to minimize doses to the liver and kidneys.[74–76] Patients with disseminated disease, similar to their nodal counterparts, can be adequately treated with 6–8 cycles of CHOP–R (cyclophosphosphamide, doxorubicin, vincristine, predinosone+rituximab). It is a matter of debate whether this regimen can also be applied to patients with localized stages of gastric DLBCL. In that case, consolidating RT would not be necessary. Although it has never formally been proven that CHOP-R is superior to CHOP alone in gastric DLBCL, this combination seems rational, simply because the disease is rare, and combination with chemotherapy + rituximab has resulted in excellent treatment results in nodal typical DLBCL. In addition, there are no conclusive data in favor of an outcome benefit of CHOP 14 vs the conventional CHOP 21 regimen.

Analogous to MALT lymphomas, some recent studies have demonstrated possible regression of diffuse large B-cell localized lymphomas following anti-HP therapy.[77–79] This suggests that an antigenic drive may remain present in a subset of aggressive gastric lymphomas, especially those where a simultaneous MALT lymphoma component can be detected. It is our opinion that, when an existing or a previous *H. pylori* infection is documented, antibiotics should be added to chemotherapy at a clinician's discretion. Nevertheless, cure of *H. pylori* infection as sole therapy can not be considered standard of care for gastric DLBCL and is clearly an experimental therapy.

Gastric marginal zone B-cell lymphoma of MALT type

The concept of mucosa-associated lymphoid tissue has progressively developed during the last two decades regarding the lymphoid component observed in various organs that do not correspond to peripheral sites of the immune system.[80,81] Gastric MALT lymphoma is often multifocal within the stomach but is characterized by an indolent natural history and prolonged confinement to the site of origin in most cases. Epidemiological evidence of a plausible etiological correlation between gastric MALT lymphomas and chronic *H. pylori* infection has been found; clinical studies demonstrated histological regressions of gastric MALT lymphoma after eradication of *H. pylori* in the majority of the patients who received antibiotic therapy. Nowadays, it is generally accepted that eradication of *H. pylori* with antibiotics should be the sole initial treatment of MALT lymphomas confined to the gastric wall.[82] (Table 21.3) A strict follow-up after antibiotics is highly advisable, also because it is not possible to completely exclude the presence of a concomitant aggressive DLBCL not demonstrated in the diagnostic gastric biopsies. Postantibiotic molecular follow-up studies showed in 30–50% the cases a long-term persistence of monoclonal B cell after histological regression of the lymphoma, but this event is not necessarily heralding a relapse, and its clinical significance remains unclear.[83,84] Wundisch et al 2005.[115]

For the management of the subset of *H. pylori*-negative cases and for the patients who fail antibiotic therapy a choice can be made between conventional oncological modalities, but there are no published randomized studies for this situation. Very good disease control using RT has been reported by several institutions.[85,86] Surgery has been widely and successfully used in the past, but the precise role for surgical resection should be redefined in view of the excellent results achieved with conservative approaches.[87] Patients with systemic disease should be considered for systemic treatment, but only few anticancer compounds and chemotherapy regimens have been tested specifically in MALT lymphomas. The anti-CD20 monoclonal antibody rituximab is also very active and may represent an additional option for the treatment of systemic disease.

Immunoproliferative small intestinal disease

Immunoproliferative small intestinal disease (IPSID), alpha heavy-chain disease, and Mediterranean lymphoma all refer to the same condition, which is presently considered a variant of low-grade MALT lymphoma, characterized by a diffuse lymphoplasmacytic/plasmacytic infiltrate in the small intestine.[88,89] Most of the cases have been described in the Middle East, especially in the Mediterranean area, where the disease is endemic and affects young adults. Patients usually present with poor performance status and severe malabsorption. Remissions have been described following chemotherapy, but frequently the patients cannot tolerate standard therapy and a poor prognosis has been described in most published reports. Nevertheless, the most recent data suggest that anthracycline-containing regimens, combined with nutritional support plus antibiotics to control diarrhea and malabsorption, may offer a concrete chance of cure to most patients. The role of RT and surgical resection remains to be defined. Several authors have reported that treatment with antibiotics can produce clinical, histological, and immunological remissions in early stages, but only in 2004 did Lecuit et al demonstrate the presence of a specific pathogen that linked this lymphoma to *Campylobacter jejuni*.[90]

Primary intestinal diffuse large B-cell lymphoma

DLBCLs constitute the majority of primary intestinal lymphomas, but distinct histological presentations can include intestinal MALT lymphoma or IPSID, enteropathy-associated T-cell lymphoma (ETL), mantle cell lymphoma, or follicular lymphoma, underscoring the importance of skilled histological diagnosis.[91,92]

Small bowel is by far the most common site, large bowel or rectal lymphoma being less frequent. Presenting symptoms vary from feelings of abdominal fullness, nausea, diarrhea, and abdominal pain, to bowel obstruction and perforation. Because of these non-specific presenting symptoms, many patients require laparotomy for diagnosis and have resection of bowel lesions at diagnosis.

The management of large B-cell lymphoma is usually with surgery followed by chemotherapy (which is today usually combined with rituximab). In patients where complete tumor resection is not feasible, treatment is the same as described above for the gastic localizations.[50,93] The outcome reported in the literature varies, depending on the extent of disease and histology. In a large series of intestinal lymphomas, a 60–75% 5-year survival for patients with B-cell lymphomas is reported[71,73,94] and only a 25% 5-year survival for those with T-cell tumors.[94] A poor outcome of patients with intestinal T-cell lymphoma has also been reported in the series from the British National Lymphoma Investigation (BNLI) and the Danish LYFO Study Group.[95,96] The site of involvement was also of prognostic significance, with lesions in the terminal ileum having the best survival, but this is probably due to association between site and histology, with terminal ileum lymphomas being usually of B-cell type. Other prognostic factors in primary intestinal lymphoma include age, performance status, B symptoms, and stage.[71,73,95,96] Rectal presentations are less common than other sites in the lower intestinal tract. Treatment usually includes immunochemotherapy and RT (30–40 Gy in 1.5–2 Gy daily fractions) for patients presenting with DLBCL. Involved-field RT alone (30–35 Gy in 1.5–1.75 Gy daily fractions) has been successful in providing long-term disease control for MALT lymphoma of the rectum. There is no evidence that abdominoperineal resection can improve local control or survival.

Multiple lymphomatous polyposis

This peculiar type of lymphoma presents with multiple lymphomatous polyps of the gastrointestinal tract and in most cases represents the intestinal form of mantle cell lymphoma. Unlike MALT lymphoma, multiple lymphomatous polyposis is frequently a generalized disease with blood and bone marrow involvement. Overexpression of cyclin D_1 and presence of translocation t(11;14) is typically observed. The prognosis is quite poor in spite of aggressive chemotherapy, similar to its nodal counterpart.[97] In rare instances multiple polyposis appears as a clinical syndrome produced by different histological subtypes other than mantle cell, especially follicular lymphoma.[98] Thus, the term multiple lymphomatous polyposis should not be used to define a histopathological entity.

Enteropathy-type T-cell lymphoma

According to the WHO classification, ETL is a tumor of intraepithelial T lymphocytes, usually composed of large monomorphic CD3+, CD7+, CD8−/+, CD4−, CD103+ cells that contain cytotoxic granule-associated proteins.[99] As stated previously, patients with celiac disease (gluten-sensitive enteropathy) have an increased risk of developing intestinal lymphoma. ETL occurs mostly in adults, frequently with a short history of celiac disease. Treatment with an appropriate diet may prevent ETL, and patients diagnosed with celic disease during childhood rarely progress to ETL.[100]

Most patients show the HLA DQA1∗0501, DQB1∗0201 genotypes that characterize celiac disease.[101] It occurs most often in the sixth or seventh decades, but there have been sporadic reports of cases in young adults. Abdominal pain and/or exacerbation of enteropathy-associated symptoms (malabsorption, loss of responsiveness to a gluten-restricted diet) are the most common presentation features.

Approximately 25% of cases present with an intestinal perforation. The clinical course is often very unfavorable, and most patients die due to multiple perforations of the intestine. A variety of combination chemotherapy regimens have been proposed, but responses to the therapy (which is often poorly tolerated because of the malnourished state of most patients) are in general scarce and brief.[97]

Gastrointestinal Burkitt's lymphoma

A common childhood lymphoma but rare in adults, sporadic Burkitt's lymphoma, often presents with abdominal pain and intussusception. The ileocecal region is the most common site of involvement and 60% of cases are primarily intestinal.[97,102] Other common extranodal sites are the ovaries, the kidneys, the omentum, and the breast.[102] The histological and cytogenetic features are similar to those of the classical endemic African form, as is its association with the Epstein–Barr virus. Endemic (i.e. African-form) Burkitt's lymphoma occurs in African children and involves the facial bones as well as the GI tract, and other extranodal sites.[102] The non-endemic Burkitt's lymphoma frequently arises from abdominal lymph nodes and shows massive ascites with intestinal involvement. In addition, central nervous system (CNS), testes, ovary, breast, and bone marrow are frequently contaminated. The primary treatment modality is intensive combination chemotherapy. Very important is intensive liquor prophylaxis using i.th. (intra thecal) therapy as well as intravenous high-dose methotrexate therapy. Local and locoregional therapy (i.e. surgery and RT) is no adequate treatment, even for patients with localized disease. Surgery remains important for establishing the diagnosis and, in certain circumstances, surgical resection may be beneficial (acute abdominal emergencies, resection of intussuscepted bowel).

Primary lymphomas of the esophagus, gallbladder, and biliary ducts

Primary malignant lymphoma of the gallbladder is exceedingly rare; less than 20 well-documented cases have been reported in the literature. The histology can be variable, and occasional cases of MALT lymphomas have been reported.[103] The possible growth of malignant lymphoma in the biliary ducts has also been described.[104] Although lymphoma may involve any part of the GI tract, either primarily or secondarily, esophageal involvement is exceedingly rare. Clinical and endoscopic findings are unspecific and the diagnosis is generally biopsy-related.[105] No exact therapeutic rules have been established, but combined RT together with chemotherapy seems advisable.

ACKNOWLEDGMENTS

Acknowledges support of Wilhelm Sander Stiftung and EZ acknowledges support of Oncosuisse.

REFERENCES

1. Freeman C, Berg JW, Cutler SJ. Occurrence and prognosis of extranodal lymphomas. Cancer 1972; 29: 252–60.
2. Otter R, Gerrits WB, vd Sandt MM, et al. Primary extranodal and nodal non-Hodgkin's lymphoma. A survey of a population-based registry. Eur J Cancer Clin Oncol 1989; 25: 1203–10.
3. Otter R, Willemze R. Extranodal non-Hodgkin's lymphoma. Neth J Med 1988; 33: 49–51.
4. d'Amore F, Brincker M, Gronbaek K, et al. Non-Hodgkin's lymphoma of the gastrointestinal tract: a population-based analysis of incidence, geographic distribution, clinicopathologic presentation features, and prognosis. J Clin Oncol 1994; 12: 1673–84.
5. Herrmann R, Panahon AM, Barcos MP, et al. Gastrointestinal involvement in non-Hodgkin's lymphoma. Cancer 1980; 46: 215–22.
6. Hockey MS, Powell J, Crocker J, et al. Primary gastric lymphoma. Br J Surg 1987; 74: 483–7.
7. Jaffe ES, Harris NL, Stein H, et al. World Health Organization Classification of Tumours. Pathology and Genetics of Tumours of Haematopoietic and Lymphoid Tissues. Lyon: IARC Press, 2001: 1–351.
8. Shenkier TN, Connors JM. Primary extranodal non-Hodgkin's lymphomas. In: Canellos GP, Lister TA, Young BD, eds. The Lymphomas, 2nd edn. Philadelphia: Saunders Elsevier, 2006: 325–47.
9. Nakamura S, Matsumoto T, Iida M, et al. Primary gastrointestinal lymphoma in Japan: a clinicopathologic analysis of 455 patients with special reference to its time trends. Cancer 2003; 97: 2462–73.

10. Koch P, del Valle F, Berdel WE, et al. Primary gastrointestinal non-Hodgkin's lymphoma: I. Anatomic and histologic distribution, clinical features, and survival data of 371 patients registered in the German Multicenter Study GIT NHL 01/92. J Clin Oncol 2001; 19: 3861–73.

11. Severson RK, Davis S. Increasing incidence of primary gastric lymphoma. Cancer 1990; 66: 1283–7.

12. Doglioni C, Wotherspoon AC, Moschini A, et al. High incidence of primary gastric lymphoma in northeastern Italy. Lancet 1992; 339: 834–5.

13. Gurney KA, Cartwright RA, Gilman EA. Descriptive epidemiology of gastrointestinal non-Hodgkin's lymphoma in a population-based registry. Br J Cancer 1999; 79: 1929–34.

14. Catassi C, Bearzi I, Holmes GK. Association of celiac disease and intestinal lymphomas and other cancers. Gastroenterology 2005; 128: S79–86.

15. Cellier C, Delabesse E, Helmer C, et al. Refractory sprue, coeliac disease, and enteropathy-associated T-cell lymphoma. French Coeliac Disease Study Group. Lancet 2000; 356: 203–8.

16. Daum S, Weiss D, Hummel M, et al. Frequency of clonal intraepithelial T lymphocyte proliferations in enteropathy-type intestinal T cell lymphoma, coeliac disease, and refractory sprue. Gut 2001; 49: 804–12.

17. Wright DH, Jones DB, Clark H, et al. Is adult-onset coeliac disease due to a low-grade lymphoma of intraepithelial T lymphocytes? Lancet 1991; 337: 1373–4.

18. Carbonnel F, Grollet-Bioul L, Brouet JC, et al. Are complicated forms of celiac disease cryptic T-cell lymphomas? Blood 1998; 92: 3879–86.

19. Mearin ML, Catassi C, Brousse N, et al. European multi-centre study on coeliac disease and non-Hodgkin lymphoma. Eur J Gastroenterol Hepatol 2006; 18: 187–94.

20. Smedby KE, Hjalgrim H, Askling J, et al. Autoimmune and chronic inflammatory disorders and risk of non-Hodgkin lymphoma by subtype. J Natl Cancer Inst 2006; 98: 51–60.

21. Catassi C, Fabiani E, Corrao G, et al. Risk of non-Hodgkin lymphoma in celiac disease. JAMA 2002; 287: 1413–19.

22. Smedby KE, Akerman M, Hildebrand H, et al. Malignant lymphomas in coeliac disease: evidence of increased risks for lymphoma types other than enteropathy-type T cell lymphoma. Gut 2005; 54: 54–9.

23. Krol AD, Hermans J, Kramer MH, et al. Gastric lymphomas compared with lymph node lymphomas in a population-based registry differ in stage distribution and dissemination patterns but not in patient survival. Cancer 1997; 79: 390–7.

24. Thieblemont C, Bastion Y, Berger F, et al. Mucosa-associated lymphoid tissue gastrointestinal and non-gastrointestinal lymphoma behavior: analysis of 108 patients. J Clin Oncol 1997; 15: 1624–30.

25. Zucca E, Cavalli F. Gut lymphomas. Baillières Clin Haematol 1996; 9: 727–41.

26. Raderer M, Vorbeck F, Formanek M, et al. Importance of extensive staging in patients with mucosa-associated lymphoid tissue (MALT)-type lymphoma. Br J Cancer 2000; 83: 454–7.

27. Radaszkiewicz T, Dragosics B, Bauer P. Gastrointestinal malignant lymphomas of the mucosa-associated lymphoid tissue: factors relevant to prognosis. Gastroenterology 1992; 102: 1628–38.

28. Koch P, del Valle F, Berdel WE, et al. Primary gastrointestinal non-Hodgkin's lymphoma: II. Combined surgical and conservative or conservative management only in localized gastric lymphoma – Results of the prospective German Multicenter Study GIT NHL 01/92. J Clin Oncol 2001; 19: 3874–83.

29. Cogliatti SB, Schmid U, Schumacher U, et al. Primary B-cell gastric lymphoma: a clinicopathological study of 145 patients. Gastroenterology 1991; 101: 1159–70.

30. Rohatiner A, d'Amore F, Coiffier B, et al. Report on a workshop convened to discuss the pathological and staging classifications of gastrointestinal tract lymphoma. Ann Oncol 1994; 5: 397–400.

31. Ruskone-Fourmestraux A, Dragosics B, Morgner A, et al. Paris staging system for primary gastrointestinal lymphomas. Gut 2003; 52: 912–13.

32. de Jong D, Aleman BM, Taal BG, et al. Controversies and consensus in the diagnosis, work-up and treatment of gastric lymphoma: an international survey. Ann Oncol 1999; 10: 275–80.

33. Eidt S, Stolte M, Fischer R. Factors influencing lymph node infiltration in primary gastric malignant lymphoma of the mucosa-associated lymphoid tissue. Pathol Res Pract 1994; 190: 1077–81.

34. Taal BG, Boot H, van Heerde P, et al. Primary non-Hodgkin lymphoma of the stomach: endoscopic pattern and prognosis in low versus high grade malignancy in relation to the MALT concept. Gut 1996; 39: 556–61.

35. Nakamura S, Matsumoto T, Suekane H, et al. Predictive value of endoscopic ultrasonography for regression of gastric low grade and high grade MALT lymphomas after eradication of Helicobacter pylori. Gut 2001; 48: 454–60.

36. Caletti G, Zinzani PL, Fusaroli P, et al. The importance of endoscopic ultrasonography in the management of low-grade gastric mucosa-associated lymphoid tissue lymphoma. Aliment Pharmacol Ther 2002; 16: 1715–22.

37. Fischbach W, Goebeler-Kolve ME, Greiner A. Diagnostic accuracy of EUS in the local staging of primary gastric lymphoma: results of a prospective, multicenter study comparing EUS with histopathologic stage. Gastrointest Endosc 2002; 56: 696–700.

38. Fusaroli P, Buscarini E, Peyre S, et al. Interobserver agreement in staging gastric malt lymphoma by EUS. Gastrointest Endosc 2002; 55: 662–8.

39. Sackmann M, Morgner A, Rudolph B, et al. Regression of gastric MALT lymphoma after eradication of Helicobacter pylori is predicted by

endosonographic staging. MALT Lymphoma Study Group. Gastroenterology 1997; 113: 1087–90.

40. Steinbach G, Ford R, Glober G, et al. Antibiotic treatment of gastric lymphoma of mucosa-associated lymphoid tissue. An uncontrolled trial. Ann Intern Med 1999; 131: 88–95.

41. Ruskone-Fourmestraux A, Lavergne A, Aegerter PH, et al. Predictive factors for regression of gastric MALT lymphoma after anti-*Helicobacter pylori* treatment. Gut 2001; 48: 297–303.

42. Elstrom R, Guan L, Baker G, et al. Utility of FDG-PET scanning in lymphoma by WHO classification. Blood 2003; 101: 3875–6.

43. Hoffmann M, Kletter K, Diemling M, et al. Positron emission tomography with fluorine-18-2-fluoro-2-deoxy-D-glucose (F18-FDG) does not visualize extranodal B-cell lymphoma of the mucosa-associated lymphoid tissue (MALT)-type. Ann Oncol 1999; 10: 1185–9.

44. Beal KP, Yeung HW, Yahalom J. FDG-PET scanning for detection and staging of extranodal marginal zone lymphomas of the MALT type: a report of 42 cases. Ann Oncol 2005; 16: 473–80.

45. Ambrosini V, Rubello D, Castellucci P, et al. Diagnostic role of 18F-FDG PET in gastric MALT lymphoma. Nucl Med Rev Cent East Eur 2006; 9: 37–40.

46. Bertoni F, Sanna P, Tinguely M, et al. Association of gastric and Waldeyer's ring lymphoma: a molecular study. Hematol Oncol 2000; 18: 15–19.

47. Thirlby RC. Gastrointestinal lymphoma: a surgical perspective. Oncology 1993; 7: 29–32.

48. Sano T. Treatment of primary gastric lymphoma: experience in the National Cancer Center Hospital, Tokyo. Recent Results Cancer Res 2000; 156: 104–7.

49. Gospodarowicz MK, Bush RS, Brown TC, et al. Curability of gastrointestinal lymphoma with combined surgery and radiation. Int J Radiat Oncol Biol Phys 1983; 9: 3–9.

50. Gospodarowicz MK, Sutcliffe SB, Clark RM, et al. Outcome analysis of localized gastrointestinal lymphoma treated with surgery and postoperative irradiation. Int J Radiat Oncol Biol Phys 1990; 19: 1351–5.

51. Gospodarowicz MK, Pintilie M, Tsang R, et al. Primary gastric lymphoma: brief overview of the recent Princess Margaret Hospital experience. Recent Results Cancer Res 2000; 156: 108–15.

52. Shepherd FA, Evans WK, Kutas G, et al. Chemotherapy following surgery for stages IE and IIE non-Hodgkin's lymphoma of the gastrointestinal tract. J Clin Oncol 1988; 6: 253–60.

53. Maor MH, Velasquez WS, Fuller LM, et al. Stomach conservation in stages IE and IIE gastric non-Hodgkin's lymphoma. J Clin Oncol 1990; 8: 266–71.

54. Salles G, Herbrecht R, Tilly H, et al. Aggressive primary gastrointestinal lymphomas: review of 91 patients treated with the LNH-84 regimen. A study of the Groupe d'Etude des Lymphomes Agressifs. Am J Med 1991; 90: 77–84.

55. Gobbi PG, Ghirardelli ML, Cavalli C, et al. The role of surgery in the treatment of gastrointestinal lymphomas other than low-grade MALT lymphomas. Haematological 2000; 85: 372–80.

56. Gobbi PG, Dionigi P, Barbieri F, et al. The role of surgery in the multimodal treatment of primary gastric non-Hodgkin's lymphomas. A report of 76 cases and review of the literature. Cancer 1990; 65: 2528–36.

57. Taal BG, Burgers JM, van Heerde P, et al. The clinical spectrum and treatment of primary non-Hodgkin's lymphoma of the stomach [see comments]. Ann Oncol 1993; 4: 839–46.

58. Taal BG, Burgers JM. Primary non-Hodgkin's lymphoma of the stomach: endoscopic diagnosis and the role of surgery. Scand J Gastroenterol 1991; 188: 33–7.

59. Koch P, Probst A, Berdel WE, et al. Treatment results in localized primary gastric lymphoma: data of patients registered within the German multicenter study (GIT NHL 02/96). J Clin Oncol 2005; 23: 7050–9.

60. Popescu RA, Wotherspoon AC, Cunningham D, et al. Surgery plus chemotherapy or chemotherapy alone for primary intermediate- and high-grade gastric non-Hodgkin's lymphoma: the Royal Marsden Hospital experience. Eur J Cancer 1999; 35: 928–34.

61. Ferreri AJ, Cordio S, Ponzoni M, et al. Non-surgical treatment with primary chemotherapy, with or without radiation therapy, of stage I-II high-grade gastric lymphoma. Leuk Lymphoma 1999; 33: 531–41.

62. Schmidt WP, Schmitz N, Sonnen R. Conservative management of gastric lymphoma: the treatment option of choice. Leuk Lymphoma 2004; 45: 1847–52.

63. Raderer M, Valencak J, Osterreicher C, et al. Chemotherapy for the treatment of patients with primary high grade gastric B-cell lymphoma of modified Ann Arbor Stages IE and IIE. Cancer 2000; 88: 1979–85.

64. Raderer M, Chott A, Drach J, et al. Chemotherapy for management of localised high-grade gastric B-cell lymphoma: how much is necessary? Ann Oncol 2002; 13: 1094–8.

65. Aviles A, Nambo MJ, Neri N, et al. The role of surgery in primary gastric lymphoma: results of a controlled clinical trial. Ann Surg 2004; 240: 44–50.

66. Yoon SS, Coit DG, Portlock CS, et al. The diminishing role of surgery in the treatment of gastric lymphoma. Ann Surg 2004; 240: 28–37.

67. Tondini C, Giardini R, Bozzetti F, et al. Combined modality treatment for primary gastrointestinal non-Hodgkin's lymphoma: the Milan Cancer Institute experience. Ann Oncol 1993; 4: 831–7.

68. Tondini C, Balzarotti M, Santoro A, et al. Initial chemotherapy for primary resectable large-cell lymphoma of the stomach. Ann Oncol 1997; 8: 497–9.

69. Sutcliffe SB, Gospodarowicz MK. Localized extranodal lymphomas. In: Keating A, Armitage J, Burnett A, et al, eds. Hematological Oncology. Cambridge: Cambridge University Press, 1992: 189–222.

70. Ibrahim EM, Ezzat AA, Raja MA, et al. Primary gastric non-Hodgkin's lymphoma: clinical features, management, and prognosis of 185 patients with diffuse large B-cell lymphoma. Ann Oncol 1999; 10: 1441–9.

71. Ibrahim EM, Ezzat AA, El-Weshi AN, et al. Primary intestinal diffuse large B-cell non-Hodgkin's lymphoma: clinical features, management, and prognosis of 66 patients. Ann Oncol 2001; 12: 53–8.

72. Cortelazzo S, Rossi A, Roggero F, et al. Stage-modified international prognostic index effectively predicts clinical outcome of localized primary gastric diffuse large B-cell lymphoma. International Extranodal Lymphoma Study Group (IELSG). Ann Oncol 1999; 10: 1433–40.

73. Cortelazzo S, Rossi A, Oldani E, et al. The modified International Prognostic Index can predict the outcome of localized primary intestinal lymphoma of both extranodal marginal zone B-cell and diffuse large B-cell histologies. Br J Haematol 2002; 118: 218–28.

74. Gospodarowicz M, Tsang R. Radiation therapy of mucosa-associated lymphoid tissue (MALT) lymphomas. In: Zucca E, ed. MALT Lymphomas. Georgetown, TX: Landes Bioscience/Kluwer Academic, 2004: 104–29.

75. Tsang RW, Gospodarowicz MK, Pintilie M, et al. Localized mucosa-associated lymphoid tissue lymphoma treated with radiation therapy has excellent clinical outcome. J Clin Oncol 2003; 21: 4157–64.

76. Wirth A, Teo A, Wittwer H, et al. Gastric irradiation for MALT lymphoma: reducing the target volume, fast! Australas Radiol 1999; 43: 87–90.

77. Chen LT, Lin JT, Tai JJ, et al. Long-term results of anti-Helicobacter pylori therapy in early-stage gastric high-grade transformed MALT lymphoma. J Natl Cancer Inst 2005; 97: 1345–53.

78. Montalban C, Santon A, Boixeda D, et al. Regression of gastric high grade mucosa associated lymphoid tissue (MALT) lymphoma after Helicobacter pylori eradication. Gut 2001; 49: 584–7.

79. Morgner A, Miehlke S, Fischbach W, et al. Complete remission of primary high-grade B-cell gastric lymphoma after cure of Helicobacter pylori infection. J Clin Oncol 2001; 19: 2041–8.

80. Zucca E, Bertoni F, Roggero E, et al. The gastric marginal zone B-cell lymphoma of MALT type. Blood 2000; 96: 410–19.

81. Isaacson PG, Du MQ. MALT lymphoma: from morphology to molecules. Nat Rev Cancer 2004; 4: 644–53.

82. Zucca E, Cavalli F. Are antibiotics the treatment of choice for gastric lymphoma? Curr Hematol Rep 2004; 3: 11–16.

83. Bertoni F, Conconi A, Capella C, et al. Molecular follow-up in gastric mucosa-associated lymphoid tissue lymphomas: early analysis of the LY03 cooperative trial. Blood 2002; 99: 2541–4.

84. Thiede C, Wundisch T, Alpen B, et al. Persistence of monoclonal B cells after cure of Helicobacter pylori infection and complete histologic remission in gastric mucosa-associated lymphoid tissue B-cell lymphoma. J Clin Oncol 2001; 19: 1600–9.

85. Tsang RW, Gospodarowicz MK. Radiation therapy for localized low-grade non-Hodgkin's lymphomas. Hematol Oncol 2005; 23: 10–17.

86. Schechter NR, Yahalom J. Low-grade MALT lymphoma of the stomach: a review of treatment options. Int J Radiat Oncol Biol Phys 2000; 46: 1093–103.

87. Bertoni F, Zucca E. State-of-the-art therapeutics: marginal-zone lymphoma. J Clin Oncol 2005; 23: 6415–20.

88. Al-Saleem T, Al-Mondhiry H. Immunoproliferative small intestinal disease (IPSID): a model for mature B-cell neoplasms. Blood 2005; 105: 2274–80.

89. Isaacson PG, Muller-Hermelink HK, Piris MA, et al. Extranodal marginal zone B-cell lymphoma of mucosa-associated lymphoid tissue (MALT lymphoma). In: Jaffe ES, Harris NL, Stein H, et al, eds. World Health Organization Classification of Tumours. Pathology and Genetics of Tumours of Haematopoietic and Lymphoid Tissues. Lyon: IARC Press, 2001: 157–60.

90. Lecuit M, Abachin E, Martin A, et al. Immunoproliferative small intestinal disease associated with Campylobacter jejuni. N Engl J Med 2004; 350: 239–48.

91. Foss HD, Stein H. Pathology of intestinal lymphomas. Recent Results Cancer Res 2000; 156: 33–41.

92. Isaacson PG. Gastrointestinal lymphomas of T- and B-cell types. Mod Pathol 1999; 12: 151–8.

93. Gospodarowicz MK, Ferry JA, Cavalli F. Unique aspects of primary extranodal lymphomas. In: Mauch PM, Armitage JO, Harris NL, et al, eds. Non-Hodgkin's Lymphomas. Philadelphia: Lippincott Williams & Wilkins, 2003: 685–707.

94. Domizio P, Owen RA, Shepherd NA, et al. Primary lymphoma of the small intestine: a clinicopathological study of 119 cases. Am J Surg Pathol 1993; 17: 429–42.

95. Morton JE, Leyland MJ, Vaughan Hudson G, et al. Primary gastrointestinal non-Hodgkin's lymphoma: a review of 175 British National Lymphoma Investigation cases. Br J Cancer 1993; 67: 776–82.

96. d'Amore F, Christensen BE, Brincker H, et al. Clinicopathological features and prognostic factors in extranodal non-Hodgkin lymphomas. Danish LYFO Study Group. Eur J Cancer 1991; 27: 1201–8.

97. Zucca E, Roggero E, Bertoni F, et al. Primary extranodal non-Hodgkin's lymphomas. Part 1: gastrointestinal, cutaneous and genitourinary lymphomas. Ann Oncol 1997; 8: 727–37.

98. Hashimoto Y, Nakamura N, Kuze T, et al. Multiple lymphomatous polyposis of the gastrointestinal tract

is a heterogenous group that includes mantle cell lymphoma and follicular lymphoma: analysis of somatic mutation of immunoglobulin heavy chain gene variable region. Hum Pathol 1999; 30: 581–7.

99. Isaacson PG, Wright DH, Ralfkiaer E, et al. Enteropathy-type T-cell lymphoma. In: Jaffe ES, Harris NL, Stein H, et al, eds. World Health Organization Classification of Tumours. Pathology and Genetics of Tumours of Haematopoietic and Lymphoid Tissues. Lyon: IARC Press, 2001: 208–9.

100. Silano M, Volta U, Vincenzi AD, et al. Effect of a gluten-free diet on the risk of enteropathy-associated T-cell lymphoma in celiac disease. Dig Dis Sci 2007 (Epub ahead of print Oct 13, 2007)

101. Howell WM, Leung ST, Jones DB, et al. HLA-DRB, -DQA, and -DQB polymorphism in celiac disease and enteropathy-associated T-cell lymphoma. Common features and additional risk factors for malignancy. Hum Immunol 1995; 43: 29–37.

102. Ferry JA. Burkitt's lymphoma: clinicopathologic features and differential diagnosis. Oncologist 2006; 11: 375–83.

103. Jelic TM, Barreta TM, Yu M, et al. Primary, extranodal, follicular non-Hodgkin lymphoma of the gallbladder: case report and a review of the literature. Leuk Lymphoma 2004; 45: 381–7.

104. Chiu KW, Changchien CS, Chen L, et al. Primary malignant lymphoma of common bile duct presenting as acute obstructive jaundice: report of a case. J Clin Gastroenterol 1995; 20: 259–61.

105. Gupta NM, Goenka MK, Jindal A, et al. Primary lymphoma of the esophagus. J Clin Gastroenterol 1996; 23: 203–6.

106. Dragosics B, Bauer P, Radaszkiewicz T. Primary gastrointestinal non-Hodgkin's lymphomas. A retrospective clinicopathologic study of 150 cases. Cancer 1985; 55: 1060–73.

107. Liang R, Todd D, Chan TK, et al. Prognostic factors for primary gastrointestinal lymphoma. Hematol Oncol 1995; 13: 153–63.

108. Amer MH, el-Akkad S. Gastrointestinal lymphoma in adults: clinical features and management of 300 cases. Gastroenterology 1994; 106: 846–58.

109. Isikdogan A, Ayyildiz O, Buyukcelik A, et al. Non-Hodgkin's lymphoma in southeast Turkey: clinicopathologic features of 490 cases. Ann Hematol 2004; 83: 265–9.

110. List AF, Greer JP, Cousar JC, et al. Non-Hodgkin's lymphoma of the gastrointestinal tract: an analysis of clinical and pathologic features affecting outcome. J Clin Oncol 1988; 6: 1125–33.

111. Pinotti G, Zucca E, Roggero E, et al. Clinical features, treatment and outcome in a series of 93 patients with low-grade gastric MALT lymphoma. Leuk Lymphoma 1997; 26: 527–37.

112. Neubauer A, Thiede C, Morgner A, et al. Cure of Helicobacter pylori infection and duration of remission of low-grade gastric mucosa-associated lymphoid tissue lymphoma. J Natl Cancer Inst 1997; 89: 1350–5.

113. Nobre-Leitao C, Lage P, Cravo M, et al. Treatment of gastric MALT lymphoma by *Helicobacter pylori* eradication: a study controlled by endoscopic ultrasonography. Am J Gastroenterol 1998; 93: 732–6.

114. Montalban C, Santon A, Boixeda D, et al. Treatment of low grade gastric mucosa-associated lymphoid tissue lymphoma in stage I with *Helicobacter pylori* eradication. Long-term results after sequential histologic and molecular follow-up. Haematologica 2001; 86: 609–17.

115. Wundisch T, Thiede C, Morgner A, et al. Long-term follow-up of gastric MALT lymphoma after *Helicobacter pylori* eradication. J Clin Oncol 2005; 23: 8018–24.

Cutaneous lymphomas

22

Reinhard Dummer and Elaine S Jaffe

INTRODUCTION

Cutaneous lymphomas (CLs) belong to the group of extranodal non-Hodgkin's lymphomas; they are the second most common member of this group. Their incidence is estimated at 1 in 100 000 yearly.[1] Primary CLs develop by definition in the skin and remain confined to the skin for a long period of time in most cases, while secondary CLs reflect cutaneous spread from disseminated primary nodal or extranodal lymphomas. Primary CL includes a wide spectrum of clinically and histologically heterogeneous lymphoproliferative neoplasms: 65% of CL are cutaneous T-cell lymphomas (CTCLs); 25% are cutaneous B-cell lymphomas (CBCLs); and 10% are other uncommon forms. CLs and nodal or extracutaneous lymphomas with the same cytomorphology may differ greatly not only in regard to clinical features but also with respect to therapy and prognosis. Thus, it is advisable for patients with CLs to be treated either by a specialized center or to be in close cooperation with such an institution,[2] and to have the biopsy reviewed by an expert in the salient features of cutaneous lymphomas.

Until recently, almost all common lymphoma classification schemes were based primarily on cytological criteria.[3] These classifications did not consider CLs as unique entities, and did not appropriately emphasize the distinctive clinical, therapeutic, and prognostic characteristics of CL. In 2004, a group of pathologists and dermatologists elaborated the present WHO/ EORTC (World Health Organization/ European Organization for Research and Treatment of Cancer) classification for primary lymphoproliferative disorders of the skin, which accurately reflects the specific features of cutaneous lymphomas but remains within the framework of the basic WHO classification for nodal lymphomas (Table 22.1).

This chapter discusses the most common primary cutaneous lymphomas. Adult T-cell lymphoma/leukemia, while it may present with cutaneous disease, is in essence a systemic process and is not covered. Similarly, extranodal natural killer (NK)/T-cell lymphoma, while it may present in the skin as a primary site, most often is secondary in the skin, and is covered elsewhere in this book. The CD4+ CD56+ neoplasms also are generally associated with systemic disease, with frequent involvement of bone marrow and lymph nodes, in addition to cutaneous involvement. As precursor neoplasms, they are related to the acute leukemias and are best discussed in that context. Finally, intravascular large B-cell lymphoma, while it may exhibit initial clinical manifestations in the skin, should be considered from a clinical standpoint as a systemic lymphoma requiring aggressive therapy. Those intravascular large B-cell lymphomas presenting in the skin appear to have a somewhat better prognosis, perhaps because of earlier clinical recognition and diagnosis.

CLINICAL FEATURES OF THE MOST COMMON CUTANEOUS LYMPHOMAS

Primary cutaneous T-cell lymphomas

Mycosis fungoides, including variants and subtypes

Mycosis fungoides (MF) is the most common CL (approx. 50% of CLs). It usually appears in the 4th to 7th decades and is more common in

Table 22.1   WHO-EORTC classification of cutaneous lymphomas with primary cutaneous manifestations

Cutaneous T-cell and NK-cell lymphomas

Mycosis fungoides(MF)

Mycosis fungoides variants and subtypes:
- Folliculotropic MF
- Pagetoid reticulosis
- Granulomatous slack skin

Sézary syndrome

Adult T-cell leukemia/lymphoma

Primary cutaneous CD30-positive lymphoproliferative disorders:
- Primary cutaneous anaplastic large cell lymphoma
- Lymphomatoid papulosis

Subcutaneous panniculitis-like T-cell lymphoma

Extranodal NK/T-cell lymphoma, nasal type

Primary cutaneous peripheral T-cell lymphoma, unspecified:
- Primary cutaneous aggressive epidermotropic CD8-positive T-cell lymphoma (provisional)
- Cutaneous γ/δ T-cell lymphoma (provisional)
- Primary cutaneous CD4+ small/medium-sized pleomorphic T-cell lymphoma (provisional)

Cutaneous B-cell lymphomas

Primary cutaneous marginal zone B-cell lymphoma

Primary cutaneous follicle center lymphoma

Primary cutaneous diffuse large B-cell lymphoma, leg type

Primary cutaneous diffuse large B-cell lymphoma, other:
- Primary cutaneous intravascular large B-cell lymphoma

Precursor hematological neoplasm

CD4+/CD56+ hematodermic neoplasm (formerly blastic NK cell lymphoma (represents tumors with a precursor plasmacytoid dendritic phenotype[4]

men. MF usually first presents as flat dermatitic lesions (patch stage), which after years or even decades become infiltrated and thickened (plaque stage) and later evolve into bulky nodules (tumor stage). Using routine clinical and histological methods, involvement of lymph nodes, internal organs, or bone marrow can first – if ever – be identified in late stages. In addition to patches, plaques, and tumors, some patients develop more unusual clinical findings such as follicular mucinosis and hyper- or hypopigmentation (Figures 22.9 to 22.12). MF only rarely presents as a solitary lesion. Pagetoid reticulosis is a variant of MF in which the malignant cells are confined to the epidermis.

Granulomatous slack skin (GSS) is a rare form of CTCL, nosologically related to MF, and therefore referred to as subtype of MF in the WHO/EORTC classification. GSS is clinically characterized by the development of bulky skin lesions in the major skin folds.

Histology

The hallmark of MF is a superficial, generally bandlike infiltrate in the dermis, with evidence of epidermotropism. The presence of classical intraepidermal Pautrier's microabscesses is highly characteristic but is only seen in a minority of cases.[5,6] The atypical lymphocytes may be confined to the epidermis, often in the basal

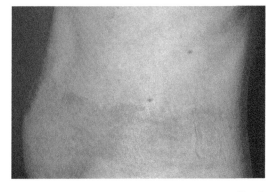

Figure 22.9   Hyperpigmented mycosis fungoides (Patch stage)

layer, with a string of pearls effect (Figure 22.1). Spongiosis is typically absent, while fibrosis of the papillary dermis is often seen. The neoplastic cells have hyperchromatic cerebriform nuclei, and vary in size and shape. Blast-like cells may be present in small numbers, and may increase with histological progression.

The folliculotropic variant of MF often spares the epidermis, but instead shows preferential involvement of the hair follicles, particularly on the face and head. Follicular mucinosis is a common feature and in most instances follicular mucinosis represents the folliculotropic variant of MF. Folliculotropic MF has a poorer prognosis than the classical plaque type of MF.[7]

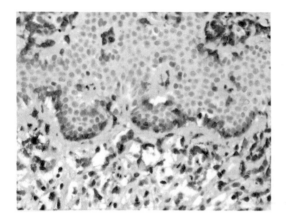

Figure 22.1 Mycosis fungoides. Neoplastic lymphoid cells are aligned in the basal layer, the "String of Pearls" effect. Neoplastic cells are highlighted with stain for CD3 (Immunoperoxi-dase, Hematoxylin counterstain).

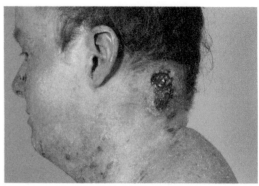

Figure 22.11   Mycosis fungoides (tumor stage)

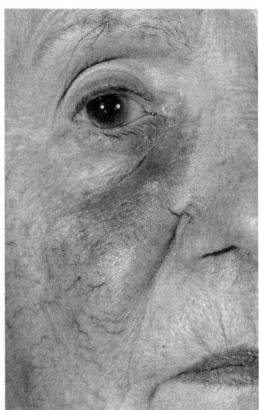

Figure 22.12   Mucinosis follicularis

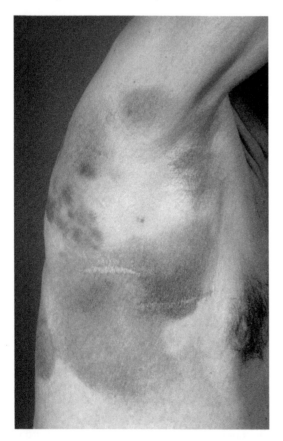

Figure 22.10   Mycosis fungoides (Plaque stage)

The neoplastic cells have a mature T-cell phenotype, expressing CD3, CD4, and typically loss of CD7. Rare CD8+ cases exist and are felt to be clinically similar. CD30 is usually negative, but with histological progression, transformation to a CD30+ or CD30− lymphoma composed of large cells may be seen. Molecular studies to identify T-cell receptor gene rearrangement are helpful in early cases, but false-positive results in reactive conditions are a potential pitfall. Additionally, in some cases of early MF, a clone may not be identified, perhaps due to low numbers of neoplastic cells. Identification of the same clone in more than one site enhances specificity.[8]

The molecular alterations in MF are diverse, but often involve deregulation of cell-cycle-related genes.[9] Additional common abnormalities include loss of tumor suppressor genes p15, p16, and p53, as well as chromosomal loss at 10q.[10]

Sézary syndrome

Sézary syndrome (SS) presents with erythroderma (redness, infiltration, and often edema with mild to marked scaling involving the entire skin), usually with prominent palmoplantar changes. In addition, there are leukemic changes in the peripheral blood and generalized lymphadenopathy.[11] The International Society for Cutaneous Lymphomas (ISCL) stated in a consensus paper that SS is defined by erythroderma and the identification of tumor cells in the peripheral blood (Figure 22.14). These findings can be identified with a variety of methods – morphological (identification of Sézary cells in blood smear or in buffy coat with electron microscopy), immunophenotypic (CD4/CD8 ratio >10 or CD4+/CD7– T cells >40%), or molecular biological (identification of a T-cell clone with Southern blot or polymerase chain reaction [PCR], chromosomal alterations).[11]

Histology

The cellular infiltrates in SS are typically more monotonous than in MF, with a uniform infiltrate of small to medium-sized atypical cells. Epidermotropism is sometimes absent. In some cases of otherwise clinically typical SS, the histopathological findings in the skin may be non-specific. Therefore, the absence of diagnosis features in the skin biopsy cannot be used to rule out the diagnosis.[12]

Primary cutaneous CD30-positive lymphoproliferative disorders

Primary cutaneous CD30+ lymphoproliferative disorders (LPDs) are the second most common group of CTCLs, accounting for approximately 30% of CTCLs. This group includes primary cutaneous anaplastic large cell lymphoma

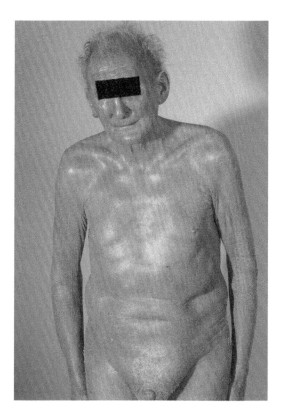

Figure 22.14 Melano-erythrodermia in a patient with Sezary syndrome

(C-ALCL), lymphomatoid papulosis (LYP), and borderline cases (Figure 22.13).

Lymphomatoid papulosis is a chronic but self-healing papulonodular disease with the histological picture of a CTCL.[13] The patients present with papular, papulonecrotic, or nodular lesions, which can be found in different stages of development. The course of the disease tends to be benign, lasting from just a few months to over 40 years. The individual lesions disappear spontaneously over weeks, usually leaving behind a small scar. About 5–20% of the patients with lymphomatoid papulosis develop another lymphoma, either before or after their lymphomatoid papulosis appears. The usual associated tumors are MF, large cell CD30+ CTCL, or Hodgkin's lymphoma. Primary cutaneous anaplastic large cell lymphomas present as nodular skin lesions varying in size from 1 to 15 cm. They are more common in adults. Typically, a single nodule or a group of nodules are found in a single anatomical region. The prognosis of this

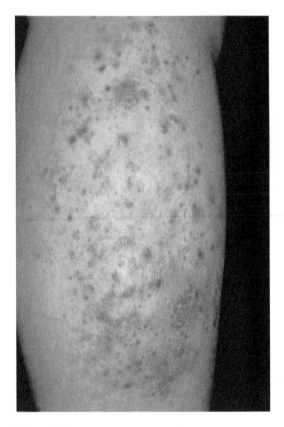

Figure 22.13 Lymphomatoide papulose

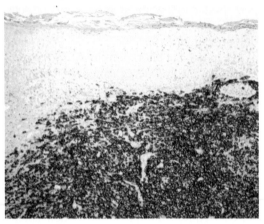

Figure 22.2 Primary cutaneous anaplastic large cell lymphoma.Neoplastic cells strongly positive for CD30 infiltrate the dermis in diffuse sheets. (Immunoperoxidase, Hematoxylin counter-stain).

disorder is excellent, in contrast to that of CD30+ nodal lymphomas. Spontaneous regression is seen in up to 25% of patients, but in some patients the regional lymph nodes become involved. This event is not associated with a worse prognosis.[13]

Histology
The hallmark of primary cutaneous CD30+ LPDs is the atypical CD30+ T cell, usually large in size, and sometimes with pleomorphic and Hodgkin-like features (Figure 22.2). The CD30+ cells are generally present in a polymorphous inflammatory background. In LYP inflammatory cells predominate, whereas in C-ALCL they may be sparse or absent. Neutrophils or other inflammatory cells may be so abundant as to mask the presence of the neoplastic cells.[14] The epidermis usually shows pseudoepitheliomatous hyperplasia, with ulceration in the later stages of evolution of individual lesions. It has been emphasized that correct categorization of

CD30+ LPDs requires integration of histological and clinical features.[15]

Subcutaneous panniculitis-like T-cell lymphoma

Subcutaneous panniculitis-like T-cell lymphoma (SPTCL) is a rare form of lymphoma, representing less than 1% of all non-Hodgkin's lymphomas. It is slightly more common in females than in males and has a broad age range.[16] Approximately 20% of patients are under the age of 20 years old, with a median age at presentation of 35 years old. Up to 20% of patients may have associated autoimmune disease, most commonly systemic lupus erythematosus.[17] Patients present with multiple subcutaneous nodules, usually in the absence of other sites of disease. The most common sites of localization are the extremities and trunk. The nodules range in size from 0.5 cm to several centimeters in diameter. Larger nodules may become necrotic; however, ulceration is rare.

Clinical symptoms are primarily related to the subcutaneous nodules. Systemic symptoms may be seen in up to 50% of patients. Laboratory abnormalities, including cytopenias and elevated liver function tests, are common, and a frank hemophagocytic syndrome is seen in 15–20%.[18] Lymphadenopathy is usually absent, but hepatosplenomegaly are more frequent.

Histology

The infiltrate involves the fat lobules, usually with sparing of septae. The overlying dermis and epidermis are typically uninvolved. The neoplastic cells range in size, but in any given case, cell size is relatively constant. The neoplastic cells have irregular and hyperchromatic nuclei. The lymphoid cells have a rim of pale-staining cytoplasm. A helpful diagnostic feature is the rimming of the neoplastic cells surrounding individual fat cells (Figure 22.3). Admixed reactive histiocytes are frequently present, particularly in areas of fat infiltration and destruction. The histiocytes are frequently vacuolated, due to ingested lipid material. Other inflammatory cells are typically absent, notably plasma cells, which are common in lupus panniculitis. Vascular invasion may be seen in some cases, and necrosis and karyorrhexis are common. The latter feature is helpful in the differential diagnosis from other lymphomas involving skin and subcutaneous tissue. Cutaneous gamma-delta (γ/δ) T-cell lymphomas may show panniculitis-like features, but commonly involve the dermis and epidermis, and may show epidermal ulceration.

The cells have a mature alpha-beta T-cell phenotype, usually CD8-positive, with expression of cytotoxic molecules including granzyme B, perforin, and T-cell intracellular antigen (TIA-1). The cells express betaF1 and are negative for CD56, helping in the distinction from cutaneous gamma-delta T-cell lymphoma.[16,19–21] The neoplastic cells show rearrangement of T-cell receptor genes, and are negative for Epstein–Barr viral (EBV) sequences. No specific cytogenetic features have been reported.

SPTCL has a much better prognosis than morphologically similar lymphomas of gamma-delta derivation.[22] For this and other reasons, gamma-delta T-cell lymphomas with panniculitis-like features are excluded from SPTCL in the WHO/EORTC classification and are included in a separate entity, termed cutaneous gamma-delta T-cell lymphoma, as discussed below. Recent studies suggest that the 5-year survival of SPTCL restricted to the alpha-beta (α/β) lineage is approximately 80%.

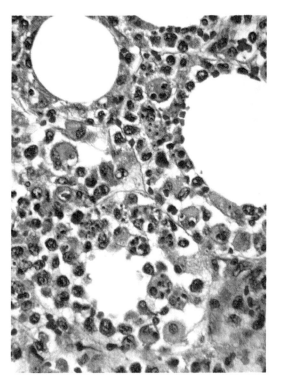

Figure 22.3 Subcutaneous panniculitis-like T-cell lymphoma. Neoplastic cells rim fat spaces. Histiocytes are abundant and show phagocytosis of apoptotic debris. (Hematoxylin and eosin).

Primary cutaneous peripheral T-cell lymphoma, unspecified

Primary cutaneous peripheral T-cell lymphoma (C-PTLU) is a diagnosis of exclusion. It is by definition a heterogeneous category. It also includes three provisional entities in the WHO/EORTC classification: primary cutaneous aggressive epidermotropic CD8-positive T-cell lymphoma; cutaneous gamma-delta T-cell lymphoma; and primary cutaneous CD4+ small/medium-sized pleomorphic T-cell lymphoma. For the parent group of C-PTLU, these lymphomas are histologically and clinically diverse. By definition, they are mainly CD30-negative, or CD30 is expressed in only a small percentage of the tumor cells. They are typically dermal in localization, without epidermotropism, as distinguished from mycosis fungoides.

Primary cutaneous gamma-delta T-cell lymphoma (CGDTCL) can present with plaques, nodules, or cutaneous tumors with ulceration.

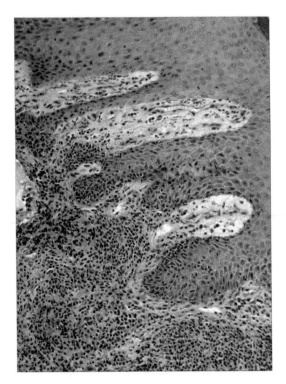

Figure 22.4 Primary cutaneous gamma delta T-cell lymphoma. Neoplastic cells infiltrate the dermis and show epidermotropism. In this case the features resemble pagetoid reticulosis. (Hematoxylin and eosin).

The tumors may extend to the subcutaneous tissue. However, in contrast to SPTCL, dermal and epidermal involvement is common in these lesions. Three major histological patterns of involvement can be present in the skin: epidermotropic, dermal, and subcutaneous (Figure 22.4). Often more than one histological pattern is present in the same patient in different biopsy specimens or within a single biopsy specimen.[21] The neoplastic cells are generally medium to large in size, with coarsely clumped chromatin. Large blastic cells with vesicular nuclei and prominent nucleoli are infrequent. Apoptosis and necrosis are common, often with angioinvasion. The subcutaneous cases may show rimming of fat cells, similar to SPTCL of gamma-delta origin.

The tumor cells characteristically have a betaF1−, CD3+, CD2+, CD5−, CD7+/−, CD56+ phenotype with strong expression of cytotoxic proteins. Most cases lack both CD4 and CD8, although CD8 may be expressed in some cases. In frozen sections, the cells are strongly

positive for TCR-delta. If only paraffin sections are available, the absence of betaF1 may be used to infer a gamma-delta origin.[23] Thus, in paraffin sections, the distinction between SPTCL and CGDTCL usually relies on the presence or absence of betaF1 and CD56, the other markers showing considerable overlap.

Gamma-delta T-cell lymphomas often show involvement of mucosa-associated sites, such as the intestine, stomach, or upper respiratory tract.[20] Skin may be a primary or secondary site of localization. Whether cutaneous and mucosal gamma-delta TCL are part of a single entity remains to be determined. All of these tumors are clinically aggressive and respond poorly to anthracycline-containing regimens.

Primary cutaneous aggressive epidermotropic CD8+ T-cell lymphoma is characterized an aggressive clinical course, and shows overlapping clinical features with cutaneous gamma-delta T-cell lymphoma. It is characterized by generalized patches, plaques, papulonodules, and tumors, spread to unusual sites but not to the lymph nodes, and an aggressive course (median survival = 32 months).[24] Histologically, it shows an often superficial infiltrate of epidermotropic T cells with necrosis (Figure 22.5). The lesions may resemble pagetoid reticulosis. The neoplastic cells express CD3, CD8, CD7, CD45RA, betaF1, and TIA-1, whereas CD2 and CD5 are frequently absent.

Primary cutaneous CD4+ small/medium-sized pleomorphic T-cell lymphoma is the last of the provisional entities included in the WHO/EORTC classification.[25] Many, if not most, of these patients present with a single skin lesion. The upper extremities, face, neck, or upper trunk are common sites of involvement. Lesions infrequently involve the lower extremities. The cells are generally small with only slight atypia. The infiltrates are typically dermal without epidermal infiltration. The infiltrates are dense and confluent, often producing nodules clinically. By definition, this is a CD3+, CD4+, CD8−, CD30− infiltrate. The lesions may contain variable numbers of reactive B cells. The differential diagnosis includes an atypical reactive lesion, and molecular studies are needed to confirm monoclonality. In patients with a single lesion, the prognosis is excellent, even with only simple

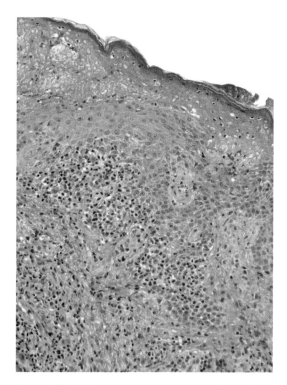

Figure 22.5 Primary cutaneous aggressive epidermotropic CD8+ T-cell lymphoma. Neoplastic cells infiltrate the epidermis and there is also epidermal necrosis. (Hematoxylin and eosin).

local excision. In patients with multiple lesions, the process is clinically more aggressive, although still more indolent than most other cutaneous T-cell lymphomas. The benign course seen in many of these patients raises the issue as to whether this is a true neoplastic process. Clonal T-cell populations may be identified in some histologically and clinically benign disorders, especially in the skin.[26,27]

Primary cutaneous B-cell lymphomas

Primary cutaneous follicle center lymphoma

Primary cutaneous follicle center lymphomas (C-FCLs) usually present with localized disease. These patients have nodular cutaneous or subcutaneous infiltrates that rarely ulcerate. Typical sites are the scalp, nape, and trunk. Extracutaneous manifestations are uncommon. The lesions are variable in size and often >2 cm in diameter. Larger lesions may be surrounded by smaller satellite nodules (Figure 22.15). The lymphoma may recur locally, but rarely disseminates. Most

patients can be treated with local approaches, surgical or radiation therapy.

In a series of patients treated in the Department of Dermatology in Zurich, the median age at diagnosis was 59 years old. In most patients the disease started with a solitary lesion. The most commonly affected sites were the head and neck region and the upper back. Tumors were not found on the extremities in any of the patients.[111]

Histology

Primary C-FCLs are composed of follicle-center-type cells, and may exhibit a follicular, follicular and diffuse, or totally diffuse growth pattern (Figure 22.6). The epidermis is uninvolved, and usually unremarkable. The infiltrate typically involves the superficial dermis, and may extend at some depth to the subcutaneous tissue in larger lesions. However, necrosis is generally absent. The cytological composition is quite variable, but the cytological 'grade' does not appear to influence the clinical behavior. Large centrocytes are a relatively prominent component in comparison with nodal follicular lymphomas (FLs). Some lesions may be composed predominantly of larger cells, but usually the cytological composition is variable. Fibrosis is often associated with the infiltrate. Immunophenotypically, the infiltrates show expression of the B-cell-associated antigens CD20 and CD79a. BCL-6 is usually positive, but CD10 is less frequently expressed than in nodal FLs. Additionally, BCL-2 protein is often negative in the atypical follicles.

Biological and clinical data suggest that primary C-FCLs are distinct from the usual nodal FLs. While the *BCL-2* translocation is found in approximately 85% of nodal FLs, evidence of *BCL-2* deregulation, based on either translocation or expression of the BCL-2 protein, is much less common in primary C-FCLs.[28,29] The data based on molecular studies appear to show some differences from the results by fluorescent in-situ hybridization (FISH), which have shown a somewhat higher incidence of BCL-2 translocation.[30]

Primary cutaneous marginal zone B-cell lymphoma

Primary cutaneous marginal zone B-cell lymphomas (PCMZLs) typically affect trunk and

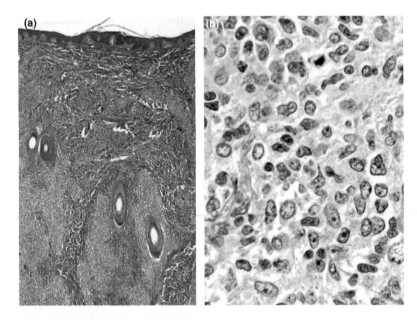

Figure 22.6 Cutaneous follicle center lymphoma. Biopsy of scalp lesion. A. Neoplastic cells are arranged in poorly defined follicles in the dermis. B. At high power cells are a mixture of large centrocytes and centroblasts. (Hematoxylin and eosin).

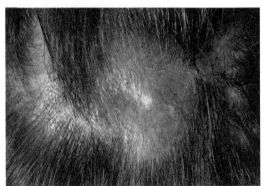

Figure 22.15 Primary cutaneous follicle center lymphoma

upper extremities. They typically present as multiple small (1–2 cm) reddish papules (Figure 22.16) Whereas patients may have multiple lesions, with recurrence over time, the prognosis is still generally excellent. Cutaneous involvement can occur in patients with a mucosal-associated lymphoma or autoimmune disease in other sites, but the typical PCMZL is a disease restricted to the skin.

The median age at diagnosis is typically lower than in primary C-FCL. In our recent series the median age of patients at diagnosis was 39 years old, and 40% of our patients had initially a solitary lesion. The most common affected sites were the upper back und upper arms; however, there are also lesions in the head and neck regions.[111]

An association with *Borrelia burgdorferi* infection has been reported in some series from European centers, but not in studies from the USA or Asia.[31,32]

Histology

Cutaneous MZL share cytological and architectural features with other extranodal mucosa-associated lymphoid tissue (MALT) lymphomas. Histologically, reactive lymphoid follicles are surrounded by a heterogeneous cellular infiltrate composed of centrocyte-like cells, monocytoid B cells, plasma cells, lymphoplasmacytoid cells, and small lymphocytes (Figure 22.7). Epidermal infiltration is absent, as is infiltration of other adnexal structures.

The immunophenotype of cutaneous MZL is similar to that seen in other sites. The B-cell associated antigens CD20 and CD79a are generally expressed. The cells are negative for the germinal center-associated markers CD10 and BCL-6. Plasmacytic differentiation correlates with the expression of cytoplasmic immunoglobulin. The plasma cells may be monotypic and in cutaneous lesions monotypic plasma cells are most readily identified in the very superficial dermis. Cases in which the light-chain class changes over time have been observed. In some cases, restricted light-chain expression may be identified in the absence of clonality by immunoglobulin heavy-chain PCR. Whether such lesions are truly lymphomas is difficult to establish with certainty.[33]

The molecular alterations identified in MALT lymphomas in other extranodal sites have generally been absent in cutaneous MZL, or seen with much lower frequency.[34–36]

Primary cutaneous large B-cell lymphoma, leg-type

This disease usually involves elderly patients who present with red-blue nodules or tumors, most often on the legs.

In our recent series the median age at diagnosis was 78 years old. The disease became apparent due to a solitary lesion (T1) in 3 of 7 patients (43%) and with multiple, but regional tumors (T2) in the remaining 4 patients (57%). None of the patients showed multiple disseminated lesions at diagnosis. The predilection sites were the legs, but tumors were also found on the head and neck and on the upper arm in 1 of the 7 patients. Ulceration was not uncommon in this CBCL subset.[111]

Histology

The large B-cell lymphomas of the leg type are composed of a monotonous population of large transformed lymphoid cells (Figure 22.8). The cells are typically round to oval, with little nuclear irregularity. The chromatin is coarse, with or without prominent nucleoli. The monotonous cytological composition contrasts with the heterogeneity seen in cutaneous FCL. There is usually minimal stromal reaction, and the infiltrate may extend into

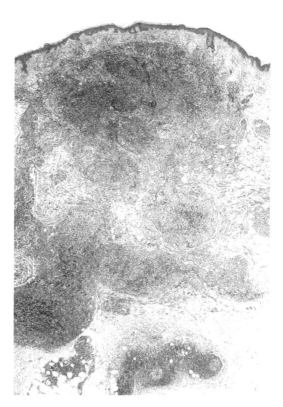

Figure 22.7 Cutaneous marginal zone B-cell lymphoma. Atypical lymphoid cells surround re-sidual reactive follicles. (Hematoxylin and eosin).

the subcutaneous tissue. Background inflammatory cells are generally absent.

The large B-cell lymphomas of the leg type have an immunophenotype similar to that seen in the activated B-cell (ABC) type of nodal diffuse large B-cell lymphoma (DLBCL).[37] They are frequently positive for MUM-1/IRF-4 and show strong positivity for the BCL-2 protein in the absence of the BCL-2/JH translocation.[38,39] BCL-6 is usually positive but CD10 is negative.[40]

Gene expression studies have confirmed an activated B-cell pattern of expression in these lymphomas, in contrast to primary C-FCL.[41] Inactivation of tumor suppressor genes has also has been identified.[41]

DIAGNOSTIC APPROACH

The diagnosis of CL requires extensive clinical experience and relies upon a detailed history, clinical observation, histological analysis (including the appropriate immunohistochemical

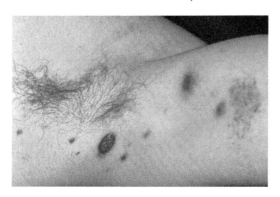

Figure 22.16 Primary cutaneous marginal zone b-cell lymphoma

studies based on the working diagnosis), and proof of clonality in lesional skin (and when SS is suspected, in the peripheral blood), as well as on various laboratory and imaging studies to exclude extranodal manifestations (Table 22.2). If the molecular biological and histological findings are weighted too heavily without adequate consideration of the clinical picture, overtreatment of the patient often results. Many inflammatory skin diseases may reveal clonality, especially when investigated with PCR.[42]

STAGING

The TMN classification is used to stage CTCL.[44,45] This classification poorly reflects the biological course and prognosis for many CTCL because it was developed primarily for MF. This classification includes categories such as N2, which do not appear in daily clinical practice, because lymph nodes that are not clinically enlarged are not biopsied (Table 22.3).

During the recent meetings of the ISCL and the Cutaneous Lymphoma Task Force of the EORTC, the representatives have established a consensus proposal of a TNM classification system applicable for all primary cutaneous lymphomas other than MF and SS.[46]

T Classification

Consistent with the definition of 'T classification' by the AJCC/UICC (American Joint Committee on Cancer/International Union Against Cancer), the T classification for cutaneous lymphoma reflects the extent/distribution of primary cutaneous involvement. A circular area is selected to define size/area criteria of T categories, since a circular area (vs a square area) may be more biological and relevant to radiation therapy planning. The size criteria of 5 and 15 cm were chosen arbitrarily to distinguish small or limited tumor involvement from the greater or more extensive involvement within the T1 and T2 categories, respectively. The T1 (solitary lesion) category is intended for the skin involvement with a single discrete tumor without morphological appearance of coalescence (merging of more than 1 lesion). The definitions of body regions are given below. For extremities,

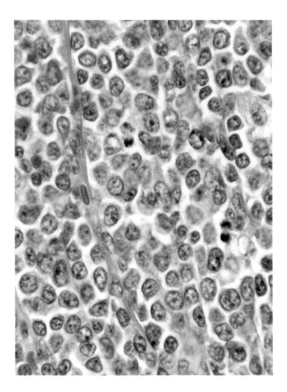

Figure 22.8 Primary cutaneous large B-cell lymphoma, leg-type. Neoplastic cells are primarily round, very uniform in appearance, and infiltrate in diffuse, cohesive sheets. (Hematoxylin and eosin).

left and right serve as separate body sites to define the specific regions. Thus, involvement of left and right arms defines 2 non-contiguous body regions (T3a). The 'regional, T2' designation is intended to describe the skin presentations where the tumors are confined in 1 or 2 contiguous body regions, whereas the 'T3' designation is intended for skin presentations that are more generalized with either extensive (3 or more body regions) or distant (2 *non*-contiguous body regions) skin involvement. In the cases of T2 and T3 designations, the morphological distribution of tumor lesions can be either discrete/separate or clustered/grouped/coalescent. It is recommended to track the type of morphological distribution and the specific body regions that are involved for prospective analysis of survival and treatment outcome.

T1 Solitary skin lesions:
T1a a solitary lesion ≤5 cm diameter

Table 22.2   Diagnostic approach for cutaneous lymphomas

Procedure	Technique	Comments
History	Type, duration and extent of cutaneous lesions	
Clinical examination	Exact cutaneous examination (perhaps with evaluation form, photo documentation or use of Tumor Burden Index[43]), lymph node evaluation, palpation of liver and spleen	
Imaging studies	Abdominal and lymph node sonography Chest X-ray or CT	Not needed for MF (stage I) or lymphomatoid papulosis
Laboratory examination	Complete routine examination (ESR, CBC with differential, LFT, renal values, LDH, electrolytes)	*For B-cell lymphomas:* • Bone marrow biopsy • Serum and urine immunoelectrophoresis *For T-cell lymphomas:* • Blood smear searching for Sézary cells • If SS is suspected: CD4/CD8 ratio, number of CD4+CD7– cells, clonality studies in blood (Southern blot or PCR) • Bone marrow biopsy usually not indicated
Biopsy	Routine histology Immunohistology As needed, biopsies of enlarged lymph nodes or internal organs where involvement is suspected	Molecular biological studies: *For B-cell lymphomas:* • IgH PCR using consensus primers for Fr I, II, & III *For T-cell lymphomas:* • PCR for the T-cell receptor γ-chain

Table 22.3   TNM staging[44] for mycosis fungoides and Sézary syndrome

Category	Definition
T: Skin	
T0	Clinically and/or histologically suspicious changes
T1	Dermatitic patches, plaques: <10% of body surface
T2	Dermatitic patches, plaques: >10% of body surface
T3	Tumors (more than one)
T4	Erythroderma
N: Lymph nodes	
N0	Non-palpable lymph nodes
N1	Palpable lymph nodes; histologically no suggestion of T-cell lymphoma
N2	Non-palpable lymph nodes; histologically T-cell lymphoma
N3	Palpable lymph nodes; histologically T-cell lymphoma
B: Peripheral blood	
B0	No atypical lymphocytes in peripheral blood (<5%)
B1	Atypical lymphocytes in peripheral blood (>5%)
M: Visceral organs	
M0	No involvement of visceral organs
M1	Histologically proven involvement of visceral organs

T1b   a solitary lesion >5 cm diameter

T2   Regional skin involvement: Multiple lesions limited to one body region or two contiguous body regions (see Definitions of body regions below)

T2a   all disease encompassing in a ≤15 cm diameter circular area

T2b   all disease encompassing in a >15 and ≤30 cm diameter circular area

T2c   all disease encompassing in a >30 cm diameter circular area

T3   Generalized skin involvement:
Multiple lesions involving 2 non-contiguous or ≥3 body regions
T3a   multiple lesions involving 2 non-contiguous body regions
T3b   multiple lesions involving ≥3 body regions

Definition of body regions

Head & Neck
Inferior border – superior border of clavicles, T1 spinous process

Chest
Superior border – superior border of clavicles
Inferior border – inferior margin of rib cage
Lateral borders – mid-axillary lines, gleno-humeral joints (inclusive of axillae)

Abdomen/genitals
Superior border – inferior margin of rib cage
Inferior border – inguinal folds, anterior perineum
Lateral borders – mid-axillary lines

Upper back
Superior border – T1 spinous process
Inferior border – inferior margin of rib cage
Lateral borders – mid-axillary lines

Lower back/buttocks
Superior border – inferior margin of rib cage
Inferior border – inferior gluteal fold, anterior perineum (inclusive of perineum)
Lateral borders – mid-axillary lines

Each upper arm
Superior borders – gleno-humeral joints (exclusive of axillae)
Inferior borders – ulnar/radial-humeral (elbow) joint

Each lower arm/hand
Superior borders – ulnar/radial-humeral (elbow) joint

Each upper leg (thigh)
Superior borders – inguinal folds, inferior gluteal folds
Inferior borders – mid-patellae, mid-popliteal fossae

Each lower leg/foot
Superior borders – mid-patellae, mid-popliteal fossae

N Classification

Since it is implicit in the definition of primary cutaneous lymphoma that extracutaneous disease (lymph node or visceral) is absent, all patients are N0 at presentation. However, to permit application of the staging system at the time of relapse (as a relapse-stage designation) or disease progression, the N classification is defined as follows: it is required that lymph node involvement be documented by histological evaluation (fine needle aspiration [FNA] or biopsy) from at least one site of clinical involvement whenever feasible.

N0   No clinical or pathological lymph node involvement

N1   Involvement of one peripheral lymph node region (see Definition of lymph node regions below) that drains an area of current or prior skin involvement

N2   Involvement of two or more peripheral lymph node regions (see Definition of lymph node regions below) or involvement of any lymph node region that does not drain an area of current or prior skin involvement

N3   Involvement of central lymph nodes

Definition of lymph node regions is consistent with the Ann Arbor system47

Peripheral sites = antecubital, cervical, supraclavicular, axillary, inguinal-femoral, and popliteal
Central sites = mediastinal, pulmonary hilar, para-aortic, iliac

M Classification

Since it is implicit in the definition of primary cutaneous lymphoma that extracutaneous disease (lymph node or visceral) is absent, all patients are M0 at presentation. However, to permit application of the staging system at the time of relapse (as a relapse-stage designation) or disease progression, the M classification is defined as follows: it is strongly recommended that visceral involvement be documented by histological evaluation from at least one site of clinical involvement whenever feasible.

M0 No evidence of extracutaneous non-lymph node disease

M1 Extracutaneous non-lymph node disease present

THERAPY

Most CLs are indolent neoplasms with a very wide variation in clinical presentations. In early stages, they affect the quality of life due to their impact on skin appearance and annoying symptoms such as pruritus. In some cases, depending on the quality of skin involvement and the areas involved, they can already be disfiguring in early disease stages. In advanced stages, local skin problems are accompanied by systemic deviations of the immune reaction pattern, which result in an increased risk of infections and secondary malignancies. It is important to note that some of the late-stage problems in CL patients might have been aggravated by earlier therapeutic interventions. For example, radiotherapy or phototherapy may contribute to mutations that increase the proliferative and invasive capacity of the tumor cell populations. Cytotoxic drugs favor infectious complications. Most patients with advanced disease do not die due to lymphoma manifestations but due to secondary problems such as infections.

The patient population suffering from CL is of advanced age. These patients have many concomitant medical problems such as hypertension, heart failure, diabetes, and other diseases. Since the current literature does not demonstrate any curative treatment options, a realistic goal for CL treatment is to achieve long-lasting remissions in a significant percentage of patients with drugs that can be safely used over a certain period of time without long-term toxicity. Many clinical studies dealing with the therapy of CL are difficult, if not impossible, to evaluate because of changing classification schemes and staging systems which are not appropriate for cutaneous disease. For these reasons, high-quality prospective randomized therapeutic trials using generally accepted diagnostic criteria and uniform description of skin involvement and staging are urgently needed.

Based on the current knowledge, initial therapy should be skin-directed. If the disease is not sufficiently controlled, systemic biological therapy can be added. Aggressive polychemotherapy is rarely adequate.

Therapy of cutaneous T-cell lymphomas

Mycosis fungoides, follicular mucinosis, and pagetoid reticulosis

A stage-adjusted, conservative therapeutic approach is recommended for MF and its variants (level of evidence III). In a prospective study, 103 patients with MF were randomized to receive either total skin electron beam therapy (TSEBT) in a dosage of 30 Gy combined with chemotherapy or various topical treatments, adjusted to the stage of disease, including phototherapy and mechlorethamine (nitrogen mustard; HN2). In more advanced stages, both radiation therapy and methotrexate (MTX) were employed. This study showed, as expected, a higher response rate in the group treated with TSEBT and chemotherapy, but also identified serious side effects and showed no difference in the overall survival rate.[48]

In earlier studies, favored treatments were topical measures such as topical corticosteroids, PUVA (psoralen plus UVA), topical cytostatic agents such as mechlorethamine (HN2)[49] and BCNU (carmustine),[50] or radiation therapy with electron beam or soft X-rays.[51] The topical cytostatic agents are popular in the USA and Scandinavia, but not often used in central Europe, where PUVA is the favored option.

In advanced stages, combined topical and systemic therapy is often employed; e.g. a combination of PUVA with systemic retinoids or recombinant interferon-α (IFN-α) (Table 22.4).

In another randomized multicenter study, patients with stage I and II MF and pleomorphic TCL were treated with IFN-α (9 million units 3× weekly) combined with PUVA or with acitretin (Neotigason) (25 mg daily in the first week, then 50 mg daily). Both the rate of complete remission (70%) as well as the time for remission were better for the IFN-α and PUVA group. The IFN-α and acitretin groups achieved 38% complete remission[52] (Table 22.4). In the follow-up randomized study, PUVA plus IFN-α was compared with

Table 22.4 Therapy recommendations for MF, MF variants, and pagetoid reticulosis

Stage	Recommended therapy		Comments
	First-line therapy	Second-line therapy	
I A	PUVA[54] Topical corticosteroids class III-IV[55] Topical HN2/BCNU[49,50] UVB/UVB narrow band[56-58]	Bexarotene gel[59] Hexadecylphosphocoline solution[60] methotrexate	PUVA favored in Europe
Unilesional MF	Radiation therapy (soft X-rays or electron beam, total dose 30–40 Gy; 2 Gy 5× weekly)[61-64]	Topical PUVA Intralesional IFN Topical corticosteroids class III-IV	These disorders represent special presentation forms of CTCL in stage IA
Pagetoid reticulosis			
I B–II A	PUVA Topical HN2/BCNU[49,50]	PUVA + IFN-α[52,65-67] Oral bexarotene[68]	
II B	PUVA + IFN-α[52,65-67] and radiation therapy for tumors Topical HN2/BCNU[49,50]	Low-dose methotrexate Oral bexarotene[69] Total body electron beam[70,71] Denileukin diftitox[72]	
III[a]	PUVA + IFN-α[52,65-67] Topical HN2/BCNU[49,50] Extracorporeal photopheresis[73-78]	Low-dose methotrexate[79] Oral bexarotene[69] Total body electron beam[70,71] Chlorambucil/corticosteroids[80] Low-dose long-distance (2 m) soft X-rays[63]	
IV A	PUVA + IFN-α[52,65-67] Extracorporeal photopheresis[73-78] Perhaps combined with IFN or methotrexate	Low-dose methotrexate[79] Oral bexarotene[69] Total body electron beam[70,71] Chlorambucil /corticosteroids[80] Low-dose long-distance (2 m) soft X-rays[63]	
IV B	PUVA + IFN-α[52,65-67] Chlorambucil/corticosteroids[80] Liposomal doxorubicin[81] Soft X-rays or electron beam for tumors	Oral bexarotene[69], gemcitabine[82] CHOP polychemotherapy[83] Denileukin diftitox[72]	Maintenance therapy with PUVA+IFN-α when remission is achieved

[a] Erythrodermic MF.

PUVA alone. The group receiving retinoids required significantly less UVA and had longer remission times. The response rate for stage I-IIa CTCL was around 80%. Whereas the combination of PUVA with IFN-α does not increase the remission rate, it produces quicker healing and a longer remission time.

Localized forms of MF such as pagetoid reticulosis are best treated with radiation therapy – soft X-rays (12–20 Gy total dose, 2 Gy 2× weekly for 3–5 weeks) or electron beam (30–40 Gy) (see Table 22.4).[53]

Lymphomatoid papulosis and large cell CD30+ CTCL

Primary cutaneous CD30+ lymphoproliferative disorders have an excellent prognosis, in contrast to nodal CD30+ lymphomas.[84] Both lymphomatoid papulosis and the nodules of large cell CD30+ CTCL often spontaneously regress, healing with scarring. The therapeutic recommendations are given in Tables 22.5 and 22.6. Although the use of PUVA in these disorders has not been examined in a large study, various centers have had success with small numbers of patients using this modality.

Sézary syndrome

Many retrospective studies on the treatment of SS contain inadequate information on the diagnostic criteria and staging of the disease,[11] making a comparison of the therapeutic options impossible (Table 22.7).

Table 22.5 Therapy recommendations for lymphomatoid papulosis

Degree of involvement	First-line therapy	Second-line therapy
Solitary or localized lesions	Excision Observation[13] Observation PUVA[85–89] Methotrexate up to 20 mg/weekly[13,90]	IFN[91,92] IFN + retinoid[93] Bexarotene[94]

Table 22.6 Therapy recommendations for large cell CD30+ CTCL (level of evidence III)[13]

Degree of involvement	First-line therapy	Second-line therapy
Solitary or localized lesions	Excision Radiation therapy	Methotrexate[13, 90] perhaps IFN
Multifocal lesions without spontaneous remission	Methotrexate[13, 90]	Radiation therapy, perhaps IFN

Table 22.7 Therapy recommendations for Sézary syndrome

First-line therapy	Second-line therapy
PUVA + IFN[65, 66] Extracorporeal photopheresis[74–78] HN2[49]	Bexarotene[69] Chlorambucil/corticosteroids[80] Low-dose methotrexate[79] CHOP polychemotherapy[83] Denileukin diftitox[72] Total skin electron beam therapy[71]

Therapy of CBCL

Low-grade primary cutaneous B-cell lymphoma (follicular lymphoma, marginal zone lymphoma)

The low-grade CBCL are morphologically similar to MALT lymphomas and therefore described by some authors as SALT (skin-associated lymphoid tissue) lymphomas. The prognosis of these tumors is in general very favorable.[95,96] In those cases in which infectious agents (such as *Borrelia burgdorferi* DNA) can be identified, an initial therapeutic try with broad-spectrum antibiotics is recommended.[97] Since the identification of borrelial DNA can give false-negative results and is ery time-consuming, we recommend giving each patient in this group a trial of doxycycline (100 mg twice a day for 3 weeks) and assessing the clinical response. Distinguishing between low-grade CBCL and reactive B-cell pseudolymphomas can be quite difficult; even clonality studies cannot separate the two entities with

certainty. The therapeutic recommendations are given in Table 22.8. Rituximab should only be employed in those cases in which CD20 expression has been proven histologically.

Large cell B-cell lymphoma

This group of CBCL has a worse prognosis than those with follicular differentiation.[108] There are no large studies dealing with these tumors, making the formulation of guidelines difficult. Our suggestions are given in Table 22.9.

Therapy of non-T- and non-B-cell lymphomas

In general, aggressive polychemotherapy regimens are recommended, although no large studies or therapeutic comparisons are available.

Experimental approaches

Since there are few therapeutic approaches accepted by the authorities and due to the rareness of the disease, CTCLs are promising model neoplasias for new drugs.

Most CTCLs are characterized by immune deviations. There is a proven shift of T-cell responses to a so-called T helper-2 type. Consequently, immunomodulation will correct this immunological dysbalance. Currently, several drugs are used, including retinoids (e.g. bexarotene) and interferons (conventional interferons or pegylated interferons).

Table 22.8 Therapy recommendations for low-grade primary cutaneous B-cell lymphoma (follicular lymphoma, marginal zone lymphoma)

Degree of involvement	First-line therapy	Second-line therapy
Solitary lesions	Excision[98] Antibiotics[98] Radiation therapy[99,100]	Intralesional rituximab[101,102] Intralesional corticosteroids
Multiple lesions	Antibiotics[98] Radiation therapy[99,100,103]	Intralesional IFN-α[104] Intralesional rituximab[101,102] Intravenous rituximab[105-107]

Table 22.9 Therapy recommendations for large cell CBCL

Degree of involvement	First-line therapy	Second-line therapy
Solitary or localized lesions	Radiation therapy Excision	
Multiple lesions	Monochemotherapy (for example, liposomal doxorubicin) Polychemotherapy (for example, CHOP)	Chemotherapy + rituximab

In addition, the toll-like receptor agonist imiquimod can be used locally. A more modern approach is the application of gene therapy approaches. There is substantial experience using a recombinant adenoviral vector encoding for the cytokine interferon-γ. This substance induced the regression of very various CTCL lesions after intralesional injection.[109] Another promising substance is the heterodimeric cytokine interleukin-12, which can be used systemically or locally.[110]

Histone deacetylases increase gene transcription and are promising targets for therapy. Two histone deacetylase inhibitors are currently being studied in CTCL: FR-901228, a cyclic peptide; and suberanilohydroxamic acid (SAHA). Both compounds are undergoing phase II investigation. SAHA has recently been registered for advanced CTCL.

Currently, a number of other new substances, including forodesine (a purine nucleoside phosphorylase inhibitor) and APO 866 (a specific inhibitor of niacinamide phosphoribosyltransferase), have shown significant efficacy in animal models and early trials. CTCL are model tumors for other lymphoproliferative malignancies.

FOLLOW-UP

The interval between visits for patients with CLs must be adjusted to the clinical findings. In those with early disease (stage Ia, Ib), evaluation every 6–12 months is reasonable. In advanced disease (stage III-IV), the patient must often be checked every 4–6 weeks to assess the therapeutic response.

REFERENCES

1. Weinstock MA. Epidemiology of mycosis fungoides. Semin Dermatol 1994; 13(3): 154–9.
2. Kempf W, Dummer R, Burg G. Klinische und therapeutische Besonderheiten kutaner Lymphome. Dt Ärztebl 2001; 98(11): A697–703.
3. Burg G, Dummer R, Kerl H. Classification of cutaneous lymphomas. Derm Clinics 1994; 12: 213–17.
4. Urosevic M, Conrad C, Kamarashev J, et al. CD4+CD56+ hematodermic neoplasms bear a plasmacytoid dendritic cell phenotype. Hum Pathol 2005; 36(9): 1020–4.
5. Massone C, Kodama K, Kerl H, Cerroni L. Histopathologic features of early (patch) lesions of mycosis fungoides: a morphologic study on 745 biopsy specimens from 427 patients. Am J Surg Pathol 2005; 29(4): 550–60.
6. Pimpinelli N, Olsen EA, Santucci M, et al. Defining early mycosis fungoides. J Am Acad Dermatol 2005; 53(6): 1053–63.

7. Bonta MD, Tannous ZS, Demierre MF, et al. Rapidly progressing mycosis fungoides presenting as follicular mucinosis. J Am Acad Dermatol 2000; 43(4): 635–40.

8. Thurber SE, Zhang B, Kim YH, et al. T-cell clonality analysis in biopsy specimens from two different skin sites shows high specificity in the diagnosis of patients with suggested mycosis fungoides. J Am Acad Dermatol 2007; 57(5): 789–90.

9. Mao X, Orchard G, Vonderheid EC, et al. Heterogeneous abnormalities of CCND1 and RB1 in primary cutaneous T-cell lymphomas suggesting impaired cell cycle control in disease pathogenesis. J Invest Dermatol 2006; 126(6): 1388–95.

10. Smoller BR, Santucci M, Wood GS, Whittaker SJ. Histopathology and genetics of cutaneous T-cell lymphoma. Hematol Oncol Clin North Am 2003; 17(6): 1277–311.

11. Vonderheid EC, Bernengo MG, Burg G, et al. Update on erythrodermic cutaneous T-cell lymphoma: report of the International Society for Cutaneous Lymphomas. J Am Acad Dermatol 2002; 46(1): 95–106.

12. Trotter MJ, Whittaker SJ, Orchard GE, Smith NP. Cutaneous histopathology of Sézary syndrome: a study of 41 cases with a proven circulating T-cell clone. J Cutan Pathol 1997; 24(5): 286–91.

13. Bekkenk MW, Geelen FA, van Voorst Vader PC, et al. Primary and secondary cutaneous CD30(+) lymphoproliferative disorders: a report from the Dutch Cutaneous Lymphoma Group on the long-term follow-up data of 219 patients and guidelines for diagnosis and treatment. Blood 2000; 95(12): 3653–61.

14. Burg G, Kempf W, Kazakov DV, et al. Pyogenic lymphoma of the skin: a peculiar variant of primary cutaneous neutrophil-rich CD30+ anaplastic large-cell lymphoma. Clinicopathological study of four cases and review of the literature. Br J Dermatol 2003; 148(3): 580–6.

15. Paulli M, Berti E, Rosso R, et al. CD30/Ki-1-positive lymphoproliferative disorders of the skin – clinicopathologic correlation and statistical analysis of 86 cases: a multicentric study from the European Organization for Research and Treatment of Cancer Cutaneous Lymphoma Project Group. J Clin Oncol 1995; 13(6): 1343–54.

16. Kumar S, Krenacs L, Medeiros J, et al. Subcutaneous panniculitic T-cell lymphoma is a tumor of cytotoxic T lymphocytes. Hum Pathol 1998; 29(4): 397–403.

17. Magro CM, Crowson AN, Kovatich AJ, Burns F. Lupus profundus, indeterminate lymphocytic lobular panniculitis and subcutaneous T-cell lymphoma: a spectrum of subcuticular T-cell lymphoid dyscrasia. J Cutan Pathol 2001; 28(5): 235–47.

18. Gonzalez CL, Medeiros LJ, Braziel RM, Jaffe ES. T-cell lymphoma involving subcutaneous tissue. A clinicopathologic entity commonly associated with hemophagocytic syndrome. Am J Surg Pathol 1991; 15(1): 17–27.

19. Salhany KE, Macon WR, Choi JK, et al. Subcutaneous panniculitis-like T-cell lymphoma: clinicopathologic, immunophenotypic, and genotypic analysis of alpha/beta and gamma/delta subtypes. Am J Surg Pathol 1998; 22(7): 881–93.

20. Arnulf B, Copie-Bergman C, Delfau-Larue MH, et al. Nonhepatosplenic gammadelta T-cell lymphoma: a subset of cytotoxic lymphomas with mucosal or skin localization. Blood 1998; 91(5): 1723–31.

21. Toro JR, Beaty M, Sorbara L, et al. Gamma delta T-cell lymphoma of the skin: a clinical, microscopic, and molecular study. Arch Dermatol 2000; 136(8): 1024–32.

22. Toro JR, Liewehr DJ, Pabby N, et al. Gamma-delta T-cell phenotype is associated with significantly decreased survival in cutaneous T-cell lymphoma. Blood 2003; 101(9): 3407–12.

23. Jones D, Vega F, Sarris AH, Medeiros LJ. CD4-CD8-"Double-negative" cutaneous T-cell lymphomas share common histologic features and an aggressive clinical course. Am J Surg Pathol 2002; 26(2): 225–31.

24. Berti E, Tomasini D, Vermeer MH, et al. Primary cutaneous CD8-positive epidermotropic cytotoxic T cell lymphomas. A distinct clinicopathological entity with an aggressive clinical behavior. Am J Pathol 1999; 155(2): 483–92.

25. Bekkenk MW, Vermeer MH, Jansen PM, et al. Peripheral T-cell lymphomas unspecified presenting in the skin: analysis of prognostic factors in a group of 82 patients. Blood 2003; 102(6): 2213–19.

26. Lee SC, Berg KD, Racke FK, Griffin CA, Eshleman JR. Pseudo-spikes are common in histologically benign lymphoid tissues. J Mol Diagn 2000; 2(3): 145–52.

27. Weiss LM, Wood GS, Ellisen LW, Reynolds TC, Sklar J. Clonal T-cell populations in pityriasis lichenoides et varioliformis acuta (Mucha–Habermann disease). Am J Pathol 1987; 126(3): 417–21.

28. Mirza I, Macpherson N, Paproski S, et al. Primary cutaneous follicular lymphoma: an assessment of clinical, histopathologic, immunophenotypic, and molecular features. J Clin Oncol 2002; 20(3): 647–55.

29. Goodlad JR, Krajewski AS, Batstone PJ, et al. Primary cutaneous follicular lymphoma: a clinicopathologic and molecular study of 16 cases in support of a distinct entity. Am J Surg Pathol 2002; 26(6): 733–41.

30. Kim BK, Surti U, Pandya A, et al. Clinicopathologic, immunophenotypic, and molecular cytogenetic fluorescence in situ hybridization analysis of primary and secondary cutaneous follicular lymphomas. Am J Surg Pathol 2005; 29(1): 69–82.

31. Cerroni L, Zochling N, Putz B, Kerl H. Infection by Borrelia burgdorferi and cutaneous B-cell lymphoma. J Cutan Pathol 1997; 24(8): 457–61.

32. Li C, Inagaki H, Kuo TT, et al. Primary cutaneous marginal zone B-cell lymphoma: a molecular and clinicopathologic study of 24 Asian cases. Am J Surg Pathol 2003; 27(8): 1061–9.

33. Schmid U, Eckert F, Griesser H, et al. Cutaneous follicular lymphoid hyperplasia with monotypic plasma cells. A clinicopathologic study of 18 patients. Am J Surg Pathol 1995; 19(1): 12–20.

34. Gronbaek K, Ralfkiaer E, Kalla J, Skovgaard GL, Guldberg P. Infrequent somatic Fas mutations but no evidence of Bcl10 mutations or t(11;18) in primary cutaneous MALT-type lymphoma. J Pathol 2003; 201(1): 134–40.

35. Hallermann C, Kaune KM, Gesk S, et al. Molecular cytogenetic analysis of chromosomal breakpoints in the IGH, MYC, BCL6, and MALT1 gene loci in primary cutaneous B-cell lymphomas. J Invest Dermatol 2004; 123(1): 213–19.

36. Palmedo G, Hantschke M, Rutten A, et al. Primary cutaneous marginal zone B-cell lymphoma may exhibit both the t(14;18)(q32;q21) IGH/BCL2 and the t(14;18) (q32;q21) IGH/MALT1 translocation: an indicator for clonal transformation towards higher-grade B-cell lymphoma? Am J Dermatopathol 2007; 29(3): 231–6.

37. Hans CP, Weisenburger DD, Greiner TC, et al. Confirmation of the molecular classification of diffuse large B-cell lymphoma by immunohistochemistry using a tissue microarray. Blood 2004; 103(1): 275–82.

38. Grange F, Petrella T, Beylot-Barry M, et al. Bcl-2 protein expression is the strongest independent prognostic factor of survival in primary cutaneous large B-cell lymphomas. Blood 2004; 103(10): 3662–8.

39. Paulli M, Viglio A, Vivenza D, et al. Primary cutaneous large B-cell lymphoma of the leg: histogenetic analysis of a controversial clinicopathologic entity. Hum Pathol 2002; 33(9): 937–43.

40. Senff NJ, Hoefnagel JJ, Jansen PM, et al. Reclassification of 300 primary cutaneous B-cell lymphomas according to the new WHO-EORTC classification for cutaneous lymphomas: comparison with previous classifications and identification of prognostic markers. J Clin Oncol 2007; 25(12): 1581–7.

41. Hoefnagel JJ, Dijkman R, Basso K, et al. Distinct types of primary cutaneous large B-cell lymphoma identified by gene expression profiling. Blood 2005; 105(9): 3671–8.

42. Wood GS, Tung RM, Haeffner AC, et al. Detection of clonal T-cell receptor gamma gene rearrangements in early mycosis fungoides/Sézary syndrome by polymerase chain reaction and denaturing gradient gel electrophoresis (PCR/DGGE). J Invest Dermatol 1994; 103: 34–41.

43. Dummer R, Nestle F, Wiede J, et al. Coincidence of increased soluble interleukin-2 receptors, diminished natural killer cell activity and progressive disease in cutaneous T-cell lymphomas. Eur J Dermatol 1991; 1: 135–8.

44. Bunn PA Jr, Lamberg SI. Report of the Committee on Staging and Classification of Cutaneous T-Cell Lymphomas. Cancer Treat Rep 1979; 63(4): 725–8.

45. Kerl H, Sterry W. Classification and staging. In: Burg G, Sterry W, eds. EORTC/BMFT Cutaneous Lymphoma Project Group: Recommendations for Staging and Therapy of Cutaneous Lymphomas. Brussels: European Organization for Research in Treatment of Cancer, 1987: 1–10.

46. Kim YH, Willemze R, Pimpinelli N, et al. TNM classification system for primary cutaneous lymphomas other than mycosis fungoides and Sézary syndrome: a proposal of the International Society for Cutaneous Lymphomas (ISCL) and the Cutaneous Lymphoma Task Force for the European Organization for Research and Treatment of Cancer (EORTC). Blood 2007; 110(2): 479–84.

47. American Joint Committee on Cancer (AJCC). AJCC Cancer Staging Manual, 6th edn. New York: Springer, 2002.

48. Kaye FJ, Bunn PJ, Steinberg SM, et al. A randomized trial comparing combination electron-beam radiation and chemotherapy with topical therapy in the initial treatment of mycosis fungoides. N Engl J Med 1989; 321(26): 1784–90.

49. Vonderheid EC, Tan ET, Kantor AF, et al. Long-term efficacy, curative potential, and carcinogenicity of topical mechlorethamine chemotherapy in cutaneous T cell lymphoma. J Am Acad Dermatol 1989; 20(3): 416–28.

50. Zackheim HS, Epstein EJ, Crain WR. Topical carmustine (BCNU) for cutaneous T cell lymphoma: a 15-year experience in 143 patients. J Am Acad Dermatol 1990; 22: 802–10.

51. Dummer R, Häffner AC, Hess M, Burg G. A rational approach to the therapy of cutaneous T-cell lymphomas. Onkologie 1996; 19: 226–30.

52. Stadler R, Otte HG, Luger T, et al. Prospective randomized multicenter clinical trial on the use of interferon-2a plus acitretin versus interferon-2a plus PUVA in patients with cutaneous T-cell lymphoma stages I and II. Blood 1998; 92(10): 3578–81.

53. Trautinger F, Knobler R, Willemze R, et al. EORTC consensus recommendations for the treatment of mycosis fungoides/Sézary syndrome. Eur J Cancer 2006; 42(8): 1014–30.

54. Honigsmann H, Brenner W, Rauschmeier W, Konrad K, Wolff K. Photochemotherapy for cutaneous T cell lymphoma. A follow-up study. J Am Acad Dermatol 1984; 10(2 Pt 1): 238–45.

55. Zackheim HS, Kashani Sabet M, Amin S. Topical corticosteroids for mycosis fungoides. Experience in 79 patients. Arch Dermatol 1998; 134(8): 949–54.

56. Ramsay DL, Lish KM, Yalowitz CB, Soter NA. Ultraviolet-B phototherapy for early-stage cutaneous T-cell lymphoma. Arch Dermatol 1992; 128(7): 931–3.

57. Hofer A, Cerroni L, Kerl H, Wolf P. Narrowband (311-nm) UV-B therapy for small plaque parapsoriasis and early-stage mycosis fungoides. Arch Dermatol 1999; 135(11): 1377–80.

58. Clark C, Dawe RS, Evans AT, Lowe G, Ferguson J. Narrowband TL-01 phototherapy for patch-stage mycosis fungoides. Arch Dermatol 2000; 136(6): 748–52.

59. Breneman D, Duvic M, Kuzel T, et al. Phase 1 and 2 trial of bexarotene gel for skin-directed treatment of patients with cutaneous T-cell lymphoma. Arch Dermatol 2002; 138(3): 325–32.

60. Dummer R, Krasovec M, Röger J, Sindermann H, Burg G. Topical application of hexadecylphosphocholine in patients with cutaneous lymphomas: results of a phase I/II study. J Am Acad Dermatol 1993; 29(12): 963–70.

61. Hodak E, Phenig E, Amichai B, et al. Unilesional mycosis fungoides: a study of seven cases. Dermatology 2000; 201(4): 300–6.

62. Heald PW, Glusac EJ. Unilesional cutaneous T-cell lymphoma: clinical features, therapy, and follow-up of 10 patients with a treatment-responsive mycosis fungoides variant. J Am Acad Dermatol 2000; 42(2 Pt 1): 283–5.

63. Goldschmidt H. Radiation therapy of other cutaneous tumors. In: Goldschmidt H, Panizzon R, eds. Modern Dermatologic Radiation Therapy. New York: Springer Verlag, 1991: 123–32.

64. Cerroni L, Fink Puches R, El Shabrawi Caelen L, et al. Solitary skin lesions with histopathologic features of early mycosis fungoides. Am J Dermatopathol 1999; 21(6): 518–24.

65. Rajan G, Seifert B, Prümmer O, et al. Incidence and in-vivo relevance of anti-interferon antibodies during treatment of low-grade cutaneous T-cell lymphomas with interferon-alpha2a combined with acetretin or PUVA. Arch Derm Res 1996; 288: 543–8.

66. Kuzel TM, Roenigk HH Jr, Samuelson E, et al. Effectiveness of interferon alfa-2a combined with phototherapy for mycosis fungoides and the Sézary syndrome. J Clin Oncol 1995; 13(1): 257–63.

67. Roenigk H, Kuzel TM, Skoutelis AP, et al. Photochemotherapy alone or combined with interferon alpha-2a in the treatment of cutaneous T-cell lymphoma. J Invest Dermatol 1990; 95: 198S-205S.

68. Duvic M, Martin AG, Kim Y, et al. Phase 2 and 3 clinical trial of oral bexarotene (Targretin capsules) for the treatment of refractory or persistent early-stage cutaneous T-cell lymphoma. Arch Dermatol 2001; 137(5): 581–93.

69. Duvic M, Hymes K, Heald P, et al. Bexarotene is effective and safe for treatment of refractory advanced-stage cutaneous T-cell lymphoma: multinational phase II-III trial results. J Clin Oncol 2001; 19(9): 2456–71.

70. Chinn DM, Chow S, Kim YH, Hoppe RT. Total skin electron beam therapy with or without adjuvant topical nitrogen mustard or nitrogen mustard alone as initial treatment of T2 and T3 mycosis fungoides. Int J Radiat Oncol Biol Phys 1999; 43(5): 951–8.

71. Jones GW, Rosenthal D, Wilson LD. Total skin electron radiation for patients with erythrodermic cutaneous T-cell lymphoma (mycosis fungoides and the Sézary syndrome). Cancer 1999; 85(9): 1985–95.

72. Olsen E, Duvic M, Frankel A, et al. Pivotal phase III trial of two dose levels of denileukin diftitox for the treatment of cutaneous T-cell lymphoma. J Clin Oncol 2001; 19(2): 376–88.

73. Kirova YM, Piedbois Y, Pan Q, Guo L, Le Bourgeois JP. [Radiotherapy of cutaneous lymphomas]; Cancer Radiother 1999; 3(2): 105–11. [in French]

74. Fraser Andrews E, Seed P, Whittaker S, Russell Jones R. Extracorporeal photopheresis in Sézary syndrome. No significant effect in the survival of 44 patients with a peripheral blood T-cell clone. Arch Dermatol 1998; 134(8): 1001–5.

75. Heald P, Rook A, Perez M, et al. Treatment of erythrodermic cutaneous T-cell lymphoma with extracorporeal photochemotherapy. J Am Acad Dermatol 1992; 27(3): 427–33.

76. Knobler R, Girardi M. Extracorporeal photochemoimmunotherapy in cutaneous T cell lymphomas. Ann N Y Acad Sci 2001; 941: 123–38.

77. Russell Jones R. Extracorporeal photopheresis in cutaneous T-cell lymphoma. Inconsistent data underline the need for randomized studies. Br J Dermatol 2000; 142(1): 16–21.

78. Stevens SR, Bowen GM, Duvic M, et al. Effectiveness of photopheresis in Sézary syndrome. Arch Dermatol 1999; 135(8): 995–7.

79. Zackheim HS, Epstein EH Jr. Low-dose methotrexate for the Sézary syndrome. J Am Acad Dermatol 1989; 21(4 Pt 1): 757–62.

80. Coors EA, von den Driesch P. Treatment of erythrodermic cutaneous T-cell lymphoma with intermittent chlorambucil and fluocortolone therapy. Br J Dermatol 2000; 143(1): 127–31.

81. Wollina U, Graefe T, Kaatz M. Pegylated doxorubicin for primary cutaneous T cell lymphoma: a report on ten patients with follow-up. Ann N Y Acad Sci 2001; 941: 214–16.

82. Bunn PJ, Hoffman SJ, Norris D, Golitz LE, Aeling JL. Systemic therapy of cutaneous T-cell lymphomas (mycosis fungoides and the Sézary syndrome). Ann Intern Med 1994; 121(8): 592–602.

83. Fierro MT, Quaglino P, Savoia P, Verrone A, Bernengo MG. Systemic polychemotherapy in the treatment of primary cutaneous lymphomas: a clinical follow-up study of 81 patients treated with COP or CHOP. Leuk Lymphoma 1998; 31(5–6): 583–8.

84. Willemze R, Kerl H, Sterry W, et al. EORTC classification for primary cutaneous lymphomas: a proposal

from the Cutaneous Lymphoma Study Group of the European Organization for Research and Treatment of Cancer. Blood 1997; 90(1): 354–71.

85. Wantzin GL, Thomsen K. PUVA-treatment in lymphomatoid papulosis. Br J Dermatol 1982; 107(6): 687–90.

86. Volkenandt M, Kerscher M, Sander C, Meurer M, Rocken M. PUVA-bath photochemotherapy resulting in rapid clearance of lymphomatoid papulosis in a child. Arch Dermatol 1995; 131(9): 1094.

87. Kowalzick L, Ott A, Waldmann T, Suckow M, Ponnighaus JM. [Therapy of lymphomatoid papulosis with balneo-PUVA-photochemotherapy]. Hautarzt 2000; 51(10): 778–80. [in German]

88. Gambichler T, Maushagen E, Menzel S. Foil bath PUVA in lymphomatoid papulosis. J Eur Acad Dermatol Venereol 1999; 13(1): 63–5.

89. Blondeel A, Knitelius AC, De Coninck A, De Dobbeleer G, Achten G. [Lymphomatoid papulosis improved with PUVA therapy]. Dermatologica 1982; 165(5): 466–8. [in French]

90. Vonderheid EC, Sajjadian A, Kadin ME. Methotrexate is effective therapy for lymphomatoid papulosis and other primary cutaneous CD30-positive lymphoproliferative disorders. J Am Acad Dermatol 1996; 34(3): 470–81.

91. Proctor SJ, Jackson GH, Lennard AL, Marks J. Lymphomatoid papulosis: response to treatment with recombinant interferon alfa-2b. J Clin Oncol 1992; 10(1): 170.

92. Schmuth M, Topar G, Illersperger B, et al. Therapeutic use of interferon-alpha for lymphomatoid papulosis. Cancer 2000; 89(7): 1603–10.

93. Wyss M, Dummer R, Dommann SN, et al. Lymphomatoid papulosis – treatment with recombinant interferon alfa-2a and etretinate. Dermatology 1995; 190: 288–91.

94. Krathen RA, Ward S, Duvic M. Bexarotene is a new treatment option for lymphomatoid papulosis. Dermatology 2003; 206: 142–7.

95. Berti E, Alessi E, Caputo R, et al. Reticulohistiocytoma of the dorsum. J Am Acad Dermatol 1988; 19: 259–272.

96. Burg G, Hess M, Küng E, Dommann S, Dummer R. Semimalignant ("Pseudolymphomatous") cutaneous B-cell lymphomas. Derm Clinics 1994; 12: 399–407.

97. Cerroni L, Zochling N, Putz B, Kerl H. Infection by Borrelia burgdorferi and cutaneous B-cell lymphoma. J Cutan Pathol 1997; 24(8): 457–61.

98. Zenahlik P, Fink Puches R, Kapp KS, Kerl H, Cerroni L. [Therapy of primary cutaneous B-cell lymphoma]. Hautarzt 2000; 51(1): 19–24. [in German]

99. Kirova YM, Piedbois Y, Le Bourgeois JP. Radiotherapy in the management of cutaneous B-cell lymphoma. Our experience in 25 cases. Radiother Oncol 1999; 52(1): 15–18.

100. Piccinno R, Caccialanza M, Berti E. Dermatologic radiotherapy of primary cutaneous follicle center cell lymphoma. Eur J Dermatol 2003; 13: 49–52.

101. Heinzerling L, Dummer R, Kempf W, Hess-Schmid M, Burg G. Intralesional therapy with anti-CD20-antibody in primary cutaneous B-cell lymphoma. Arch Dermatol 2000; 136(3): 374–8.

102. Paul T, Radny P, Krober SM, et al. Intralesional rituximab for cutaneous B-cell lymphoma. Br J Dermatol 2001; 144(6): 1239–43.

103. Voss N, Kim Sing C. Radiotherapy in the treatment of dermatologic malignancies. Dermatol Clin 1998; 16(2): 313–20.

104. Kutting B, Bonsmann G, Metze D, Luger TA, Cerroni L. Borrelia burgdorferi-associated primary cutaneous B cell lymphoma: complete clearing of skin lesions after antibiotic pulse therapy or intralesional injection of interferon alfa-2a. J Am Acad Dermatol 1997; 36(2): 311–14.

105. Heinzerling ML, Urbanek M, Funk JO, et al. Reduction of tumor burden and stablization of disease by systemic therapy with anti-CD20 antibody (rituximab) in patients with primary cutaneous B-cell lymphomas. Cancer 2000; 89: 1835–44.

106. Gellrich S, Muche JM, Pelzer K, Audring H, Sterry W. [Anti-CD20 antibodies in primary cutaneous B-cell lymphoma. Initial results in dermatologic patients]. Hautarzt 2001; 52(3): 205–10. [in German]

107. Sabroe RA, Child FJ, Woolford AJ, Spittle MF, Russell Jones R. Rituximab in cutaneous B-cell lymphoma: a report of two cases. Br J Dermatol 2000; 143(1): 157–61.

108. Grange F, Bekkenk MW, Wechsler J, et al. Prognostic factors in primary cutaneous large B-cell lymphomas: a European multicenter study. J Clin Oncol 2001; 19(16): 3602–10.

109. Dummer R, Hassel JC, Fellenberg F, et al. Adenovirus-mediated intralesional interferon-gamma gene transfer induces tumor regressions in cutaneous lymphomas. Blood 2004; 104(6): 1631–8.

110. Dummer R, Cozzio A, Meier S, et al. Standard and experimental therapy in cutaneous T-cell lymphomas. J Cutan Pathol 2006; 33(Suppl 1): 52–7.

111. Golling P, Cozzio A, Dummer R, French L, Kempf W. Primary cutaneous B-cell lymphoma. Leukemia and Lymphoma 2008 – in press.

Primary extranodal head and neck lymphomas

23

Richard W Tsang, Atto Billio, and Sergio Cortelazzo

INTRODUCTION

Although the head and neck region is identified as a distinct extranodal location in this chapter, it consists of many different organs and tissues that are functionally and embryologically diverse but yet are anatomically close to one another. Therefore, for the purpose of this chapter, this term is applied to stage I and II lymphomas arising from the Waldeyer's ring (lymphoid tissue of the nasopharynx, oropharygeal, and lingual tonsils), salivary glands, nasal and paranasal sinuses, thyroid gland, oral cavity, larynx, and trachea.

Waldeyer's ring is considered in Ann Arbor classification[1] as a lymphatic tissue, and therefore its involvement was not defined as extralymphatic. However, most clinicians distinguish a nodal from an extranodal presentation, rather than lymphatic and extralymphatic sites. Thus, we have included Waldeyer's ring lymphomas within primary extranodal head and neck lymphomas (PEHNL), even if they are not extralymphatic, because their presentation is outside lymph node areas.

The head and neck region is one of the most common sites of extranodal non-Hodgkin's lymphoma (NHL), accounting for 10–20% of all cases of NHL.[2,3] Most cases occur in Waldeyer's ring[4] and the majority of patients are elderly males, with the exception of thyroid lymphomas, in which women predominate. More than half of the patients are in an early stage at presentation and diffuse large B-cell lymphoma (DLBCL) is the most common. The majority of lymphomas are of B-cell origin, but natural killer (NK)/T-cell lymphomas are also found in the nasal cavity or nasopharynx. These lymphomas appear exceedingly rare in Western countries, but are relatively common among Asians and Native Americans of Central and South America.[5]

Epstein–Barr virus (EBV) infection plays a role in the neoplastic transformation, particularly in human immunodeficiency virus (HIV)-infected patients[6] and in other immunocompromised patients.

The majority of PEHNL patient present with symptoms of a local mass or pain. Less commonly, the presentation is in cervical lymph nodes and, rarely, systemic symptoms. The presenting complaints are often indistinguishable from those of patients with epithelial (squamous-type) cancer, which is a more common tumor of this region. A complete clinical evaluation, including direct or indirect laryngoscopy, imaging (computed tomography [CT], and magnetic resonance imaging [MRI]), bone marrow biopsy, and lumbar puncture (paranasal sinuses with unfavorable histology) is essential for defining the extent of the disease and for planning treatment.

Several studies showed that PEHNL prognosis is influenced by age, histological subtype, location of disease, disease bulk, and stage. Recently, it has been reported that a prognostic model, which included stage II within the adverse prognostic factors of International Prognostic Index (IPI), was effective in predicting survival of a large series of patients with aggressive PEHNL.[7]

Long-term results in patients presenting with PEHNL have shown that the prognosis is affected by the site of presentation. Tonsil lymphoma has the best prognosis.[4,8] In another series from Stanford University, the 5-year overall survival varied from 61% for salivary gland location, to 12% for lymphoma arising in paranasal sinuses.[9]

Regarding treatment, the general approach has been based on the standard for nodal lymphomas, which in turn is largely determined by histology and stage. For localized low-grade lymphomas (follicular lymphoma, and mucosa-associated lymphoid tissue [MALT] lymphoma), the widely adopted standard practice is radiation therapy (RT), either given alone or as the main modality of therapy.[10–12] For aggressive-histology lymphoma, the standard treatment is an anthracycline-based chemotherapy regimen followed by involved field radiation therapy.[13] For B-cell lymphomas, promising results have been reported with the use of immunotherapy with anti-CD20 antibody alone or in combination with chemotherapy. Moreover, central nervous system (CNS) prophylaxis appears to be indicated only in patients with localiztion in proximity to meninges (e.g. base of the skull and paranasal sinuses), or for unfavorable histology (lymphoblastic, Burkitt's). In other head and neck locations, it remains a matter of controversy.

WALDEYER'S RING LYMPHOMAS

Waldeyer's ring structures includes the tonsils in the lateral oropharyngeal wall (palatine tonsil), the nasopharyngeal lymphatic tissue, and the lingual tonsil. Waldeyer's ring is the most common head and neck site of involvement by lymphoma, accounting for 50–60% of cases.[3,8,14,15] Involvement of palatine tonsils is more common than the other two locations. B-cell lymphoma predominates, with the most frequent being DLBCL,[3] while follicular lymphoma is uncommon, and MALT lymphoma rare. In a large series of low-grade lymphomas of the Waldeyer's ring, MALT lymphoma accounted for less than 4% of all cases.[16] T-cell lymphomas of the Waldeyer's ring are equally rare. Clinically, median age at presentation varied from 55 to 67 years old[4,8] and patients tend to have a local mass effect causing odynophagia and dysphagia. In the nasopharynx, there is usually nasal or eustachian tube obstruction. Occasionally, cervical lymphadenopathy is the first sign and, if involved, ipsilateral level 2 (high jugular chain) is the most common. Weight loss is often seen, but is usually a consequence of dysphagia rather than a constitutional symptom of the lymphoma, and fever and sweats are rare. In addition to the standard physical examination, direct or indirect visualization of the whole Waldeyer's ring is important, to define the extent of the disease, specifically noting infiltration of surrounding tissues such as the palate, gingiva, larynx, hypopharynx, the laterality of the disease, and adequacy of the airway. In addition to imaging with CT, MRI is often useful to define the extent of involvement. There have been reports of association with gastrointestinal tract involvement,[17] specifically the stomach, and some centers routinely perform gastroscopy as part of staging. The majority of patients, however, will prove to have localized disease, with stage IIE (cervical lymph node involvement) outnumbering stage IE (tonsil involvement only).[8,17]

Although local RT alone (35–50 Gy) results in a high rate of local control, recurrences are frequent and they typically occur in distant sites, with some predilection for the gastrointestinal tract.[17,18] Combined modality therapy (CMT) – anthracycline-based, in combination with rituximab, followed by RT – is the standard treatment for stage I-IIE DLBCL. Previous CMT, before the routine use of rituximab, results in local control rates in excess of 85% and survival rates of 60–75%, depending upon the stage and tumor bulk.[4,8,14,17] With the addition of rituximab, further improvements are expected, as for nodal DLBCL. Location of disease in the tonsil only is a favorable prognostic attribute,[8] as is low bulk disease.[14] A prospective randomized trial by Aviles et al in 316 patients demonstrated the superiority of CMT in this disease, with 5-year failure-free survival rates of 48% for RT alone, 45% for CHOP (cyclophosphamide, doxorubicin, vincristine, prednisone) chemotherapy alone, and 83% for CMT (p <0.001), and confirms CMT as the standard therapeutic approach.[19] It is likely that a small stage IE tonsil lymphoma (<3 cm), without any IPI adverse factors, will be adequately treated with abbreviated (3 cycles) CHOP-R (CHOP+rituximab) chemotherapy, followed by local RT (30–35 Gy) to the ipsilateral tonsil and cervical lymph nodes. Although unproven, this follows the paradigm for equally favorable stage I nodal lymphomas.[20,21]

Low-grade lymphomas consist of follicular lymphomas, and MALT lymphomas, both being B-cell lymphomas. A localized tonsillar presentation is very uncommon but, if confirmed, local RT alone is the treatment of choice (30–35 Gy). Similar to localized nodal follicular lymphomas, local control is expected, but a high rate of sytemic disease recurrence (50% in 5–10 years) is observed.

The traditional radiation target volume includes bilateral tonsillar fossa, nasopharynx, posterior tongue, and bilateral cervical lymph nodes. This can be accomplished with a conventional four-field technique with lateral fields to treat the Waldeyer's ring and upper cervical lymph nodes, matched to two anterior–posterior fields to treat the lower neck. Acute morbidity of irradiation (35–40 Gy) includes xerostomia, loss of taste, mucositis, and dysphagia, which are usually mild to moderate in degree, and recovery in a few weeks. For traditional treatment fields, including most of the parotid salivary glands, some degree of permanent xerostomia is common.[22,23] The use of highly precise intensity-modulated radiation therapy (IMRT) is a preferred alternative, as this allows sparing of the major salivary glands from high-dose radiation and leads to less xerostomia (Figure 23.1). For stage IE, non-bulky involvement of the palatine tonsil where the disease is lateralized and away from the midline structures, following a complete response to 3–6 cycles of chemotherapy, a more limited RT volume may be appropriate. In such cases, a volume to cover just the initially involved tonsil, and its immediate drainage lymph node area on the ipsilateral side is generally accomplished best with an IMRT technique. Radiation doses of 35–40 Gy given in 1.8–2 Gy fractions are within the tolerance of all the critical head and neck tissues such as the spinal cord, neurovascular structures, larynx, trachea, esophagus, and soft tissues. Serious long-term side effects are rare, although hypothyroidism can occur in up to one-third of patients where the thyroid gland may be exposed to radiation directed at lower cervical lymph nodes.

SALIVARY GLAND LYMPHOMAS

Salivary gland lymphomas are the second most common head and neck lymphoma location, and can involve the parotid gland (most frequent), and the submandibular or lingual glands (less frequent). Patients with Sjögren's syndrome are at increased risk, particularly for MALT lymphoma.[24,25] Myoepithelial sialadenitis (MESA) is the characteristic lesion of Sjögren's syndrome, and this histologically benign feature forms the benign counterpart of the morphological spectrum of findings which characterize salivary gland MALT lymphoma: centrocyte-like cells, hyperplastic nodules, and lymphoepithelial lesions. In a study conducted by the International Extranodal Lymphoma Study Group (IELSG), 78% are stage IE at presentation and lymph node involvement is uncommon.[26] There is a tendency for multifocal, and hence bilateral involvement, either at the time of presentation, or metachronously after initial treatment in the subsequent follow-up.[27] These MALT lymphomas generally follow an indolent course and tend to remain localized for prolonged periods of time. A variety of treatment approaches have been used, ranging from surgical excision (superficial parotidectomy), RT, chemotherapy, and rituximab. The 5-year progression-free survival rate was 67%, with overall survival rate of 97% in a series of 46 patients.[26] RT offers excellent local control, with a complete remission rate of 100% and a 5-year survival of 90%,[28] and a randomized trial demonstrated no advantage for chemotherapy with cyclophosphamide, vincristine, and prednisone.[28] Equally good results with local therapy were obtained by other investigators.[27,29] Therefore, there is a limited role for systemic treatment initially in the management of localized disease. However, the treatment strategy should be individualized, weighing the relative toxicities of RT, chiefly

(a)

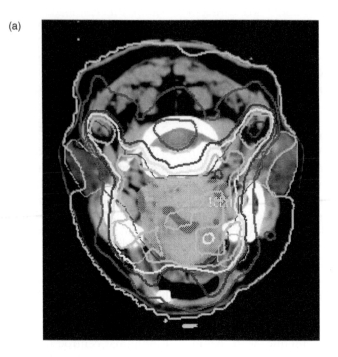

(b)

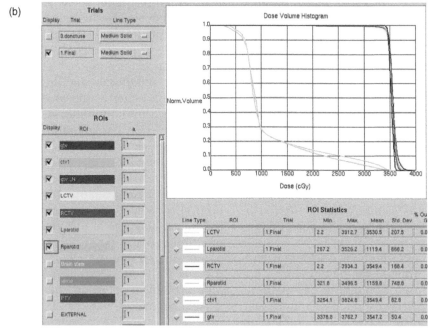

Figure 23.1   A 68-year-old man with stage II diffuse large B-cell lymphoma (DLBCL) of the left tonsil; partial response after chemotherapy. (a) Intensity-modulated radiation therapy (IMRT – 6 MV photons, 9 fields) with isodose distribution shown from a transverse perspective, with the main objective to spare the parotid salivary glands. The clinical target volume is shaded green. Note the concavity of the isodose lines around the contours of the parotid glands. Dose lines are shown in Gy, from outermost to innermost: 10, 25, 31.5 (blue), 33.25 (yellow), 35 (green), 37.45 (red). (b) Dose volume histogram for the target tissues and organs at risk. Note the bilateral parotid sparing with mean dose <12 Gy, and less that 30% of the right and left parotid glands receiving a dose of >10 Gy, for a prescribed dose to the target of 35 Gy.

increased xerostomia particularly in the presence of Sjögren's syndrome, vs surgical excision, or a trial of systemic therapy (oral chemotherapy, or rituximab).[30,31] Surgery may put the facial nerve at risk, and also results in a moderately high local relapse rate. The RT of salivary MALT lymphomas is best achieved with IMRT, or a conventional ipsilateral wedge pair of fields to spare the contralateral neck tissues. Elective cervical nodal irradiation is not required, although conventional techniques in the past have frequently included the level 2 (high jugular) lymph nodes. Since many patients will have Sjögren's syndrome, the care of patients with salivary gland MALT lymphoma includes meticulous dental care and maintainence of good oral hygiene, and joint management and follow-up by the dentist and rheumatology specialist. Occasionally, localized follicular lymphoma, usually not associated with autoimmune disease, may present in the salivary gland and the management is similar to MALT lymphoma, with RT.[32]

Infrequently, aggressive DLBCL will present de novo in the salivary gland, or following a history of MALT lymphoma (transformation). The use of CMT, using an anthracycline-based regimen, is standard for these aggressive B-cell lymphomas. The prognosis is poorer than MALT lymphoma,[33] but comparable to nodal lymphomas of similar stage and prognostic attributes.

NASAL AND PARANASAL SINUSES

In the Western population, primary lymphomas originating in the nasal cavity and paranasal sinuses (PNSL) are uncommon neoplasms, accounting for 3–4% of extranodal lymphomas, but contributing to 8–16% of the lymphomas of the head and neck region.[7,34] Among malignant tumors of the paranasal sinuses, the proportion of lymphomas is also low, representing less than 8%. However, in some Asian countries, nasal and PNSL lymphomas are the second most frequent extranodal lymphoma and the majority of them have NK/T-cell histology.[5] Their clinical characteristics and outcome are unique and are discussed in Chapter 14.

The following discussion focuses on B-cell lymphomas.

Most cases of PNSL occur in the maxillary sinus, while isolated localization in the ethmoid sinus, sphenoid sinus, or frontal sinuses is rare.[35] In immunocompetent patients, B-cell lymphomas are generally not associated with EBV infection.[36] On the contrary, in HIV-infected patients, evidence of past EBV infection is found frequently, similar to other HIV-associated B-cell lymphomas from other extranodal locations.[6]

The majority of nasal and PNSL cases are aggressive B-cell lymphomas, dominated by DLBCL (77%), followed by low-grade lymphomas (MALT type and follicular lymphomas – 18%), with the remainder being Burkitt's and mantle cell lymphomas (5%).[7] Presenting symptoms and signs are related to histology. Patients with low-grade lymphomas generally have masses in paranasal sinuses associated with obstructive symptoms, whereas histologically aggressive lymphomas present with more invasive features such as cranial nerve palsies, facial swelling, non-healing ulcer on the skin or palate, epistaxis, or pain.[37] Soft tissue or bone destruction, particularly of the orbit, with associated proptosis, was identified only in the aggressive B-cell lymphomas. Cervical lymph node involvement is uncommon.

Patients tend to be elderly males with bulky localized disease. Thus, the age and sex distribution, as well as the presenting symptoms of lymphomas, are similar to squamous cancers, a more common tumor of this region, and they can only be distinguished by biopsy specimens. A complete clinical evaluation, including laryngoscopy, bone marrow biopsy, and lumbar puncture, in patients with aggressive histological subtypes (DLBCL, lymphoblastic, and Burkitt's lymphomas) is essential for defining the extent of the disease and treatment planning. As in other head and neck sites, MRI is the best imaging method in evaluating the extent of soft tissue tumor, whereas CT is better for bony changes. Most cases will turn out to have Ann Arbor stage I or II disease. Systemic symptoms are notably absent, and laboratory profiles are usually normal, but elevation of lactate dehydrogenase (LDH)

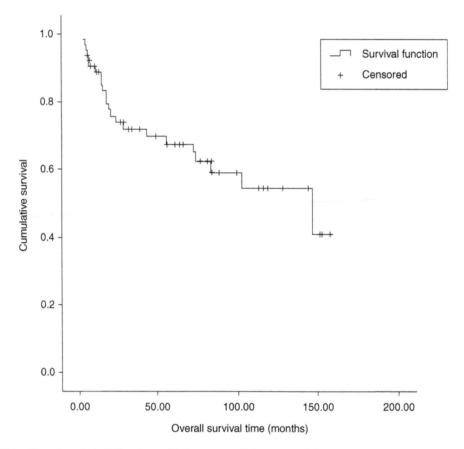

Figure 23.2 Overall survival of 32 patients with lymphoma of the paranasal sinuses.

can be found. Since patients are often assessed by physicians experienced in the management of epithelial cancers initially, some investigators also employ the TNM staging system,[38] with also a belief that tumor size may additionally influence the prognosis.

The modified IPI system proposed by Miller et al[39] was effective in predicting survival of a large series of patients with head and neck DLBCL, including 32 cases with PNSL.[7] The relatively small cohorts of patients reported in the literature received heterogeneous treatment modalities. Consequently, a broad variation in survival rate has been reported, with two larger series demonstrating a 5-year survival of about 50%.[40,41] There is a tendency for aggressive lymphomas to relapse in noncontiguous nodal and extranodal sites after

radiation therapy given alone, suggesting the necessity of systemic therapy to eliminate occult systemic disease. Most centers currently treat localized aggressive lymphoma with anthracycline-based chemotherapy followed by involved field RT (30–40 Gy).[13,40,42] In a series of 32 patients with DLBCL of the sinonasal tract, treated with anthracycline-containing chemotherapy with or without involved-field RT (IFRT), the 5-year overall survival was 68%[7] (Figure 23.2). When chemotherapy is contraindicated, radiation therapy is a reasonable alternative for patients with stage IE (T1-2) disease, but it is insufficient for patients with more advanced or bulky disease (stage IIE, or T3-4). Precision of RT target volume delineation and sparing of surrounding organs (e.g. eyes, brain, brainstem, spinal cord, salivary glands), where appropriate,

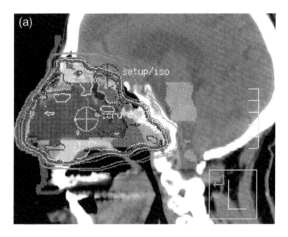
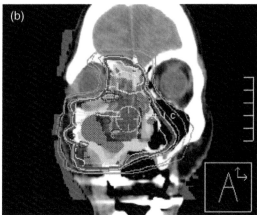

Figure 23.3   Intensity-modulated radiation therapy (IMRT – 6 MV photons, 6 fields) plan for nasal and right maxillary sinus lymphoma. Prescribed dose 35 Gy in 20 fractions. (a) Isodose distribution in midline sagittal perspective, demonstrating coverage of the entire nasal cavity and ethmoid sinus. Prechemotherapy gross tumor volume, shaded red; planning target volume, shaded green. (b) Isodose distribution in coronal perspective, showing the 'carving out' sparing of the left eye, and partially the right eye from high-dose radiation, achieved with IMRT. The two outermost isodose lines are 17.5 Gy (green) and 21 Gy (orange).

is required to achieve the best results. IMRT is very useful, and an example is illustrated in Figure 23.3.

Several series indicate that patients with aggressive lymphomas of paranasal sinuses are at high risk for leptomeningeal relapse,[34,40,43] particularly those with erosion of the base of the skull. As a result, some authors had recommended CNS prophylaxis with intrathecal chemotherapy for all patients with PNSL.[40] This is relevant even when rituximab is combined with anthracycline-based chemotherapy.[44] Not every study, however, has found a predilection for CNS spread.[7,37,41] It seems likely that the development of CNS disease is a reflection of advanced disease with a poor prognosis, systemic lymphoma progression, and/or chemotherapy-resistant disease.[43–45] CNS prophylaxis is indicated only for PNSL patients who are at high risk of CNS failure based on histology (lymphoblastic and Burkitt's lymphomas) or with disease invading or in proximity to the meninges in the base of the skull. In other cases it remains a matter of controversy.

For localized low-grade lymphomas (stage I–II) it has been suggested that RT (30–40 Gy over 4–5 weeks) should be given alone or as the main modality of therapy, and follow-up should be continued over a long period.[10]

THYROID LYMPHOMAS

The median age of presentation is over 60 years old, and women are affected more commonly than men.[46–49] B-cell lymphomas predominate, and are either MALT lymphomas or DLBCL. Preexisting Hashimoto's thyroiditis is usually present, and may or may not have been clinically diagnosed prior to the presentation of lymphoma.[50,51] Follicular lymphomas are rare. MALT lymphomas are usually indolent and may have a prolonged history of a slowly growing mass, or a diffuse goiter at the time of presentation, and have a better prognosis than non-MALT tumors.[52] MALT lymphoma is usually localized, with 60% of patients in stage IE, and 40% in stage IIE (cervical lymph node involvement).[26] A total thyroidectomy is not required, although some patients might be treated with a total or near-total thyroidectomy as the diagnostic procedure. If complete excision of the MALT lymphoma is achieved and there is no regional nodal involvement, further therapy is not required. For patients diagnosed with a lesser procedure, where there is residual lymphoma, RT alone is the standard therapy, with an expected local control rate of 95–100%.[27] Adequately treated MALT lymphoma of the thyroid gland rarely relapses systemically.[27,53] The 5-year cause-specific survival approaches 100%,[26,27] with a variety of treatment options.

Patients with DLBCL often present with a rapidly enlarging, bulky neck mass causing local aerodigestive obstructive symptoms. Extrathyroidal extension of the disease to surrounding neck structures is common. Integrity of the airway must be maintained, and some patients require a tracheostomy. Surgery is a diagnostic procedure and thyroidectomy is not indicated for clinically evident lymphoma diagnosed by fine needle or core biopsy.[54] CMT has become the standard treatment approach for DLBCL. With chemotherapy (anthracycline-containing regimen with rituximab, full 6 cycles) and locoregional RT (35–40 Gy), local control is achieved in the majority of patients, and survival and relapse-free survival should exceed 75%.[46–49,55]

The RT target volume includes the thyroid bed, bilateral cervical, and superior mediastinal lymph nodes.[46,49] A modified mantle field will cover this volume with sparing of the axilla, heart, and minimize lung exposure. Alternatively, IMRT can be used. Most if not all patients will eventually require thyroid hormone therapy.

ORAL CAVITY LYMPHOMA

Lymphoma arising within the oral cavity represents <10% of the extranodal head and neck lymphomas,[56–58] but is the most frequent non-epithelial malignant tumor of this region, accounting for 3.5% of all oral malignancies.[58] There is paucity of data on the relative frequency of the anatomical subsite involved. The palate appears to be the most frequent localization

compared to the maxilla, the mandible, the gum, the oral vestibule, and the mucosal lip.[59,60] More often, the lesions arise in the soft tissues or mucosa, as opposed to the bone.[56]

The majority are B-cell lymphomas (approximately 90%), with DLBCL being the most frequent histology.[61] Whereas most oral cavity lymphomas in an immunocompetent host are not associated with EBV infection, in those immunosuppressed, specifically by HIV infection, a high frequency of EBV is found, suggesting a pathogenetic role of EBV in the neoplastic transformation.[59] Plasmablastic lymphoma, a relatively new entity recognized by the World Health Organization (WHO) classification,[62] is a CD20-negative and CD138-positive large B-cell lymphoma with a predilection of the gums and palatal mucosa. There is a strong association with HIV infection.[63,64]

Localization in the palate is significantly associated with low-grade histology, in contrast to aggressive histology that predominates in the remaining oral sites. Marginal zone B-cell lymphoma of MALT type has been described in a few cases in the mucosal surface of the palate, buccal membrane, and the lip, which are sites containing minor salivary glands. These lymphomas arose from minor salivary glands and are often associated with Sjögren's syndrome, as in MALT lymphoma of major salivary glands.

The mean age of the patients is 60 years old, with higher prevalence in males in most series.[56–58,61] Clinical presentation is that of a local swelling, usually soft, elastic, with or without ulceration. Mucosal discoloration (red or red-blue) may be present.[58] Gingival lymphoma may be nodular and plaque-like, or papillary and exophytic. Lymphomas arising in the jaw typically present with non-specific signs and symptoms such as swelling with or without pain. Constitutional symptoms are rare.

Differential diagnosis includes odontogenic inflammatory process, periodontal disease, squamous cell carcinoma, and other malignancies of oral soft tissue. In the palate, follicular hyperplasia is a rare, benign, but potentially misleading lymphoproliferative lesion, presenting as a firm painless, non-fluctuating, slowly growing mass or swelling usually on one side of the palate.[65] A high index of suspicion is required and a thorough history and an oral and dental examination should be obtained as a first step of the diagnostic work-up. In cases with bone involvement, standard radiographic investigations usually show either diffuse bone destruction with obliteration of the lamina dura of the teeth or a solitary radiolucent defect. Some lymphomas may show osteoblastic activity and bone reabsorption, resulting in a mixed radiolucent–radiopaque appearance.[57,66] These cases should probably be considered primary bone lymphomas, although it may be clinically impossible to distinguish the origin for tumors that involve the bone with ulceration on the oral cavity mucosa. A CT scan is useful for detection of bone destruction involving the mandible or the maxilla, whereas MRI is preferred for the assessment of soft tissues.

In prognostication, the general approach is to apply the traditional methods such as stage, histology, and the IPI, but the relevance to primary oral cavity lymphomas is not known. However, early stages compared with more disseminated disease showed statistically significant differences both for overall survival and recurrence-free survival in a series of 34 cases of the oral cavity, with mean survival time and mean recurrence-free survival time of 38 and 31 months for the whole group, respectively.[56] In the same series, bone vs soft tissue localization of the lymphoma was not associated with differences in survival time. In contrast, 3-year disease-specific survival rates for NHL of the mandible were 90.5% and 47.6% in stage I and II, respectively.[67] Plasmablastic lymphoma associated with HIV infection has the worst prognosis, with a median survival time of 6 months.[63]

The guide to therapy in oral cavity lymphomas is based on experience with other limited-stage lymphomas. For histologically aggressive lymphomas, CMT is the main therapeutic strategy. An anthracycline-containing regimen, with addition of rituximab (for CD20-positive B-cell lymphoma) for 3–6 cycles is followed by RT. The optimal RT total dose is 30–40 Gy, as is the practice for nodal lymphomas. RT alone is probably adequate for stage I-II low-grade lymphomas (follicular lymphoma or MALT lymphoma), although further data are needed to confirm the long-term efficacy of this strategy.[11,68]

LARYNX LYMPHOMA AND TRACHEAL LYMPHOMA

Lymphomas of the larynx are rare tumors that represent <1% of primary malignant laryngeal cancers.[69] The median age of diagnosis is in the sixth decade, with a male predominance of 1.4:1.[70] Due to the local distribution of lymphatic tissue, the supraglottic larynx is the most common subsite involved.[70,71] Most tumors are B-cell lymphomas, and low-grade MALT lymphoma predominates.[70] No association with a specific chronic inflammatory process and laryngeal MALT lymphoma has been found to date.[72] On laryngoscopy, the lymphoma appears characteristically as a submucosal mass. Dysphagia and dysphonia are the most frequent presenting symptoms, with more than 90% of cases confirming to have limited-stage disease (IE or IIE), without B symptoms.[70]

Primary lymphoma of the trachea is an extremely rare entity.[73] The clinical presentation is one of a localized disease without dissemination. Bronchoscopic appearance consists of a localized nodular or polypoid mass, producing narrowing of the trachea associated with dyspnea and wheezing.[74] Because symptoms are early, the diagnosis is often made when the disease is not bulky. Lymphocytic lymphoma, MALT lymphoma, and large cell types have been described in the few reported cases.[74-76] Local control of the disease can be obtained by surgery, RT, or chemotherapy.[74]

It must be emphasized that, due to its rarity, specific evidence-based therapeutic guidelines of laryngeal and tracheal lymphomas with respect to effectiveness and toxicity are still lacking, and the general principles of managing stage I-II lymphomas are followed. IFRT could be employed for stage I-II low-grade lymphomas (including MALT lymphomas and follicular lymphomas). Histologically aggressive lymphomas are best approached with CMT.[13,39]

REFERENCES

1. Carbone PP, Kaplan HS, Musshoff K, Smithers DW, Tubiana M. Report of the Committee on Hodgkin's Disease Staging Classification. Cancer Res 1971; 31: 1860–1.
2. Otter R, Gerrits WB, Sandt MM, Hermans J, Willemze R. Primary extranodal and nodal non-Hodgkin's lymphoma. A survey of a population-based registry. Eur J Cancer Clin Oncol 1989; 25(8): 1203–10.
3. Shima N, Kobashi Y, Tsutsui K, et al. Extranodal non-Hodgkin's lymphoma of the head and neck. A clinicopathologic study in the Kyoto-Nara area of Japan. Cancer 1990; 66(6): 1190–7.
4. López-Guillermo A, Colomo L, Jiménez M, et al. Diffuse large B-cell lymphoma: clinical and biological characterization and outcome according to the nodal or extranodal primary origin. J Clin Oncol 2005; 23(12): 2797–804.
5. Jaffe ES, Chan J, Su IJ, et al. Report of the workshop on nasal and related extranodal angiocentric T/natural killer cell lymphomas: definitions, differential diagnosis, and epidemiology. Am J Surg Pathol 1996; 20(1): 103–11.
6. Finn DG. Lymphoma of the head and neck and acquired immunodeficiency syndrome: clinical investigation and immunohistological study. Laryngoscope 1995; 105(4 Pt 2 Suppl 68): 1–18.
7. Cortelazzo S, Rossi A, Federico M, et al. The stage modified IBI (MIPI), histology, and combined treatment influence the clinical outcome of 401 patients with primary extranodal head and neck lymphomas (PHNBCL). Blood 2005; 106(S3): Abstract 927.
8. Ezzat AA, Ibrahim EM, El Weshi AN, et al. Localized non-Hodgkin's lymphoma of Waldeyer's ring: clinical features, management, and prognosis of 130 adult patients. Head Neck 2001; 23(7): 547–58.
9. Jacobs C, Hoppe RT. Non-Hodgkin's lymphomas of head and neck extranodal sites. Int J Radiat Oncol Biol Phys 1985; 11(2): 357–64.
10. Ikeda H, Inoue T, Teshima T, et al. Treatment of indolent non-Hodgkin's lymphoma localized in the head and neck. Am J Clin Oncol 1993; 16(1): 72–6.
11. MacDermed D, Thurber L, George TI, Hoppe RT, Le QT. Extranodal nonorbital indolent lymphomas of the head and neck: relationship between tumor control and radiotherapy. Int J Radiat Oncol Biol Phys 2004; 59(3): 788–95.
12. Frata P, Buglione M, Grisanti S, et al. Localized extranodal lymphoma of the head and neck: retrospective analysis of a series of 107 patients from a single institution. Tumori 2005; 91(6): 456–62.
13. Horning SJ, Weller E, Kim K, et al. Chemotherapy with or without radiotherapy in limited-stage diffuse aggressive non-Hodgkin's lymphoma: Eastern Cooperative Oncology Group Study 1484. J Clin Oncol 2004; 22(15): 3032–8.
14. Oguchi M, Ikeda H, Isobe K, et al. Tumor bulk as a prognostic factor for the management of localized aggressive non-Hodgkin's lymphoma: a survey of the Japan Lymphoma Radiation Therapy Group. Int J Radiat Oncol Biol Phys 2000; 48(1): 161–8.
15. Jacobs C, Hoppe R. Non-Hodgkin's lymphomas of the head and neck: prognosis and patterns of recurrence. Int J Radiat Oncol Biol Phys 1985; 11: 357–64.
16. Paulsen J, Lennert K. Low-grade B-cell lymphoma of mucosa-associated lymphoid tissue type in Waldeyer's ring. Histopathology 1994; 24(1): 1–11.
17. Liang R, Ng RP, Todd D, et al. Management of Stage I-II diffuse aggressive non-Hodgkin's lymphoma of the Waldeyer's ring: combined modality therapy versus radiotherapy alone. Hematol Oncol 1987; 5: 223–30.
18. Krol AD, Le Cessie S, Snijder S, et al. Waldeyer's ring lymphomas: a clinical study from the Comprehensive Cancer Center West population based NHL registry. Leuk Lymphoma 2001; 42(5): 1005–13.
19. Avilés A, Delgado S, Ruiz H, et al. Treatment of non-Hodgkin's lymphoma of Waldeyer's ring: radiotherapy versus chemotherapy versus combined therapy. Eur J Cancer B Oral Oncol 1996; 32B(1): 19–23.
20. Shenkier TN, Voss N, Fairey R, et al. Brief chemotherapy and involved-region irradiation for limited-stage diffuse large-cell lymphoma: an 18-year experience from the British Columbia Cancer Agency. J Clin Oncol 2002; 20(1): 197–204.
21. Miller T, Unger J, Spier C, et al. Effect of adding rituximab to three cycles of CHOP plus involved field radiotherapy for limited stage aggressive diffuse large B-cell lymphoma (SWOG-0014). Blood 2004; 104(11): 48a–9 (Abstract 158).
22. Liu RP, Fleming TJ, Toth BB, Keene HJ. Salivary flow rates in patients with head and neck cancer 0.5 to 25 years after radiotherapy. Oral Surg Oral Med Oral Pathol 1990; 70: 724–9.
23. Cooper JS, Fu K, Marks J, Silverman S. Late effects of radiation therapy in the head and neck region. Int J Radiat Oncol Biol Phys 1995; 31: 1141–64.
24. Pariente D, Anaya JM, Combe B, et al. Non-Hodgkin's lymphoma associated with primary Sjögren's syndrome. Eur J Med 1992; 1(6): 337–42.
25. Royer B, Cazals-Hatem D, Sibilia J, et al. Lymphomas in patients with Sjögren's syndrome are marginal zone B-cell neoplasms, arise in diverse extranodal and nodal sites, and are not associated with viruses. Blood 1997; 90(2): 766–75.
26. Zucca E, Conconi A, Pedrinis E, et al. Nongastric marginal zone B-cell lymphoma of mucosa-associated lymphoid tissue. Blood 2003; 101(7): 2489–95.
27. Tsang RW, Gospodarowicz MK, Pintilie M, et al. Localized mucosa-associated lymphoid tissue lymphoma treated with radiation therapy has excellent clinical outcome. J Clin Oncol 2003; 21(22): 4157–64.
28. Avilés A, Delgado S, Huerta-Guzmán J. Marginal zone B cell lymphoma of the parotid glands: results of a randomised trial comparing radiotherapy to combined therapy. Eur J Cancer B Oral Oncol 1996; 6: 420–2.
29. Olivier KR, Brown PD, Stafford SL, Ansell SM, Martenson JA Jr. Efficacy and treatment-related

toxicity of radiotherapy for early-stage primary non-Hodgkin lymphoma of the parotid gland. Int J Radiat Oncol Biol Phys 2004; 60(5): 1510–14.

30. Conconi A, Martinelli G, Thieblemont C, et al. Clinical activity of rituximab in extranodal marginal zone B-cell lymphoma of MALT type. Blood 2003; 102(8): 2741–5.

31. Raderer M, Jager G, Brugger S, et al. Rituximab for treatment of advanced extranodal marginal zone B cell lymphoma of the mucosa-associated lymphoid tissue lymphoma. Oncology 2003; 65(4): 306–10.

32. Nakamura S, Ichimura K, Sato Y, et al. Follicular lymphoma frequently originates in the salivary gland. Pathol Int 2006; 56(10): 576–83.

33. Voulgarelis M, Dafni UG, Isenberg DA, Moutsopoulos HM. Malignant lymphoma in primary Sjögren's syndrome: a multicenter, retrospective, clinical study by the European Concerted Action on Sjögren's Syndrome. Arthritis Rheum 1999; 42(8): 1765–72.

34. Jacobs C, Weiss L, Hoppe RT. The management of extranodal head and neck lymphomas. Arch Otolaryngol Head Neck Surg 1986; 112(6): 654–8.

35. Neves MC, Lessa MM, Voegels RL, Butugan O. Primary non-Hodgkin's lymphoma of the frontal sinus: case report and review of the literature. Ear Nose Throat J 2005; 84(1): 47–51.

36. Bahnassy AA, Zekri AR, Asaad N, et al. Epstein–Barr viral infection in extranodal lymphoma of the head and neck: correlation with prognosis and response to treatment. Histopathology 2006; 48(5): 516–28.

37. Abbondanzo SL, Wenig BM. Non-Hodgkin's lymphoma of the sinonasal tract. A clinicopathologic and immunophenotypic study of 120 cases. Cancer 1995; 75(6): 1281–91.

38. Mill WB, Lee FA, Franssila KO. Radiation therapy treatment of stage I and II extranodal non-Hodgkin's lymphoma of the head and neck. Cancer 1980; 45(4): 653–61.

39. Miller T, Dahlberg S, Cassady J, et al. Chemotherapy alone compared with chemotherapy plus radiotherapy for localized intermediate- and high-grade non-Hodgkin's lymphoma. N Engl J Med 1998; 339: 21–6.

40. Laskin JJ, Savage KJ, Voss N, Gascoyne RD, Connors JM. Primary paranasal sinus lymphoma: natural history and improved outcome with central nervous system chemoprophylaxis. Leuk Lymphoma 2005; 46(12): 1721–7.

41. Logsdon MD, Ha CS, Kavadi VS, et al. Lymphoma of the nasal cavity and paranasal sinuses: improved outcome and altered prognostic factors with combined modality therapy. Cancer 1997; 80(3): 477–88.

42. Hausdorff J, Davis E, Long G, et al. Non-Hodgkin's lymphoma of the paranasal sinuses: clinical and pathological features, and response to combined-modality therapy. Cancer J Sci Am 1997; 3(5): 303–11.

43. Liang R, Chiu E, Loke SL. Secondary central nervous system involvement by non-Hodgkin's lymphoma: the risk factors. Hematol Oncol 1990; 8(3): 141–5.

44. Feugier P, Virion JM, Tilly H, et al. Incidence and risk factors for central nervous system occurrence in elderly patients with diffuse large-B-cell lymphoma: influence of rituximab. Ann Oncol 2004; 15(1): 129–33.

45. Haioun C, Besson C, Lepage E, et al. Incidence and risk factors of central nervous system relapse in histologically aggressive non-Hodgkin's lymphoma uniformly treated and receiving intrathecal central nervous system prophylaxis: a GELA study on 974 patients. Groupe d'Etudes des Lymphomes de l'Adulte. Ann Oncol 2000; 11(6): 685–90.

46. Harrington KJ, Michalaki VJ, Vini L, et al. Management of non-Hodgkin's lymphoma of the thyroid: the Royal Marsden Hospital experience. Br J Radiol 2005; 78(929): 405–10.

47. DiBiase SJ, Grigsby PW, Guo C, Lin HS, Wasserman TH. Outcome analysis for stage IE and IIE thyroid lymphoma. Am J Clin Oncol 2004; 27(2): 178–84.

48. Ha CS, Shadle KM, Medeiros LJ, et al. Localized non-Hodgkin lymphoma involving the thyroid gland. Cancer 2001; 91(4): 629–35.

49. Tsang R, Gospodarowicz MK, Sutcliffe SB, et al. Non-Hodgkin's lymphoma of the thyroid gland: prognostic factors and treatment outcome. Int J Radiat Oncol Biol Phys 1993; 27: 599–604.

50. Aozasa K. Hashimoto's thyroiditis as a risk factor of thyroid lymphoma. Acta Pathol Jpn 1990; 40(7): 459–68.

51. Thieblemont C, Mayer A, Dumontet C, et al. Primary thyroid lymphoma is a heterogeneous disease. J Clin Endocrinol Metab 2002; 87(1): 105–11.

52. Laing RW, Hoskin P, Hudson BV, et al. The significance of MALT histology in thyroid lymphoma: a review of patients from the BNLI and Royal Marsden Hospital. Clin Oncol 1994; 6(5): 300–4.

53. Thieblemont C, Bastion Y, Berger F, et al. Mucosa-associated lymphoid tissue gastrointestinal and non-gastrointestinal lymphoma behavior: analysis of 108 patients. J Clin Oncol 1997; 15(4): 1624–30.

54. Cha C, Chen H, Westra WH, Udelsman R. Primary thyroid lymphoma: can the diagnosis be made solely by fine-needle aspiration? Ann Surg Oncol 2002; 9(3): 298–302.

55. Belal AA, Allam A, Kandil A, et al. Primary thyroid lymphoma: a retrospective analysis of prognostic factors and treatment outcome for localized intermediate and high grade lymphoma. Am J Clin Oncol 2001; 24(3): 299–305.

56. van der Waal RI, Huijgens PC, van der Valk P, van der Waal I. Characteristics of 40 primary extranodal non-Hodgkin lymphomas of the oral cavity in perspective of the new WHO classification and the International Prognostic Index. Int J Oral Maxillofac Surg 2005; 34(4): 391–5.

57. Kolokotronis A, Konstantinou N, Christakis I, et al. Localized B-cell non-Hodgkin's lymphoma of oral cavity and maxillofacial region: a clinical study. Oral Surg Oral Med Oral Pathol Oral Radiol Endod 2005; 99(3): 303–10.

58. Epstein JB, Epstein JD, Le ND, Gorsky M. Characteristics of oral and paraoral malignant lymphoma: a population-based review of 361 cases. Oral

Surg Oral Med Oral Pathol Oral Radiol Endod 2001; 92(5): 519–25.

59. Leong IT, Fernandes BJ, Mock D. Epstein–Barr virus detection in non-Hodgkin's lymphoma of the oral cavity: an immunocytochemical and in situ hybridization study. Oral Surg Oral Med Oral Pathol Oral Radiol Endod 2001; 92(2): 184–93.

60. Rinaggio J, Aguirre A, Zeid M, Hatton MN. Swelling of the nasolabial area. Oral Surg Oral Med Oral Pathol Oral Radiol Endod 2000; 89(6): 669–73.

61. Regezi JA, Zarbo RJ, Stewart JC. Extranodal oral lymphomas: histologic subtypes and immunophenotypes (in routinely processed tissue). Oral Surg Oral Med Oral Pathol 1991; 72(6): 702–8.

62. Jaffe ES, Harris NL, Stein H, Vardiman JW, eds. Pathology and Genetics of Tumours of Haematopoietic and Lymphoid Tissues. Lyon, France: IARC Press, 2001.

63. Delecluse HJ, Anagnostopoulos I, Dallenbach F, et al. Plasmablastic lymphomas of the oral cavity: a new entity associated with the human immunodeficiency virus infection. Blood 1997; 89(4): 1413–20.

64. Colomo L, Loong F, Rives S, et al. Diffuse large B-cell lymphomas with plasmablastic differentiation represent a heterogeneous group of disease entities. Am J Surg Pathol 2004; 28(6): 736–47.

65. Kolokotronis A, Dimitrakopoulos I, Asimaki A. Follicular lymphoid hyperplasia of the palate: report of a case and review of the literature. Oral Surg Oral Med Oral Pathol Oral Radiol Endod 2003; 96(2): 172–5.

66. Mealey BL, Tunder GS, Pemble CW 3rd. Primary extranodal malignant lymphoma affecting the periodontium. J Periodontol 2002; 73(8): 937–41.

67. Someya M, Sakata K, Nagakura H, et al. Three cases of diffuse large B-cell lymphoma of the mandible treated with radiotherapy and chemotherapy. Radiat Med 2005; 23(4): 296–302.

68. Nathu RM, Mendenhall NP, Almasri NM, Lynch JW. Non-Hodgkin's lymphoma of the head and neck: a 30-year experience at the University of Florida. Head Neck 1999; 21(3): 247–54.

69. Franzen A, Kurrer MO. Malignant lymphoma of the larynx: a case report and review of the literature. Laryngorhinootologie 2000; 79(10): 579–83.

70. Horny HP, Kaiserling E. Involvement of the larynx by hemopoietic neoplasms. An investigation of autopsy cases and review of the literature. Pathol Res Pract 1995; 191(2): 130–8.

71. Morgan K, MacLennan KA, Narula A, Bradley PJ, Morgan DA. Non-Hodgkin's lymphoma of the larynx (stage IE). Cancer 1989; 64(5): 1123–7.

72. Kania RE, Hartl DM, Badoual C, Le Maignan C, Brasnu DF. Primary mucosa-associated lymphoid tissue (MALT) lymphoma of the larynx. Head Neck 2005; 27(3): 258–62.

73. Allen MS. Malignant tracheal tumors. Mayo Clin Proc 1993; 68(7): 680–4.

74. Fidias P, Wright C, Harris NL, Urba W, Grossbard ML. Primary tracheal non-Hodgkin's lymphoma. A case report and review of the literature. Cancer 1996; 77(11): 2332–8.

75. Wiggins J, Sheffield E, Green M. Primary B cell malignant lymphoma of the trachea. Thorax 1988; 43(6): 497–8.

76. Kaplan MA, Pettit CL, Zukerberg LR, Harris NL. Primary lymphoma of the trachea with morphologic and immunophenotypic characteristics of low-grade B-cell lymphoma of mucosa-associated lymphoid tissue. Am J Surg Pathol 1992; 16(1): 71–5.

Lymphoma of the liver

24

Christoph Loddenkemper and Thomas Longerich

INTRODUCTION

The liver is the third most frequently involved extranodal site in malignant lymphoma, following the spleen and bone marrow. Liver infiltration by lymphoma is usually secondary and represents advanced disease.[1,2] Regarding the exact definition of primary hepatic lymphoma, no final consensus has been achieved, but most commonly the criteria of Caccamo and co-workers are applied.[3] Accordingly, primary hepatic lymphoma is defined as an extranodal lymphoma with main tumor burden within the liver and without any evidence of lymphadenopathy or splenomegaly; in addition, the peripheral blood count should be normal for at least 6 months.

INCIDENCE AND EPIDEMIOLOGY

Approximately 200 cases of primary hepatic lymphoma have been published so far. Primary hepatic lymphoma represents 0.016% of all non-Hodgkin's lymphomas (NHL) and 0.4% of all extranodal lymphomas.[4–6] Primary hepatic lymphomas occur more often in males than in females (2:1). They are mainly observed in adolescents or adults, whereas occurrence in childhood is rare.[7–10] Owing to the lack of large cohort analyses, it is impossible to determine the precise incidence of primary hepatic lymphoma. Overall, it seems that most cases belong to the group of diffuse large B-cell lymphoma (DLBCL), followed by extranodal marginal zone lymphoma of the mucosa-associated lymphoid tissue (MALT) and follicular lymphoma.[11–13] Primary hepatic T-cell lymphomas seem to be more prevalent in Asia than in Western countries.[14–17] In autopsies, secondary liver involvement is seen in 30–50% of patients suffering from advanced disease.[18,19] Data on the frequency of associated chronic liver disease with primary hepatic lymphoma are contradicting. Whereas the prevalence of associated liver diseases was 7% in one series,[12] including 4 cases of hepatitis B virus (HBV) infection, 1 case of hepatitis C virus (HCV) infection, 1 'cryptogenic' liver cirrhosis, and 1 genetic hemochromatosis, other studies report an association in up to 40% (Asia) or 10% (Western countries) of cases, respectively.[20] Following liver transplantation, hepatic involvement is seen in 84% of cases with post-transplant lymphoproliferative disorder (PTLD).[21]Overall, the incidence of PTLD following liver transplantation is reported to be 4%.[22]

ETIOLOGY AND BIOLOGICAL FEATURES

Primary hepatic lymphomas have been described in association with chronic liver diseases, although there is no direct experimental evidence supporting a pathogenic link. Beside their hepatotropism, the HBV as well as the HCV have been demonstrated to be also lymphotropic.[23,24] Epidemiological data show an increased prevalence (9–50%) of chronic HBV and HCV infection in patients suffering from NHL.[11,15,25–27] Similar to hepatocarcinogenesis, both HBV integration and HBx-mediated transactivation may be involved in HBV-associated lymphogenesis, but experimental evidence is missing. HCV-associated lymphomagenesis has been attributed to chronic B-cell stimulation and some authors have hypothesized that HCV-associated cryoglobulinemia may be a precursor stage in this regard. Additionally, a translocation t(14;18) involving the *BCL2* gene has been detected in some chronically HCV-infected patients.[28-30] Casuistically, primary hepatic lymphomas have been described in association with genetic hemochromatosis.[31,32]

Immunocompromised patients represent a subgroup of patients with hepatic lymphoma involvement, especially those infected with the human immunodeficiency virus (HIV). Following Kaposi's sarcoma, malignant lymphomas are the second most frequent malignancies in acquired immunodeficiency syndrome (AIDS) patients and usually involve the gastrointestinal tract or the central nervous system. AIDS-associated primary hepatic lymphomas were first described in an autopsy series in 1983.[33] Pathogenetically, they reflect a heterogeneous group. Cytokine-mediated transformation and herpes viruses such as Epstein–Barr virus (EBV) or Kaposi sarcoma herpes virus (KSHV/HHV8 [human herpes virus 8]) have been attributed to act as causative agents.[34] A second group of lymhomas associated with immunodeficiency represent malignant lymphomas following organ transplantation and, similar to HIV-associated lymphomas, EBV is often involved in these cases.

Primary hepatic lymphomas (e.g. marginal zone lymphomas) have also been observed in association with autoimmune diseases such as primary biliary cirrhosis, Sjögren's syndrome, systemic lupus erythematosus, and celiac disease. Pathogenetically, chronic antigen-mediated B-cell proliferation is discussed.[35-41]

PATHOLOGY

Hepatic manifestations of B-cell lymphomas usually exhibit characteristic infiltration patterns, allowing the use of restricted immunohistochemical analyses to reach a final diagnosis. In contrast, the diagnosis of hepatic T-cell lymphomas is more challenging due to the lack of a typical morphology.[13,42] Furthermore, the differentiation of T-cell lymphomas from reactive non-neoplastic conditions (e.g. EBV infection) may be very difficult, and additional molecular analysis evaluating T-cell receptor (TCR) rearrangement may be required.

In contrast, the hepatosplenic T-cell lymphoma (HSTCL), which usually affects young men and is presumed to evolve from immature cytotoxic T cells mostly of γδ T-cell receptor type, can often be diagnosed based on its typical sinusoidal infiltration pattern. HSTCL represents less than 5% of peripheral T-cell lymphomas.[43] Clinically, HSTCL is characterized by severe thrombocytemia, anemia, leukocytosis, and marked hepatosplenomegaly without lymphadenopathy.[44] Bone marrow involvement is nearly always seen, but may be difficult to detect without additional immunohistochemical demonstration.[43] Since γδ T-cell lymphomas are more often seen in immunocompromised patients following organ transplantation, chronic immune stimulation has been proposed to be involved in its pathogenesis.[45,46] Genetically, neoplastic cells have rearranged TCRγ genes, whereas TCRβ may be germline or rearranged. Isochromosome 7 is typically observed and may be associated with other abnormalities, most frequently trisomy 8. EBV positivity has not been demonstrated.[47-49] The course of HSTCL is usually aggressive with a median survival of less than 2 years despite initial response to chemotherapy.[50] In contrast to γδ T-cell lymphomas, the infrequent αβ type is more often observed in female patients.[51]

In B-cell lymphomas, four major infiltration patterns can be distinguished: (1) diffuse-nodular growth, predominance of portal infiltrates (2) either with dense sheets of neoplastic cells or (3) scattered neoplastic cells in a background of reactive bystander cells, and (4) sinusoidal spread.

Diffuse-nodular lymphoma infiltrates are usually seen in high-grade B-cell NHL such as DLBCL or Burkitt's lymphoma. The application of an immunohistochemical algorithm (proposed by Hans et al[52]), using antibodies against CD10, BCL6, and IRF4/MUM1, may allow the discrimination of DLBCL into germinal center B-cell (GCB) type from the activated B-cell (ABC) type. Gene expression profiling has demonstrated a significantly better overall survival for patients with DLBCL of GCB type compared with the ABC type[53] (Figure 24.1A–F).

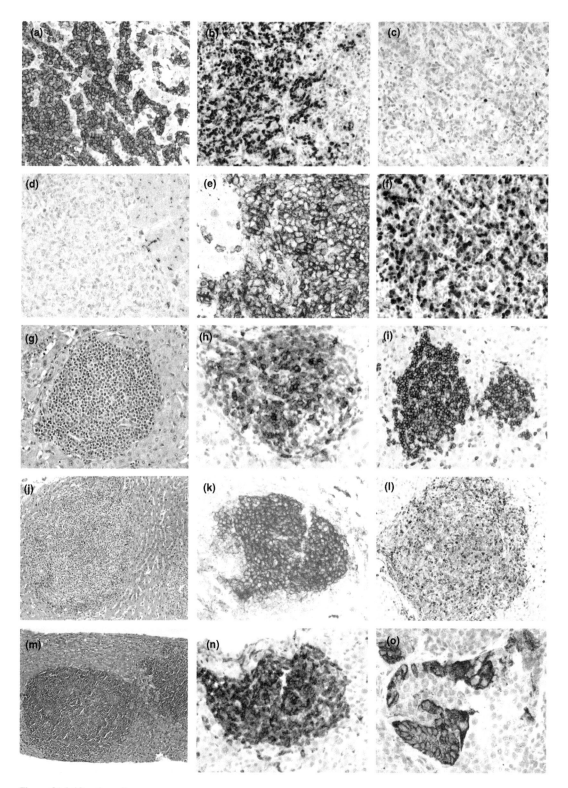

Figure 24.1 (Continued)

Figure 24.1 Diffuse large B-cell lymphoma (DLBCL) of germinal center B-cell (GCB) type with nodular pattern and expression of CD10 (**A**) and BCL6 (**B**), while being negative for MUM1 (**C**). DLBCL of activated B-cell (ABC) type without expression of CD10 (positive bile canaliculi serve as intrinsic control) (**D**), being positive for CD5 (**E**) and MUM1 (**F**). Chronic lymphocytic leukemia (B-CLL) with a predominantly portal infiltrate of small lymphocytes (**G**) with expression of CD23 (**H**) and CD5 (**I**). Follicular lymphoma (FL) (**J**) with expression of CD10 (**K**) and BCL2 (**L**). Marginal zone B-cell lymphoma with portal involvement following liver transplantation (**M**) showing expression of memory B-cell marker CD27 (**N**) and a lymphoepithelial lesion of a CK7-positive bile duct (**O**). (Reproduced from Loddenkemper et al,[13] with permission of *Virchows Archive* [Springer, Heidelberg].)

A recently published study on a series of 205 liver biopsies with lymphoma showed that this distinction can be made even in needle biopsies and, out of 80 DLBCL, 35% of the cases were of GCB and 65% of non-GCB type.[13]

The T-cell rich variant of DLBCL (TCRBL), in which the majority of cells are non-neoplastic T cells and histiocytes (Figure 24.2A–C), is found more frequently in the liver than in the lymph node (up to 14% of DLBCL in the liver compared to 2% of nodal DLBCL). Thus, this phenomenon should be kept in mind to prevent misdiagnosis of TCRBCL as a reactive condition or a T-cell lymphoma.[54,55] It may be hypothesized that the hepatic immune response leads to the strong T-cell reaction in TCRBCL.

Dense portal tract-associated infiltrates are seen in most cases of chronic lymphocytic leukemia (B-CLL), follicular lymphoma, marginal zone lymphoma, and mantle cell lymphoma. In extranodal marginal zone lymphoma of MALT type, typical lymphoepithelial lesions are seen in the bile duct epithelium and may be highlighted by cytokeratin staining (Figure 24.1G–O). Reliable immunohistochemical markers for the differentiation of these B-NHL include CD5, CD23, CD10, BCL6, and cyclin D_1.[42] Whereas tumor cells in B-CLL express CD5 and CD23, labeling with the germinal center markers CD10 and BCL6 is seen in follicular lymphoma. Mantle cell lymphoma is usually CD5- and cyclin D_1-positive. Diagnostic limitations are encountered in accurate grading of follicular lymphoma in liver needle biopsy. Loose portal infiltrates with scattered neoplastic cells in a reactive background are seen in Hodgkin lymphoma and TCRBCL. Especially in liver biopsy specimens, the diagnosis of Hodgkin lymphoma may be difficult and require additional immunohistochemical analyses. The scattered Hodgkin and Reed–Sternberg (HRS) cells have to be differentiated from tumor cells in anaplastic large cell lymphoma (ALCL), which can resemble HRS cells. As the neoplastic cells in both entities express CD30, additional immunohistochemical stainings (e.g. T-cell markers, cytotoxic molecules like perforin or the B-cell specific transcription factor pax-5) are needed to distinguish these lymphomas (Figure 24.2D–I). Sometimes ALCL or the anaplastic variant of DLBCL may pose problems in the differential diagnosis with metastatic undifferentiated carcinoma, histiocytic sarcoma, or follicular dendritic cell tumor, which can be resolved by further immunohistochemical characterization.

A predominantly sinusoidal infiltrate is observed in plasmacytoma, hairy cell leukemia, precursor lymphoblastic leukemia (ALL), and HSTCL. In HSTCL, typically medium-sized, monomorphic tumor cells are found with a rim of pale cytoplasm. Nuclei have loosely condensed chromatin with small inconspicuous nucleoli and may show irregular nuclear contours. Immunohistochemically, neoplastic T cells of HSTCL express CD3, cytotoxic molecules (e.g. T-cell intracellular antigen 1 [TIA-1]) and sometimes CD56, whereas CD4, CD8, and CD5 are negative in most cases (Figure 24.2J–L). In contrast, sinusoidal infiltration of plasmacytoma frequently shows concomitant extramedullary hematopoiesis, which may be explained by the fact that most cases in the liver represent a leukemic phase of plasma cell myeloma with extensive bone marrow infitration. Until now, only 2 cases of primary hepatic plasmacytoma have been described.[56] Sinusoidal infiltrates of ALL are characterized by the expression of terminal desoxynucleotidyl transferase (TdT). In hairy cell

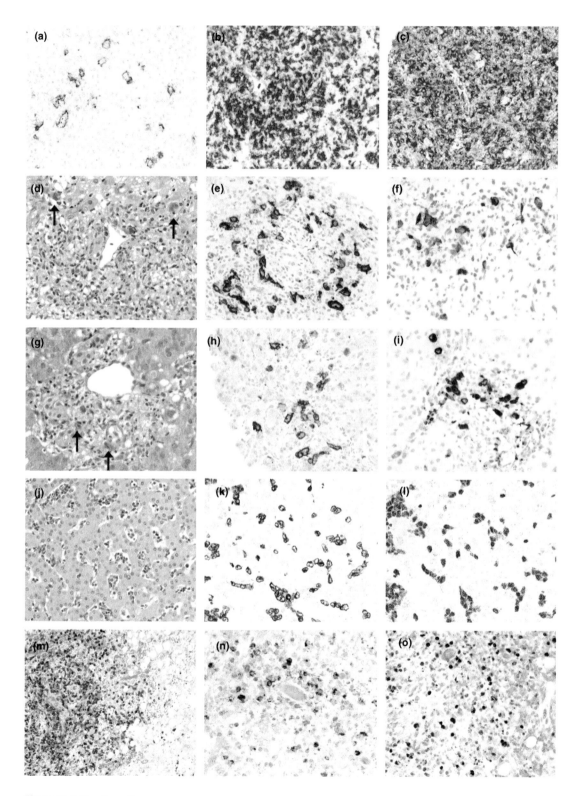

Figure 24.2 (Continued)

Figure 24.2 T-cell/histiocyte-rich B-cell lymphoma (TCRBCL) with less than 10% large CD20-positive neoplastic B cells (**A**) associated with numerous CD3-positive T cells (**B**) and CD68-positive histiocytes (**C**). Classical Hodgkin's lymphoma (cHL) with portal infiltrates of Hodgkin and Reed–Sternberg (HRS) cells (arrows) in a background rich in eosinophils (**D**). The HRS cells strongly express CD30 (**E**) and the EBV-encoded latent membrane protein 1 (LMP1) (**F**). Anaplastic large cell lymphoma (ALCL) with portal infiltrates of pleomorphic large cells resembling HRS cells (arrows) (**G**) and strong positivity for CD30 (**H**) and the cytotoxic molecule perforin (**I**). Hepatosplenic T-cell lymphoma (HSTCL) with a sinusoidal infiltrate of monotonous neoplastic cells (**J**) with expression of CD3 (**K**) and the cytotoxic granule associated protein TIA-1 (**L**). Post-transplant lymphoproliferative disorder (PTLD) with CD79a-positive B-cell infiltrates (**M**) and EBV association demonstrated by the expression of LMP1 (**N**) and the nuclear antigen of the EBV EBNA2 (**O**). (**A–L** are reproduced from Loddenkemper et al,[13] with permission of *Virchows Archive* [Springer, Heidelberg].)

leukemia (HCL), liver involvement is regularly seen, but may be clinically inert. Similar to HSTCL, the neoplastic cells show single file rowing, but have a wider rim of cytoplasm. Immunohistochemically, they express B-cell markers, DBA.44, CD25, and sometimes cyclin D_1, but are negative for CD5, CD10, and CD23. Characteristically, HCL is associated with pelio-sis-like alterations of the hepatic architecture, congestion or so-called angiomatoid lesions, which represent blood-filled sinusoids surrounded by neoplastic B cells. These lesions may be a clue for the diagnosis of HCL but have to be differentiated from hemangiomas.

Diagnosis of most T-cell lymphomas in the liver, most commonly unspecified peripheral T-cell lymphomas, may be challenging due to the lack of a typical infiltration pattern. Additionally, the differential diagnosis often includes reactive conditions and infectious diseases, especially EBV hepatitis. Frequently, final diagnosis may rely on confirmation by molecular analysis demonstrating a clonal TCR rearrangement (Figure 24.3). The distribution and frequency of hepatic lymphoma manifestations compared to other extranodal sites are summarized in Table 24.1.

CLINICAL AND RADIOGRAPHIC PRESENTATION

Diagnosis of primary hepatic lymphoma may evolve incidentally during the evaluation of abnormal liver values or during follow-up of chronic liver disease.[57] Symptoms are usually non-specific and include (upper) abdominal pain, hepatomegaly, weight loss, fever, nausea, and vomiting. Serologically, transaminase and

lactate dehydrogenase (LDH) elevation may be observed, whereas α-fetoprotein and carcino-embryonic antigen (CEA) are usually normal.[4] Occasionally, hepatic lymphoma involvement may mimic hepatitis or cholangitis and eventually acute hepatic failure may occur.[58–62]

Macroscopically, primary hepatic lymphomas are usually observed as solitary focal liver lesions (60–70%), whereas multiple lesions or diffuse enlargement involving both liver lobes is seen in the remaining cases.[20,63]

Using imaging techniques, nodular lymphoma infiltrates are hypoechogenic in ultrasound examination, hypodense in computed tomography (CT) scans, and usually do not show enhancement following contrast media application (Figure 24.4). Angiographically, they present as hypovascularized lesions in most cases. On magnetic resonance imaging (MRI), they are hypointense in T1-weighted images, whereas T2-weighted images show hyperintense lesions in most cases.[64]

PROGNOSTIC FACTORS

Owing to their rare occurrence, prognostic factors have not been worked out in detail for most primary hepatic lymphomas. In general, prognosis depends largely on the histological subtype and, especially, HSTCL usually shows an aggressive course, with a medium survival time of less than 2 years.[4,5,20,43] Prognostic factors in PTLD are largely stage-dependent and include increased age, high LDH activity, severe organ dysfunction, and B symptoms.[65] Additionally, involvement of the central nervous system, monoclonality, as well as T-cell PTLD have been shown to indicate worse

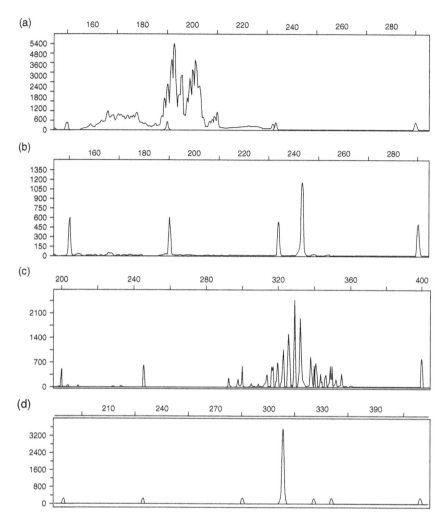

Figure 24.3 Size fragment analyses (GeneScan) of the amplificates in needle biopsies of the liver after TCR-γ polymerase chain reaction (PCR) in parallel to a size standard indicating (**A**) a polyclonal (reactive) T-cell pattern as compared to (**B**) the presence of a clonal T-cell population in a case of peripheral T-cell lymphoma. IgH PCR (FR1) showing a polyclonal (reactive) pattern (**C**) as compared to (**D**) a monoclonal pattern in a case of B-NHL infiltrating the liver. (Courtesy of Michael Hummel, Department of Pathology, Reference Center for Hematopathology (Professor H Stein), Charité – Campus Benjamin Franklin.)

prognosis.[66] Prognosis of secondary hepatic lymphoma involvement depends largely on the stage and the histological subtype of the primary lymphoma.

DIAGNOSTIC AND STAGING PROCEDURES

Diagnostic procedures include physical examination, laboratory evaluation of the peripheral blood, and serology, including transaminases, cholestasis parameters, LDH, and uric acid, as well as serum electrophoresis and immune fixation. Additionally, EBV serology should be performed. Radiological staging procedures include thoracic, abdominal, and cervical CT or MRI scans and, in case of PTLD, cranial imaging. Pathological staging has to consider a liver and a bone marrow biopsy and, in case of enlarged lymph nodes,

Table 24.1 Distribution and frequency of extranodal lymphoma at different sites

	Liver (n = 135)	Brain (n = 31)	Testis (n = 61)	Lung (n = 79)	Bone marrow (n = 1996)	Stomach (n = 855)	Small intestine (n = 71)	Large intestine (n = 102)	Spleen (n = 128)	Skin (n = 427)
DLBCL	52	25	57	22	66	238	30	32	21	78
TCRBCL	9	–	–	–	7	–	–	–	3	–
FL	11	1	–	2	168	16	3	3	20	91
B-CLL	13	1	–	2	656	12	–	4	10	7
PL	4	3	–	–	473	–	–	–	1	2
MZL	6	–	–	40	17	577	4	12	18	12
MCL	3	–	–	3	107	7	7	41	19	6
LPL	–	–	–	3	122	–	–	2	13	5
HCL	1	–	–	–	112	–	–	–	6	–
B-ALL	2	–	1	–	78	–	–	–	1	–
BL	5	–	1	–	4	–	3	2	–	2
cHL	10	–	–	3	52	–	–	–	3	10
B-NHL total (%)	116/135 (86%)	30/31 (97%)	59/61 (97%)	75/79 (95%)	1862/1996 (93%)	850/855 (99%)	47/71 (66%)	96/102 (94%)	115/128 (90%)	213/427 (50%)
pTCL	13	1	1	3	93	4	6	6	12	94
NK/T	–	–	1	–	–	–	2	–	–	2
T-ALL	–	–	1	–	29	–	–	–	–	9
ALCL	5	–	–	1	8	1	6	–	–	26
Enteropathy-type TCL	–	–	–	–	–	–	10	–	–	–
HSTCL	1	–	–	–	5	–	–	–	1	–
MF	–	–	–	–	–	–	–	–	–	83
T-NHL total (%)	19/135 (14%)	1/31 (3%)	2/61 (3%)	4/79 (5%)	134/1996 (7%)	5/855 (1%)	24/71 (34%)	6/102 (6%)	13/128 (10%)	214/427 (50%)

Reference Center for Hematopathology 1994–2003, Charité – Campus Benjamin Franklin.

NHL, non-Hodgkin lymphoma; DLBCL, diffuse large B-cell lymphoma; cHL, classical Hodgkin's lymphoma; TCRBCL, T-cell-rich B-cell lymphoma; ALCL, anaplastic large cell lymphoma; HSTCL, hepatosplenic T-cell lymphoma; BL, Burkitt's lymphoma; PL, plasmacytoma; B-CLL, B-cell chronic lymphocytic leukemia; FL, follicular lymphoma; MZL, marginal zone lymphoma; MCL, mantle cell lymphoma; B-ALL, precursor B lymphoblastic leukemia; pTCL, peripheral T-cell lymphoma, unspecified; HCL, hairy cell leukemia; MF, mycosis fungoides; LPL, lymphoplasmacytic lymphoma; NK/T, extranodal natural killer T-cell lymphoma; T-ALL, precursor T lymphoblastic leukemia.

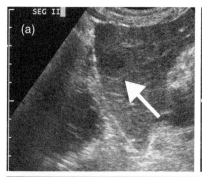
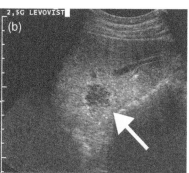
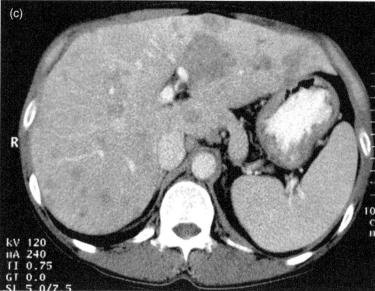

Figure 24.4 (**A**) Unenhanced sonogram of the liver in a patient with focal lymphoma infiltration showing an ill-defined hypoechoic lesion (arrow). (**B**) After contrast medium injection (Levovist, Schering AG, Germany), the lesion is shown as a well-defined enhancement defect (arrow) relative to normal parenchyma and surrounded by a thin hyperenhancing rim. (**C**) Contrast-enhanced CT scan with multiple hypodense nodular hepatic infiltrates in a patient with classical Hodgkin lymphoma. (Courtesy of Thomas Albrecht, Department of Radiology, Charité – Campus Benjamin Franklin.)

a respective biopsy should also be considered for diagnostic purposes.

TREATMENT AND OUTCOME

Whereas secondary hepatic lymphoma involvement is treated with therapy schemes according to the respective primary lymphoma, sustained remission or cure may be attempted by surgery, radiotherapy, or trans-arterial chemoembolization in some cases of localized primary hepatic lymphomas. Further treatment options include adjuvant chemotherapy or, in cases of B-cell lymphoma, anti-CD20 antibody therapy. Prognosis depends largely on the histological subtype and, as already mentioned, HSTCL usually shows an aggressive course, with a medium survival time of less than 2 years.[4,5,20,43,67–70] In primary lymphomas associated with chronic viral hepatitis, antiviral therapy may result in complete regression of the hepatic lymphoma.[71–73] Treatment of PTLD is stage-dependent. In early lesions like plasma cell hyperplasia or mononucleosis-like PTLD, reduction of immunosuppression may be sufficient.[65] Antiviral therapy may result in complete or sustained remission in cases of PTLD, where EBV expression has been proven by histology (Figure 24.2M–O). Since the latently infected B cells of PTLD usually do not express the viral thymidine kinase, recommended antivirals include direct inhibitors of the viral DNA polymerase such as cidofovir and foscarnet.[74]

In advanced disease, anti-CD20 antibody therapy and/or CHOP (cyclophosphamide, doxorubicin, vincristine, prednisone)-based chemotherapy may result in good response rates.[75]

REFERENCES

1. Kim H, Dorfman RF. Morphological studies of 84 untreated patients subjected to laparotomy for the staging of non-Hodgkin's lymphomas. Cancer 1974; 33(3): 657–74.

2. Jaffe ES. Malignant lymphomas: pathology of hepatic involvement. Semin Liver Dis 1987; 7(3): 257–68.

3. Caccamo D, Pervez NK, Marchevsky A. Primary lymphoma of the liver in the acquired immunodeficiency syndrome. Arch Pathol Lab Med 1986; 110(6): 553–5.

4. Avlonitis VS, Linos D. Primary hepatic lymphoma: a review. Eur J Surg 1999; 165(8): 725–9.

5. Noronha V, Shafi NQ, Obando JA, Kummar S. Primary non-Hodgkin's lymphoma of the liver. Crit Rev Oncol Hematol 2005; 53(3): 199–207.

6. Osborne BM, Butler JJ, Guarda LA. Primary lymphoma of the liver. Ten cases and a review of the literature. Cancer 1985; 56(12): 2902–10.

7. Collins MH, Orazi A, Bauman M, et al. Primary hepatic B-cell lymphoma in a child. Am J Surg Pathol 1993; 17(11): 1182–6.

8. Huang CB, Eng HL, Chuang JH, Cheng YF, Chen WJ. Primary Burkitt's lymphoma of the liver: report of a case with long-term survival after surgical resection and combination chemotherapy. J Pediatr Hematol Oncol 1997; 19(2): 135–8.

9. Miller ST, Wollner N, Meyers PA, et al. Primary hepatic or hepatosplenic non-Hodgkin's lymphoma in children. Cancer 1983; 52(12): 2285–8.

10. Ramos G, Murao M, de Oliveira BM, de Castro LP, Viana MB. Primary hepatic non-Hodgkin's lymphoma in children: a case report and review of the literature. Med Pediatr Oncol 1997; 28(5): 370–2.

11. Bronowicki JP, Bineau C, Feugier P, et al. Primary lymphoma of the liver: clinical-pathological features and relationship with HCV infection in French patients. Hepatology 2003; 37(4): 781–7.

12. Lei KI. Primary non-Hodgkin's lymphoma of the liver. Leuk Lymphoma 1998; 29(3–4): 293–9.

13. Loddenkemper C, Longerich T, Hummel M, et al. Frequency and diagnostic patterns of lymphomas in liver biopsies with respect to the WHO classification. Virchows Arch 2007; 450(5): 493–502.

14. Andreola S, Audisio RA, Mazzaferro V, et al. Primary lymphoma of the liver showing immunohistochemical evidence of T-cell origin. Successful management by right trisegmentectomy. Dig Dis Sci 1988; 33(12): 1632–6.

15. Eom DW, Huh JR, Kang YK, Lee YS, Yu E. Clinicopathological features of eight Korean cases of primary hepatic lymphoma. Pathol Int 2004; 54(11): 830–6.

16. Lee SS, Cho KJ, Kim CW, Kang YK. Clinicopathological analysis of 501 non-Hodgkin's lymphomas in Korea according to the revised European-American classification of lymphoid neoplasms. Histopathology 1999; 35(4): 345–54.

17. Stancu M, Jones D, Vega F, Medeiros LJ. Peripheral T-cell lymphoma arising in the liver. Am J Clin Pathol 2002; 118(4): 574–81.

18. Scheimberg IB, Pollock DJ, Collins PW, et al. Pathology of the liver in leukemia and lymphoma. A study of 110 autopsies. Histopathology 1995; 26(4): 311–21.

19. Walz-Mattmuller R, Horny HP, Ruck P, Kaiserling E. Incidence and pattern of liver involvement in haematological malignancies. Pathol Res Pract 1998; 194(11): 781–9.

20. Ohsawa M, Aozasa K, Horiuchi K, et al. Malignant lymphoma of the liver. Report of five cases and review of the literature. Dig Dis Sci 1992; 37(7): 1105–9.

21. Penn I. Primary malignancies of the hepato-biliary-pancreatic system in organ allograft recipients. J Hepatobiliary Pancreat Surg 1998; 5(2): 157–64.

22. Rostaing L, Suc B, Fourtanier G, et al. Liver B cell lymphoma after liver transplantation. Transplant Proc 1995; 27(2): 1781–2.

23. Romet-Lemonne JL, McLane MF, Elfassi E, et al. Hepatitis B virus infection in cultured human lymphoblastoid cells. Science 1983; 221(4611): 667–9.

24. Zignego AL, Macchia D, Monti M, et al. Infection of peripheral mononuclear blood cells by hepatitis C virus. J Hepatol 1992; 15(3): 382–6.

25. Luppi M, Grazia Ferrari M, Bonaccorsi G, et al. Hepatitis C virus infection in subsets of neoplastic lymphoproliferations not associated with cryoglobulinemia. Leukemia 1996; 10(2): 351–5.

26. Silvestri F, Pipan C, Barillari G, et al. Prevalence of hepatitis C virus infection in patients with lymphoproliferative disorders. Blood 1996; 87(10): 4296–301.

27. Wands JR, Chura CM, Roll FJ, Maddrey WC. Serial studies of hepatitis-associated antigen and antibody in patients receiving antitumor chemotherapy for myeloproliferative and lymphoproliferative disorders. Gastroenterology 1975; 68(1): 105–12.

28. Zignego AL, Giannelli F, Marrocchi ME, et al. T(14;18) translocation in chronic hepatitis C virus infection. Hepatology 2000; 31(2): 474–9.

29. Kitay-Cohen Y, Amiel A, Hilzenrat N, et al. Bcl-2 rearrangement in patients with chronic hepatitis C associated with essential mixed cryoglobulinemia type II. Blood 2000; 96(8): 2910–12.

30. Zuckerman E, Zuckerman T, Sahar D, et al. bcl-2 and immunoglobulin gene rearrangement in patients with hepatitis C virus infection. Br J Haematol 2001; 112(2): 364–9.

31. Andres E, Perrin AE, Maloisel F, Marcellin L, Goichot B. Primary hepatic anaplastic large cell Ki-1 non-Hodgkin's lymphoma and hereditary hemochromatosis: a fortuitous association? Clin Lab Haematol 2003; 25(3): 185–6.

32. Ferluga D, Luzar B, Gadzijev EM. Follicular lymphoma of the gallbladder and extrahepatic bile ducts. Virchows Arch 2003; 442(2): 136–40.

33. Reichert CM, O'Leary TJ, Levens DL, Simrell CR, Macher AM. Autopsy pathology in the acquired immune deficiency syndrome. Am J Pathol 1983; 112(3): 357–82.

34. Jaffe ES, Harris NL, Stein H, Vardiman JW, eds. World Health Organisation of Tumours. Pathology and Genetics of Tumours of Haematopoietic and Lymphoid Tissues. Lyon: IARC Press, 2001.

35. Freeman HJ. Hepatobiliary tract and pancreatic disorders in celiac disease. Can J Gastroenterol 1997; 11(1): 77–81.

36. Sato S, Masuda T, Oikawa H, et al. Primary hepatic lymphoma associated with primary biliary cirrhosis. Am J Gastroenterol 1999; 94(6): 1669–73.

37. Sutton E, Malatjalian D, Hayne OA, Hanly JG. Liver lymphoma in systemic lupus erythematosus. J Rheumatol 1989; 16(12): 1584–8.

38. Tsuruta S, Enjoji M, Nakamuta M, et al. Primary hepatic lymphoma in a patient with Sjögren's syndrome. J Gastroenterol 2002; 37(2): 129–32.

39. Tsutsumi Y, Deng YL, Uchiyama M, Kawano K, Ikeda Y. OPD4-positive T-cell lymphoma of the liver in systemic lupus erythematosus. Acta Pathol Jpn 1991; 41(11): 829–33.

40. Ye MQ, Suriawinata A, Black C, et al. Primary hepatic marginal zone B-cell lymphoma of mucosa-associated lymphoid tissue type in a patient with primary biliary cirrhosis. Arch Pathol Lab Med 2000; 124(4): 604–8.

41. Yoshimoto T, Araki Y, Kawano K, et al. [Primary hepatic lymphoma in a patient with autoimmune hemolytic anemia and SLE]. Rinsho Ketsueki 1990; 31(11): 1878–83. [in Japanese]

42. Longerich T, Schirmacher P, Dienes HP, Stein H, Loddenkemper C. [Malignant lymphomas of the liver: new diagnostic algorithms]. Pathologe 2006; 27(4): 263–72. [in German]

43. Cooke CB, Krenacs L, Stetler-Stevenson M, et al. Hepatosplenic T-cell lymphoma: a distinct clinicopathologic entity of cytotoxic gamma delta T-cell origin. Blood 1996; 88(11): 4265–74.

44. Farcet JP, Gaulard P, Marolleau JP, et al. Hepatosplenic T-cell lymphoma: sinusal/sinusoidal localization of malignant cells expressing the T-cell receptor gamma delta. Blood 1990; 75(11): 2213–19.

45. Arnulf B, Copie-Bergman C, Delfau-Larue MH, et al. Nonhepatosplenic gammadelta T-cell lymphoma: a subset of cytotoxic lymphomas with mucosal or skin localization. Blood 1998; 91(5): 1723–31.

46. Ross CW, Schnitzer B, Sheldon S, Braun DK, Hanson CA. Gamma/delta T-cell posttransplantation lymphoproliferative disorder primarily in the spleen. Am J Clin Pathol 1994; 102(3): 310–15.

47. Alonsozana EL, Stamberg J, Kumar D, et al. Isochromosome 7q: the primary cytogenetic abnormality in hepatosplenic gammadelta T cell lymphoma. Leukemia 1997; 11(8): 1367–72.

48. Colwill R, Dube I, Scott JG, et al. Isochromosome 7q as the sole abnormality in an unusual case of T-cell lineage malignancy. Hematol Pathol 1990; 4(1): 53–8.

49. Wang CC, Tien HF, Lin MT, et al. Consistent presence of isochromosome 7q in hepatosplenic T gamma/delta lymphoma: a new cytogenetic-clinicopathologic entity. Genes Chromosomes Cancer 1995; 12(3): 161–4.

50. Belhadj K, Reyes F, Farcet JP, et al. Hepatosplenic gammadelta T-cell lymphoma is a rare clinicopathologic entity with poor outcome: report on a series of 21 patients. Blood 2003; 102(13): 4261–9.

51. Macon WR, Levy NB, Kurtin PJ, et al. Hepatosplenic alphabeta T-cell lymphomas: a report of 14 cases and comparison with hepatosplenic gammadelta T-cell lymphomas. Am J Surg Pathol 2001; 25(3): 285–96.

52. Hans CP, Weisenburger DD, Greiner TC, et al. Confirmation of the molecular classification of diffuse large B-cell lymphoma by immunohistochemistry using a tissue microarray. Blood 2004; 103(1): 275–82.

53. Alizadeh AA, Eisen MB, Davis RE, et al. Distinct types of diffuse large B-cell lymphoma identified by gene expression profiling. Nature 2000; 403(6769): 503–11.

54. Dargent JL, De Wolf-Peeters C. Liver involvement by lymphoma: identification of a distinctive pattern of infiltration related to T-cell/histiocyte-rich B-cell lymphoma. Ann Diagn Pathol 1998; 2(6): 363–9.

55. Khan SM, Cottrell BJ, Millward-Sadler GH, Wright DH. T-cell-rich B-cell lymphoma presenting as liver disease. Histopathology 1993; 23(3): 217–24.

56. Ng P, Slater S, Radvan G, Price A. Hepatic plasmacytomas: case report and review of imaging features. Australas Radiol 1999; 43(1): 98–101.

57. Scoazec JY, Degott C, Brousse N, et al. Non-Hodgkin's lymphoma presenting as a primary tumor of the liver: presentation, diagnosis and outcome in eight patients. Hepatology 1991; 13(5): 870–5.

58. Castroagudin JF, Gonzalez-Quintela A, Fraga M, Forteza J, Barrio E. Presentation of T-cell-rich B-cell lymphoma mimicking acute hepatitis. Hepatogastroenterology 1999; 46(27): 1710–13.

59. Harris AC, Kornstein MJ. Malignant lymphoma imitating hepatitis. Cancer 1993; 71(8): 2639–46.

60. Harris AC, Ben-Ezra JM, Contos MJ, Kornstein MJ. Malignant lymphoma can present as hepatobiliary disease. Cancer 1996; 78(9): 2011–19.

61. Myszor MF, Record CO. Primary and secondary malignant disease of the liver and fulminant hepatic failure. J Clin Gastroenterol 1990; 12(4): 441–6.

62. Smith MS, Nguyen GK. Primary hepatic non-Hodgkin's lymphoma manifested initially as acute hepatitis. Diagn Cytopathol 1996; 14(2): 191–3.

63. Memeo L, Pecorello I, Ciardi A, et al. Primary non-Hodgkin's lymphoma of the liver. Acta Oncol 1999; 38(5): 655–8.

64. Maher MM, McDermott SR, Fenlon HM, et al. Imaging of primary non-Hodgkin's lymphoma of the liver. Clin Radiol 2001; 56(4): 295–301.

65. Tsai DE, Hardy CL, Tomaszewski JE, et al. Reduction in immunosuppression as initial therapy for post-transplant lymphoproliferative disorder: analysis of prognostic variables and long-term follow-up of 42 adult patients. Transplantation 2001; 71(8): 1076–88.

66. Leblond V, Dhedin N, Mamzer Bruneel MF, et al. Identification of prognostic factors in 61 patients with posttransplantation lymphoproliferative disorders. J Clin Oncol 2001; 19(3): 772–8.

67. Gockel HR, Heidemann J, Lugering A, et al. Stable remission after administration of rituximab in a patient with primary hepatic marginal zone B-cell lymphoma. Eur J Haematol 2005; 74(5): 445–7.

68. Ho SJ, Manoharan A. Progressive hepatic lymphoma successfully treated with regional chemotherapy through a hepatic artery catheter. Intern Med J 2006; 36(8): 538–9.

69. Kirk CM, Lewin D, Lazarchick J. Primary hepatic B-cell lymphoma of mucosa-associated lymphoid tissue. Arch Pathol Lab Med 1999; 123(8): 716–19.

70. Shin SY, Kim JS, Lim JK, et al. Longlasting remission of primary hepatic mucosa-associated lymphoid tissue (MALT) lymphoma achieved by radiotherapy alone. Korean J Intern Med 2006; 21(2): 127–31.

71. Zuckerman E, Zuckerman T, Sahar D, et al. The effect of antiviral therapy on t(14; 18) translocation and immunoglobulin gene rearrangement in patients with chronic hepatitis C virus infection. Blood 2001; 97(6): 1555–9.

72. Iannitto E, Ammatuna E, Tripodo C, et al. Long-lasting remission of primary hepatic lymphoma and hepatitis C virus infection achieved by the alpha-interferon treatment. Hematol J 2004; 5(6): 530–3.

73. Levine AM, Shimodaira S, Lai MM. Treatment of HCV-related mantle-cell lymphoma with ribavirin and pegylated interferon alfa. N Engl J Med 2003; 349(21): 2078–9.

74. Oertel SH, Anagnostopoulos I, Hummel MW, Jonas S, Riess HB. Identification of early antigen BZLF1/ZEBRA protein of Epstein–Barr virus can predict the effectiveness of antiviral treatment in patients with post-transplant lymphoproliferative disease. Br J Haematol 2002; 118(4): 1120–3.

75. Oertel SH, Verschuuren E, Reinke P, et al. Effect of anti-CD 20 antibody rituximab in patients with post-transplant lymphoproliferative disorder (PTLD). Am J Transplant 2005; 5(12): 2901–6.

Extranodal lymphomas in patients with HIV infection

25

Michele Spina and Umberto Tirelli

INTRODUCTION

Approximately 30–40% of patients with human immunodeficiency virus (HIV) infection are likely to develop malignancies during the course of their disease. With the improved survival of HIV patients, due to the better prevention and treatment of infectious complications, as well as the development of more effective antiretroviral therapies, there may be an increase of malignant tumors, in particular those non-diagnostic of acquired immunodeficiency syndrome (AIDS).[1]

Three malignancies are considered to be AIDS-defining conditions:

- Kaposi's sarcoma (KS)
- intermediate or high-grade B-cell non-Hodgkin's lymphoma (NHL)
- invasive cervical cancer (ICC).

In addition, Hodgkin's disease (HD) has been increasingly described in HIV.

NON-HODGKIN'S LYMPHOMA

The incidence of NHL in HIV-infected individuals (HIV-NHLs) is over 100 times that among the general population.[2] It is the second most common HIV-associated cancer, and represents AIDS-defining illness in approximately 3% of patients in the USA and 3.6% in Europe.[3] Since 1996, the use of combination antiretroviral therapy, consisting of protease inhibitors and nucleoside analogs, to achieve maximal viral burden reduction, a treatment strategy known as highly active antiretroviral therapy (HAART),

has been followed by a reduction in morbidity and mortality secondary to HIV infection. Moreover, the use of HAART has reduced the incidence of HIV-NHLs.[4,5]

HIV-NHLs are generally a late event in the course of HIV infection. Risk factors for its development include a low CD4 cell count, a high HIV viral load, and increased age. According to the World Health Organization (WHO,) HIV-NHLs are divided into three categories:

- lymphomas also occurring in immunocompetent patients such as Burkitt's lymphoma (BL) (40% of cases) and diffuse large B-cell lymphoma (DLBCL) (60% of cases) that includes centroblastic (25%), immunoblastic (25%), and anaplastic variants (10%)
- lymphomas occurring more specifically in HIV patients, such as primary effusion lymphoma (PEL) and plasmablastic lymphoma (PBL)
- lymphomas also occurring in other immunodeficiency states, such as polymorphic or post-transplant lymphoproliferative disorder-like B-cell lymphoma associated with HIV infection.[6]

BL typically occurs at relatively higher CD4 cell counts (>200 cells/mm^3), whereas immunoblastic lymphomas occurs in a more severe immunodeficiency (CD4 <50 cells/mm^3).[7,8] Clinical features and natural history of HIV-NHLs differ greatly from those observed in the general population. Extranodal involvement is more common in the NHL affecting HIV-infected patients and some primary extranodal localizations (central nervous system [CNS], serous body cavities, oral cavity) are typical of HIV-associated lymphoma entities. Indeed, at the onset, HIV-NHLs fall within stages III and IV in over 70% of the cases, with extranodal involvement in 70–98%. The most common extranodal sites of involvement are the gastrointestinal tract, the bone marrow, and the CNS. The most common symptoms at diagnosis are fever, night sweats, and weight loss (75%). Typically, HIV-NHLs are often bulky (nodal masses >10 cm in diameter), have a rapid growth rate, and serum lactate dehydrogenase (LDH) levels well above normal range.[9–12]

Primary CNS lymphoma (PCNSL) is a distinct extranodal presentation of DLBCL in HIV infection, usually of the immunoblastic type, that is associated with severe immunosuppression (CD4 <50 cells/mm³), Epstein–Barr virus (EBV) positivity, and a poor prognosis. Leptomeningeal involvement by lymphoma occurs in approximately 20% of patients with newly diagnosed HIV-NHLs.[13,14]

PEL is associated with infection by human herpes virus 8 (HHV8) and frequent coinfection with EBV. Two variants have been described: the classic PEL, or 'body cavity-based lymphoma', which has a unique tropism for serous body cavities (pleura, pericardium, peritoneum); the extracavitary or solid PEL, which is an extraserous lymphoma reported in HIV-positive patients with or without associated effusions. Prognosis is poor, as PEL presents in advanced AIDS and seems to be resistant to chemotherapy.[15–18]

PBL is another subtype of DLBCL, with plasmacytoid differentiation that typically involves the jaw and oral cavity of HIV patients. The neoplasm is highly associated with EBV infection. Pathological findings are large plasmablasts cells that retain the blastoid morphology of immunoblasts but have otherwise acquired immunophenotypic features of plasma cells.[19–21] HHV-8 may play a role in HIV-associated PBL, although it is still unclear if that role is causative or whether HHV-8 infection of PBL tumor cells is secondary.[22,23] HIV-related PBL has been documented in sites other than the oral cavity, such as the anorectum, nasal and paranasal regions, skin, testes, bones, and lymph nodes.[24] Prognosis is poor, despite the use of HAART and chemotherapy. In recent years a huge amount of data have demonstrated the beneficial effect of HAART on the clinical presentation of HIV-NHLs. A comparison between the clinical features of the disease in HAART-treated and HAART-naive patients has actually shown that the patients who develop NHLs while taking HAART are older and present with a minor degree of extranodal involvement, especially of bone marrow and meninges.[9]

Unfortunately, a comparison with aggressive NHLs in the general population still produces a negative effect. In fact, in HIV patients, BL is more frequent and they present with more advanced disease, more extensive extranodal involvement (most commonly gastrointestinal tract), higher International Prognostic Index (IPI), and frequently higher LDH levels. Interestingly, HAART has a positive impact on the outcome of antiretroviral-receiving patients, with significantly improved survival and disease-free progression vs HAART-naive patients; and, above all, a significantly improved disease-free survival (DFS) rate (possibly a result of the improved immune deficit) has been reported. When the outcome of patients with HIV-NHL is compared to that of HIV-negative patients with NHL, overall survival (OS) is shorter in the first group, may be because of the lower complete remission (CR) rate, even if response-adjusted OS is similar in both groups. Hence, it has to be recognized that in the HAART era a curative care takes priority over a palliative approach in all patients, as in the general population.[25]

There is still much controversy regarding treatment of HIV-NHLs. Based on pathology and clinical features, aggressive chemotherapy treatment would be required, which is often incompatible with the complications related to the underlying HIV infection.

The prospective studies on the treatment of HIV-NHLs that were performed in the pre-HAART era or that were started before the introduction of the new antiretroviral agents belong to three major research lines:

- The first approach, followed by American investigators, comprises low-dose chemotherapy protocols that are administered indistinctively to all patients.

- The second research approach is supported by European investigators and consists of different dose–intensity treatment protocols stratified by outcome (good, intermediate, and poor prognosis).
- The third research line is again an American approach and includes the administration by continuous infusion chemotherapy to patients that have not been stratified by outcome.

Low-dose M-BACOD (methotrexate, bleomycin, doxorubicin, cyclophosphamide, vincristine, dexamethasone) is associated with CR rates (46–56%) and median survival (6.5–8 months) that are comparable with those achieved with standard doses (CR >50%; median survival 7–8 months), but severe toxicity (G3-G4 according to WHO) is significantly lower with the administration of lower doses (51% vs 70%, p <0.008).[26]

In May 1993, the European Intergroup NHL-HIV Study started the first randomized study on the effectiveness of different dose–intensity chemotherapy regimens in the treatment of NHL with patients stratified by presence/absence of certain prognostic factors (CD4 <100 cells/µl, prior AIDS diagnosis, and performance status ≥2). A total of 485 patients were enrolled. In the low-risk group (no unfavorable prognostic factors), patients were randomized between the intensive ACVBP (doxorubicin, cyclophosphamide, vindesine, bleomycin, prednisone) regimen and the less aggressive CHOP (cyclophosphamide, doxorubicin, vincristine, prednisone) therapy with granulocyte colony- stimulating factor (G-CSF) support. In the intermediate-risk group (only one unfavorable prognostic factor), randomization was between CHOP and low-dose CHOP (reduced by 50%). In the high-risk group (two or three unfavorable prognostic factors), patients were randomized between low-dose CHOP reduced to 50% and palliative vincristine + prednisone. In the low-risk group both ACVBP and CHOP arms reached similar CR (66% vs 60%) and 5-year survival rates (51% vs 47%). In the

intermediate-risk group, CR rate was significantly higher after the standard CHOP arm than with low-dose CHOP (49% vs 32%, p <0.05), even if 5-year OS rates are similar (28% vs 24%).

In the high-risk group the CR rate was much higher in the low-dose CHOP arm than in the group that had received vincristine + prednisone (20% vs 5%). The 5-year OS rates were similar (11% for low-dose CHOP vs 3% for vincristine + prednisone). The only factors influencing survival rates were the administration of HAART, HIV score, and the IPI score. Investigators concluded that the study, which was terminated before monoclonal antibodies became available, showed that CHOP was the standard chemotherapy regimen for HIV-NHLs, as for NHLs in the general population, and that increasing the treatment dose–intensity in patients with good prognosis had no effect on outcome.[27]

Continuous infusional CDE (cyclophosphamide, doxorubicin, etoposide) for 4 days is the first study protocol within the third research line concerning treatment of HIV-NHLs. With the CDE regimen, the following rates were achieved: CR = 45%, 2-year OS = 43%, and 2-year failure-free rate = 36%. The prevalence of severe opportunistic infections during chemotherapy and follow-up was 14% and, once again, HAART had a positive impact on the patient outcome, with improved survival and, lower toxicity rates.[28] The new continuous infusional 'dose-modified' EPOCH (etoposide, prednisone, vincristine, cyclophosphamide, doxorubicin) regimen has been used so far to treat good-prognosis patients (median CD4 >200 cells/µl). Preliminary results are very satisfactory both in terms of CR (74%), progression-free survival (PFS) (92%), and OS (60%) rates at 53 months.[29]

In recent years, the introduction of rituximab (R-CHOP) has significantly improved the survival of NHL of the general population as against patients receiving CHOP alone.[30–32] Based on these data, several authors have explored the feasibility and effectiveness of rituximab in combination with chemotherapy in patients with HIV-NHL. The Italian Cooperative Group on AIDS and Tumors

Table 25.1 Comparison between CDE and R-CDE

	CDE (95% CI)	R-CDE (95% CI)
No. of patients	55	74
Median age (years)	40	38
Median CD4 count (cells/ml)	227	161
Histology:		
Burkitt or Burkitt'-like	22%	28%
Diffuse large cell or variants	78%	72%
Age-adjusted IPI:		
Low or low-intermediate	42%	43%
High or high-intermediate	58%	57%
Complete remission rate	45% (30%–58%)	70% (59%–81%)
Disease-free survival at 2 years	38% (25%–51%)	59% (47%–71%)
Overall survival at 2 years	45% (20%–58%)	64% (52%–76%)

CDE = cyclophosphamide, doxorubicin, etoposide;
R = rituximab.

(GICAT) performed a study on the administration of rituximab (375 mg/m^2 on day 1) + infusional CDE (cyclophosphamide 187.5 mg/m^2/day, doxorubicin 12.5 mg/m^2/day, etoposide 60 mg/m^2/day administered by continuous intravenous infusion for 4 days) every 4 weeks for a total of 6 cycles with concomitant HAART. In total, 74 patients were enrolled, and 75% of them responded to treatment, of which 70% reached CR and 5% partial remission (PR). Treatment-related toxicity was acceptable for this patient setting, except for infectious events. Actually, 19 non-opportunistic infections developed in 23% of the patients during neutropenia; 14% of the patients were diagnosed with AIDS-defining opportunistic infections during chemotherapy or in the first 3 months after conclusion of the treatment plan. After a median follow-up of 16 months (range 1–57 months), median survival has not yet been reached, and 2-year OS rate is 62%, DFS is 89%, and PFS is 86%. Univariate analysis identified Burkitt histotype, homosexual lifestyle, and positive viremia at the end of

chemotherapy as negative prognostic factors, whereas multivariate analysis showed that only Burkitt histotype and homosexual lifestyle had unchanged statistical significance.[33] Table 25.1 compares the R-CDE regimen to CDE without monoclonal antibody.

Other studies have evaluated the effectiveness of rituximab in combination with chemotherapy in the treatment of HIV-NHL. The first trial took place in France and used R-CHOP to treat 61 patients (Table 25.2). A 77% CR rate was reported. After a median follow-up of 33 months, the 2-year OS was 75%, and PFS was 69%.[34] A phase II study was performed in Spain using the same treatment regimen. Out of 60 patients, the following rates were achieved: CR = 66%, 2-year OS = 63%.[35] Another trial carried out in the USA is currently the only existing randomized study comparing CHOP to R-CHOP. One hundred and fifty patients were enrolled (of which 99 received R-CHOP and 50 received CHOP alone). No differences were observed in CR (58% in the group that received R-CHOP vs 47% in the CHOP group) and OS rates. In the authors' opinion, the toxic death rate attributed to infection was significantly higher in the R-CHOP group than in the group treated with CHOP alone (14% vs 2%), above all in patients with a CD4 count lower than 50 cells/µl at the time of enrolment. Moreover, the CR rate reported in the combination treatment arm is much lower than that recorded by other post-HAART studies with or without rituximab (58% vs 74% for EPOCH vs 76% or 66% for others R-CHOP studies).[36]

HAART has improved the immune status of HIV-positive patients, thereby reducing the incidence of opportunistic infections and improving NHL course; the only exception is BL, which has turned out to be clinically more aggressive than DLCL. This is related to the strong positive effect HAART has on the outcome of DLCLs, whereas the outcome for BL is unchanged.[37,38] Since this lymphoma subtype affects survival, a question has arisen of whether it should be treated more aggressively. A retrospective analysis has been conducted on the feasibility of intensive aggressive chemotherapy regimens

Table 25.2   Rituximab and chemotherapy in HIV-related non-Hodgkin's lymphomas: review of the literature

	R-CDE[33]	R-CHOP[34]	R-CHOP[36]	R-CHOP[35]
No. of patients	74	61	95	60
Stage III-IV (%)	70	69	80	63
IPI ≥2 (%)	57	48	58	64
Median CD4 (cells/dl)	161	172	128	152
Complete remission rate	70%	77%	57%	66%
Febrile neutropenia	31%	25%	32%	NA
Deaths from infections	7%	2%	11%	5%

R-CDE = rituximab + cyclophosphamide, doxorubicin, etoposide; R-CHOP = rituximab + cyclophosphamide, vincristine, doxorubicin, prednisone.

(i.e. CODOX-M/IVAC or PETHEMA-LAL3/97), which are usually used in the treatment of BL in the general population, and also in HIV patients. The results have been published recently: American and Spanish investigators report a 63–68% CR rate, a 46–60% failure-free survival rate at 2 years, and the same toxicity as in the general population, which confirms the feasibility of the above regimens also in the HIV setting.[39,40]

Lymphoma progression is the leading cause of death in 35–55% of the patients with HIV-NHL receiving chemotherapy, of whom around 50% of patients need second-line chemotherapy following progression or relapse of the disease. To date, the results achieved by salvage therapies that do not include a standard high-dose chemotherapy regimen with peripheral blood stem cell transplant have been very frustrating (median survival = 2–4 months).[41] The results of treatment regimens incorporating experimental drugs such as mitoguazone have been just as disappointing, with a 11% CR rate and median survival <3 months.[42] With the introduction of HAART into clinical practice, more aggressive treatment protocols, whose effectiveness has already been documented in HIV-negative lymphoma patients, can be taken into consideration. Preliminary studies support the feasibility of high-dose chemotherapy in combination with autologous stem cell transplant in patients with HIV-NHLs, chemosensitive recurrence, or PR after first-line chemotherapy.

Preliminary findings prove that peripheral blood stem cell collections are adequate, anchoring rates are similar to those recorded in HIV-negative patients, and high-dose chemotherapy is well tolerated with no increase in the incidence of opportunistic infections, at least on a short term.[43–53] Within the GICAT, a study has been performed on a group of patients with NHL or refractory or recurrent Hodgkin's disease: the results support the feasibility of an adequate peripheral blood stem cell collection, with no transplant-related mortality and a very good outcome – 60% of the patients being alive and disease-free.[54]

In HIV-NHLs the conventional prognostic factors influencing survival in lymphoma patients in the general population (age, disease stage, extranodal involvement, performance status, LDH levels) have been used together with HIV-specific factors. In the pre-HAART era, the main unfavorable prognostic factors were presence of a severe immune deficit (CD4+ <100/μl), prior AIDS diagnosis, and poor general health. The advent of HAART into clinical practice has changed outcome significantly: conventional survival-influencing lymphoma-related factors have a stronger impact on survival than factors associated with the underlying HIV infection. In particular, in the most extensive surveys, the IPI score is the most discriminating negative prognostic factor in patients with HIV-NHLs together with Burkitt subtype.[10,27]

HODGKIN'S DISEASE

In Western countries, HD has been the non-AIDS-defining disease that in very recent years has reached the most consistently increasing incidence rate among HIV-positive patients. The largest epidemiological studies demonstrate that HIV-positive patients have a 8–16 times higher risk for developing HD than the general population.[55-64]

Pathological features of HIV-related HD (HIV-HD) are different from those observed in the general population. HIV-HD is associated with poor-prognosis histological subtypes, especially mixed-cellularity and lymphocyte depletion disease, and a very high number of Reed–Sternberg cells, which are unusual in immunocompetent hosts with HD.[65] The association with EBV is observed more frequently in HIV-positive patients (80–100% of the cases) than in the immunocompetent population. The EBV genome is clonal, even when detected in multiple lesions.[66-70] As for natural history, HIV-HD differs greatly from non-HIV-related disease. Over 70% of the patients present with systemic symptoms and 85–90% have advanced disease, with frequent extranodal involvement (most often of the bone marrow, liver, and spleen). As already mentioned for BL, in HIV-HD the infection stage is usually earlier than in other lymphomas, with a median CD4+ count between 275 and 300 cells/dl.[71]

The most indicated therapy for HIV-HD is not yet known. At the beginning of the pandemic, the same treatments as those used for the general population were applied: i.e. the MOPP (mechlorethamine, vincristine, procarbazine, and prednisone) or ABVD (doxorubicin, bleomycin, vinblastine, dacarbazine) protocols, but CR rates were much lower than those achieved in HIV-negative patients, with median survival being around 18 months.[71] So far, no randomized trials but only prospective phase II studies have been performed on HIV-HD.

A GICAT prospective trial enrolled 17 patients to test a combined chemotherapy regimen based on epirubicin, bleomycin, and vinblastine. Overall, the CR rate was 53% with an 11-month median survival and a 2-year DFS of 55%.[72] In an attempt to improve the above findings, another trial was performed on the feasibility of the EBVP (epirubicin, bleomycin, vinblastine, and prednisone) combination. Thirty-five patients were admitted. The results showed a CR rate of 74%, but a recurrence was observed after 2 years in 38% of the cases. Survival and 3-year DFS were 32% and 53%, respectively.[73] The AIDS Clinical Trial Group (ACTG) reported the findings of a phase II study on 21 patients receiving 6 cycles of ABVD regimen. Antiretroviral therapy was not administered concomitantly, but at the end of chemotherapy. A CR rate of 43% was observed, with a 18-month median survival.[74]

As with NHLs, in the HAART era a more aggressive protocol, similar to the treatment regimen given to HIV-negative patients, has also been used in HD.

The GICAT has reported the final results of a prospective phase II study to determine the feasibility of a 12-week chemotherapy with classical Stanford V regimen and adjuvant radiotherapy in 59 patients. Overall, 89% of the patients had an objective response, with CR and PR rates of 81% and 8%, respectively. The estimated 3-year OS, DFS, and time-to-progression rates are 51%, 68%, and 60%, respectively.[75]

Recently, the results of the combined BEACOPP (bleomycin, etoposide, doxorubicin, cyclophosphamide, vincristine, procarbazine, and prednisone) regimen on a small group of patients with HD and HIV infection have been reported. All patients have achieved CR, and 9 patients are still alive and disease-free after a median follow-up of 49 months.[76] At the present time, a prospective phase II study with VEBEP (vinorelbine, cyclophosphamide, bleomycin, epirubicin, and prednisone) has enrolled 27 patients, with an overall response rate of 82% and a 2-year OS and DFS of 86% and 90%, respectively.[77] Table 25.3 summarizes the results of these prospective studies.

CONCLUSIONS

Involvement of extranodal sites (either primary or secondary) is exceedingly common in HIV-associated NHL. Following the introduction of

Table 25.3 Results of the main studies published in the literature on the therapy of Hodgkin's disease in HIV-infected patients

Regimen	No. of patients	OR (%)	CR (%)	Overall survival	Disease-free survival
EBVP	35	91	74	16 months	53% at 2 years
ABVD	21	62	43	18 months	57 weeks
Stanford V	59	89	81	68% at 2 years	70% at 2 years
BEACOPP	12	100	100	83% at 2 years	83% at 2 years
VEBEP	27	82	75	86% at 2 years	90% at 2 years

CR = complete remission; OR = objective response; EBVP = epirubicin, bleomycin, vinblastine, prednisone; ABVD = doxorubicin, bleomycin, vinblastine, dacarbazine; Stanford V = doxorubicin, vinblastine, mecloretamine, etoposide, vincristine, bleomycin, prednisone; BEACOPP = cyclophosphamide, doxorubicin, etoposide, procarbazine, prednisone, vincristine, bleomycin; VEBEP = vinorelbine, epiribicin, bleomycin, cyclophosphamide, prednisone.

HAART, the incidence of AIDS-related CNS lymphoma has dramatically declined.

Prognosis for HIV-associated lymphoma patients, with or without extranodal involvement, could be improved by using better combined chemotherapy protocols incorporating anticancer treatments and antiretroviral drugs. The administration of the newly available effective antiretroviral drugs (protease inhibitors) during chemotherapy, together with nucleoside analogues, can improve control of the underlying HIV infection. A reduction in the viral load to indeterminable levels and an increased CD4+ count may lower the risk for opportunistic infections during chemotherapy. The inclusion of hematopoietic growth factors in the treatment of this patient group makes it possible to increase chemotherapy doses and prolong the administration of antiretroviral drugs with an intent to improve survival. At the present time, we strongly recommend that patients with lymphoma and HIV infection should be treated the same as patients with lymphoma in the general population.

REFERENCES

1. Spina M, Vaccher E, Carbone A, Tirelli U. Neoplastic complications of HIV infection. Ann Oncol 1999; 10: 1271–86.
2. Goedert JJ, Cote TR, Virgo P, et al. Spectrum of AIDS-associated malignant disorders. Lancet 1998; 351: 1833–9.
3. Franceschi S, Dal Maso L, La Vecchia C. Advances in the epidemiology of HIV-associated non-Hodgkin's lymphoma and other lymphoid neoplasms. Int J Cancer 1999; 83: 481–5.
4. Dal Maso L, Tirelli U, Polesel J, Franceschi S. Trends in cancer incidence rates among HIV-infected patients. Clin Infect Dis 2005; 41(1): 124–6.
5. Clifford GM, Polesel J, Rickenbach M, et al. Cancer risk in the Swiss HIV Cohort Study: associations with immunodeficiency, smoking, and highly active antiretroviral therapy. J Natl Cancer Inst 2005; 97(6): 425–32.
6. Harris NL, Jaffe ES, Diebold J, et al. World Health Organization classification of neoplastic diseases of the hematopoietic and lymphoid tissues: report of the Clinical Advisory Committee meeting – Airlie House, Virginia, November 1997. J Clin Oncol 1999; 17: 3835–49.
7. Gabarre J, Lepage E, Thyss A, et al. Chemotherapy combined with zidovudine and GM-CSF in human immunodeficiency virus-related non-Hodgkin's lymphoma. Ann Oncol 1995; 6: 1025–32.
8. Powles T, Matthews G, Bower M. AIDS related systemic non-Hodgkin's lymphoma. Sex Transm Infect 2000; 76: 335–41.
9. Vaccher E, Spina M, Talamini R, et al. Improvement of systemic human immunodeficiency virus-related non-Hodgkin's lymphoma outcome in the era of highly active antiretroviral therapy. Clin Infect Dis 2003; 37: 1556–64.
10. Vaccher E, Tirelli U, Spina M, et al. Age and serum lactate dehydrogenase level are independent prognostic factors in human immunodeficiency virus-related non-Hodgkin's lymphomas: a single-institute study of 96 patients. J Clin Oncol 1996; 14: 2217–33.
11. Tirelli U, Spina M, Vaccher E, et al. Clinical evaluation of 451 patients with HIV related non-Hodgkin's lymphoma: experience of the Italian Cooperative Group

on AIDS and tumors (GICAT). Leuk Lymphoma 1995; 20: 91–6.

12. Sparano JA. Clinical aspects and management of AIDS-related lymphoma. Eur J Cancer 2001; 37: 1296–305.

13. Cingolani A, Fratino L, Scoppettuolo G, Antinori A. Changing pattern of primary cerebral lymphoma in the highly active antiretroviral therapy era. J Neurovirol 2005; 11(Suppl 3): 38–44.

14. Cinque P, Cingolani A, Bossolasco S, Antinori A. Positive predictive value of Epstein–Barr virus DNA detection in HIV-related primary central nervous system lymphoma. Clin Infect Dis 2004; 39(9): 1396–7.

15. Simonelli C, Spina M, Cinelli R, et al. Clinical features and outcome of primary effusion lymphoma in HIV-infected patients: a single-institution study. J Clin Oncol 2003; 21(21): 3948–54.

16. Boulanger E, Gerard L, Gabarre J, et al. Prognostic factors and outcome of human herpesvirus 8-associated primary effusion lymphoma in patients with AIDS. J Clin Oncol 2005; 23: 4372–80.

17. Carbone A, Gloghini A. HHV-8-associated lymphoma: state-of-the-art review. Acta Haematol 2006; 117(3): 129–31.

18. Klein A, Gloghini A, Gaidano G, et al. Gene expression profile analysis of AIDS-related primary effusion lymphoma (PEL) suggests a plasmablastic derivation and identifies PEL-specific transcripts. Blood 2003; 101(10): 4115–21.

19. Delecluse HJ, Anagnostopoulos I, Dallenbach F, et al. Plasmablastic lymphomas of the oral cavity: a new entity associated with the human immunodeficiency virus infection. Blood 1997; 89: 1413–20.

20. Carbone A. Emerging pathways in the development of AIDS-related lymphomas. Lancet Oncol 2003; 4(1): 22–9.

21. Gaidano A, Cerri M, Capello D, et al. Molecular histogenesis of plasmablastic lymphoma of the oral cavity. Br J Haematol 2002; 119(3): 622–8.

22. Carbone A, Gloghini A, Gaidano G. Is plasmablastic lymphoma of the oral cavity an HHV-8-associated disease? Am J Surg Pathol 2004; 28(9): 1251–2.

23. Cioc AM, Allen C, Kalmar JR, et al. Oral plasmablastic lymphomas in AIDS patients are associated with human herpesvirus 8. Am J Surg Pathol 2004; 28: 41–6.

24. Schichman SA, McClure R, Schaefer RF, Mehta P. HIV and plasmablastic lymphoma manifesting in sinus, testicles, and bones: a further expansion of the disease spectrum. Am J Hematol 2004; 77: 291–5.

25. Spina M, Carbone A, Vaccher E, et al. Outcome in patients with non-Hodgkin lymphoma and with or without human immunodeficiency virus infection. Clin Infect Dis 2004; 38(1): 142–4.

26. Kaplan LD, Straus DJ, Testa MA, et al. Low-dose compared with standard-dose m-BACOD chemotherapy for non-Hodgkin's lymphoma associated with human immunodeficiency virus infection. National Institute

of Allergy and Infectious Diseases AIDS Clinical Trials Group. N Engl J Med 1997; 336: 1641–8.

27. Mounier N, Spina M, Gabarre J, et al. AIDS-related non-Hodgkin lymphoma: final analysis of 485 patients treated with risk-adapted intensive chemotherapy. Blood 2006; 107: 3832–40.

28. Sparano JA, Lee S, Chen MG, et al. Phase II trial of infusional cyclophosphamide, doxorubicin, and etoposide in patients with HIV-associated non-Hodgkin's lymphoma: an Eastern Cooperative Oncology Group Trial (E1494). J Clin Oncol 2004; 22: 1491–500.

29. Little RF, Pittaluga S, Grant N, et al. Highly effective treatment of acquired immunodeficiency syndrome-related lymphoma with dose-adjusted EPOCH: impact of antiretroviral therapy suspension and tumor biology. Blood 2003; 101: 4653–9.

30. Coiffier B, Lepage E, Briere J, et al. CHOP chemotherapy plus rituximab compared with CHOP alone in elderly patients with diffuse large-B-cell lymphoma. N Engl J Med 2002; 346: 235–42.

31. Habermann TM, Weller EA, Morrison VA, et al. Rituximab-CHOP versus CHOP alone or with maintenance rituximab in older patients with diffuse large B-cell lymphoma. J Clin Oncol 2006; 24(19): 3121–7.

32. Pfreundschuh M, Trumper L, Osterborg A, et al. CHOP-like chemotherapy plus rituximab versus CHOP-like chemotherapy alone in young patients with good-prognosis diffuse large-B-cell lymphoma: a randomised controlled trial by the MabThera International Trial (MInT) Group. Lancet Oncol 2006; 7(5): 379–91.

33. Spina M, Jaeger U, Sparano JA, et al. Rituximab plus infusional cyclophosphamide, doxorubicin, and etoposide (R-CDE) in HIV-associated non-Hodgkin's lymphoma: pooled results from three phase II trials. Blood 2005; 105(5): 1891–7.

34. Boue F, Gabarre J, Gisselbrecht C, et al. Phase II trial of CHOP plus rituximab in patients with HIV-associated non-Hodgkin's lymphoma. J Clin Oncol 2006; 24: 4123–8.

35. Ribera JM, Oriol A, Morgades M, et al. Treatment with rituximab, CHOP and highly active antiretroviral therapy (HAART) in AIDS-related diffuse large B-cell lymphomas (DLBCL). Study of 60 patients. Procedings of the 47th annual meeting of the American Society of Hematology, Atlanta, GA, December 10–13, 2005; 228a abstract #774.

36. Kaplan LD, Lee JY, Ambinder RF, et al. Rituximab does not improve clinical outcome in a randomized phase 3 trial of CHOP with or without rituximab in patients with HIV-associated non-Hodgkin lymphoma: AIDS-Malignancies Consortium Trial 010. Blood 2005; 106: 1538–43.

37. Lim ST, Karim R, Nathwani BN, et al. AIDS-related Burkitt's lymphoma versus diffuse large-cell lymphoma in the pre-highly active antiretroviral therapy (HAART) and HAART eras: significant differences in survival with standard chemotherapy. J Clin Oncol 2005; 23: 4430–8.

38. Spina M, Simonelli C, Talamini R, Tirelli U. Patients with HIV with Burkitt's lymphoma have a worse outcome than those with diffuse large-cell lymphoma also in the highly active antiretroviral therapy era. J Clin Oncol 2005; 23(31): 8132–3.

39. Wang ES, Straus DJ, Teruya-Feldstein J, et al. Intensive chemotherapy with cyclophosphamide, doxorubicin, high-dose methotrexate/ifosfamide, etoposide, and high-dose cytarabine (CODOX-M/IVAC) for human immunodeficiency virus-associated Burkitt lymphoma. Cancer 2003; 98: 1196–205.

40. Oriol A, Ribera JM, Esteve J, et al. Lack of influence of human immunodeficiency virus infection status in the response to therapy and survival of adult patients with mature B-cell lymphoma or leukemia. Results of the PETHEMA-LAL3/97 study. Haematologica 2003; 88(4): 445–53.

41. Spina M, Vaccher E, Juzbasic S, et al. Human immunodeficiency virus-related non-Hodgkin lymphoma: activity of infusional cyclophosphamide, doxorubicin and etoposide as second-line chemotherapy in 40 patients. Cancer 2001; 1(92): 200–6.

42. Levine AM, Tulpule A, Tessman D, et al. Mitoguazone therapy in patients with refractory or relapsed AIDS-related lymphoma: results from a multicenter phase II trial. J Clin Oncol 1997; 15(3): 1094–103.

43. Gabarre J, Leblond V, Sutton L, et al. Autologous bone marrow transplantation in relapsed HIV-related non-Hodgkin's lymphoma. Bone Marrow Transplant 1996; 18(6): 1195–7.

44. Huzicka I. Could bone marrow transplantation cure AIDS?: review. Med Hypotheses 1999; 52: 247–57.

45. Gabarre J, Azar N, Autran B, Katlama C, Leblond V. High-dose therapy and autologous haematopoietic stem-cell transplantation for HIV-1-associated lymphoma. Lancet 2000; 355(9209): 1071–2.

46. Molina A, Krishnan AY, Nademanee A, et al. High dose therapy and autologous stem cell transplantation for human immunodeficiency virus-associated non-Hodgkin lymphoma in the era of highly active antiretroviral therapy. Cancer 2000; 89(3): 680–9.

47. Krishnan AY, Molina A, Zaia J, et al. Autologous stem cell transplantation for HIV-associated lymphoma. Blood 2001; 98(13): 3857–9.

48. Bi J, Espina BM, Tulpule A, Boswell W, Levine AM. High-dose cytosine-arabinoside and cisplatin regimens as salvage therapy for refractory or relapsed AIDS-related non-Hodgkin's lymphoma. J Acquir Immune Defic Syndr 2001; 28(5): 416–21.

49. Krishnan AY, Molina A, Zaia J, et al. Stem cell transplantation and gene therapy for HIV-related lymphomas. J Hematother Stem Cell Res 2002; 11: 765–75.

50. Molina A, Zaia J, Krishnan AY. Treatment of human immunodeficiency virus-related lymphoma with haematopoietic stem cell transplantation. Blood Rev 2003; 17(4): 249–58.

51. Krishnan AY, Zaia J, Forman SJ. Should HIV-positive patients with lymphoma be offered stem cell transplants? Bone Marrow Transplant 2003; 32(8): 741–8.

52. Gabarre J, Marcelin AG, Azar N. High-dose therapy plus autologous hematopoietic stem cell transplantation for human immunodeficiency virus (HIV)-related lymphoma: results and impact on HIV disease. Haematologica 2004; 89(9): 1100–8.

53. Krishnan AY, Molina A, Zaia J, et al. Durable remissions with autologous stem cell transplantation for high-risk HIV-associated lymphomas. Blood 2005; 105(2): 874–8.

54. Re A, Cattaneo C, Michieli M, et al. High-dose therapy and autologous peripheral-blood stem-cell transplantation as salvage treatment for HIV-associated lymphoma in patients receiving highly active antiretroviral therapy. J Clin Oncol 2003; 21(23): 4423–7.

55. Hessol NA, Katz MH, Liu JY, et al. Increased incidence of Hodgkin disease in homosexual men with HIV infection. Ann Intern Med 1992; 117: 309–11.

56. Goedert JJ, Cote TR, Virgo P, et al. Spectrum of AIDS-associated malignant disorders. Lancet 1998; 351: 1833–9.

57. Serraino D, Boschini A, Carrieri P, et al. Cancer risk among men with, or at risk of, HIV infection in southern Europe. AIDS 2000; 14: 553–9.

58. Frisch M, Biggar RJ, Engels EA, Goedert JJ, for the AIDS-Cancer Match Registry Study Group. Association of cancer with AIDS-related immunosuppression in adults. JAMA 2001; 285: 1736–45.

59. Grulich AE, Li Y, McDonald A, et al. Rates of non-AIDS-defining cancers in people with HIV infection before and after AIDS diagnosis. AIDS 2002; 16: 1155–61.

60. Franceschi S, Dal Maso L, Pezzotti P, et al. Cancer and AIDS Registry Linkage Study. Incidence of AIDS-defining cancers after AIDS diagnosis among people with AIDS in Italy, 1986–1998. J Acquir Immune Defic Syndr 2003; 34: 84–90.

61. Biggar RJ, Kirby KA, Atkinson J, McNeel TS, Engels E, for the AIDS Cancer Match Study Group. Cancer risk in elderly persons with HIV/AIDS. J Acquir Immune Defic Syndr 2004; 36: 861–8.

62. Dal Maso L, Tirelli U, Polesel J, Franceschi S. Trends in cancer incidence rates among HIV-infected patients. Clin Infect Dis 2005; 41(1): 124–6.

63. Clifford GM, Polesel J, Rickenbach M, et al. Cancer risk in the Swiss HIV Cohort Study: associations with immunodeficiency, smoking, and highly active antiretroviral therapy. J Natl Cancer Inst 2005; 97(6): 425–32.

64. Biggar RJ, Jaffe ES, Goedert JJ, et al. Hodgkin lymphoma and immunodeficiency in persons with HIV/AIDS. Blood 2006; 108(12): 3786–91.

65. Carbone A, Gloghini A, Larocca LM, et al. Human immunodeficiency virus-associated Hodgkin's disease derives from post-germinal center B cells. Blood 1999; 93(7): 2319–26.

66. De Re V, Boiocchi M, De Vita S, et al. Subtypes of Epstein–Barr virus in HIV-1-associated and HIV-1-unrelated Hodgkin's disease cases. Int J Cancer 1993; 54(6): 895–8.

67. De Re V, De Vita S, Dolcetti R, Boiocchi M. Association between B-type Epstein-Barr virus and Hodgkin's disease in immunocompromised patients. Blood 1993; 82(1): 328–30.

68. Dolcetti R, Zancai P, De Re V, et al. Epstein-Barr virus strains with latent membrane protein-1 deletions: prevalence in the Italian population and high association with human immunodeficiency virus-related Hodgkin's disease. Blood 1997; 89(5): 1723–31.

69. Dolcetti R, Boiocchi M, Gloghini A, Carbone A. Pathogenetic and histogenetic features of HIV-associated Hodgkin's disease. Eur J Cancer 2001; 37(10): 1276–87.

70. Guidoboni M, Ponzoni M, Caggiari L, et al. Latent membrane protein 1 deletion mutants accumulate in Reed–Sternberg cells of human immunodeficiency virus-related Hodgkin's lymphoma. J Virol 2005; 79(4): 2643–9.

71. Tirelli U, Errante D, Dolcetti R, et al. Hodgkin's disease and human immunodeficiency virus infection: clinicopathologic and virologic features of 114 patients from the Italian Cooperative Group on AIDS and Tumors. J Clin Oncol 1995; 13(7): 1758–67.

72. Errante D, Tirelli U, Gastaldi R, et al. Combined antineoplastic and antiretroviral therapy for patients with Hodgkin's disease and human immunodeficiency virus infection. A prospective study of 17 patients. The Italian Cooperative Group on AIDS and Tumors (GICAT). Cancer 1994; 73(2): 437–44.

73. Errante D, Gabarre J, Ridolfo AL, et al. Hodgkin's disease in 35 patients with HIV infection: an experience with epirubicin, bleomycin, vinblastine and prednisone chemotherapy in combination with anti-retroviral therapy and primary use of G-CSF. Ann Oncol 1999; 10(2): 189–95.

74. Levine AM, Li P, Cheung T, et al. Chemotherapy consisting of doxorubicin, bleomycin, vinblastine, and dacarbazine with granulocyte-colony-stimulating factor in HIV-infected patients with newly diagnosed Hodgkin's disease: a prospective, multi-institutional AIDS clinical trials group study (ACTG 149). J Acquir Immune Defic Syndr 2000; 24(5): 444–50.

75. Spina M, Gabarre J, Rossi G, et al. Stanford V regimen and concomitant HAART in 59 patients with Hodgkin disease and HIV infection. Blood 2002; 100(6): 1984–8.

76. Hartmann P, Rehwald U, Salzberger B, et al. BEACOPP therapeutic regimen for patients with Hodgkin's disease and HIV infection. Ann Oncol 2003; 14(10): 1562–9.

77. Spina M, Rossi G, Antinori A, et al. VEBEP regimen and highly active antiretroviral therapy (HAART) in patients (pts) with HD and HIV infection. Proceedings of the 47th annual meeting of the American Society of Hematology, Atlanta, GA, December 10–13, 2005; 100a abstract #329.

Primary effusion lymphoma

26

Annarita Conconi and Antonino Carbone

INTRODUCTION

First described during the last decade as a late manifestation of the acquired immunodeficiency syndrome (AIDS) related to human immunodeficiency virus (HIV) infection,[1] the primary effusion lymphoma (PEL) is a B-cell neoplasm recognized as a distinct disease entity in the World Health Organization (WHO) classification of neoplastic diseases of the hematopoietic and lymphoid tissues.[2] The clonal tumor infection by the human herpes virus 8 (HHV-8) is a consistent feature of the disease, as well as a preferential distribution into the fluid-filled spaces, usually the serous cavities, in the context of an underlying immunodeficiency status.

EPIDEMIOLOGY

The low incidence of PEL and its identification as a disease entity of advanced AIDS has hampered for a long time a precise evaluation of the epidemiological features of the disease. Nevertheless, based on available information, PEL is a rare entity that accounts for about 0.3% of all aggressive non-Hodgkin's lymphomas (NHLs) and 1–5% of AIDS-related lymphomas.[3,4] PEL development is consistently associated with the immunodeficiency status of the host, most cases occurring in the course of an HIV infection as a manifestation of an advanced disease with severe immunological compromise. An increasing number of cases are being described in the context of iatrogenic immunodeficiencies, in particular the immunosuppression following a solid organ transplantation.[5–7] Cases of PEL not related to an overt immunodeficiency have been reported in elderly individuals, usually in the 8th and 9th decades, mostly from geographical areas that have a high prevalence of HHV-8 infection in the general population, such as the Mediterranean region.[8–10]

PATHOGENESIS

Since the first recognition of PEL as a distinct disease entity, a great number of investigations have been focused on the pathogenetic role of HHV-8 in its development, and HHV-8 tumor infection is now considered a sine qua non for the diagnosis of PEL.[11]

HHV-8 is a γ-herpes virus with a peculiar tropism for lymphocytes, endothelial cells, keratinocytes, and marrow stromal cells. A number of HHV-8 genes, expressed during latency or lytic life cycle, have effects on cell binding, proliferation, angiogenesis, and inflammation. The number of HHV-8 DNA copies in PEL cells is high. PEL tumor cells are latently infected by HHV-8, with consistent expression of the latency-associated nuclear antigen (LANA). LANA protein can act as transcriptional regulator, modulating both viral and cellular gene expression,[12] and displays transforming action in primary rodent cells. HHV-8-encoded FAS-associated death domain-like interleukin (IL)-1β-converting enzyme inhibitory protein (vFLIP) is responsible for activation of the alternative nuclear factor kappa B (NF-κB) pathway, playing a key role in growth and proliferation of PEL cells.[13] The viral *bcl-2* contains conserved domains for interaction with other *bcl-2* members, and has been shown to inhibit apoptosis in vitro.[14] A latent HHV-8 gene product, kaposin B, increases the expression of cytokines by blocking the degradation of their messenger RNAs (mRNAs) through the p38/MK2 pathway.[15]

Viral cyclin can be responsible for deregulated pRB inactivation escaping mechanisms of cell cycle control.[16,17] HHV-8-encoded cytokines, such as viral IL-6 or viral macrophage inhibitory protein (vMIP), can activate mitogen-induced intracellular cascades.[18] Signaling via viral G-protein coupled receptor (vGPCR),[19] homologous to the human IL-8 receptor, leads to the up-regulation of vascular endothelial growth factor (VEGF) expression, inducing angiogenesis via paracrine mechanisms.[20] HHV-8 encodes a homologue of the human interferon response factors (IRFs), transcriptional factors that inhibit interferon-mediated effects.[21] In summary, HHV-8 seems to have elaborated a complex of tools aimed at overcomimg the physiological cellular antiviral responses; some of these mechanisms could have a role in PEL pathogenesis, since some of these viral genes are homologous to cellular oncogenes, possibly modulating the cell cycle, cell death, and signal transduction.[22]

The tumor infection by Epstein–Barr virus (EBV), a γ-herpes virus causally associated with several lymphoproliferative disorders, is reported in a large proportion of PEL cases, suggesting that EBV is an important pathogenetic cofactor. EBV infection in PEL is generally monoclonal:[23] the virus infects the tumor cells from the early phases of clonal expansion, and is typically latent, with a latency I pattern.[10] Analysis of the rearranged immunoglobulin (Ig) variable region (IgV) genes in EBV-positive PEL is consistent with a derivation from germinal centre or post germinal center B cells (the cell population targeted by EBV), whereas EBV-negative PEL may originate from either naive or germinal/post-germinal center B cells.[24] EBV-positive cells are more susceptible to HHV-8 infection; thus, EBV infection dictates the cell population targeted by HHV-8. Gene expression profile studies have shown that many genes, including cell cycle and signal transduction regulators, are differentially expressed between HHV-8-positive and HHV-8 negative PEL, confirming the pathogenetic role of HHV-8, but also that the presence of EBV in HHV-8-positive PEL is associated with a distinct gene expression signature, different from that of EBV-negative

Table 26.1 HHV-8-associated lymphomas: morphological and phenotypical features[33]

Immunoblast-like cells
Anaplastic large cells
Immunoblast-like cells/anaplastic large cells
Plasmablastic
Irrespective of morphological type, tumor cells usually express a plasma cell-related phenotypic profile.

cases.[25] In EBV-negative cases, the expression of a set of genes, either directly or indirectly involved in the mitogen-activated protein kinase pathway, could represent a compensation for the lack of EBV infection.

Molecular studies performed on PEL have failed (to date) to reveal genetic lesions or cellular cancer-related genes consistently associated with all cases of disease. Moreover, PEL are devoid of the chromosomal translocations associated with other aggressive B-cell non-Hodgkin's lymphomas, including BCL-6, BCL-2, and c-MYC.[10,26,27] Approximately 70% of PEL cases bear somatic mutations of BCL-6, suggesting the origin of the tumor clone from the germinal center, with unclear pathogenetic implications.[28] An aberrant somatic hypermutation mechanism could have a role in the pathogenesis of PEL.[29] Few data on the karyotypic profile of PEL suggest the possible presence of recurrent anomalies such as trisomy 7, trisomy 12, and chromosomal aberrations of bands 1q21-25.[30] Other cases display complex karyotypes without recurrent abnormalities.[31] Gene expression profiling studies in PEL have demonstrated the overexpression of genes involved in inflammation, cell adhesion, and invasion, which may be responsible for their presence in body cavities.[32]

PATHOLOGY AND HISTOGENESIS

PEL present morphological features common to either large cell immunoblastic plasmacytoid lymphoma and/or anaplastic large cell lymphoma (Table 26.1, Figure 26.1).[26,27,33] The classic pathological feature of PEL is a diffuse spreading along the serous membranes without markedly infiltrative or destructive growth

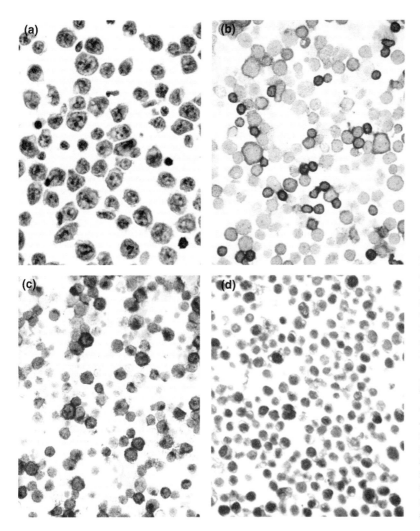

Figure 26.1 (a) Cytomorphology of PEL. The tumor cells are characterized by nuclei that are irregularly shaped and variably chromatic, with prominent, often multiple nucleoli. Cytospin preparation, hematoxylin–eosin stain (H&E), ×630. b–d) Immunophenotypic features of PEL. Tumor cells express leukocyte common antigen (b). Among plasma cell-associated markers, PEL cells score positive for CD138/syndecan-1 (the staining is cytoplasmic) (c) and for MUM1/IRF4 (the staining is nuclear) (d). Cytospin preparations, hematoxylin counterstain, ×400.

patterns.[11] A preferential distribution in the body cavities is a distinctive clinical feature of PEL, but extension into tissues underlying the serous membranes, as well as nodal and extranodal non-serous involvement, have been reported.[33–36]

PEL have a non-B, non-T immunophenotype, since they lack expression of surface immunoglobulin and of B- and T-cell associated antigens.[10,26,27,37] The hematolymphoid derivation of PEL cells is confirmed by the expression of CD45; the CD138 expression indicates an advanced stage of B-cell differentiation.[38] A variety of activation antigens, including CD30, CD38, CD71, and epithelial membrane antigen (EMA), are usually present.[2]

Infection by HHV-8 represents a sine qua non genetic hallmark of the disease, whereas EBV infection is often present but not necessarily required for diagnosis. The diagnosis of tumor infection by HHV-8 can be documented by immunohistochemistry, in-situ hybridization (ISH) (Figure 26.2), and polymerase chain reaction (PCR) studies.[11]

Immunogenotypical studies have documented the monoclonal nature of the PEL cell population.[26,27] Moreover, mRNA ISH techniques have demonstrated restriction in the expression pattern of immunoglobulin light chains.[10] The mutational status of IgV genes and *BCL-6* protooncogene are consistent with an origin from germinal center-related B cells,

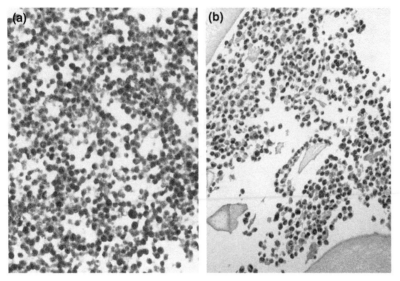

Figure 26.2 (a) HHV-8 viral sequence in PEL. HHV-8 is present in the nuclei of PEL tumor cells, as evidenced by in-situ hybridization (ISH). Cell block from CRO-AP/6 PEL cell line, hematoxylin counterstain, ×250. (b) HHV-8 viral antigen expression in PEL. Tumor cells express latency-associated nuclear antigen (LANA, also called ORF73). The staining is nuclear. Cell block from CRO-AP/2 PEL cell line, hematoxylin counterstain, ×250.

since PEL frequently harbors somatic mutations of both genes.[28,39,40] The origin of PEL from postgerminal center, preterminal B cells is supported by immunohistochemical investigations demonstrating a bcl-6-/MUM1+/CD138+ phenotype.[41] Gene expression profiling studies have identified a distinct pattern of gene expression and features common to plasma cells.[32,42]

CLINICAL PRESENTATION AND DIAGNOSIS

The classical description of PEL refers to a clinical entity characterized by the elective involvement of serous cavities, with the development of effusions in the absence of tumor masses spreading along serous membranes and without infiltrative growth patterns.[11] The increased knowledge about PEL has led to the identification of cases with contemporary nodal involvement and extranodal non-serous sites of localization.[4,33–36] Morphological, immunophenotypical and virological features consistent with the diagnosis of PEL have been recognized in cases with no lymphoma localization in serous cavities at diagnosis, but subsequent cavitary involvement in the setting of relapsed disease.[33,35,36,43] Extracavitary lymphomas have also been reported following resolution of PEL.[36,44] The common biopathological

Table 26.2   HHV-8-associated lymphomas: Clinical and pathological presentation, and HIV viral status[33]

Primary effusion lymphomas (PEL) – in the absence of tumor masses
mainly found in the HIV setting
'Solid' lymphomas
commonly found in the HIV setting
– prior to the development of PEL
– following resolution of PEL
'Solid' lymphomas without serous effusions
irrespective of the HIV status
– extranodal tissue based
– lymph node based

and clinical features of HHV-8-related lymphomas, in their liquid and solid presentation, allow the recognition of these entities as part of the spectrum of PEL (Table 26.2).[33]

Among HIV-infected patients, PEL usually represents a manifestation of advanced AIDS, related to deep immunodepression and severe depletion of circulating CD4+ lymphocytes.[4,34,36] An extremely variable time interval between AIDS and PEL diagnosis has been reported in both patient groups treated with highly active antiretroviral therapy (HAART) and non-treated with HAART.[36]

Signs and symptoms of disease largely depend on the distribution of sites of the disease. The presence of constitutional or B symptoms is common[36] and reflects the disease aggressiveness and the frequent pre-existent compromise of general conditions of the affected patients.

The relationship between PEL and other HHV-8-related diseases such as multicentric Castleman disease (MCD) and Kaposi's sarcoma is not well understood. PEL development in MCD-affected patients could be promoted by the cytokine-rich environment of the MCD lesions and involve a B-cell subset outside MCD lesions.[45] In only a minority of cases reported in the IELSG (International Extranodal Lymphoma Study Group) series has been reported a previous or concomitant diagnosis of Kaposi's sarcoma and the Castleman disease was not frequent and exclusively described in the subset of HIV-positive patients.[36]

DIAGNOSTIC AND STAGING PROCEDURES

The heterogeneous pattern of clinical presentation translates into heterogeneous aspects in the field of radioimaging. The computed tomography (CT) finding of diffuse slight thickening of the serous membranes reflects a typical PEL feature of lymphomatous infiltration of serosal surfaces adjacent to the site of primary malignant effusion.[46] A consistent radiological finding associated with the demonstrated presence of other HHV-8-related diseases should raise the diagnostic suspicion of PEL. Nevertheless, the diagnosis of PEL requires the integrated analysis of morphological, immunophenotypical, genotypical, virological, and clinical features in order to distinguish PEL from other lymphoma subtypes primarily involving the serous body cavities and from node-based AIDS-related non-Hodgkin's lymphomas often characterized by the secondary spread to serous body cavities.

The differential diagnosis of PEL from pyothorax-associated lymphoma (PAL) is based on the presence of a tumor mass localized in the serous cavity without effusion in patients with a clinical history of long-standing pyothorax,[47] representing a late sequelae of a persistent inflammatory status. PAL

tumor tissues are consistently EBV-positive but devoid of HHV-8 infection. Burkitt's lymphoma, which is frequently characterized by serous involvement in immunocompromised patients, can be differentiated from PEL since it is HHV-8 negative and characterized by the translocation of the *c-MYC* protooncogene.

The staging work-up of PEL is common to other subtypes of non-Hodgkin's lymphomas and includes radioimaging based on CT scans, bone marrow biopsy, and endoscopic investigations if clinically required.

PROGNOSTIC FACTORS

The low number of published clinical series and their small size prevent the proper definition of reproducible prognostic factors.

The strongest predictor of poor clinical outcome in the population of HIV-infected individuals is the absence of HAART before PEL diagnosis.[4,34,36] The HAART effect probably relies on a favorable impact on patients' clinical conditions and on the reversion of severe immunodeficiency: the enhanced tolerance to chemotherapy toxicity reduces the risk of treatment–related mortality. Moreover, the control of HIV replication and the subsequent immunological recovery induced by HAART could negatively affect the PEL progression.[4]

Poor performance status has also prognostic significance, representing the main variable defining the relevance of comorbidities and limiting the intensity of treatments to be delivered.

Interestingly, the application of the International Prognostic Index (IPI)[48] score did not display any significant impact on clinical outcome of PEL.[36] The prognostic model, whose clinical relevance has also been validated in a large cohort of AIDS-related non-Hodgkin's lymphomas,[49] probably met a severe limitation in the definition of the clinical stage according to Ann Arbor criteria, which may be not useful for this mainly extranodal entity.

TREATMENT AND OUTCOME

PEL prognosis is poor. Median survival in most series ranges from 2 months up to 6 months.[4,34,36,50] Anecdotal cases characterized by an indolent clinical course have been reported that suggesting a possible heterogeneity of the clinical spectrum of disease.[36,51]

In the cohorts of HIV-positive patients, prior to introduction of HAART, the therapeutic results were unsatisfactory despite the use of aggressive polychemotherapy regimens including anthracyclines. The significant improvement of the prognosis of AIDS-related lymphomas observed in the HAART era also applies to the PEL setting. As mentioned before, clinical series report the prognostic impact of HAART, in association with chemotherapy, on PEL outcome.[4,34,36] HAART positively affects patients' performance status and reverses severe immunodeficiency with indirect effects on the course of PEL tightly dependent on a severe immunological compromise.[52] According to this hypothesis, complete remissions of PEL have been reported after implementation of the sole HAART, without antiblastic drugs.[4,36,53,54]

Despite the improvement in therapeutical strategies during the last few years, there is no evidence of cure of PEL patients with conventional systemic chemotherapy addressed to aggressive non-Hodgkin's lymphomas. The suggested benefit of high-dose methotrexate[55] in association with CHOP (cyclophosphamide, doxorubicin, vincristine prednisone)-like regimens is hampered by the toxicity of methotrexate in the presence of serous effusions.[34] Autologous transplantation in the setting of relapsed disease has been reported as feasible and effective.[56] Anti-CD20 immunotherapy with rituximab represents a therapeutic tool in the rare cases expressing the CD20 antigen.[36,57]

Antitumor activity of antiviral therapy directed against HHV-8 infection has been reported. Patients with a diagnosis of PEL, related or not to HIV infection, experienced prolonged complete remission after the intracavitary administration of cidofovir,[54,58,59] an antiviral agent with a broad activity against multiple DNA viruses and one of the most effective agents for inhibiting HHV-8 replication in vitro.[60] The inhibition of viral replication and a direct proapoptotic effect on lymphoma cells by the high concentration of

cidofovir achieved through the intracavitary administration probably explain this relevant clinical effect. Intracavitary cidofovir, as well as interferon-α,[54] may represent a reasonable choice in patients refractory to conventional chemotherapy or in frail, elderly patients not eligible for more toxic systemic therapies.

Interesting perspectives for the use of a therapeutic immunomodulatory approach have been recently raised by investigations suggesting a potential role for natural killer cells in controlling growth and infiltration of AIDS-associated PEL cells.[61]

REFERENCES

1. Knowles DM, Inghirami G, Ubriaco A, Dalla-Favera, Molecular genetic analysis of three AIDS-associated neoplasms of uncertain lineage demonstrates their B-cell derivation and the possibile pathogenetic role of the Epstein–Barr virus. Blood 1989; 73: 792–9.
2. Banks PM, Warnke RA. Primary effusion lymphoma. In: Jaffe, ES, Harris NL, Stein H, Vardiman JW, eds, World Health Organization Classification of Tumours. Pathology and Genetics. Tumours of Haematopoietic and Lymphoid Tissues, Lyon: International Agency for Research on Cancer Press, 2001: 260–3.
3. Navarro WH, Kaplan LD. AIDS-related lymphoproliferative disease. Blood 2006; 107: 13–20.
4. Simonelli C, Spina M, Cinelli R, et al. Clinical features and outcome of primary effusion Lymphoma in HIV-infected patients: a single-institution study. J Clin Oncol 2003; 21: 3948–54.
5. Dotti G, Fiocchi R, Motta T, et al. Primary effusion lymphoma after heart transplantation: a new entity associated with human herpesvirus-8. Leukemia 1999; 13: 664–70.
6. Jones D, Ballestas M, Kaye KM, et al. Primary-effusion lymphoma and Kaposi's sarcoma in a cardiac-transplant recipient. N Eng J Med 1998; 339: 444–9.
7. Kapelushnik J, Ariad S, Benharroch D, et al. Post renal transplantation human herpesvirus-8 associated lymphoproliferative disorder and Kaposi's sarcoma. Br J Haematol 2001; 113: 425–8.
8. Ascoli V, Scalzo CC, Danese C, et al. Human herpes virus-8 associated primary effusion lymphoma of the pleural cavity in HIV-negative elderly men. Eur Respir J 1999; 14: 1231–4.
9. Boulanger E, Hermine O, Fermand JP, et al. Human herpesvirus 8 (HHV-8)-associated peritoneal primary effusion lymphoma (PEL) in two HIV-negative elderly patients. Am J Hematol 2004; 76: 88–91.
10. Carbone A, Gloghini A, Vaccher E, et al. Kaposi's sarcoma-associated herpesvirus DNA sequences in AIDS-related and AIDS-unrelated lymphomatous effusions. Br J Haematol 1996; 94: 533–43.

11. Gaidano G, Carbone A. Primary effusion lymphoma: a liquid phase lymphoma of fluid-filled body cavities. Adv Cancer Res 2001; 80: 115–46.

12. Renne R, Barry C, Dittmer D, et al. Modulation of cellular and viral gene expression by the latency-associated nuclear antigen of Kaposi's sarcoma-associated herpesvirus. J Virol 2001; 75: 458–68.

13. Matta H, Chaudhary PM. Activation of alternative NF-κB pathway by human herpes virus 8-encoded Fas-associated death domain-like IL-1-β-converting enzyme inhibitory protein (vFLIP). Proc Natl Acad Sci USA 2004; 101: 9399–404.

14. Sarid R, Sato T, Bohenzky RA, Russo JJ, Chan Y. Kaposi's sarcoma-associated herpesvirus encodes a functional bcl-2 homologue. Nat Med 1997; 3: 293–8.

15. McCormick C, Ganem D. The kaposin B protein of KSHV activates the p38/MK2 pathway and stabilizes cytokine mRNAs. Science 2005; 307: 739–41.

16. Li M, Lee H, Yoon DW, et al. Kaposi's sarcoma-associated herpesvirus encodes a functional cyclin. J Virol 1997; 71: 1984–91.

17. Carbone A, Gloghini A, Bontempo D, et al. Proliferation in HHV-8-positive primary effusion lymphoma is associated with expression of HHV-8 cyclin but independent of p21(kip1). Am J Pathol 2000; 156: 1209–15.

18. Boshoff C, Endo Y, Collins PD, et al. Angiogenic and inhibitory functions of KSHV-encoded chemokines. Science 1997; 278: 290–4.

19. Cannon M, Cesarman E, Boshoff C. KSHV G-protein-coupled receptor inhibits lytic gene transcription in primary-effusion lymphoma cells via p21-mediated inhibition of Cdk2. Blood 2006; 107: 277–84.

20. Cesarman E. The role of Kaposi's sarcoma-associated herpesvirus (KSHV/HHV-8) in lymphoproliferative diseases. Recent Results Cancer Res 2002; 159: 27–37.

21. Gao SJ, Boshoff C, Jayachandra S, et al. KSHV ORF K9 (vIRF) is an oncogene which inhibits the interferon signaling pathway. Oncogene 1997; 15: 1979–85.

22. Hengge UR, Ruzicka T, Tyring SK, et al. Update on Kaposi's sarcoma and other HHV8 associated diseases. Part 2: pathogenesis, Castleman's disease, and pleural effusion lymphoma. Lancet Infect Dis 2002; 2: 281–92.

23. Fassone L, Bhatia K, Gutierrez M, et al. Molecular profile of Epstein–Barr virus infection in HHV-8-positive primary effusion lymphoma. Leukemia 2000; 14: 271–7.

24. Hamoudi R, Diss TC, Oksenhendler E, et al. Distinct cellular origins of primary effusion lymphoma with and without EBV infection. Leuk Res 2004; 28: 333–8.

25. Fan W, Bubman D, Chadburn A, et al. Distinct subsets of primary effusion lymphoma can be identified based on their cellular gene expression profile and viral association. J Virol 2005; 79: 1244–51.

26. Cesarman E, Chang Y, Moore PS, Said JW, Knowles DM. Kaposi's sarcoma-associated herpesvirus-like DNA sequences in AIDS-related body cavity-based lymphomas. N Engl J Med 1995; 332: 1186–91.

27. Nador, RG, Cesarman E, Chadburn A, et al. Primary effusion lymphoma: a distinct clinicopathologic entity associated with the Kaposi's sarcoma-associated herpes virus. Blood 1996; 88: 645–56.

28. Gaidano G, Capello D, Cilia AM, et al. Genetic characterization of HHV-8/KSHV-positive primary effusion lymphoma reveals frequent mutations of BCL6: implications for disease pathogenesis and histogenesis. Genes Chromosomes. Cancer 1999; 24: 16–23.

29. Gaidano G, Pasqualucci L, Capello D, et al. Aberrant somatic hypermutation in multiple subtypes of AIDS-associated non-Hodgkin lymphoma, Blood 2003; 102: 1833–41.

30. Gaidano G, Capello D, Fassone L, et al. Molecular characterization of HHV-8 positive primary effusion lymphoma reveals pathogenetic and histogenetic features of the disease. J Clin Virol 2000; 16: 215–24.

31. Boulanger E, Agbalika F, Maarek O, et al. A clinical, molecular and cytogenetic study of 12 cases of human herpesvirus 8 associated primary effusion lymphoma in HIV-infected patients. Hematol J 2001; 2: 172–9.

32. Jenner RG, Maillard K, Cattini N, et al, Kaposi's sarcoma-associated herpesvirus-infected primary effusion lymphoma has a plasma cell gene expression profile. Proc Natl Acad Sci USA 2003; 100: 10399–404.

33. Carbone A, Gloghini A. HHV-8-associated lymphoma: state-of-the-art review. Acta Haematol 2006; 117: 129–31.

34. Boulanger E, Gerard L, Gabarre J, et al. Prognostic factors and outcome of human herpesvirus 8-associated primary effusion lymphoma in patients with AIDS. J Clin Oncol 2005; 23: 4372–80.

35. Carbone A, Gloghini A, Vaccher E, et al. Kaposi's sarcoma-associated herpesvirus/human herpesvirus type 8-positive solid lymphoma. A tissue-based variant of primary effusion lymphoma. J Mol Diagn 2005; 7: 17–27.

36. Conconi A, Spina M, Ascoli V, et al. An IELSG international survey on primary effusion lymphoma (PEL). Blood 2004; 104: 3265 (abstract).

37. Ansari MQ, Dawson DB, Nador R, et al. Primary body cavity-based AIDS-related lymphomas. Am J Clin Pathol 1996; 105: 221–9.

38. Gaidano G, Gloghini A, Gattei V, et al. Association of Kaposi's sarcoma-associated herpesvirus-positive primary effusion lymphoma with expression of the CD138/syndecan-1 antigen, Blood 1997; 90: 4894–900.

39. Gaidano G, Capello D, Gloghini A. BCL-6 in AIDS-related lymphomas: pathogenetic and histogenetic implications. Leuk Lymphoma 1998; 31: 39–46.

40. Fais F, Gaidano G, Capello D, et al. Immunoglobulin V region gene use and structure suggest antigen selection in AIDS-related primary effusion lymphoma. Leukemia 1999; 13: 1093–9.

41. Carbone A, Gloghini A, Larocca LM, et al. Expression profile of MUM1/IRF4, BCL-6, and

CD138/syndecan-1 defines novel histogenetic subsets of human immunodeficiency virus-related lymphomas. Blood 2001; 97: 744–51.

42. Klein U, Gloghini A, Gaidano G, et al. Gene expression profile analysis of AIDS-related primary effusion lymphoma (PEL) suggests a plasmablastic derivation and identifies PEL-specific transcripts. Blood 2003; 101: 4115–21.

43. Chadburn A, Hyjek E, Mathew S, et al. KSHV-positive solid lymphomas represent an extra-cavitary variant of primary effusion lymphoma. Am J Surg Pathol 2004; 28: 1401–16.

44. Huang Q, Chang KL, Gaal K, Arber DA. Primary effusion lymphoma with subsequent development of a small bowel mass in a HIV-seropositive patient: a case report and literature review. Am J Surg Pathol 2002; 26: 1363–7.

45. Oksenhendler E, Boulanger E, Galicier L, et al. High incidence of Kaposi sarcoma-associated herpesvirus-related non-Hodgkin lymphoma in patients with HIV infection and multicentric Castleman disease, Blood 2002; 99: 2331–6.

46. Morassut S, Vaccher E, Balestrieri L, et al. HIV-associated human herpesvirus 8-positive primary lymphomatous effusions: radiologic findings in six patients, Radiology 1997; 205: 459–63.

47. Nakatsuka S, Yao M, Hoshida Y, et al. Pyothorax-associated lymphoma: a review of 106 cases. J Clin Oncol 2002; 20: 4255–60.

48. The International Non-Hodgkin's Lymphoma Prognostic Factors Project. A predictive model for aggressive non-Hodgkin's lymphoma. N Engl J Med 1993; 329: 987–94.

49. Bower M, Gazzard B, Mandalia S, et al. A prognostic index for systemic AIDS-related non-Hodgkin lymphoma treated in the era of highly active antiretroviral therapy. Ann Intern Med 2005; 143: 265–73.

50. Valencia ME, Martinez P, Moreno V, Laguna F, Lahoz JG. AIDS-related body cavity-based lymphomas, herpesvirus-8 and HIV infection: a study of seven cases. AIDS 1999; 13: 2603–5.

51. Ascoli V, Lo Coco F, Torelli G, et al. Human herpesvirus 8-associated primary effusion lymphoma in HIV-patients: a clinicopidemiologic variant resembling classic Kaposi's sarcoma, Haematologica 2002; 87: 339–43.

52. Simonelli C, Tedeschi R, Gloghini A, et al. Characterization of immunologic and virological parameters in HIV-infected patients with primary effusion lymphoma during antiblastic therapy and highly active antiretroviral therapy. Clin Infec Dis 2005; 40: 1022–7.

53. Oksenhendler E, Clauvel JP, Jouveshomme S, Davi F, Mansour G. Complete remission of a primary effusion lymphoma with antiretroviral therapy. Am J Hematol 1998; 57: 266.

54. Hocqueloux L, Agblika F, Oksenhendler E, Molina JM Long-term remission of an AIDS-related primary effusion lymphoma with antiviral therapy. AIDS 2001; 15: 280–2.

55. Boulanger E, Daniel MT, Agbalika F, Oksenhend E. Combined chemotherapy including high-dose methotrexate in KSHV/HHV8-associated primary effusion lymphoma. Am J Hematol 2003; 73: 143–8.

56. Won JH, Han SH, Bae SB, et al. Successful eradication of relapsed primary effusion lymphoma with high-dose chemotherapy and autologous stem cell transplantation in a patient seronegative for human immunodeficiency virus. Int J Hematol 2006; 83: 328–30.

57. Klepfish A, Sarid R, Shtalrid M, et al. Primary effusion lymphoma (PEL) in HIV-negative patients – a distinct clinical entity. Leuk Lymphoma 2001; 41: 439–43.

58. Luppi M, Trovato R, Barozzi P, et al. Treatment of herpesvirus associated primary effusion lymphoma with intracavity cidofovir. Leukemia 2005; 19: 473–6.

59. Halfdanarson TR, Markovic SN, Kalokhe U, Luppi M. A non-chemotherapy treatment of a primary effusion lymphoma: durable remission after intracavitary cidofovir in HIV negative PEL refractory to chemotherapy. Ann Oncol 2006; 17: 1849–50.

60. De Clercq E. Clinical potential of the acyclic nucleoside phosphonates cidofovir, adefovir, and tenofovir in treatment of DNA virus and retrovirus infections. Clin Microbiol Rev 2003; 16: 569–96.

61. Dewan MZ, Terunuma H, Toi M, et al. Potential role of natural killer cells in controlling growth and infiltration of AIDS-associated primary effusion lymphoma cells. Cancer Sci 2006; 97: 1 381–7.

Rare primary extranodal sites (genitourinary, adrenal, cardiac, meningeal, esophageal, pancreatic, gall bladder, and soft tissue lymphomas)

27

Luciano Wannesson and Armando López-Guillermo

INTRODUCTION

Extranodal lymphomas have been found in virtually all the extranodal organs.[1–3] However, while some sites, such as stomach, are very frequent sites of primary extranodal lymphomas, this event is rare in other locations. The aim of this chapter is to review the current knowledge on rare extranodal presentations of non-Hodgkin's lymphomas (NHL), particularly those not addressed in other chapters. The incidence of primary lymphomas appearing in rare extranodal sites showed a significant increase after the AIDS (acquired immuno-deficiency syndrome) epidemics, especially regarding aggressive lymphomas; nevertheless, their incidence is still considered very low.

The infrequency of these lymphomas has some important limitations. First, most publications refer to a single or a few cases of every particular primary site, large series being almost inexistent. For this reason, the treatments used have been very heterogeneous; precluding the possibility of drawing strong conclusions on this topic. Moreover, it is hard to find a consistent histological assessment of those cases diagnosed before the introduction of the World Health Organization (WHO) classification of lymphoid malignancies for which immunophenotyping and genetics studies are seldom available.

A major issue in the context of primary extranodal lymphomas is to distinguish between a real primary extranodal lymphoma from a secondary involvement by systemic disease, which is particularly important in rare sites. Thus, the rules to diagnose a case as primarily extranodal should be very strict, including the absence of lymph node involvement outside local areas.

An overview of primary lymphoma of rare sites is given in Table 27.1.

PRIMARY GENITOURINARY LYMPHOMA

Primary lymphoma of the female reproductive organs

The relative frequency of primary lymphomas involving the female genital tract in a large series of 1467 patients was 1%.[1] In order of frequency, primary lymphomas of the cervix and ovaries are at first place, followed by the corpus and vagina, and those of the vulva and fallopian tubes are the rarest.

Ovary

Primary ovarian lymphoma remains a rare form of ovarian tumor even in young patients in whom epithelial tumors are uncommon, estimated at about 0.6% in females younger than 20 years old.[2] However, in areas in which Burkitt's lymphoma is endemic, lymphoma accounts for over one-half of the ovarian tumors in young patients. Remarkably, testicular lymphoma is 10 times more common than its ovarian counterpart.[1]

Diffuse large B-cell lymphoma (DLBCL) is most common in the fourth and fifth decades

Table 27.1 Overview of primary lymphoma of rare sites

Site	Predominant histology	Prognosis	Observations	Suggested treatment
Ovary	• DLBCL • Burkitt (endemic)	• Favorable	• 75% long-term survival rate	• Systemic chemotherapy according to histology
Uterine corpus	• DLBCL • Burkitt • T-cell lymphomas	• Probably similar to nodal counterpart		• Systemic chemotherapy according to histology
Uterine cervix	• DLBCL • FL and other low-grade	• Probably similar to nodal counterpart		• Systemic chemotherapy according to histology, with or without radiation
Prostate	• DLBCL • Various low-grade variants	• Probably similar to nodal counterpart	• Enlarged prostate with normal PSA	• Systemic chemotherapy according to histology, with or without radiation
Kidney	• Lymphoblastic lymphoma of B- or T-cell type • DLBCL	• Poor	• Usually bilateral and infiltrative • High incidence of CNS involvement	• Intensive chemotherapy according to histology • CNS prophylaxis
Bladder	• MALT-type lymphoma • DLBCL	• Favorable		• Systemic chemotherapy according to histology • Low-grade cases: radiation or surgery alone as options
Adrenal	• DLBCL	• Poor	• Usually bilateral and infiltrative • High incidence of CNS involvement	• Intensive chemotherapy according to histology • CNS prophylaxis
Cardiac	• DLBCL	• Poor	• High-rate of complications: arrhythmia, cardiac tamponade, cardiac failure, embolic stroke • High mortality before CT can be initiated	• Systemic chemotherapy according to histology • Cardiovascular surgery reserved for cases with hemodynamic compromise
Dura mater	• MALT-type lymphoma	• Favorable	• Outside blood-brain barrier; although CSF may be invaded by contiguity	• Patient tailored: surgery, radiation, or chemotherapy
Esophagus	• DLBCL • MALT-type lymphoma	• Probably similar to nodal counterpart		• Systemic chemotherapy according to histology, with or without radiation
Gallbladder	• MALT-type lymphoma • DLBCL	• Probably similar to nodal counterpart		• Systemic chemotherapy according to histology, with or without radiation • Surgery alone may eradicate a localized low-grade disease
Pancreas	• DLBCL • MALT-type lymphoma	• Probably similar to nodal counterpart		• Systemic chemotherapy according to histology, with or without radiation
Soft tissues	• DLBCL	• Probably similar to nodal counterpart		• Systemic chemotherapy according to histology

of life, whereas follicular lymphoma and small lymphocytic lymphoma are more often found in older women. First presentation may occur during pregnancy. Endemic primary Burkitt's lymphoma of the ovary typically affects children, with some cases reported in adults.[3]

Presentation is similar to that of other ovarian tumors, with an abdominal or pelvic mass often accompanied by pain.[4] Ascites has occasionally been present at diagnosis, whereas less commonly, these tumors are incidental findings at routine pelvic examination or surgery for other indications.

About 90% of primary lymphomas of the ovary are B-cell neoplasms.[5,6] The lymphomas encountered most often in the ovary are DLBCL and Burkitt's lymphoma.[5,6] The proportion of these two tumors reflects the age of the patient population in the study, because Burkitt's lymphoma is common in patients under <20 years old and DLBCL in older patients.[7] Ovarian follicular lymphomas constitute about 15% of ovarian lymphomas in the older patient population.[6] Lymphoblastic lymphoma, usually of T-cell origin, occurs in younger patients and even infants.[8] Other T-cell lymphomas such as anaplastic large cell lymphoma (ALCL) are rarely seen.[4]

Systemic therapy is recommended, even if the disease is apparently localized. The selection of the chemotherapy regimen should be based on histology; primary ovarian lymphomas treated with anthracycline-based combinations have a favorable prognosis, with 75% of the patients achieving long-term survival.[9] Failure-free survival of ovarian DLBCL treated with chemotherapy is similar to nodal NHL.[10] On the other hand, the outcome of ovarian lymphoma treated with radical surgery was usually dismal, whereas only limited success was reported in cases treated with radiotherapy after surgery.[6,7]

Fallopian tube

A few cases of primary lymphoma from this location were reported, with an age range of 30–70 years old,[11] but the tubes may be involved in up to 25% of cases of primary ovarian lymphoma.[7] The predominant presenting symptom is a pelvic pain that can resemble a chronic salpingitis and is due to the adnexal mass. Sometimes it

is an unexpected finding during hysterectomy performed for other reasons.[11] Given the rarity of the disease, standards of treatment are yet to be defined, although observing the guidelines for nodal lymphoma (based on histology, stage, and risk factors) could be a rational approach.

Uterus

Uterine corpus

The relative frequency of cervical vs endometrial lymphoma varies among different series. In some studies, the cervix is involved nearly 10 times more often than the endometrium,[4,12] but other clinicians have found equal rates.[1,5,13]

Most cases of primary endometrial lymphoma occur in postmenopausal women, usually in the fifth or sixth decades of life.[6] Bleeding is the most common presenting symptom. Rare cases are discovered during work-up for cervical dysplasia. The clinical diagnosis is established mainly by cervical biopsy, curetting, conization, or hysterectomy.[5]

Aggressive endometrial lymphomas show a polypoid growth pattern, whereas a diffuse thickening is more common in low-grade cases.[6] The myometrium is usually spared. DLBC, Burkitt's and T-cell lymphomas account for most of the cases.[5] Mucosa-associated lymphoid tissue (MALT)-type and intravascular lymphomas are less frequently found. A case of plasmablastic lymphoma was described in a patient infected by human immunodeficiency virus HIV.[5,6]

Uterine cervix

Three-quarters of the cases of primary lymphoma of the uterine cervix occur in premenopausal women, with most patients being 20–50 years old.[6] Affected women usually have a progeny, but cases in nulliparous women do occur. The condition presents with bleeding in 70% of the patients, sometimes accompanied by dyspareunia or pelvic pain.[6] Hematuria caused by bladder involvement is less common. The disease is sometimes discovered incidentally in the course of a routine gynecological assessment, or when atypical lymphoid cells are detected on a routine PAP (Papanicolaou) smear. Cervical lymphoma can clinically resemble a squamous cell carcinoma and thus, risks to be approached therapeutically with a radical surgery, emphasizing the need for a careful preoperative evaluation since surgery is usually not necessary for lymphoma. Cervical lymphoma presents also as an obstructing mass in pregnant women, impeding the delivery. Rare cases were discovered during the work-up of autoimmune hemolytic anemia.[6]

The outcome for patients with primary cervical lymphoma treated according to actual standards are equivalent to what is expected for lymphoma 'overall', according to histology and stage.[14] Cases of primary cervical lymphoma with central nervous system (CNS) progression are a rarity, and hence, routine cerebrospinal fluid (CSF) screening or CNS chemoprophylaxis may not be necessary unless specific risk factors for this are present.[14,15]

Vagina and vulva

There is evidence that vaginal lymphoma occurs at a frequency similar to, or somewhat higher than, the endometrium, which is higher than that of the vulva and fallopian tubes.[12]

Patients with vaginal lymphoma may present with a mass at the introitus, vaginal bleeding, or urinary complaints.[4,12]

Patients with vulvar lymphoma are usually older than those with lymphomas of any other gynecological organ, with a mean age of 60 years old at diagnosis.[4] The finding of a mass is the most common complaint.

Primary lymphoma of the male reproductive organs

Penis

Primary penile lymphoma is one of the rarest neoplastic disorders of this organ. Macroscopically, it could appear as a mass or an ulcer located on the shaft, glans penis, or prepuce.[16] Metastatic disease to the penis is very rare, and most reported cases of penile lymphoma are assumed to be primary.[17] Time from presentation to definitive diagnosis ranges from 3 to 6 months. B-cell lymphoma is the most common type, with reported cases of ALCL and T-cell-rich B-cell lymphoma.

The advantage of chemotherapy in the management of this disease is the preservation of the structure and function of the penis.[16] There are no reported cases of systemic dissemination, although patients with long-term follow-up are scarce. Of note, some early-stage extranodal lymphomas from specific sites have a poor prognoses (e.g. CNS versus gastrointestinal); however, penile lymphomas have not been associated with unfavorable outcomes thus far.

Prostate

Primary prostate lymphoma occurs in men with a median age of 60 years old. The most frequent presentation includes obstructive urinary symptoms that can progress to renal failure.[18] Fever or weight loss, hepatosplenomegaly, inguinal lymphadenopathy, or changes in laboratory tests are uncommon. The digital rectal examination can reveal a very large prostate with normal consistency in the context of a prostate-specific antigen (PSA) level in the normal range.

In a series of 22 patients with primary prostate lymphoma, a variety of histological subtypes were described, including 4 patients with small lymphocytic lymphoma; 2 patients with follicular center cell, diffuse, small cell; 1 patient with follicular center cell grade 1 and another grade 2; 12 patients with DLBC, and finally, high-grade B-cell lymphoma, Burkitt-like in two additional cases.[18]

Several therapeutic modalities have been reported, including prostatectomy, radiotherapy, chemotherapy, and even cystoprostatectomy. However, the best therapeutic approach for primary lymphoma of the prostate is chemotherapy.[19] Among the 23 cases of primary lymphoma of the prostate from Japan, 3 of 5 cases treated with radiotherapy or radical prostatectomy resulted in death or progression. On the other hand, 11 out of 16 cases (69%) that received chemotherapy alone or associated with other treatments achieved complete remission.[19]

Primary lymphoma of the kidney and urinary tract

Kidney

Renal involvement is a common finding in patients with advanced NHL and the reported frequency is very high, ranging from 37 to

47%.[20,21] However, primary renal lymphoma (PRL) is extremely rare, the kidney being one of the extranodal organs usually not containing lymphoid tissue.[22] It accounts for 0.7% of all extranodal lymphomas in North America.[1]

Acute renal failure is a common manifestation of primary renal NHL and its prognosis is generally poor, mainly conditioned by a frequent involvement of the CNS, either at presentation or at relapse.[23-29] PRL mostly affects adults[30,31] and is usually a lymphoblastic B- or T-cell lymphoma or DLBCL.[29] One of the most common presenting symptoms is flank pain; other symptoms include abdominal mass, hematuria, and systemic symptoms such as fever, weight loss, and fatigue. The mechanism of renal failure secondary to diffuse infiltration has not been clearly established. The most likely explanation is that dense tumor infiltration of the renal parenchyma may cause compressive alteration of tubules and impairment of the renal vascularization.[31,32] The infiltration of the renal interstitium, causing obliteration of the intertubular capillary network (without interstitial fibrosis), might explain several specific clinical characteristics of PRL, including the absence of significant proteinuria, absence of cells in the urine, markedly elevated serum creatinine, and usually, a rapid restoration of normal renal function after chemotherapy.[33] The presentation as a delimitated renal mass has been rarely reported.[34]

Treatment should be selected according to the standards for the corresponding histology, which is almost invariably aggressive.[23,29,31] Even primary DLBCL of the kidney tends to have a poor prognosis, with early progression or relapse, especially if presented as infiltrative parenchymal disease.[25] Prophylactic therapy of CNS relapses is therefore recommended.[23-29]

Bladder

Primary bladder lymphoma (PBL) is a rare condition, accounting for only 0.2% of extranodal lymphomas.[1] Unlike most extranodal lymphomas, a female to male ratio of 2:1 is reported. The disease usually presents with urinary symptoms, with hematuria present in 3 out of 4 patients at diagnosis. Weight loss, fever, or night sweats are rare.[35,36]

Similar to MALT-type lymphomas arising from some specific locations such as the stomach or the ocular adnexa, an association of PBL of MALT type with chronic local immunological stimuli has been proposed based upon the observation that up to one-third of the patients diagnosed with this entity refer a history of cystitis and even some cases have been cured with antibiotic therapy alone.[36]

Definitive diagnosis can be performed through a cystoscopic biopsy. MALT-type lymphomas account for a ≥50% of the cases, depending on the series, with DLBCL as the second most frequent type.[35-37] Small lymphocytic lymphoma,[38] ALK-1(+) ALCL,[36] and other peripheral T-cell variants have also been reported.[39,40] Treatment of primary bladder lymphoma has, in general, a favorable outcome. Most, if not all, patients with low-grade variants are cured regardless of the treatment modality, including surgery, radiation therapy, chemotherapy, or a combination of them.[36,37] Those few patients who are not cured often become long-term survivors.[35] Primary intermediate-grade lymphomas (DLBCL and ALCL), which are by definition a localized disease, also attains high cure rates, with survival outcomes that are comparable to their nodal counterparts at equivalent disease stages if a cyclophosph-amide, doxorubicin, vincristine, and prednisone (CHOP)-based chemotherapy regimen is used.[36] Interestingly, one case of primary bladder DLBCL associated with *Chlamydia* infection was eradicated with oral doxycycline as the sole therapy.[36] Given that PBL is not associated with a high incidence of CNS failures, intrathecal prophylaxis may not be routinely necessary unless other traditional risk factors are present.

Urethra

The urethra is the second most common localization of primary urinary tract lymphoma after the bladder, with about 15 cases published.[41] Primary urethral lymphomas show similar clinical and pathological findings to primary bladder lymphomas, including:

- female predominance
- presentation as a polypoid mass

- history of chronic cystitis or urethral caruncle
- predominance of a B-cell phenotype.

MALT-type lymphoma is the most common histological type of primary urethral lymphoma. Presenting symptoms include urinary urgency or hesitancy, hematuria, duplicated urine steam, and vaginal spotting, whereas systemic B symptoms are seldom present.[41] A definitive cure can be achieved with the resection of small lesions of MALT-type lymphoma, but chemotherapy should be part of the therapeutic plan in cases of aggressive histology such as DLBCL.[41]

Upper urinary tract

Primary lymphomas of the renal pelvis and ureters are a rarity among rare diseases. Isolated cases of low-grade follicular or MALT-type lymphoma have been reported.[42–44] A higher likelihood of chronic infections in the lower portions of the urinary tract (bladder and urethra) with respect to the higher ones (renal pelvis and ureters), together with the fact that the most frequent histology is represented by MALT-type lymphomas, may explain the differences in incidence.

PRIMARY ADRENAL LYMPHOMA

Primary adrenal lymphoma is uncommon, with less than 90 cases described in the medical literature.[45] It is a disorder affecting older patients in their sixth decade of life, with male predominance. Most patients have bilateral involvement and bulky disease at presentation, with a median maximum diameter of 8 cm.[46] Lumbar pain is often present and may be accompanied of fever and weight loss. Symptoms of adrenal insufficiency such as vomiting, fatigue, skin hyperpigmentation, and hypotension are also frequent. Uncommon presentations include autoimmune hemolytic anemia, hypercalcemia, and concomitant involvement of other extranodal sites.[45]

Imaging studies that better characterize the lesions are computed tomography (CT) scan and magnetic resonance imaging (MRI), and the main differential diagnosis is metastatic carcinoma. Tissue can be obtained by a CT- or ultrasound-guided biopsy or by surgical excision biopsy. Fine-needle aspiration (FNA) is discouraged, since it is not possible to ascertain the tissue architecture by means of the analysis of individual cells, with the potential of a misleading diagnosis. DLBCL accounts for most of the cases of primary adrenal lymphoma; other types described are ALCL, intravascular, follicular, and T-cell lymphomas.[45]

For staging purposes, it is important to note that involvement of unusual extranodal sites has been described at presentation in patients with adrenal lymphoma, including the testis, thyroid, eyes, and the pituitary gland. The disease appears to have a propensity for CNS involvement at diagnosis, but mainly at relapse, with many series reporting on cases of brain or meningeal relapse.[45]

Primary adrenal lymphoma is an aggressive disease and should be approached accordingly. The mainstay of therapy is chemotherapy, as for DLBCL from other sites. The utilization of modern CHOP-like regimens associated with rituximab and the use of CNS prophylaxis could probably improve the poor outcomes achieved so far, with reported long-term overall survival rates not higher than 30%.[45]

PRIMARY CARDIAC LYMPHOMA

Primary cardiac lymphoma (PCL) account for 1.3% of the tumors originating in the heart.[47] The mean age at presentation for cardiac lymphoma is 38 years old, with a slight predominance in men. Patients with cardiac lymphomas present with various symptoms, including cardiac tamponade, heart failure, exertional dyspnea, atrial fibrillation, and right-sided heart obstruction.[47] Cardiac lymphomas are more common in immunodeficient patients,[48] A predominant involvement of right-sided chambers has been observed.[49] The high mortality and morbidity of PCL is due to arrhythmia, cardiac failure, pericardial effusions, or embolic stroke. Late diagnosis appears to be a major contributor to its poor outcome.[50,51]

PCLs can be detected by a variety of imaging modalities, such as angiography, transthoracic echocardiography (TTE), transesophageal echocardiography (TEE), CT, and MRI. In addition, contrast perfusion echocardiography with TEE has been used to differentiate a thrombus from a vascular mass.[52] Biopsy specimens can be obtained via an endomyocardial sampling, by TEE-guided or even open biopsies.[53] With regard to the histology, DLBCL was observed in up to 80% of the cases.[50] Other rarely reported types are non-cleaved small cell, diffuse mixed small and large cell, and small cleaved cell lymphoma.

The mainstay of treatment is chemotherapy, which should be started immediately after the diagnosis is confirmed. This is supported by the observation that most reported patients died before chemotherapy could be initiated.[50,51] Surgical treatment is associated with a high rate of complications, and is discouraged as a front-line therapy, although, it can be reserved for cases with hemodynamic compromise due to heart inflow or outflow obstruction or cardiac tamponade.

DURA MATER PRIMARY LYMPHOMA

Primary lymphoma of the dura is infrequent, representing less than 3% of CNS lymphomas.[54,55] The biological behavior of primary dural lymphoma is different from other CNS lymphomas, mainly because of the predominant histological subtype (MALT-type in dural lymphomas) and, particularly, because dura mater is outside the blood–brain barrier.[54,55] As for other primary extranodal lymphomas, three conditions are required to diagnose properly a primary dural lymphoma:

- no evidence of systemic involvement
- no evidence of primary brain parenchymal infiltration
- evidence of an extra-axial mass arising from the dura mater.

From the histological point of view, the vast majority of dural lymphomas are marginal zone B-cell MALT-type lymphomas.[55–61] It has been suggested that meningoepithelial cells in the dura mater may have the same role as epithelial tissue in other sites with MALT-type lymphoma. Morphological features are similar to MALT-type lymphomas of other sites. Tumor cells have B-cell markers, including CD20, and are usually negative for CD5, CD10, and CD23. Little information is available regarding specific genetic features of dural MALT-type lymphomas.[62] Although it is very rare, primary DLBCL of the dura has also been described.[63]

Dural lymphomas are more frequent in middle-aged women. They usually present as single or multiple extra-axial masses showing diffuse enhancement after gadolinium at the cranial MRI. En plaque thickening of the meninges can sometimes be observed. Clinical symptoms depend on the location of the tumor and include headache (50% of cases), seizure (50%), focal paresthesias and other sensorial symptoms (40%), visual symptoms (40%), and other symptoms such as dizziness or motor deficits. Clinical presentation and imaging often suggest the diagnosis of meningioma. In fact, differential diagnosis is usually difficult only with the imaging techniques. The presence of vasogenic edema as well as parenchymal brain invasion, very rare in meningioma, is suggestive of dural lymphoma.[55] The biopsy of the mass is mandatory to make diagnosis and characterize the disease. In fact, cases diagnosed as plasmocytomas or other lymphomas in old series have been reclassified as MALT-type lymphomas in subsequent pathology reviews. Staging should be performed as in systemic lymphomas, in order to rule out systemic involvement. Moreover, the importance of assessing the CSF status among these patients has been recently addressed: leptomeningeal involvement was observed in 5 of 8 cases (62%) of MALT-type lymphoma of the dura in one series.[55] This event may be due to contiguity and, of course, has important implications for the treatment.

Given that the available literature on primary dural lymphoma is sparse, it is difficult to establish a standard treatment for these patients. In cases with localized disease, surgery may be the best option, with a very favorable prognosis when the lymphoma is completely removed.[55,59] However, complete resection of the tumor is often difficult, owing to the presence of multifocal disease, brain infiltration, or an en plaque growth pattern. Therefore, if residual disease is present after surgery, radiation or chemotherapy is necessary. Radiation therapy is a good option, because MALT-type lymphoma is a highly radiosensitive tumor; relatively low doses of focal radiotherapy (20–30 Gy) can eradicate the tumor with minimal neurotoxicity. When leptomeninges are involved, intrathecal chemotherapy must be administered. Of note, even those cases with meningeal infiltration may be cured.[55] High-dose methotrexate seems to be unnecessary, since tumors arising from the dura are outside the blood–brain barrier. Overall, the prognosis of primary dural lymphomas is favorable, and the majority of patients are cured.[55,57–59] The cure rate seems to be lower than that observed for gastric MALT-type cases, mainly due to a higher risk of relapse, which often occurs outside the meninges. No data are available on the role of initial chemotherapy in the prevention of late systemic relapses.

RARE PRIMARY LYMPHOMAS OF THE DIGESTIVE TRACT

Esophagus

Primary gastrointestinal (GI) lymphoma is the most common extranodal presentation of NHL; however, most cases involve the stomach, small intestine and colon.[1] Esophageal involvement is the rarest, representing <1% of all GI lymphomas.[64] Even after the AIDS epidemics, primary involvement of these sites is still exceptional.[65] Secondary lymphomatous infiltration of the esophagus from the stomach or the mediastinum is relatively common, whereas primary esophageal lymphoma is exceptional, with only a few cases published.[65–83] According to the Dawson criteria,[84] a primary extranodal lymphoma requires the absence of peripheral or mediastinal adenopathy, splenic or hepatic infiltration, whereas a regional adenopathy is acceptable. DLBCL is the predominant diagnosis, although other histologies have been described, including MALT-type, T-cell, and Hodgkin's lymphomas.

Primary esophageal lymphoma affects adult patients of all ages (17–86 years old), with a slightly predominance in males. The dominant presenting symptom is dysphagia, followed by chest pain, weight loss, and hematemesis.[64] The disease has been found in all segments of the organ, adopting various morphological appearances (nodular, polypoidal, ulcerated, or stenotic). The main differential diagnoses are squamous cell carcinoma and adenocarcinoma, entities that constitute more than 95% of the esophageal tumors. Although imaging techniques could be of help, the diagnosis is usually performed by means of gastroscopy with biopsy of the tumor. Treatment of primary esophageal lymphoma is extremely variable in the literature and depends on the histology. Patients with DLBCL should be treated with anthracycline-based regimens in association with rituximab. Therapy for MALT-type lymphoma is similar to that of the helicobacter-negative gastric case.

Gallbladder

The lymphomatous involvement of the gallbladder is an unusual event, mainly secondary to a systemic dissemination of an aggressive lymphoma. Primary lymphoma of the gallbladder is even rarer, with only about 20 cases published in the literature so far.[85–100] The origin of primary gallbladder lymphoma is controversial, since the lymphoid tissue in the normal mucosa of the gallbladder is scant. However, lymphoid hyperplasia after chronic cholecystitis has been described.[94] About one-half of the patients have a marginal zone B-cell MALT-type lymphoma,[82,85,88,93–95,101] followed in frequency by DLBCL,[98,100] and more rarely by follicular and peripheral T-cell lymphomas.[89] The relationship between MALT-type gallbladder lymphoma and chronic infection of the organ by Gram-negative bacteria has been suggested but not yet proven.

The most frequent symptoms of patients with gallbladder lymphoma are abdominal pain, nausea and vomiting, jaundice, and a palpable mass. In most cases, the diagnosis is done after surgery. The differential diagnosis includes adenocarcinoma and adenomyomatosis, both entities that are far more frequent than lymphoma.

Surgery is usually sufficient to eradicate localized MALT-type lymphomas. The treatment of DLBCL of the gallbladder is similar to any other systemic lymphoma. The prognosis depends on the histological subtype: it is excellent in localized MALT-type cases, whereas it is less favorable in aggressive lymphomas.

Pancreas

Secondary invasion of the pancreas from the retroperitoneal lymph nodes, especially when a bulky mass is present, is a well-known feature often seen in aggressive as well as in some indolent lymphomas. Pancreatic infiltration from peripancreatic lymph nodes or from the duodenum is less frequent. Primary pancreatic lymphoma is very rare, and this diagnosis needs the exclusion of evidence of extrapancreatic lesions.[84,102–111] Very little is known regarding the etiology of these lymphomas.[1] Immunosuppressed patients, including HIV-related and post-transplantation cases, may have a higher risk of lymphoma; however, primary pancreatic lymphoma is uncommon, even among these patients.[106] No relationship with *Helicobacter pylori* or other infectious agents has been established for pancreatic MALT-type lymphomas. Finally, a familial pancreatic lymphoma has been reported.[112] The histological spectrum is very wide. About two-thirds of the cases are DLBCLs, but indolent lymphomas (mainly MALT-type) and T-cell lymphomas, including anaplastic ALK-negative and unspecified peripheral T-cell lymphomas, have been reported.

Primary pancreatic lymphoma affects patients aged 35–75 years old, with a strong male predominance.[109] A single tumor, ranging from 2–15 cm in diameter, located at the head of the pancreas (80% of cases), is the usual presentation. Clinical symptoms usually mimic a carcinoma of the head of the pancreas. Abdominal pain is the most common symptom (80% of cases), followed by abdominal mass, weight loss, jaundice, acute pancreatitis, small bowel obstruction, or diarrhea.[109] Obstructive jaundice seems to be less frequent than in adenocarcinoma. B symptoms other than weight loss

are infrequent. Abdominal CT scan, MRI, and endoscopic retrograde cholangiopancreatography could be of help to detect the mass in the pancreas, but they cannot do the diagnosis of lymphoma. On a contrast-enhanced CT scan, most primary pancreatic lymphomas show a homogeneous uptake. CT, ultrasound, or endoscopy-guided FNA may be diagnostic if sufficient tissue is obtained and flow cytometry is performed.[113] Limitations of this technique are evident and, in fact, open surgery is carried out in the majority of patients without a preoperative diagnosis of lymphoma. Surgery, radiotherapy, and chemotherapy have been the standard therapeutic approach in patients with pancreatic lymphoma, with an overall poor prognosis. At present, total pancreatectomy is not a standard procedure because its role is doubtful in the treatment of these patients.[114,115] Thus, patients with DLBCL should be treated with anthracycline-based chemotherapy in combination with rituximab, according to the treatment guidelines for aggressive lymphomas. The role of radiotherapy is also controversial. Prognosis depends on standard prognostic factors, being similar to that of other locations.

PRIMARY LYMPHOMAS OF SOFT TISSUES

Primary soft tissue lymphoma (PSTL) is an infrequent clinical entity that represents about 0.1% of all the lymphomas[116–118] and less than 2% of all soft tissues tumors (mainly constituted by sarcomas[119]). In a recent study, primary DLBCL of the soft tissue represented 4.5% of all the primary extranodal DLBCLs.[120] The occurrence of PSTL has been associated with previous injury or surgery; however, this association remains controversial.[121,122] In addition to DLBCL, almost all the spectrum of lymphoma have been reported. The clinical presentation is usually as a mass growing within the connective or adipose tissue or skeletal muscle in a region in which lymph nodes are not usually present, but it varies depending on the histological subtype and the location of the disease.[117,123–125] In fact, several categories of soft tissue involvement by lymphoma have been recognized, including the primary extranodal soft tissue lymphomas, intramuscular lymphoma, and subcutaneous lymphoma. The latter stresses the difficulties in distinguishing between 'soft tissue' and other organs such as skin or bone. The main differential diagnosis is sarcoma. Biopsy is mandatory to establish the diagnosis. Management decisions depend on the histological subtype and the location of the disease. In most cases, along with local measures, rituximab in combination with CHOP-like regimens is the treatment of choice.

REFERENCES

1. Freeman C, Berg JW, Cutler SJ. Occurrence and prognosis of extranodal lymphomas. Cancer 1972; 29: 252–60.

2. Norris HJ, Jensen RD. Relative frequency of ovarian neoplasms in children and adolescents. Cancer 1972; 30: 713–19.

3. Konje JC, Otolorin EO, Odukoya OA, et al. Burkitts lymphoma of the ovary in Nigerian adults – a 27-year review. Afr J Med Med Sci 1989; 18: 301–5.

4. Vang R, Medeiros LJ, Ha CS, Deavers M. Non-Hodgkin's lymphomas involving the uterus: a clinicopathologic analysis of 26 cases. Mod Pathol 2000; 13: 19–28.

5. Kosari F, Daneshbod Y, Parwaresch R, et al. Lymphomas of the female genital tract: a study of 186 cases and review of the literature. Am J Surg Pathol 2005; 29: 1512–20.

6. Lagoo AS, Robboy SJ. Lymphoma of the female genital tract: current status. Int J Gynecol Pathol 2006; 25: 1–21.

7. Osborne BM, Robboy SJ. Lymphomas or leukemia presenting as ovarian tumors. An analysis of 42 cases. Cancer 1983; 52: 1933–43.

8. Turken A, Ciftci AO, Akcoren Z, et al. Primary ovarian lymphoma in an infant: report of a case. Surg Today 2000; 30: 305–7.

9. Monterroso V, Jaffe ES, Merino MJ, Medeiros LJ. Malignant lymphomas involving the ovary. A clinicopathologic analysis of 39 cases. Am J Surg Pathol 1993; 17: 154–70.

10. Dimopoulos MA, Daliani D, Pugh W, et al. Primary ovarian non-Hodgkin's lymphoma: outcome after treatment with combination chemotherapy. Gynecol Oncol 1997; 64: 446–50.

11. Ferry JA, Young RH. Malignant lymphoma, pseudolymphoma, and hematopoietic disorders of the female genital tract. Pathol Annu 1991; 26 (Pt 1): 227–63.

12. Harris NL, Scully RE. Malignant lymphoma and granulocytic sarcoma of the uterus and vagina. A clinicopathologic analysis of 27 cases. Cancer 1984; 53: 2530–45.

13. el Omari-Alaoui H, Kebdani T, Benjaafar N, et al. [Non-Hodgkin's lymphoma of the uterus: apropos of 4 cases and review of the literature]. Cancer Radiother 2002; 6: 39–45. [in French]

14. Wannesson L. Primary lymphoma of the uterine cervix: an approach to management. Gynecol Oncol 2006; 100: 626–7; author reply 627–8.

15. Dursun P, Gultekin M, Bozdag G, et al. Primary cervical lymphoma: report of two cases and review of the literature. Gynecol Oncol 2005; 98: 484–9.

16. Lin DW, Thorning DR, Krieger JN. Primary penile lymphoma: diagnostic difficulties and management options. Urology 1999; 54: 366.

17. Arena F, di Stefano C, Peracchia G, et al. Primary lymphoma of the penis: diagnosis and treatment. Eur Urol 2001; 39: 232–5.

18. Bostwick DG, Iczkowski KA, Amin MB, et al. Malignant lymphoma involving the prostate: report of 62 cases. Cancer 1998; 83: 732–8.

19. Fukutani K, Koyama Y, Fujimori M, Ishida T. [Primary malignant lymphoma of the prostate: report of a case achieving complete response to combination chemotherapy and review of 22 Japanese cases]. Nippon Hinyokika Gakkai Zasshi 2003; 94: 621–5. [in Japanese]

20. Miyake O, Namiki M, Sonoda T, Kitamura H. Secondary involvement of genitourinary organs in malignant lymphoma. Urol Int 1987; 42: 360–2.

21. Richmond J, Sherman RS, Diamond HD, Craver LF. Renal lesions associated with malignant lymphomas. Am J Med 1962; 32: 184–207.

22. Paganelli E, Arisi L, Ferrari ME, et al. Primary non-Hodgkin's lymphoma of the kidney. Haematologica 1989; 74: 301–4.

23. Arranz Arija JA, Carrion JR, Garcia FR, et al. Primary renal lymphoma: report of 3 cases and review of the literature. Am J Nephrol 1994; 14: 148–53.

24. Becker AM, Bowers DC, Margraf LR, et al. Primary renal lymphoma presenting with hypertension. Pediatr Blood Cancer 2007; 48: 711–13.

25. Guilpain P, Delarue R, Matignon M, et al. Primary bilateral diffuse renal lymphoma. Am J Hematol 2006; 81: 804–5.

26. Harris GJ, Lager DJ. Primary renal lymphoma. J Surg Oncol 1991; 46: 273–7.

27. Kandel LB, McCullough DL, Harrison LH, et al. Primary renal lymphoma. Does it exist? Cancer 1987; 60: 386–91.

28. Malbrain ML, Lambrecht GL, Daelemans R, et al. Acute renal failure due to bilateral lymphomatous infiltrates. Primary extranodal non-Hodgkin's lymphoma (p-EN-NHL) of the kidneys: does it really exist? Clin Nephrol 1994; 42: 163–9.

29. Stallone G, Infante B, Manno C, et al. Primary renal lymphoma does exist: case report and review of the literature. J Nephrol 2000; 13: 367–72.

30. Ferry JA, Harris NL, Papanicolaou N, Young RH. Lymphoma of the kidney. A report of 11 cases. Am J Surg Pathol 1995; 19: 134–44.

31. Okuno SH, Hoyer JD, Ristow K, Witzig TE. Primary renal non-Hodgkin's lymphoma. An unusual extranodal site. Cancer 1995; 75: 2258–61.

32. Truong LD, Soroka S, Sheth AV, et al. Primary renal lymphoma presenting as acute renal failure. Am J Kidney Dis 1987; 9: 502–6.

33. Yasunaga Y, Hoshida Y, Hashimoto M, et al. Malignant lymphoma of the kidney. J Surg Oncol 1997; 64: 207–11.

34. Ahmad AH, MacLennan GT, Listinsky C. Primary renal lymphoma: a rare neoplasm that may present as a primary renal mass. J Urol 2005; 173: 239.

35. Bates AW, Norton AJ, Baithun SI. Malignant lymphoma of the urinary bladder: a clinicopathological study of 11 cases. J Clin Pathol 2000; 53: 458–61.

36. Hughes M, Morrison A, Jackson R. Primary bladder lymphoma: management and outcome of 12 patients with a review of the literature. Leuk Lymphoma 2005; 46: 873–7.

37. Kempton CL, Kurtin PJ, Inwards DJ, et al. Malignant lymphoma of the bladder: evidence from 36 cases that low-grade lymphoma of the MALT-type is the most common primary bladder lymphoma. Am J Surg Pathol 1997; 21: 1324–33.

38. Carver JD, Calverley D, Shen P. Chronic lymphocytic leukemia/small lymphocytic lymphoma presenting in urinary bladder without peripheral blood lymphocytosis: case report and literature review. Leuk Lymphoma 2006; 47: 1163–5.

39. Choi JH, Jeong YY, Shin SS, et al. Primary calcified T-cell lymphoma of the urinary bladder: a case report. Korean J Radiol 2003; 4: 252–4.

40. Mourad WA, Khalil S, Radwi A, et al. Primary T-cell lymphoma of the urinary bladder. Am J Surg Pathol 1998; 22: 373–7.

41. Masuda A, Tsujii T, Kojima M, et al. Primary mucosa-associated lymphoid tissue (MALT) lymphoma arising from the male urethra. A case report and review of the literature. Pathol Res Pract 2002; 198: 571–5.

42. Bozas G, Tassidou A, Moulopoulos LA, et al. Non-Hodgkin's lymphoma of the renal pelvis. Clin Lymphoma Myeloma 2006; 6: 404–6.

43. Lebowitz JA, Rofsky NM, Weinreb JC, Friedmann P. Ureteral lymphoma: MRI demonstration. Abdom Imaging 1995; 20: 173–5.

44. Mita K, Ohnishi Y, Edahiro T, et al. Primary mucosa-associated lymphoid tissue lymphoma in the renal pelvis. Urol Int 2002; 69: 241–3.

45. Grigg AP, Connors JM. Primary adrenal lymphoma. Clin Lymphoma 2003; 4: 154–60.

46. Wang J, Sun NC, Renslo R, et al. Clinically silent primary adrenal lymphoma: a case report and review of the literature. Am J Hematol 1998; 58: 130–6.

47. Butany J, Nair V, Naseemuddin A, et al. Cardiac tumours: diagnosis and management. Lancet Oncol 2005; 6: 219–28.

48. Holladay AO, Siegel RJ, Schwartz DA. Cardiac malignant lymphoma in acquired immune deficiency syndrome. Cancer 1992; 70: 2203–7.

49. Gowda RM, Khan IA. Clinical perspectives of primary cardiac lymphoma. Angiology 2003; 54: 599–604.

50. Ceresoli GL, Ferreri AJ, Bucci E, et al. Primary cardiac lymphoma in immunocompetent patients: diagnostic and therapeutic management. Cancer 1997; 80: 1497–506.

51. Rolla G, Bertero MT, Pastena G, et al. Primary lymphoma of the heart. A case report and review of the literature. Leuk Res 2002; 26: 117–20.

52. Jang JJ, Danik S, Goldman M. Primary cardiac lymphoma: diagnosis and treatment guided by transesophageal echocardiogram perfusion imaging. J Am Soc Echocardiogr 2006; 19: 1073 e7–9.

53. Gosev I, Siric F, Gasparovic H, et al. Surgical treatment of a primary cardiac lymphoma presenting with tamponade physiology. J Card Surg 2006; 21: 414–16.

54. Iwamoto FM, Abrey LE. Primary dural lymphomas: a review. Neurosurg Focus 2006; 21: E5.

55. Iwamoto FM, DeAngelis LM, Abrey LE. Primary dural lymphomas: a clinicopathologic study of treatment and outcome in eight patients. Neurology 2006; 66: 1763–5.

56. Benouaich A, Delord JP, Danjou M, et al. [Primary dural lymphoma: a report of two cases with review of the literature]. Rev Neurol (Paris) 2003; 159: 652–8. [in French]

57. Goetz P, Lafuente J, Revesz T, et al. Primary low-grade B-cell lymphoma of mucosa-associated lymphoid tissue of the dura mimicking the presentation of an acute subdural hematoma. Case report and review of the literature. J Neurosurg 2002; 96: 611–14.

58. Kambham N, Chang Y, Matsushima AY. Primary low-grade B-cell lymphoma of mucosa-associated lymphoid tissue (MALT) arising in dura. Clin Neuropathol 1998; 17: 311–17.

59. Kumar S, Kumar D, Kaldjian EP, et al. Primary low-grade B-cell lymphoma of the dura: a mucosa associated lymphoid tissue-type lymphoma. Am J Surg Pathol 1997; 21: 81–7.

60. Rottnek M, Strauchen J, Moore F, Morgello S. Primary dural mucosa-associated lymphoid tissue-type lymphoma: case report and review of the literature. J Neurooncol 2004; 68: 19–23.

61. Tu PH, Giannini C, Judkins AR, et al. Clinicopathologic and genetic profile of intracranial marginal zone lymphoma: a primary low-grade CNS lymphoma that mimics meningioma. J Clin Oncol 2005; 23: 5718–27.

62. Zucca E, Conconi A, Pedrinis E, et al. Nongastric marginal zone B-cell lymphoma of mucosa-associated lymphoid tissue. Blood 2003; 101: 2489–95.

63. Miranda RN, Glantz LK, Myint MA, et al. Stage IE non-Hodgkin's lymphoma involving the dura: a clinicopathologic study of five cases. Arch Pathol Lab Med 1996; 120: 254–60.

64. Herrmann R, Panahon AM, Barcos MP, et al. Gastrointestinal involvement in non-Hodgkin's lymphoma. Cancer 1980; 46: 215–22.

65. Bernal A, del Junco GW. Endoscopic and pathologic features of esophageal lymphoma: a report of four cases in patients with acquired immune deficiency syndrome. Gastrointest Endosc 1986; 32: 96–9.

66. Berman MD, Falchuk KR, Trey C, Gramm HF. Primary histiocytic lymphoma of the esophagus. Dig Dis Sci 1979; 24: 883–6.

67. Bolondi L, De Giorgio R, Santi V, et al. Primary non-Hodgkin's T-cell lymphoma of the esophagus. A case with peculiar endoscopic ultrasonographic pattern. Dig Dis Sci 1990; 35: 1426–30.

68. Chung JJ, Kim MJ, Kie JH, Kim KW. Mucosa-associated lymphoid tissue lymphoma of the esophagus coexistent with bronchus-associated lymphoid tissue lymphoma of the lung. Yonsei Med J 2005; 46: 562–6.

69. Doki T, Hamada S, Murayama H, et al. Primary malignant lymphoma of the esophagus. A case report. Endoscopy 1984; 16: 189–92.

70. Gelb AB, Medeiros LJ, Chen YY, et al. Hodgkin's disease of the esophagus. Am J Clin Pathol 1997; 108: 593–8.

71. George MK, Ramachandran V, Ramanan SG, Sagar TG. Primary esophageal T-cell non-Hodgkin's lymphoma. Indian J Gastroenterol 2005; 24: 119–20.

72. Hosaka S, Nakamura N, Akamatsu T, et al. A case of primary low grade mucosa associated lymphoid tissue (MALT) lymphoma of the oesophagus. Gut 2002; 51: 281–4.

73. Kitamoto Y, Hasegawa M, Ishikawa H, et al. Mucosa-associated lymphoid tissue lymphoma of the esophagus: a case report. J Clin Gastroenterol 2003; 36: 414–16.

74. Maipang T, Panjapiyakul C, Sriplung H. Primary lymphoma of the esophagus: a case report. J Med Assoc Thai 1992; 75: 299–303.

75. Matsuura H, Saito R, Nakajima S, et al. Non-Hodgkin's lymphoma of the esophagus. Am J Gastroenterol 1985; 80: 941–6.

76. Mengoli M, Marchi M, Rota E, et al. Primary non-Hodgkin's lymphoma of the esophagus. Am J Gastroenterol 1990; 85: 737–41.

77. Miyazaki T, Kato H, Masuda N, et al. Mucosa-associated lymphoid tissue lymphoma of the esophagus: case report and review of the literature. Hepatogastroenterology 2004; 51: 750–3.

78. Nagrani M, Lavigne BC, Siskind BN, et al. Primary non-Hodgkin's lymphoma of the esophagus. Arch Intern Med 1989; 149: 193–5.

79. Oguzkurt L, Karabulut N, Cakmakci E, Besim A. Primary non-Hodgkin's lymphoma of the esophagus. Abdom Imaging 1997; 22: 8–10.

80. Stein HA, Murray D, Warner HA. Primary Hodgkin's disease of the esophagus. Dig Dis Sci 1981; 26: 457–61.

81. Taal BG, Van Heerde P, Somers R. Isolated primary oesophageal involvement by lymphoma: a rare cause of dysphagia: two case histories and a review of other published data. Gut 1993; 34: 994–8.

82. Tsukada T, Ohno T, Kihira H, et al. Primary esophageal non-Hodgkin's lymphoma. Intern Med 1992; 31: 569–72.

83. Williams MR, Chidambaram M, Salama FD, Ansell ID. Tracheo-oesophageal fistula due to primary lymphoma of the oesophagus. J R Coll Surg Edinb 1984; 29: 60–1.

84. Dawson IM, Cornes JS, Morson BC. Primary malignant lymphoid tumours of the intestinal tract. Report of 37 cases with a study of factors influencing prognosis. Br J Surg 1961; 49: 80–9.

85. Bickel A, Eitan A, Tsilman B, Cohen HI. Low-grade B cell lymphoma of mucosa-associated lymphoid tissue (MALT) arising in the gallbladder. Hepatogastroenterology 1999; 46: 1643–6.

86. Botha JB, Kahn LB. Primary lymphoma of the gall bladder. Case report and review of the literature. S Afr Med J 1974; 48: 1345–8.

87. Chatila R, Fiedler PN, Vender RJ. Primary lymphoma of the gallbladder; case report and review of the literature. Am J Gastroenterol 1996; 91: 2242–4.

88. Chim CS, Liang R, Loong F, Chung LP. Primary mucosa-associated lymphoid tissue lymphoma of the gallbladder. Am J Med 2002; 112: 505–7.

89. Ferluga D, Luzar B, Gadzijev EM. Follicular lymphoma of the gallbladder and extrahepatic bile ducts. Virchows Arch 2003; 442: 136–40.

90. Friedman EP, Lazda E, Grant D, Davis J. Primary lymphoma of the gallbladder. Postgrad Med J 1993; 69: 585–7.

91. Jelic TM, Barreta TM, Yu M, et al. Primary, extranodal, follicular non-Hodgkin lymphoma of the gallbladder: case report and a review of the literature. Leuk Lymphoma 2004; 45: 381–7.

92. Laurino L, Melato M. Malignant angioendotheliomatosis (angiotropic lymphoma) of the gallbladder. Virchows Arch A Pathol Anat Histopathol 1990; 417: 243–6.

93. McCluggage WG, Mackel E, McCusker G. Primary low grade malignant lymphoma of mucosa-associated lymphoid tissue of gallbladder. Histopathology 1996; 29: 285–7.

94. Mitropoulos FA, Angelopoulou MK, Siakantaris MP, et al. Primary non-Hodgkin's lymphoma of the gall bladder. Leuk Lymphoma 2000; 40: 123–31.

95. Mosnier JF, Brousse N, Sevestre C, et al. Primary low-grade B-cell lymphoma of the mucosa-associated lymphoid tissue arising in the gallbladder. Histopathology 1992; 20: 273–5.

96. Pelstring RJ, Essell JH, Kurtin PJ, et al. Diversity of organ site involvement among malignant lymphomas of mucosa-associated tissues. Am J Clin Pathol 1991; 96: 738–45.

97. Tsuchiya T, Shimokawa I, Higami Y, et al. Primary low-grade MALT lymphoma of the gallbladder. Pathol Int 2001; 51: 965–9.

98. Vaittinen E. Sarcoma of the gall-bladder. Ann Chir Gynaecol Fenn 1972; 61: 185–9.

99. Yamamoto T, Kawanishi M, Yoshiba H, et al. Primary non-Hodgkin's lymphoma of the gallbladder. AJR Am J Roentgenol 2005; 184: S86–7.

100. Yasuma T, Yanaka M. Primary sarcoma of the gallbladder – report of three cases. Acta Pathol Jpn 1971; 21: 285–304.

101. Rajesh LS, Nada R, Yadav TD, Joshi K. Primary low-grade B-cell lymphoma of the mucosa-associated lymphoid tissue of the gallbladder. Histopathology 2003; 43: 300–1.

102. Arcari A, Anselmi E, Bernuzzi P, et al. Primary pancreatic lymphoma. Report of five cases. Haematologica 2005; 90: ECR09.

103. Battula N, Srinivasan P, Prachalias A, et al. Primary pancreatic lymphoma: diagnostic and therapeutic dilemma. Pancreas 2006; 33: 192–4.

104. Boni L, Benevento A, Dionigi G, et al. Primary pancreatic lymphoma. Surg Endosc 2002; 16: 1107–8.

105. Ezzat A, Jamshed A, Khafaga Y, et al. Primary pancreatic non-Hodgkin's lymphomas. J Clin Gastroenterol 1996; 23: 109–12.

106. Jones WF, Sheikh MY, McClave SA. AIDS-related non-Hodgkin's lymphoma of the pancreas. Am J Gastroenterol 1997; 92: 335–8.

107. Nayer H, Weir EG, Sheth S, Ali SZ. Primary pancreatic lymphomas: a cytopathologic analysis of a rare malignancy. Cancer 2004; 102: 315–21.

108. Nishimura R, Takakuwa T, Hoshida Y, et al. Primary pancreatic lymphoma: clinicopathological analysis of 19 cases from Japan and review of the literature. Oncology 2001; 60: 322–9.

109. Saif MW. Primary pancreatic lymphomas. JOP 2006; 7: 262–73.

110. Salvatore JR, Cooper B, Shah I, Kummet T. Primary pancreatic lymphoma: a case report, literature review, and proposal for nomenclature. Med Oncol 2000; 17: 237–47.

111. Savopoulos CG, Tsesmeli NE, Kaiafa GD, et al. Primary pancreatic anaplastic large cell lymphoma, ALK negative: a case report. World J Gastroenterol 2005; 11: 6221–4.

112. James JA, Milligan DW, Morgan GJ, Crocker J. Familial pancreatic lymphoma. J Clin Pathol 1998; 51: 80–2.

113. Faulkner JE, Gaba CE, Powers JD, Yam LT. Diagnosis of primary pancreatic lymphoma by fine needle aspiration. Acta Cytol 1998; 42: 834–6.

114. Behrns KE, Sarr MG, Strickler JG. Pancreatic lymphoma: is it a surgical disease? Pancreas 1994; 9: 662–7.

115. Koniaris LG, Lillemoe KD, Yeo CJ, et al. Is there a role for surgical resection in the treatment of early-stage pancreatic lymphoma? J Am Coll Surg 2000; 190: 319–30.

116. Krol AD, le Cessie S, Snijder S, et al. Primary extranodal non-Hodgkin's lymphoma (NHL): the impact of alternative definitions tested in the Comprehensive Cancer Centre West population-based NHL registry. Ann Oncol 2003; 14: 131–9.

117. Lanham GR, Weiss SW, Enzinger FM. Malignant lymphoma. A study of 75 cases presenting in soft tissue. Am J Surg Pathol 1989; 13: 1–10.

118. Travis WD, Banks PM, Reiman HM. Primary extranodal soft tissue lymphoma of the extremities. Am J Surg Pathol 1987; 11: 359–66.

119. Krementz ET, Muchmore JH. Soft tissue sarcomas: behavior and management. Adv Surg 1983; 16: 147–96.

120. Lopez-Guillermo A, Colomo L, Jimenez M, et al. Diffuse large B-cell lymphoma: clinical and biological characterization and outcome according to the nodal or extranodal primary origin. J Clin Oncol 2005; 23: 2797–804.

121. Radhi JM, Ibrahiem K, al-Tweigeri T. Soft tissue malignant lymphoma at sites of previous surgery. J Clin Pathol 1998; 51: 629–32.

122. Shpilberg O, Friedman B, Azaria M, et al. Primary striated muscle lymphoma presenting in an amputation stump. Isr J Med Sci 1989; 25: 116–17.

123. Bozas G, Anagnostou D, Tassidou A, et al. Extranodal non-Hodgkin's lymphoma presenting as an abdominal wall mass. A case report and review of the literature. Leuk Lymphoma 2006; 47: 329–32.

124. Salamao DR, Nascimento AG, Lloyd RV, et al. Lymphoma in soft tissue: a clinicopathologic study of 19 cases. Hum Pathol 1996; 27: 253–7.

125. Wallner RJ, Dadparvar S, Croll MN, Brady LW. Demonstration of a malignant soft-tissue lymphoma during triple-phase skeletal scintigraphy. J Nucl Med 1985; 26: 1275–7.

Extranodal involvement Hodgkin's lymphoma

28

Daniel Re, Michael Fuchs, Volker Diehl, and Franco Cavalli

INTRODUCTION

Hodgkin's lymphoma (HL) has become a highly curable disease over the last decades but attention has to be paid to late treatment-associated effects that increase mortality in long-term Hodgkin's survivors. It is therefore of utmost importance to follow strict staging procedures to avoid overtreatment of patients. Individualization of treatment using prognostic clinical and possibly biological factors might also help to tailor the amount and quality of therapy. It is the scope of this article to summarize available data on extranodal involvement in the context of risk and response adapted individualized treatment. Extranodal disease should be distinguished from extralymphatic disease extending from a lymph node or disseminated organ involvement.

SITES OF EXTRANODAL DISEASE

Staging procedures recommended for determining the extent of disease have become less invasive in recent years. Staging laparotomy and splenectomy are used only in patients with limited, often infradiaphragmatic or occult disease, for which ultrasound- or computed tomography (CT)-guided fine-needle biopsy is impossible or not informative. CT of the neck, chest, abdomen, and pelvis is routinely performed in the diagnostic evaluation of a patient with HL.

Two-thirds of patients with newly diagnosed HL have radiographic evidence of intrathoracic involvement. A large mediastinal mass has been arbitrarily defined as a mass with the ratio being greater than one-third between the largest transverse diameter of the mediastinal mass over the transverse diameter of the thorax at the diaphragm on a standing posteroanterior chest radiograph.[1] Alternatively, other clinicians have defined extensive mediastinal disease as >35% of the thoracic diameter at T5-6 or as wider than 5–10 cm. Patients with large mediastinal masses are at increased risk for relapsing in nodal and extranodal sites above the diaphragm after radiation therapy alone.[2,3]

Of note, in some of those instances it might be difficult to distinguish between true E lesions and per continuitatem invasion of adjacent anatomical regions such as the lung, pericardium, pleura, chest wall, or bone due to penetration of the capsule of a lymph node. Effusions of the pericardium, pleural cavity, or peritoneal cavity are often associated with extranodal involvement and invasive growth into neighboring structures.

Concerning isolated primary extranodal disease, there is little systematic data available. A report of clinical characteristics of all E lesions observed in over 10 000 German Hodgkin Study Group (GHSG) patients is currently in preparation. Concerning extranodal disease in combination with nodal disease in untreated patients with HL, details for organ involvement and extranodal lesions are given in Table 28.1, indicating that 10–15 % patients have extranodal disease. An unpublished analysis of GHSG data also shows that between 8% and 13% of patients in intermediate and advanced stages show extranodal manifestation. This figure corresponds well with 8% nodal involvement reported by the Groupe d'Etude des Lymphomes de l'Adulte (GELA) for patients treated in the H8 and the H9

Table 28.1 Sites of disease involvement in untreated patients with HL

Anatomical site	Involvement (%)
Waldeyer's ring	1–2
Cervical nodes	60–70
Axillary nodes	30–35
Mediastinum	50–60
Hilar nodes	15–35
Para-aortic nodes	30–40
Iliac nodes	15–20
Mesenteric nodes	1–4
Inguinal nodes	8–15
Spleen	30–35
Liver	2–6
Bone marrow	1–4
Total extranodal	10–15

Adapted from Gupta et al.[28]

European Organization for Research and Treatment of Cancer (EORTC) trials.[4]

In a preliminary analysis we found that both bone marrow and diffuse bone involvement are rare (approximately 0.7% and 0.5%, respectively) in patients that otherwise would have been classified as early favorable stage. For intermediate-stage disease, the figures are 1% and 1.3%. In other words, it is rarely necessary to classify early-stage patients as advanced stage based solely on bone or bone marrow involvement. This fits well with the literature describing bone lesions to be very rare.

Skin involvement is seen very rarely and can appear as small, opaque, or red papules or as ulcerating lesions. An unpublished analysis of more than 5000 patients treated within GHSG trials identified only 10 patients with skin lesions. Those patients had early- or advanced-stage disease. In addition, non-specific lesions such as lymphomatoid papulosis may also be found in HL patients.[5]

Involvement of the central nervous system (CNS) is similarly a very rare observation in HL patients and was reported to occur in 0.2–0.5% of

cases based on the analysis of two heterogeneous series of 780 and 2185 HL patients, respectively.[6,7] Importantly, in these two studies, all patients with assumed intracerebral HL suffered from systemic relapse of their disease. In addition, in most those cases, CNS lesions were not analyzed histopathologically. In one study, CNS involvement was reported to occur due to nodes within the para-aortic region that grow through the intervertebral foramina, manifesting as neurological symptoms and pain. In contrast, a recent analysis of GHSG data of almost 15 000 patients with untreated and relapsed HL identified only two cases of intracerebral HL in relapsed patients (0.02%).[8] In both instances, bone lesions of the skull or the orbita were also present.

Primary involvement of the intestinal wall had never been observed in GHSG patients, but secondary invasion of the gut from adjacent mesenterial lymph nodes was described anecdotally.

The spleen is involved in about 30–35% of patients at diagnosis, is less frequent with nodular sclerosis Hodgkin's lymphoma (NSHL) histology, and occurs rarely in patients with lymphocyte-predominant Hodgkin's lymphoma (LPHL). Spleen involvement is often subclinical and hard to diagnose with modern imaging techniques.

In HIV-positive patients, the pattern of extranodal involvement is somewhat different. HL is the most common non-AIDS (acquired immunodeficiency syndrome) defining tumor diagnosed in HIV (human immunodeficiency virus) infected patients but the impact of highly active antiretroviral therapy (HAART) on the epidemiology of HL remains unclear.[9] At the time of diagnosis, 70–90% of all patients with HIV-associated HL presented with advanced disease. Extranodal involvement is common (60%) in these patients and includes bone marrow, liver, and spleen. In HIV-infected patients, non-contiguous spread of lymphoma can be observed frequently, such as liver involvement without splenic disease or lung involvement without mediastinal adenopathy. In contrast to HIV-negative patients, bone marrow involvement occurs in 40–50% of patients and may be the first indicator of the presence of HL in almost 20% of cases.[10]

EXTRANODAL INVOLVEMENT AS PROGNOSTIC FACTOR IN UNTREATED PATIENTS

Despite an enormous effort to define clinically relevant and generally acceptable prognostic factors, there are still two major characteristics for dividing HL patients according to a risk- or prognosis-adapted therapeutic approach: stage and systemic symptoms. A third factor meets general trans-Atlantic acceptance: massive local tumor burden (i.e. bulky disease >10 cm in diameter). Prognostic factors are rarely the subject of specific clinical studies but are recognized and evaluated using data from large cohorts of uniformly treated, well-documented, and reliably followed patients, usually from large clinical trials. As specified below, different prognostic factors are applied by US–American centers, the EORTC, or the GHSG.

In the USA, most centers still treat HL patients according to the traditional separation of early stages (I-II, A and B), representing about 45% of newly diagnosed patients, and advanced stages (III-IV, A and B), which also might include any stage with B symptoms, bulky disease (>10 cm) or multiple E lesions, representing about 55% of newly diagnosed patients.

The EORTC identified in the H1 and H2 trials additional prognostic factors that are now used to assign clinical stage I or II patients to a more unfavorable-prognosis group. The EORTC has, since 1982, defined clinical stage I or II (supradiaphragmatic only) patients as having an early unfavorable prognosis HL if any of the following factors is present: age >50 years old, asymptomatic with an erythrocyte sedimentation rate (ESR) >50; B symptoms with an ESR >30; and a large mediastinal mass. In previous trials, stage II disease with mixed cellularity Hodgkin's lymphoma (MCHL) or lymphocyte depletion Hodgkin's lymphoma (LDHL) histology and number of involved regions had also been counted as adverse factors.[11]

The GHSG has, since 1988, assigned clinical stage I or II patients to an intermediate group if they had any of the following adverse factors: large mediastinal mass ($\geq$ one-third of maximum thoracic diameter); three or more involved lymphatic regions (which is not equivalent to lymphatic areas); elevated ESR; and localized extranodal infiltration.[12] Because of the rarity of splenectomy, massive splenic involvement was seldom reported and was abandoned for the current generation of trials. It can be difficult to distinguish consistently between E lesions and stage IV disease, and various assessments of the prognostic value of this feature have been obtained by different investigators.

In summary, the EORTC includes in its advanced-stage cohorts stage III and IV patients only, without regard to other factors, while US cooperative groups, and some European groups also include stage (I-) II patients in the advanced-stage group, if they have specific risk factors such as B symptoms, bulky disease, large mediastinal mass, or E lesions. The GHSG includes only stage IIB patients with large mediastinal mass and extranodal involvement in the advanced-stage group. The gradual shift towards more intensive therapy is thus based on the incorporation of prognostic factors into treatment algorithms.

In order to identify more conclusive and generally applicable prognostic factor analyses for the advanced-stage disease, the International Prognostic Factor Project produced an International Prognostic Score (IPS) (data from 5141 patients treated in 25 centers).[13] In the group of patients with stage IV disease, organ involvement was analyzed to determine whether the combination of stage IV disease and particular sites of involvement had additional prognostic importance (Table 28.2). There were only small differences in freedom from progression (FFP) of disease according to the site of involvement. Liver involvement was associated with poor overall survival (OS), because the survival rate among patients with such involvement is low after a relapse, regardless of their age.

All of the IPS factors were shown to be highly significant in a multivariate analysis, and their prognostic power were confirmed in an independent sample. Serum albumin and hemoglobin levels, male gender, and age of

Table 28.2 Organ involvement and clinical outcome; univariate analysis at 5 years according to Hasenclever and Diehl[13]

Organ involvement in stage IV	Number of patients (%)	Rate of FFP (%)	p value	Rate of OS (%)	p value
Liver involvement	1908		0.015		<0.001
• Absent	1339 (70)	62 ± 1		75 ± 1	
• Present	569 (30)	58 ± 2		67 ± 2	
Bone marrow involvement	1965		0.46		0.12
• Absent	1351 (69)	61 ± 1		74 ± 2	
• Present	614 (31)	60 ± 2		70 ± 2	
Lung involvement	1969		0.34		0.47
• Absent	1324 (67)	61 ± 1		72 ± 2	
• Present	645 (33)	59 ± 2		73 ± 2	

OS = overall survival; FFP = freedom from progression.

$\geq$45 years old are also prognostic factors for early-stage patients. All seven factors were associated with similar relative risks of between 1.26 and 1.49. It was recommended to combine these factors into a single score by counting the number of adverse factors and giving an integer prognostic score between 0 and 7. However, even patients with $\geq$5 factors (7% of cases) had a 5-year failure-free rate of more than 40%. A number of other factors such as pathologic gradeal in NSHL, the amount of tissue eosinophilia, inguinal involvement, serum lactic dehydrogenase (LDH) concentration, and β_2-microglobulin level have been shown to correlate with prognosis in advanced stage without being significant in that multivariate analysis. In an univariate analysis, liver involvement is a poor risk factor, whereas lung or bone marrow involvement do not have an independent prognostic importance in advanced-stage patients. Nevertheless, a more detailed analysis, taking into account both the number and specific location of E lesions, might add some information.

Other prognostic factors may subsequently be used for treatment intensification or for treatment reduction. Proctor and coworkers[14] constructed a continuous numeric index for this purpose as a weighted sum of the variables – including age, stage, lymphocyte count, hemoglobin level, and the presence of bulky disease

– and included patients with an index greater than 0.5 in the poor-prognosis subset. In contrast to the GHSG and the British National Lymphoma Investigation (BNLI), Federico and colleagues[15] included patients with E lesions in a high-risk population that might benefit from early treatment intensification. Two or more of the following factors were required: high LDH levels, very large mediastinal mass, $\geq$2 extranodal sites, inguinal involvement, low hematocrit, and bone marrow involvement. Nevertheless, results indicated that the early high-dose intensification based on these factors is unlikely to result in clinically relevant long-term survival benefit compared with conventional treatment.

EXTRANODAL INVOLVEMENT IN RELAPSED PATIENTS

The pattern of relapse and treatment strategies for relapsed patients depend mainly on prior therapy. Nowadays, high-dose chemotherapy (HDCT) followed by autologous stem cell transplantation (ASCT) is the treatment of choice for patients with relapsed or refractory HL after first-line combination chemotherapy.[16,17] However, a considerable number of good-risk patients may be overtreated with the use of HDCT.

Many prognostic factors have been described for patients relapsing after first-line chemotherapy. These include age, gender, histology, relapse sites, stage at relapse, B symptoms, performance status, and extranodal relapse. The impact of these variables is difficult to assess because of a variety of confounding factors, including small numbers of patients and inclusion of primary progressive HL. Multivariate analyses were not performed systematically. Several groups[18-20] identified good risk factors in relapsed and refractory patients, but E lesions were not of prognostic significance in these trials. In contrast, Reece and associates[21] reported an analysis of 58 patients treated with HDCT and ASCT. Four prognostic subgroups were identified according to the presence of the following parameters at relapse: B symptoms, extranodal disease, initial remission duration of <12 months, and no risk factors. Patients with no risk factors had a 3-year progression-free survival of 100%, compared with 81% of patients with one factor, 40% of those with two factors, and 0% of patients with all three adverse risk factors.

The Royal Marsden Hospital series included relapsed patients that received first-line radiation therapy without chemotherapy. Age, histology, and nodal vs extranodal involvement were found to be predictve for clinical with a relapse-free-survival of 63% at 10 years. Nodal recurrence had a 10-year survival of 74% compared with 51% for extranodal recurrence.[22] This is in accordance with earlier studies suggesting that extranodal relapse is a poor prognostic factor in patients treated with radiotherapy only.[23]

The GHSG performed a retrospective analysis that included a much larger number of relapsed patients (n = 422) than previously reported.[24] Of these patients, 59 (14%) had lung involvement, 51 (12%) had liver involvement, 38 (9%) had bone involvement, 38 (9%) had bone marrow involvement, and 21 (5%) had extranodal disease. In the multivariate analysis, patients with extranodal lesions at relapse showed a worse overall survival (p = 0.075). However, this factor was not considered in the main analysis because of the small number of cases with extranodal lesions. The most relevant factors of the main analysis were

combined into a prognostic score. This score was calculated on the basis of duration of first remission, stage at relapse, and presence of anemia at relapse. Early recurrence within 3–12 months after the completion of primary treatment, relapse with stage III or IV disease, and hemoglobin levels at relapse (<10.5 g/dl for female patients, <12 g/dl for male patients) were counted in a score, with possible values of 0, 1, 2, and 3 in order of worsening prognosis. This prognostic score allows the doctor to distinguish patients with different rates of freedom from second failure and OS. The actuarial 4-year rates for freedom from second failure and OS for patients relapsing after chemotherapy with three unfavorable factors were 17% and 27%, respectively. In contrast, patients with none of the unfavorable factors had rates of freedom from second failure and OS at 4 years of 48% and 83%, respectively. The prognostic score could also predict the major candidate groups for dose intensification: patients relapsing after radiotherapy and patients relapsing after chemotherapy who were treated with conventional therapies or with HDCT followed by ASCT.

SUMMARY

With the exception of the EORTC, most study groups consider extranodal involvement in HL to be a poor prognostic factor. This is reflected by the current classification system that classifies patients with E lesions as early unfavorable or even advanced stage. In clinical practice, differentiation between true E lesions, extralymphatic lesions extending from lymph nodes, and diffuse organ involvement might be difficult.

Based on the finding that liver involvement is a poor prognostic factor in a univariate analysis, liver lesions (in analogy to bone marrow involvement) are synonymous with diffuse organ involvement according to the GHSG. Although there is no evidence that patients with extranodal involvement are relapsing more frequently at initial extranodal sites, it appears that relapses in extranodal sites indicate poor prognosis and might need special attention.

REFERENCES

1. Lister TA, Crowther D, Sutcliffe SB, et al. Report of a committee convened to discuss the evaluation and staging of patients with Hodgkin's disease: Cotswolds meeting [J Clin Oncol 1990; 8(9):1602.] erratum appears in J Clin Oncol 1989; 7(11): 1630–6.

2. Hughes-Davies L, Tarbell NJ, Coleman CN, et al. Stage IA–IIB Hodgkin's disease: management and outcome of extensive thoracic involvement. Int J Radiat Oncol Biol Phys 1997; 39(2): 361–9.

3. Hoppe R, Coleman CN, Cox RS, Rosenberg SA, Kaplan HS. The management of stage I–II Hodgkin's disease with irradiation alone or combined modality therapy: the Stanford experience. Blood 1982; 59(3): 455–65.

4. Gisselbrecht C, Mounier N, André M, et al. How to define intermediate stage in Hodgkin's lymphoma? Eur J Haematol Suppl 2005; 66: 111–14.

5. Cavalli F. Rare syndromes in Hodgkin´s disease. Ann Oncol 1998; 9(Suppl 5): S109–13.

6. Sapozink M, Kaplan H, Intracranial Hodgkin's disease. A report of 12 cases and review of the literature. Cancer 1983; 52(7): 1301–7.

7. Akyüz C, Yakin B, Atahan IL, et al. Intracranial involvement in Hodgkin's disease. Pediatr Hematol Oncol 2005; 22: 589–96.

8. Re D, et al. CNS involvement in Hodgkin's lymphoma. J Clin Oncol 2007; 25 (21): 3182.

9. Gates AE, Kaplan LD. AIDS malignancies in the era of highly active antiretroviral therapy. Oncology (Williston Park) 2002; 16(4): 441–51, 456, 459.

10. Andrieu J, et al. Hodgkin's disease during HIV1 infection: the French registry experience. French Registry of HIV-associated Tumors. Ann Oncol 1993; 4(8): 635–41.

11. Carde P, Burger JM, Henry-Amar M. Clinical stages I and II Hodgkin's disease: a specifically tailored therapy according to prognostic factors. J Clin Oncol 1988; 6: 239–52.

12. Loeffler M, Pfreundschuh M, Rühl U. Risk factor adapted treatment of Hodgkin's lymphoma: strategies and perspectives. Recent Results Cancer Res 1989; 117: 142–62.

13. Hasenclever D, Diehl V. A prognostic score for advanced Hodgkin's disease. International Prognostic Factors Project on Advanced Hodgkin's Disease. N Engl J Med 1998; 339(21): 1506–14.

14. Proctor SJ, Taylor P, Machie MJ, et al. A numerical prognostic index for clinical use in identification of poor-risk patients with Hodgkin's disease at diagnosis. The Scotland and Newcastle Lymphoma Group (SNLG) Therapy Working Party. Leuk Lymphoma 1992; 7(Suppl): 17–20.

15. Federico M, Bellei M, Briee P, et al. High-dose therapy and autologous stem-cell transplantation versus conventional therapy for patients with advanced Hodgkin's lymphoma responding to front-line therapy. J Clin Oncol 2003; 21(12): 2320–5.

16. Linch DC, Winfield D, Goldstone AH, et al. Dose intensification with autologous bone-marrow transplantation in relapsed and resistant Hodgkin's disease: results of a BNLI randomised trial. Lancet 1993; 341(8852): 1051–4.

17. Schmitz N, Sextro M, Pfistner B. HDR-1: high-dose therapy (HDT) followed by hematopoietic stem cell transplantation (HSCT) for relapsed chemosensitive Hodgkin`s disease (HD): final results of a randomized GHSG and EBMT trial (HD-R1). Proc ASCO 1999; (Suppl 5): 18.

18. Lohri A, Barnett M, Fairey RN, et al. Outcome of treatment of first relapse of Hodgkin's disease after primary chemotherapy: identification of risk factors from the British Columbia experience 1970 to 1988. Blood 1991; 77(10): 2292–8.

19. Fermé C, Bastion Y, Lepage Y, et al. The MINE regimen as intensive salvage chemotherapy for relapsed and refractory Hodgkin's disease. Ann Oncol 1995; 6(6): 543–9.

20. Brice P, Bastion Y, Divine M, et al. Analysis of prognostic factors after the first relapse of Hodgkin's disease in 187 patients. Cancer 1996; 78(6): 1293–9.

21. Reece DE, Barnett MJ, Shepherd JD, et al. High-dose cyclophosphamide, carmustine (BCNU), and etoposide (VP16-213) with or without cisplatin (CBV +/− P) and autologous transplantation for patients with Hodgkin's disease who fail to enter a complete remission after combination chemotherapy. Blood 1995; 86(2): 451–6.

22. Horwich A, Specht L, Ashley S. Survival analysis of patients with clinical stages I or II Hodgkin's disease who have relapsed after initial treatment with radiotherapy alone. Eur J Cancer 1997; 33(6): 848–53.

23. Mauch P. Controversies in the management of early stage Hodgkin's disease. Blood 1994; 83(2): 318–29.

24. Josting A, Franklin J, May M, et al. New prognostic score based on treatment outcome of patients with relapsed Hodgkin's lymphoma registered in the database of the German Hodgkin's lymphoma study group. J Clin Oncol 2002; 20(1): 221–30.

25. Gupta RK, Gospodarowicz MK, Lister TA. Clinical evaluation and staging of Hodgkin's disease. In: Mauch PM, Armitage JO, Diehl V, et al, eds. Hodgkin's Disease. Philadelphia: Lippincott Williams & Wilkins, 1999.

Index

Printed and bound by CPI Group (UK) Ltd, Croydon, CR0 4YY
23/10/2024
01778251-0005